COMPLEMENTARY AND ALTERNATIVE MEDICINE SECRETS

WENDY KOHATSU, MD

Assistant Professor
Family Medicine
East Tennessee State University
Kingsport, Tennessee

Graduate Fellow
Program in Integrative Medicine
University of Arizona
Tucson, Arizona

HANLEY & BELFUS, INC./Philadelphia

Publisher: HANLEY & BELFUS, INC.
               Medical Publishers
               210 South 13th Street
               Philadelphia, PA 19107
               (215) 546-7293; 800-962-1892
               FAX (215) 790-9330
               Web site: http://www.hanleyandbelfus.com

Note to the reader: Although the techniques, ideas, and information in this book have been carefully reviewed for correctness, neither the authors nor the editor nor the publisher can accept any legal responsibility for any error or omissions that may be made. Neither the publisher nor the editor makes any guarantee, expressed or implied, with respect to the material contained herein.

This book is designed to provide information on the background and modalities used frequently in CAM, and how they are applied by practitioners in the field. It is not intended to be exhaustive, nor should patients use it as a substitute for the advice of their physician. It is strongly recommended that you talk with your own physician about any treatments you use personally, and to research the area further for safety as it applies to the person you are treating. Before trying/recommending any treatment, the reader should review dosages, accepted indications, and other information pertinent to the safe and effective use of the therapies described.

Library of Congress Control Number: 2002105859

COMPLEMENTARY AND ALTERNATIVE MEDICINE SECRETS   ISBN 1-56053-440-0

Last digit is the print number: 9 8 7 6 5 4 3 2 1

CONTENTS

I. GENERAL ISSUES

1. History of Complementary and Alternative Medicine in the U.S............... 1
   Wendy Kohatsu, M.D.

2. Research in Complementary and Alternative Medicine...................... 6
   Betsy S. Singh, Ph.D., S. P. Vinjamury, M.D., and V. J. Singh, B.A.

3. The Integrative Medicine Approach..................................... 16
   Wendy Kohatsu, M.D.

II. THERAPEUTIC MODALITIES

Mind-Body-Spirit Interventions

4. Placebo... 23
   Opher Caspi, M.D., M.A.

5. Creative Arts Therapy 31
   Pali Delevitt and Aga Lewelt

6. Hypnosis and Imagery 37
   Sherry Robbins, M.D., and Michael Floyd, Ph.D.

7. Meditation 43
   Shauna L. Shapiro, Ph.D.

8. Spirituality 47
   Ken Olive, M.D.

9. Yoga... 54
   Russell H. Greenfield, M.D.

Alternative Systems of Medical Practice

10. Ayurveda 59
    Robert E. Svoboda, BAMS, and Bhaswati Bhattacharya, M.P.H., M.D.

11. Traditional Chinese Medicine 67
    Julia Thie, L.Ac.

12. Acupuncture.. 74
    Julia Thie, L.Ac.

13. Homeopathy.. 79
    Malcolm Riley, B.D.S.

14. Allopathic Medicine... 84
    Reid Blackwelder, M.D.

Manual Healing and Physical Touch

15. Osteopathic Medicine 92
    David N. Grimshaw, D.O.

16. Chiropractic 101
    Robert D. Mootz, D.C., and Ian Coulter, Ph.D.

17. Massage 110
    Seth McLaughlin

Botanical Medicine

18. Botanical Medicine 116
    Roberta Lee, M.D.

Nutrition and Supplements

19. Nutrition 123
    Wendy Kohatsu, M.D., and Stefanie Shaver, M.D.

20. Supplements 134
    Wendy Kohatsu, M.D., and Matthew Flesch

Exercise and Fitness

21. Exercise and Fitness 143
    Jeffry S. Life, M.D., Ph.D.

Energy Medicine

22. Energy Medicine 153
    Joann D'Aprile, D.O.

III. DIAGNOSES

Affective Disorders

23. Anxiety 163
    Roberta Lee, M.D.

24. Attention-deficit Hyperactivity Disorder 168
    Mary Bove, N.D.

25. Depression 174
    Craig Schneider, M.D.

Cardiovascular Disease

26. Atherosclerosis 180
    Robert Bugarelli, D.O.

27. Congestive Heart Failure 191
    Russell H. Greenfield, M.D.

28. Hypertension 200
    Victoria Maizes, M.D.

Dermatology

29. Acne 205
    Roya Kohani, M.D.

30. Eczema 210
    Roya Kohani, M.D.

Endocrine/Metabolic

31. Diabetes Mellitus 215
    Scott M. Morcott, M.D., and Meg Landgraf, PA-C

32. Obesity 222
    Aubrey D. McElroy, M.D.

33. Osteoporosis 228
    Tamara Sachs, M.D.

Gastrointestinal

34. Gastroesophageal Reflux 234
    Marcey Shapiro, M.D.

35. Hepatitis 240
    Marcey Shapiro, M.D.

36. Irritable Bowel Syndrome 246
    Robert A. Weissberg, M.D.

37. Peptic Ulcer Disease 254
    Susan Hadley, M.D.

Gender-specific Care

38. Menopause 257
    Monica J. Stokes, M.D., FACOG

39. Premenstrual Syndrome 265
    Alison Levitt, M.D.

40. Pregnancy 271
    Aviva Romm, CPM, AHG

41. Benign Prostatic Hypertrophy 276
    David Rakel, M.D.

Infectious Disease

42. HIV/AIDS 281
    Benjamin Kligler, M.D., M.P.H.

43. Common Cold 286
    Jeffrey Jump, M.D.

44. Sinusitis 290
    Robert S. Ivker, D.O.

45. Urinary Tract Infection 298
    Bhaswati Bhattacharya, M.P.H., M.D.

Musculoskeletal

46. Chronic Pain Syndrome 304
    Reid Blackwelder, M.D.

47. Low Back Pain 313
    Wendy Kohatsu, M.D.

48. Osteoarthritis 322
    Stefanie L. Shaver, M.D.

49. Fibromyalgia 330
    Betsy B. Singh, Ph.D., S. P. Vinjamury, M.D., and V. J. Singh, B.A.

Neurology

50. Alzheimer's Dementia 338
    Raffaele Filice, M.D., FRCPC

51. Headache 345
    Ken Peters, M.D.

52. Multiple Sclerosis 352
    Patricia Ammon, M.D.

53. Peripheral Neuropathy 357
    Sunil Pai, M.D.

Oncology

54. Integrative Oncology: General Approach 363
    Matt Mumber, M.D.

55. Approach to Specific Cancers 377
    Matt Mumber, M.D.

Pediatrics

56. Pediatric Abdominal Pain.. 388
    Joy A. Weydert, M.D., FAAP

57. Infant Colic.. 392
    Joy A. Weydert, M.D., FAAP

58. Otitis Media 396
    Marcey Shapiro, M.D.

Respiratory

59. Allergic Rhinitis.. 403
    James Nicolai, M.D.

60. Asthma.. 409
    John D. Mark, M.D.

IV. SPECIAL TOPICS

61. Drug–Herb Interactions 417
    Monica J. Stokes, M.D., FACOG

62. The Business of Complementary and Alternative Medicine 423
    Nancy Schulman, M.S.B., and Michael J. Stuart-Shor, M.P.H.

INDEX 431

CONTRIBUTORS

Patricia Kay Ammon, MD
Clinical Instructor, Family Medicine, School of Medicine, University of Colorado Health Sciences Center, Denver, Colorado; Courtesy Privileges, St. Mary's Hospital, Grand Junction, Colorado

Bhaswati Bhattacharya, MD, MA, MPH
Assistant Professor, Weill Medical College, Cornell University; Director of CAM Education and Research, Family, Community and Preventive Medicine, Wyckoff Heights Medical Center, New York, New York

Reid Blackwelder, MD
Associate Professor, Family Medicine, East Tennessee State University, Kingsport, Tennessee

Mary Bove, ND
Neuropathic Physician, Brattleboro, Vermont

Robert Bugarelli, DO, FACR
Director of Integrative-Preventative Cardiology, Main Line Health System, Wynnewood, Pennsylvania; Associate Fellow, University of Arizona, Program in Integrative Medicine, Tucson, Arizona; Mercy Catholic Medical Center and Lankenau Hospital, Philadelphia/Wynnewood, Pennsylvania

Opher Caspi, MD, MA
Research Assistant Professor, Program in Integrative Medicine, University of Arizona, Tucson, Arizona

Ian Coulter, PhD
Professor, School of Dentistry, Division of Public Health and Community Dentistry, University of California, Los Angeles, Los Angeles, California

Joann D'Aprile, DO
Assistant Professor, Family Medicine, East Tennessee State University; Wellmont Holston Valley Medical Center, Kingsport, Tennessee

Pali Delevitt, PhD(c)
Education Coordinator, Duke Center for Integrative Medicine, Carrboro, North Carolina

Raffaele Filice, MD, FRCPC
Medical Director, Tzu Chi Institute for Complementary and Alternative Medicine, Vancouver, British Columbia, Canada

Matthew Flesch
Student, East Tennessee State University, Kingsport, Tennessee

Michael Floyd, PhD
Associate Professor of Family Medicine, Associate Clinical Professor of Psychiatry and Behavioral Medicine, Department of Family Medicine, East Tennessee State University, Kingsport, Tennessee; Family Medicine Associates of Johnson City, Johnson City, Tennessee

Russell Howard Greenfield, MD
Visiting Assistant Professor, Department of Medicine, The University of Arizona College of Medicine, Tucson, Arizona; Medical Director, Carolinas Integrative Health, Charlotte, North Carolina

David N. Grimshaw, DO
Assistant Professor, Osteopathic Manipulative Medicine, Michigan State University College of Osteopathic Medicine, East Lansing, Michigan; Ingham Regional Medical Center and Sparrow Hospital, Lansing, Michigan

Susan Hadley, MD
Faculty, Middlesex Hospital Family Practice Residency Program; Assistant Professor, University of Connecticut, Farmington, Connecticut

Robert S. Ivker, DO
Assistant Clinical Professor, Department of Family Medicine, University of Colorado, Denver, Colorado

Jeffrey Scott Jump, MD
Associate Professor, Director, Center for Integrative Medicine, Family Practice, East Tennessee State University, Chattanooga, Tennessee

Benjamin Kligler, MD, MPH
Assistant Professor, Department of Family Medicine, Albert Einstein College of Medicine, Bronx, New York; Attending Physician, Beth Israel Medical Center, New York, New York

Roya Kohani, MD
Assistant Professor of Clinical Medicine, University of Arizona Health Sciences Center; University Medical Center, Tucson, Arizona

Wendy Kohatsu, MD
Assistant Professor, Family Medicine, East Tennessee State University, Kingsport, Tennessee; Graduate Fellow, Program in Integrative Medicine, University of Arizona, Tucson, Arizona

Meg Landgraf, PA-C
Condell Hospital; Northern Illinois Association of Physician Assistants; Northshore Health and Wellness; North Shore Cardiologists, Libertyville, Illinois

Roberta Anne Lee, MD
Medical Director, Center for Health and Healing; Internal Medicine; Beth Israel Medical Center, New York, New York

Alison Levitt, MD
Family to Family, Asheville, North Carolina

Aga Lewelt, MD
Transitional Year Resident, Reading Hospital, Reading, Pennsylvania; Physical Medicine and Rehabilitation Resident, University of Utah, Salt Lake City, Utah

Jeffry S. Life, MD, PhD
Physician and Assistant Professor, Department of Nutrition, Marywood University, Scranton, Pennsylvania; Medical Staff, Tyler Memorial Hospital, Tunkhannock, Pennsylvania

Victoria Maizes, MD
Assistant Professor of Medicine and Family and Community Medicine, Executive Director, Program in Integrative Medicine, University of Arizona, Tucson, Arizona

John D. Mark, MD
Assistant Professor of Medicine, Pediatric Pulmonary and Integrative Medicine, University of Arizona, Tucson, Arizona

Aubrey D. McElroy, MD
Assistant Professor, Family Medicine, East Tennessee State University, Kingsport, Tennessee

Seth McLaughlin, LMT, CNC, CPhT
Essential Therapies, Inc., Kingsport, Tennessee

Robert D. Mootz, DC
Associate Medical Director for Chiropractic, State of Washington, Department of Labor and Industries, Olympia, Washington

Scott M. Morcott, MD
Vice Chairman, Department of Family Practice, Condell Hospital, Libertyville, Illinois; Lake Forest Hospital, Lake Forest, Illinois; American Academy of Family Physicians and Illinois Academy of Family Physicians

Matt Mumber, MD
Radiation Oncologist, Regional Radiation Oncology Center at Rome, Rome, Georgia

James P. Nicolai, MD
Fellow, Program in Integrative Medicine, University of Arizona College of Medicine, Tucson, Arizona

Kenneth E. Olive, MD
Associate Professor and Vice Chair, Department of Internal Medicine, East Tennessee State University; Attending Physician, Johnson City Medical Center, Johnson City, Tennessee

Sunil Pai, MD
President and Medical Director, Integrative Medicine, Sanjevani, Santa Fe, New Mexico

Kenneth S. Peters, MD
Director, Northern California Headache Clinic; El Camino Hospital, Mountain View, California

David Rakel, MD
Director, University of Wisconsin Center for Integrative Medicine; Assistant Professor, Department of Family Medicine, University of Wisconsin; University of Wisconsin Hospitals and Clinics and St. Mary's Hospital, Madison, Wisconsin

Malcolm Riley, BDS, FDS, MRD
Executive Director, Alzheimer's Prevention Foundation, Tucson, Arizona

Sherry L. Robbins, MD
Assistant Professor and Family Medicine Junior Clerkship Course Director, Family Medicine, East Tennessee State University (James H. Quillen College of Medicine); ETSU Family Physicians of Kingsport; Wellmont Holston Valley Hospital, Kingsport, Tennessee; Baptist Hospital, Knoxville, Tennessee

Aviva Romm, BS, CPM, AHG
President, American Herbalists Guild, Canton, Georgia

Tamara Sachs, MD
Department of Medicine, New Milford Hospital, New Milford, Connecticut

Craig Schneider, MD
Director of Integrative Medicine and Assistant Residency Director, Family Practice Residency Program, Maine Medical Center, Portland, Maine

Nancy Schulman, MSB
President, Integrative Health Solutions, LLC, Denver, Colorado

Marcey Shapiro, MD
Private Practice, Berkeley, California

Shauna L. Shapiro, PhD
Department of Psychology, University of Arizona, Tucson, Arizona

Stefanie L. Shaver, MD
Resident, Kingsport Family Practice Residency Program, East Tennessee State University, Kingsport, Tennessee

Betsy S. Singh, PhD
Professor, Dean of Research, Southern California University of Health Sciences, Whittier, California

Vijay John Singh, BA
Research Assistant, Research Division, Southern California University of Health Sciences, Whittier, California

Monica J. Stokes, MD, FACOG
Integrative Medicine Consultant (Board Certified in Obstetrics and Gynecology), San Francisco, California; Graduate, Clinical Fellowship Program in Integrative Medicine, University of Arizona Health Sciences Center, Tucson, Arizona

Michael J. Stuart-Shor, MPH
Director for Development, Marino Foundation for Integrative Medicine, Cambridge, Massachusetts

Robert Edwin Svoboda, BAMS (Ayurvedacharya)
Adjunct Faculty, Bastyr University, Kenmore, Washington; Ayurvedic Institute, Albuquerque, New Mexico

Julia M. Thie, LAc, DiplAc
Licensed Acupuncturist (CA), Nationally Certified Acupuncturist and Herbalist, Kingsport, Tennessee

Silvarama Prasad Vinjamury, MD
Associate Professor, Research Division, Southern California University of Health Sciences, Whittier, California

Robert A. Weissberg, MD
Integrative Medicine, Albany, New York; Ellis Hospital, Schenectady, New York

Joy A. Weydert, MD, FAAP
Fellow, Integrative Medicine, Pediatric Center for Complementary and Alternative Medicine, University of Arizona, Tucson, Arizona

DEDICATION

To my parents, Marge and Takeshi Kohatsu,
For always believing in me.

ACKNOWLEDGMENTS

Big heartfelt thanks to all my wonderful chapter authors and the thread of community that binds us all together as one.

Thanks to Jim Kearns and Lana McGrady for their invaluable assistance in putting all the pieces of this book together. You kept me sane.

My deepest gratitude goes to the ETSU crew—Dr. Jim Wilson, for continuous support; Reid Blackwelder, who made the time possible; and to my Kingsport colleagues and residents, who put up with my times of absence. Special thanks to Susan Dolen and Sharon Brown at Holston Valley Medical Center Library for their always-gracious research support.

Thanks to "Uncle" Bernie Siegel, for pulling me from the edge during med school, and to Andy Weil for making the integrative vision come true.

Special appreciation goes to Matthew Flesch for his talented artwork and never-ending love and support.

Wendy Kohatsu

PREFACE

Complementary and Alternative Medicine Secrets is a collaborative work based on the authors' clinical experience in this rapidly expanding field. It takes on a distinctly integrative approach, presenting a much-needed balanced view of both CAM and allopathic medicine. The book's title was chosen for its greater familiarity currently in the general populace. The first section covers foundation topics—the history of CAM, CAM research, and the integrative approach. Therapeutic modalities such as mind-body-spirit interventions, alternative systems of medicine, manual therapies, botanicals, nutrition, lifestyle and energy medicine are covered next. The majority of *Complementary and Alternative Medicine Secrets* covers the basic questions one would have on diagnoses frequently encountered in primary care practice—ranging from anxiety, cancer, diabetes, menopause, back pain, otitis media, and much more. The special section at the end includes drug-herb interactions and the business of CAM.

Although written in the same user-friendly manner as other Secrets Series® books, *Complementary and Alternative Medicine Secrets* is **referenced in detail**. This was intentionally designed in order to help readers find often difficult-to-access, solid information in the field of CAM. As use of CAM grows, it is important to have the most updated information available because there are myriad alternative therapies to choose from, and a relative lack of good resources to draw upon.

This book was also conceived, written, and produced with a consciousness of community and a sincere desire to help readers learn about integrative medicine in a fun, yet informed manner. May it serve you well.

Wendy Kohatsu, M.D.

FOREWORD

This book is more than a collection of tips about using complementary and alternative (CAM) therapies in clinical practice. It is a compendium of information about putting integrative medicine into practice. Dr. Wendy Kohatsu is a graduate fellow of the University of Arizona's Program in Integrative Medicine (PIM), and she is steeped in the philosophy of that system. Many of the people she has asked to contribute chapters to this volume are also past or present PIM fellows or are otherwise affiliated with the integrative medicine movement.

Integrative medicine does seek to combine the best ideas and practices of conventional medicine and CAM, but it also insists on recognizing the primary importance of the body's intrinsic potential for healing, on viewing patients as whole persons (minds, spirits, community members as well as physical bodies), on analyzing lifestyle factors that shape health and illness, and on valuing the doctor/patient relationship as central to the process of healing.

Increasing numbers of patients want practitioners who adhere to this philosophy. In addition, the economic collapse of the conventional healthcare system demands radical change in the nature of medical practice. The "secrets" described in these pages represent the experience of integrative practitioners and are part of the solution. They are consistent with the best scientific evidence available and in no way conflict with the accumulated experience of conventional medical practice. One day, many of them will be part of mainstream medicine. Indeed, the inevitable success of the integrative medicine movement will be marked by dropping the adjective. This will simply be good medicine—safe, effective, and backed by scientific evidence.

I am delighted that a colleague of mine has assembled such a valuable collection of information and hope that it will benefit practitioners and patients alike.

Andrew Weil, M.D.
Director
Program in Integrative Medicine
University of Arizona
Tucson, Arizona

I. General Issues

1. HISTORY OF COMPLEMENTARY AND ALTERNATIVE MEDICINE IN THE U.S.

Wendy Kohatsu, M.D.

1. Define complementary and alternative medicine (CAM.)

Many umbrella or catch-all terms that have been used to indicate the wide variety of therapies used for self-healing. The most widely used functional definition of CAM is Eisenberg's: "therapies neither taught widely in medical schools nor generally available at U.S. hospitals."[1] CAM usually includes traditional Chinese medicine (TCM), ayurveda, other cultural healing systems, botanical medicine, nutritional supplements, manual therapies, homeopathy, energy medicine, and mind-body therapies. Despite the vast range of possible CAM therapies, they share common principles. Unifying themes among CAM practices include individualized treatment plans; belief in the healing power of nature; union of mind, body and spirit; and, often, more time spent with patients.

2. How prevalent is the use of CAM in the U.S.?

Interest in CAM has been increasing in both public and professional sectors. Consumers use alternative therapies frequently, are willing to pay for them, and often do not inform their physicians. Eisenberg et al. reported that the number of Americans using an alternative therapy rose from about 33% in 1990 to more than 42%t in 1997.[1,2] These numbers shook the world of conventional medicine. Although some surveys report much lower percentages, others concur or report even higher percentages, especially in larger cities with sizable ethnic populations. The main therapies used were herbal medicine, massage, mega-vitamin therapy, and self-help groups. Of great concern is that two-thirds of these patients did not tell their doctors about the use of CAM. Because of growing data about interactions between conventional and CAM therapies, open communication is imperative for all concerned. Despite vocal criticism about the limitation and lack of scientific merit of CAM therapies, 60% of doctors recommended alternative therapies to their patients at least once, and about half have used CAM at some time for themselves.[3]

3. What other terms have been used to describe CAM?

Pejorative terms such as "fringe medicine," "quackery," and "unorthodox," "irregular" or "cult medicine" have been used, exemplifying some of the animosity between CAM and allopathic practitioners throughout the history of medicine. The term *untraditional* is used paradoxically, since traditions of healing such as TCM and ayurveda have been practiced for thousands of years, whereas "traditional" Western medicine is a relative newcomer.

The term *alternative medicine* has been used since the 1970s. The problem with this term is that it implies that one must choose between allopathic medicine and the myriad of "alternatives." For example, a patient either uses chemotherapy *or* a macrobiotic diet to treat cancer, and no middle ground exists. The term *complementary medicine* comes closer to describing what many people in reality do; they combine the two worlds by taking their megavitamins as well as visiting their M.D. But the term *complementary* has the disadvantage of isolating the two fields instead of merging and embracing the overlap of the two.

Holistic and *integrative medicine* can practically be used interchangeably. Both terms take a balanced view of conventional medicine and CAM in a whole-person centered approach. *Integrative medicine* is the term that many major medical universities now use.

4. Describe some of the early traditions of CAM in the U.S.

In the 1800s, many systems of natural healing were established in the U.S., largely as a response to the heroic practices of conventional medical doctors at the time, which included purging, bleeding, and large doses of calomel (mercuric chloride) and/or opium. Battle lines were drawn between the regular physicians and alternative practitioners based on philosophical, moral, political, and socioeconomic differences. The "irregular" practitioners successfully repealed medical licensing for M.D.s in the early 1800s by denouncing their elitist nature. In 1847, the American Medical Association (AMA) was founded to erect a barrier between orthodox medicine and irregular practitioners.[4]

Thomasonianism, a program of botanical healing named after Samuel Thomson, a charismatic New Hampshire farmer, was the first alternative system in America. Its popularity faded after Thomson's death in 1843. Homeopathy, founded in the 1790s by Hahnemann (see Chapter 13), became the most popular alternative system in the U.S. during that time as its successes via a non-toxic, whole-person approach became widely known. Hydropathy used mostly cold water baths as well as modifications in diet and sleep and was popular until the end of the Civil War. Another import from Europe was mesmerism, a system of magnetic healing taught by Franz Mesmer, who used hypnotic trance and the power of suggestion to treat his patients. Eclectic medicine, a combination of many of the above therapies, was promoted by New Yorker Wooster Beach and flourished from the early 1820's until the 1930's.

The last decade of the 1800's saw the birth of osteopathy (see Chapter 15) and chiropractic (see Chapter 16)— each with its unique focus on manual medicine and self-healing—as well as naturopathy. By this time, nearly 20% of all practitioners of medicine were alternative physicians, an increase from approximately 10% in 1850.[5]

5. How did the Flexner Report change the course of U.S. medicine?

No single document has affected both CAM and allopathic medicine as much as Abraham Flexner's *Medical Education in the United States and Canada* (1910), simply called the Flexner Report.[6] Flexner, a respected educator, was hired by the Carnegie Foundation to investigate the state of medical and healing schools in North America in order to help leading philanthropists of the day decide where to invest their support. The result was a scathing report of practically all existing institutions. Chief among his criticism were the appalling low requirements for entry (often no more than "common school" education) and graduation. Schools in Minnesota were deemed "utterly wretched," and a New Orleans school was called "a hopeless affair." He dismissed homeopaths, osteopaths, naturopaths, and other "drugless healers" as members of "medical sects" who at worst were "unconscionable quacks."[7]

The shock waves from his report resulted in the closure of more than half the medical schools in the U.S. as well as many of the alternative medical schools in the two decades after the report. Only medical schools firmly grounded in scientific medicine withstood the purge, and the large majority of these were located in large, urban centers. The medical curricula became top-heavy in biomedicine and science, and with the concurrent development of germ theory and rapid improvements in aseptic techniques and later antibiotics, the reductionism of medicine to disease eradication was firmly entrenched. The Flexner Report not only served as a necessary wake-up call to create higher standards in medical education; ultimately it also challenged alternative practices to re-examine and strengthen themselves.

6. What changes took place in the 1900s as a result of the Flexner Report?

The AMA sponsored and lobbied for state medical licensing laws to wrest power from irregular practitioners once again. Eventually such laws were enacted in all states. Competition from other schools of medical practice quickly declined.[8] The early 1900s also ushered in the age of scientific medicine. Flexner's success in prioritizing the scientific method into medicine was followed by the discovery of penicillin and sulfa drugs in the 1930s. Alternative systems fell out of favor as nearly miraculous cures were seen with scientific medicine. Antibiotics could stop the plagues of infectious disease that had claimed so many lives. The ability to image the body and further understanding of genetic principles and biochemistry for the first time allowed elucidation of the mysteries of the body as well as quantification and control of disease in a precise manner. The love affair between scientific method and medicine flourished for the rest of the 20th century.

The 1960s saw the counterculture resurgence toward natural therapies. People in the "holistic health movement" began to explore the powerful relationship between mind and body. Breast-feeding and vegetarianism were brought into the fold by dedicated advocacy groups. After Nixon opened the doors to China in the 1970s, acupuncture and TCM were introduced to the U.S. Other practices followed.

7. What is naturopathy?

Naturopathic medicine is based on the belief in the ability of the body to heal itself—*vis medicatrix naturae* (the healing force of nature, also called the vital force). Naturopathy was founded in the late 1890s by German immigrant Benedict Lust. The definition of naturopathy lists a set of guiding principles.[9]

- Respect and enhance the healing power of nature.
- Identify the causes of disease.
- First do no harm.
- Treat the whole person.
- Take on the role of teacher.
- Prevention is the best cure
- Establish health and wellness

These principles are strikingly similar to the philosophical goals of holistic and integrative medicine. Naturopaths undergo 4 years of medical education and graduate with an N.D. (Naturopathic Doctor) degree. In addition to basic biomedical sciences, naturopaths study clinical nutrition, botanical medicine, hydrotherapy, homeopathy, physiotherapy (including exercise and manual techniques), minor surgery, detoxification, counseling, and lifestyle modification. Eleven states plus Puerto Rico and the U.S. Virgin Islands license naturopathic physicians. N.D.s do not have hospital admitting privileges but in a few states have prescription privileges for some naturally derived substances. Like their allopathic counterparts, NDs can be generalists, or specialize in such fields as natural childbirth, pediatrics, or physical medicine, or emphasize a particular modality in their practice. For more information, consult the American Association of Naturopathic Physicians at www.naturopathic.org.

Naturopaths practice in most states without a license. Without formal licensing standards, people with little or no formal training or a certificate from a correspondence course can proclaim themselves naturopaths. A licensed ND has at least 4100 hours at an accredited institution and has passed appropriate board exams.

8. What is anthroposophically extended medicine?

Austrian philosopher Rudolf Steiner (1861–1925) is credited with laying the foundations for anthroposophy (*anthropos* = human, *sophy* = wisdom) as a spiritual-scientific view of human individuality. Anthroposophic theories have been applied to agriculture (biodynamics), education (Waldolf Schools), and art. In the 1920s, Ita Wegman, a Dutch physician, collaborated with Steiner to extend these unified spiritual principles into the practice of medicine with the goal of embracing the spiritual depths of human existence via natural medicine (botanicals), homeopathy, and modern science.[10]

Most anthroposophic physicians practice in Europe, where over 12 hospitals specialize in this field. One school in Germany grants M.D. degrees. The Board of the American College of Anthroposophically Extended Medicine is the overseeing institution in the U.S. Steiner stipulated that anthroposophic physicians must be rooted in Western medical training; these MDs augment their training to include a threefold model of illness: the "sense-nerve"system, which covers the nervous system and thinking; the "rhythmic" system, which governs the pulse, breathing, intestinal rhythms. and emotions; and the "metabolic-limb" system, which covers elimination, metabolism, voluntary movement, and human will.

9. What is the role of nursing in CAM?

In 1859 Florence Nightingale stated that "Nature alone cures" and that the goal of the art of nursing "is to put the patient in the best condition for nature to act upon him."[11] The nursing profession has always taken a more holistic, and nurturing whole-person approach to healing, and nurses have been among the strongest supporters of CAM. Indeed, the practices of therapeutic touch and healing touch arose solely from the nursing profession. The American Holistic Nursing Association, founded by Charlotte McGuire in 1981, offers education and training leading to certification in holistic nursing. Consult the American Holistic Nursing Association [www.ahna.org] for more information.

10. Discuss the role of CAM in other countries.

What is considered CAM in the U.S. may very well be mainstream medicine in other countries. The World Health Organization (WHO) estimates that 70% of the world still relies on traditional healers. The role of ritual in healing spans many cultures across time (e.g., shamanistic journeys, Native American sweat lodges, kava ceremonies in the South Pacific, the work of curanderas in Central America, African drumming ceremonies). All of these cultures have a common theme of deepening the connection with spirit as a powerful means to healing. These practices are considered part of life rather than CAM. Herbals, nutrition, manual healing, and acupuncture have been successfully used as the primary therapies in countries such as India and China. In 1958, communist leader Mao Tse-Tung reinstated TCM as part of his nationalistic agenda; TCM and Western medicine are now practiced side by side in large hospitals in China. European countries note use of CAM equally as high as the U.S., if not higher, and in Australia approximately 50% of people use CAM.[2]

11. What about Native American medicine?

The credit for establishing CAM in the U.S. belongs to Native Americans. French explorer Cartier and his men, trapped by ice in the St. Lawrence River, were falling victims to scurvy until local natives provided a tea made from pine needles (a source of high amounts of vitamin C). Two hundred indigenous drugs attributed to Native Americans have been introduced to the U.S. Pharmacopeia (USP). Native Americans also are credited with creating the first syringe with an animal bladder as bulb and a hollow bone or quill as the applicator.[12] Native American healing focuses on the interconnectedness of mind, body, spirit, community, and nature. The process differs among various tribes but usually involves healing rituals that are directed by a medicine person or shaman. Disease is viewed as a disruption in the natural pattern of life. Herbal remedies, body purification, prayer, chanting, and creative arts such as sand painting are often used to help gain insight into the disease process and teach the patient how to reintegrate with the path of harmony.

12. What is NCCAM? What NIH-sponsored studies of CAM are under way?

In 1992, the National Institutes of Health (NIH) created the Office of Alternative Medicine (OAM) after heavy lobbying in Congress. Its first annual operation budget was a mere $1 million, which represented 0.1% of the total NIH budget—even though widely published data indicated that one-third of the U.S. population was using some form of CAM. Despite strong resistance, the OAM continued to grow and in 1998 expanded into what is now the National Center for Complementary and Alternative Medicine (NCCAM), with a budget of $68.7 million for fiscal year 2000. The NCCAM conducts and supports basic and clinical research in CAM. Unfortunately, less of an emphasis is placed on education. Current research projects include trials of acupuncture for treatment of hypertension; borage oil and ginkgo for treatment of asthma; Chinese exercise modalities for treatment of Parkinson's disease; dietary phytoestrogens for promotion of bone; and the effect of yoga on attention in aging and multiple sclerosis, and many more. For more details, see http://nccam.nih.gov.

13. How many medical schools are looking into CAM?

According to a 1998 study,[13] 75 of 117 (approximately 65%) allopathic medical schools offer some course work in CAM. This finding does not guarantee that doctors are uniformly learning about CAM because many of these courses are elective and often are offered as third- and fourth-year rotations within primary care departments. Approximately half of these CAM courses are introductory. Of the remaining half, more specialized electives include herbal pharmacology, qi-gong, and psychoneuroimmunology. Of interest, nearly half of the specialized CAM offerings are courses in spirituality. The listing is available at http://salk.cmpc.columbia.edu/dept/rosenthal/MD_Courses.html.

14. Discuss current and future trends for CAM.

In a recent report, more than 67% of adults in a national phone survey had used at least one CAM therapy in their lifetime. The younger the cohort, the more commonly CAM was used. Half of respondents who used a CAM therapy 5 years before the interview continued to do so. People often used CAM therapies at least in part to prevent future illness or to maintain health and vitality.[14] More insurance carriers, academic institutions, and individual health care providers are exploring CAM and integrative models. In the 1993 Eisenberg study, 60% of people paid fully out of pocket for CAM therapies; the rest were covered by insurance companies to some degree. Modalities most often covered in full were imagery, energy therapies, biofeedback, and relaxation techniques.

Trends in Specific Therapies

1960s	Commercial diet programs	1980s	Massage
	Lifestyle diet therapy		Naturopathy
	Megavitamin therapy		
	Self-help groups	1990s	Aromatherapy
			Energy healing
1970s	Biofeedback		Herbal medicine
	Energy healing		Massage
	Herbal medicine		Yoga
	Imagery		

From Kessler RC, et al: Long term trends in the use of complementary and alternative medical therapies in the United States. Ann Intern Med 135:262–268, 2001.

It will be interesting to see what patterns emerge from the first decades of the second millennium. Perhaps as the field of CAM evolves and as more practical information is available, the distinctions between mainstream medicine and CAM will fade, and we will be able to make conscious decisions about how to best help our patients.

REFERENCES

1. Eisenberg DM, Davis RB, et al: Trends in CAM use in the United States 1990–1997. Results of a follow-up national survey. JAMA 280:1569–1575, 1998.
2. Eisenberg DM, Kessler RC, et al: Unconventional medicine in the United States: Prevalence, costs, and patterns of use. N Engl J Med 328:246–252, 1993.
3. Berman B, Singh BB, Hartnoll S, et al:. Primary care physicians and alternative/complementary medicine: Knowledge, attitudes, and usage. J Am Board Fam Pract 11:272–281, 1998.
4. Rothstein WG: American Physicians in the 19th Century: From Sects to Science. Baltimore, Johns Hopkins University Press, 1985.
5. Whorton JC: The History of complementary and alternative medicine. In Jonas W, Levin JS (eds): Essentials of Complementary and Alternative Medicine. Philadelphia, Lippincott Williams & Wilkins, 1999, pp 16–30.
6. Flexner A: Medical Education in the United States and Canada. New York, Carnegie Foundation for the Advancement of Teaching, 1910.
7. Whorton JC: From cultism to CAM. Comple Health Pract Rev 6:113–125, 2001.
8. Starr P: The Transformation of American Medicine. CITY, PUBLISHER, 1982.
9. Murray MT, Pizzorno JE: Naturopathic medicine. In Jonas WB, Levin JS (eds): Essentials of Complementary and Alternative Medcine. Philadelphia, Lippincott Williams & Wilkins, 1987.
10. National Institutes of Health: Alternative Medicine: Expanding Medical Horizons. Washington, DC, National Institutes of Health, Office of Alternative Medicine, 1994 [NIH publication no. 94-066].
11. Nightingale F: Notes on Nursing. New York, Dover, 1969.
12. Perrone B, Stockel HH, Krueger V: Medicine Women, Curanderas, and Women Doctors. Norman, OK, University of Oklahoma Press, 1989.
13. Wetzel MS, et al: Courses involving complementary and alternative medicine at US medical schools. JAMA 280:784–787, 1998.
14. Kessler RC, et al: Long term trends in the use of complementary and alternative medical therapies in the United States. Ann Intern Med 135:262–268, 2001.

2. RESEARCH IN COMPLEMENTARY AND ALTERNATIVE MEDICINE

Betsy S. Singh, Ph.D., S. P. Vinjamury, M.D., and V. J. Singh, B.A.

1. How popular is complementary and alternative medicine (CAM)?

CAM has been a topic of interest among physicians, residents, and medical students, who feel an increased need to have knowledge about efficacy, safety, and mechanism of action of CAM therapies. Eisenberg et al. reported that the number of Americans using an alternative therapy rose from about 33% in 1990 to more than 42% in 1997.[1,2] A survey published in 1994 reveals that more than 60% of doctors from a wide range of specialties recommended alternative therapies to their patients at least once. In addition, 47% of the doctors in the study reported personal use of alternative therapies.[3,4]

A national survey conducted to understand the perceptions of CAM users in the United States reflects no dissatisfaction with conventional care. Adults who use both appear to value both.[5]

2. Discuss the role of empiricism in CAM.

Empiricism is a philosophical doctrine that regards experience as the only source of knowledge. The empiricist draws rules of practice not from theory but from close observation and experimentation, emphasizing inductive rather than deductive processes of thought. When a traditional health system such as ayurveda or Chinese medicine observes that an herbal formula, lifestyle change, or pressure/needle applied to a specific point produces changes in the patient's perception of symptoms, this information is based on empirical knowledge. Practitioners of these traditions pass clinical case notes to each new generation of practitioners. This knowledge is no different from that gleaned from descriptive case studies published in medical journals. The act of relegating experience and observable events to quackery or tradition is unfortunate.[6]

3. Do CAM practitioners rely more on tradition than research?

The perception that CAM practitioners rely on tradition rather than research is influenced also by the fact that many CAM therapies were used for thousands of years before the scientific community took an interest in testing them for effectiveness, efficacy, safety, and mechanism of action. In comparison, the randomized controlled trial (RCT) has been around for only 50 years and has been the standard for accepting new drugs for half that time.[7] Many CAM therapies, such as massage, herbal medicine, and acupuncture, existed long before interest or acceptable methods of investigation were developed.

Arguing for "proof by longevity" runs counter to the Western pharmaceutical model, in which a chemical product is manufactured to treat a specific set of symptoms or a specific disease.[8] Whereas Western pharmaceutical trials prospectively attempt to answer questions about mechanism of action and potential collateral or side effects before the drug leaves the preclinical investigational stage, many investigations in traditional CAM therapies must answer these questions post facto—long after the CAM practice has been used clinically. For example, many studies in recent years have attempted to determine the mechanism of action in acupuncture and chiropractic. Failure or delay in answering preclinical and finite clinical questions of when, where, and for whom a therapy works best does not mean that CAM therapies are worthless.

4. Should all of medicine be evidence-based?

Evidence-based medicine is a triangulation of knowledge from education, clinical practice, and the best research available for a given condition or therapy. Evidence-based medicine is becoming more widely accepted by an increasing number of allopathic as well as CAM practitioners. The practice of evidence-based medicine utilizes clinical expertise and external clinical evidence, integrated into a practical application of treatment, knowledge, and patient-physician interaction. It must be pointed out that evidence-based medicine is not based strictly on research data, such as RCTs or sham/placebo methods.

External data refer to any synthesis of information that can be easily presented to the patient and clinician. Reductionistic data, such as data derived solely from clinical trials, may not yield the necessary information for the patient for whom a physician is planning a course of treatment. The development of evidence-based medicine as a holistic approach is an important issue for CAM therapies and CAM practitioners.

5. What are the pros and cons of evidence-based medicine?

A primary criticism is that evidence-based medicine suggests a "cookie-cutter" mentality for the treatment of illness and thus is of little practical utility. A patient is diagnosed with a disease and treated according to a specified protocol. Some believe that such an approach is rather short-sighted because it ignores the concerns of patients as well as the instincts of practitioners.[9] Some critics see the prospect of "streamlining" the patient-physician relationship as a cost-cutting measure for managed care organizations. If this belief is held, managed care organizations would reap the primary financial benefit. Obviously, these scenarios do not take the third arm of the decision-making triad seriously; patient's attitudes and beliefs also should be valued.[10]

Advocates suggest that the "bottom-to-top" approach of evidence-based medicine integrates external data with clinical expertise and also allows patients to exert more control over their treatment options. By synthesizing such information with patient input, advocates argue that a holistic approach in any form is no longer marginalized. If administered effectively, evidence-based medicine allows patients a voice in treatment options and offers patient-centered treatment with the additional integration of physician/practitioner experience and relevant scientific knowledge.[11]

6. How much of allopathic medicine is evidence-based?

Although it is true that conventional medical scientists follow basic scientific medicine, some have noted that the medical profession as a whole has behaved quite unscientifically throughout its history. In 1983, the U.S. Office of Technology stated that only 10–20% of all procedures currently used in medical practice have been shown to be efficacious by a controlled trial. Current data suggest that still only 20–37% of accepted current practices in conventional medicine have been subjected to this same standard.[12] An RCT, by design, is likely to be extremely reductionistic; although internal validity is secured by such a rigorous design, generalizability may suffer. Thus, when a larger and more heterogeneous pool of people becomes exposed to a product during the postmarketing phase, unforeseen adverse side effects may occur, prompting a hasty recall by the manufacturer (e.g., Baycol, troglitazone, Phen-Fen).

7. What is the goal of research in CAM?

Given the overwhelming interest in and patronage of alternative therapies, the primary goal of CAM research is to provide rigorous scientific evaluation of CAM treatments. CAM investigators are obliged to examine the potential efficacy, safety, reliability and validity of CAM therapies. Strong opinions, which often dominate CAM, can be a hindrance to good research. Evidence-based CAM should no longer remain a contradiction in terms. The other goals of CAM research include[13]:

- Bridging the communication gap between patients and providers about CAM usage
- Emphasizing physician education about CAM topics
- Identifying and evaluating CAM treatments that effectively complement conventional medicine
- Increasing the amount of medical literature and documentation of research in CAM
- Last but not the least, economic evaluations such as cost-effectiveness analyses are necessary to inform decision-makers about the efficiency of CAM relative to conventional therapies.[14]

8. How may CAM research become more readily accepted?

An important goal of research in CAM has been to bridge the gaps of acceptance. Traditional western medicine has always looked at CAM therapies with suspicion because they generally do not fit the existing pattern of accepted scientific thought. If energy transfer from a healer's hands seems implausible, it is not likely to receive further study or inquiry. Some modern research has opened doors of greater acceptance via a shift in the way that CAM modalities are viewed. The acceptance of acupuncture and the rapid growth of sales of St. John's wort (SJW) in the U.S. are examples that substantiate this phenomenon. Acupuncture was accepted in the West after it was proved that needling can produce measurable changes in the endogenous opioid system. A system that has effectively treated patients for thousands of years immediately became "valid" because a mechanism acceptable to Western science became apparent. When similar proof of the efficacy of SJW in mild-to-moderate depression was published in 1997, U.S sales sky-rocketed.

9. What are the barriers to research in CAM?

Barriers to research include structural barriers in CAM, publication bias, RCTs, philosophical differences, lack of knowledge, and sample size.

10. Explain the structural barriers in CAM.

Funders, including the government, initially encouraged collaborations with conventional medical institutions. As a result, the conventional medical institution often received the lion's share of the indirect benefits, which slowed the building of infrastructure in CAM-focused institutions.[15] Credentialing also becomes an issue in research study review. As recently as 2001, a chiropractor with 5 years of clinical practice in a specific musculoskeletal disorder was considered inadequately trained to do the clinical assays in a research grant application.[16] The institution must now file an application with an M.D. on board to do the clinical assays for which chiropractors are specifically trained.

11. How common is publication bias in CAM?

The authors have experienced personally the publication bias against CAM. Peer reviewers for a mainstream medical journal indicated that they liked the article about acupuncture, recommended publication, and thought that it would indeed contribute to the body of knowledge. However, accompanying the peer review was a notation from the editor in chief, stating that he did not believe in the therapy, regardless of the data. The editor officially rejected the article because it did not include a "sham" arm, without which he considered the data irrelevant. Another example is Boline's study of the use of spinal manipulation vs. medication for tension headache.[17] It was rated as a high-quality article in two systematic reviews[18,19] but was denied publication in the *New England Journal of Medicine* and other journals. It finally found a home in the *Journal of Manipulative and Physiological Therapeutics* several years later.

12. Is the RCT a barrier in CAM research?

Dependence on the RCT delays the development of the foundation necessary for scientifically rigorous research. CAM researchers do themselves an injustice when they are pushed into doing RCTs too soon. Currently, the authors are involved in collaborative work focusing on the effect of a common ayurvedic supplement on survival of stroke victims. This work is first being done at a basic science level and appears promising. However, such investigations must be made methodically and stepwise. It is foolhardy to enroll stroke patients into a clinical trial without first knowing the proper dose and range of effects of the herb under study. Important information that can guide clinical decision-making can be derived from basic investigations of mechanism of action and from determining appropriate dosing or potential side effects of therapies.[20]

13. How are philosophical differences a barrier in CAM research?

Philosophical differences may be a barrier to research in CAM, but generally they come from scientists who do not recognize the need for matching questions with appropriate investigative methods.[21] RCTs—the gold standard—require application of uniform treatment to all subjects in the active group. Although this approach is simple in pharmaceutical trials (325 mg aspirin is 325 mg aspirin), it is not so straightforward for other healing systems. Many CAM therapies (e.g., traditional Chinese medicine, ayurveda) traditionally tailor therapy to the individual patient. Thus, ten different people with diabetes may receive ten different therapies, depending on personal evaluation. This approach obviously creates a huge logistic problem in study design.

Although traditional Chinese medicine, ayurveda, and classic homeopathy may include individualized prescriptions based on results of practitioner examinations, certain homeopathic remedies are sold over the counter for specific indications; ayurvedic herbals are under investigation for effectiveness for specific diagnoses; and attempts are being made to determine appropriateness of points, use of e-stim, and certain herbal formulas in traditional Chinese medicine. All of these investigations are appropriate, given the context in which the research is collected. None of them belies the traditional underpinning of knowledge from which the formulas or diagnostic criteria were developed.

14. How is lack of knowledge a barrier?

Research in CAM requires a marriage of scientists trained to conduct rigorous research with scientists who know the therapeutic modality under study. Initially this union was a barrier to CAM research. However, more and more conventionally trained physicians are taking courses in CAM therapies. In a nationwide survey published in 1998, Berman et al. found that use of CAM practices was best predicted by attitude toward the practice and training.[3,4] As more health care providers attend seminars, more continuing medical education courses in CAM are offered, and more practitioners engage in integrative training programs, lack of knowledge will become less of a barrier.

15. How is sample size a barrier to CAM research?

Sample sizes in CAM can indeed be small; however, this fact is not a problem unless the investigator has chosen the wrong design. Matching the design to the ability of the research unit to execute a trial is essential. Conventional medicine and research methods texts have discussed the devastating effect of small sample size on RCTs for years; it is not unique to CAM but may be more highly visible as naive researchers propose clinical trial designs that require many more participants than the team is able to recruit.[22-24] Falling short of recruitment needs to show differences between groups is a disaster for all researchers, not just those in CAM.

16. Discuss the role of the National Institutes of Health (NIH) in sponsoring research in CAM.

The enormous public interest in CAM guided Congress in 1992 to mandate the creation of the Office of Alternative Medicine (OAM) within the NIH, specifically to evaluate "unconventional medical practices." OAM's primary roles were to encourage the rigorous scientific evaluation of CAM treatments, to develop a solid infrastructure to coordinate and conduct research at the NIH, and to establish a clearinghouse to provide information to the public.

As interest in CAM grew through the 1990s, so did the activity in the NIH. In October 1998, OAM expanded into the National Center for Complementary and Alternative Medicine (NCCAM). NCCAM has greater ability to initiate and fund additional research projects and to provide more information to an ever-growing interested public. Its overriding mission is to give the American public reliable information about the safety and effectiveness of CAM practices. From its beginning as OAM with a research budget of $600,000, NCCAM's budget has steadily risen from $2 million to approximately $89 million in 2001. This funding increase reflects the public's growing need for CAM information that is based on rigorous scientific research.[25] In fiscal year 2001, the research project grant (RPG) portion has expanded to 36% of the total NCCAM budget.

The same legislation also established a White House Commission on Complementary and Alternative Medicine Policy. This commission is studying issues related to research, training, and certification of CAM practitioners, insurance coverage, and other important concerns.

17. Explain the value of case studies in CAM.

Case studies have existed since the dawn of research, but when applied to CAM, they often are ridiculed as "anecdotal" evidence. Case study research provides a useful tool for investigation of unusual cases or therapies for which effectiveness data are lacking and for preliminary investigation of any factor that may influence patient outcome. Indeed, anecdotal evidence is highly criticized in both CAM and conventional medicine. However, it is unlikely that colleagues will stop sharing information about patients who improved using a new regimen, even though this type of "doctors' lounge" conversation is not formal. Case study design allows the clinician to systematize the information about an interesting case and present it to peers for their critique and edification. Case studies may be constructed retrospectively out of traditional SOAP (subjective, objective assessment and plan) notes that followed the progress of an unusual or informative case. Prospective case studies are often either descriptive or experimental in design.

In a **prospective descriptive case study**, the investigator generally decides to follow specific data from the SOAP (chart) notes. The investigator may probe information more closely than normal and may indeed confirm certain clinical findings with laboratory assays. For the most part, however, the patient's care is pragmatic and documented through standard chart format, written up, and published to share the findings with colleagues. For example, if a patient decides to practice daily meditation, the clinician observes and documents the patient's progress to see whether meditation is successful.

In a **prospective experimental case study**, the investigator collects the normal SOAP notes on the patient in as much detail as possible but determines what outcome markers will be used before beginning the data collection. In this case, the observation becomes structurally similar to an outcomes study except that the sample may be merely one person or perhaps less than 10 for a structured case series. For example, if a patient takes a certain dose of garlic for 3 months, blood pressure and lipid profiles are measured before taking garlic and serially after beginning the therapy.

These data provide important information about the feasibility of a larger study, expected percentages of improvement, and potential problems from side effects and can help tremendously in determining proper dosing needs before a larger trial can be planned.

18. How do selection and use of controls in CAM affect perception of data usefulness?

Designing appropriate control groups is the major obstacle to conducting RCTs in CAM. Many allopathic studies use waiting-list or no-treatment controls, and some designs use historical controls. Educational arms have been used in allopathic trials when indeed education can in no way be considered a placebo or sham arm of the therapy being tested. Haslam recently compared the usefulness of acupuncture vs. an exercise program, using as the sham arm education in the treatment of osteoarthritis.[26] Comparison arms used in CAM research as shams and placebos are often difficult to operationalize. However, CAM therapies have been criticized for the use of these types of control groups, even though they are still used in allopathic investigations.

19. What are the challenges of using placebo or sham controls in CAM?

RCTs are not too difficult when participants are merely randomized into treatment vs. no treatment. But when critics insist that CAM therapies must use either placebo groups or sham groups in the design, logistic problems becomes particularly difficult. Oddly enough, homeopathy is one therapy for which the placebo/sham criticism is relatively easily handled, if classical prescription is not required by the design. The typical homeopathy pellet looks identical to a placebo pellet. Homeopathic RCT trials can be handled much the same as allopathic pharmaceutical trials with double-blind controls.

However, RCT design with placebo or sham control is extremely difficult with therapies such as chiropractic, acupuncture, or massage.[20,21] When information is gleaned from trials with control arms, which are neither placebo nor sham (e.g., waiting-list control, no-treatment control,[27] or education control), it is important for the reader to recognize that the control group is more accurately called a "comparison group." Use of this terminology underscores the point that the differences in study arms must be kept in mind when the data are interpreted. Investigators who use the term "comparison group" acknowledge that both groups were offered treatments that are perceptively different.

20. Can rigorous research be done when no placebo or sham arm is available?

Research rigor does not depend on the use of a placebo or sham study arm. Many human and animal RCTs are conducted with positive controls rather than absolute control arms. A positive control is generally a product or intervention that has been shown to have some degree of efficacy for a particular diagnosis. For example, in trials of new analgesics, aspirin or ibuprofen may be used as positive controls instead of or in addition to the no-treatment control arm. Research rigor comes from (1) knowing the existing literature about a research topic and (2) understanding what is known about any mechanism of action. The literature may provide clues to potential biases in the trial design, data that inform investigators about possible side effects, and utility of the planned design. This knowledge a priori facilitates the maximization of internal study validity (precisely measuring what is stated in the design) and external study validity (generalizability of findings to target population) for the current state of the science.

21. Are placebo trials difficult to design in CAM?

A placebo is an inert substance or "fake" surgery or therapy used as a control in an experiment. In clinical practice, a placebo may be given to patients for its possible or probable beneficial effect.[28] The placebo effect may be a measurement of changed behavior affected by a belief in the treatment.[29] In the case of massage, chiropractic manipulation/adjustment, and acupuncture, for example, placebos and shams become problematic. Practitioners and researchers into these therapies have been working diligently on the development of techniques that will qualify as either placebos or shams. In chiropractic, it is difficult to have participants who have received chiropractic treatment accept a placebo such as someone placing hands on them without adjustment or manipulation. In such situations, an even more reductionistic parameter to the design must be utilized: only patients naive to the therapy can be recruited.

Unlike the placebo arm of a study in which a participant is not adjusted or is given an inert substance, a sham arm tries to create an even more believable situation. The goal is to create a situation in which the patients believe that they are in the active treatment group but the sham treatment has the least possible effectiveness on target outcome measures. The design of such an arm has been the focus of many studies. However, it is a difficult task that must utilize naive participants during the developmental phase. In trials that have lengthy treatment phases, shams may indeed be impractical. How long will a participant believe that he or she has been assigned to an active treatment arm when the pain and dysfunction do not improve over 8–12 weeks? With high dropout rates due to lack of symptom relief, the trial will be jeopardized.

In addition, it may not be possible to create sham controls for therapies that necessitate the touch of the therapist or, in the case of acupuncture, placement of needles at points not relevant to the diagnosis or at a specified distance from the standard points for treatment. Some researchers believe that, once the skin is pierced in an acupuncture study, physiologic change has occurred in the participant, possibly stimulating nonspecific healing effects. Therefore, no truly "neutral" placebo exists, and the results obtained from the study are compromised.

Until standardized shams are available, placebo arms and comparison groups can be used in clinical trials without serious detriment. If absolutely replicable sham acupuncture points are not discovered or sham chiropractic adjustment is not precisely defined, outcome studies or other clinical trial designs are acceptable.

22. How should RCTs be done in CAM?

It is no more appropriate to do RCTs as the first research step in CAM therapies than for a new allopathic drug. It is important to consider certain basic factors before determining whether an RCT is the appropriate research design. First, one usually searches the literature to determine the current state of the science for the therapy and the diagnosis of interest as well as the theoretical underpinning of each. If there are still considerable gaps in the knowledge base, the obvious next step is to address these gaps first before tackling advanced research methodologies. For example, if the question asked is "How many females in the U.S. suffer from fibromyalgia?," an RCT, no matter how well designed, will not provide the answer. An epidemiologic research design is more appropriate.[8]

If a clinical research issue relates to dosing or optimization of treatment, a series of quasi-experimental design studies, such as an outcome design, may be needed before a definitive RCT using a placebo or sham arm is attempted. Preliminary clinical trials may be conducted to compare people receiving the therapy with people receiving no treatment. The use of the no-treatment arm allows the investigator to determine the efficacy of the therapy, taking into consideration the natural history of disease/disorder progression. Then, with (1) a solid knowledge of the scientific literature about a diagnosis and proposed treatment, (2) experience in execution of studies using the diagnosis and treatment of interest, (3) knowledge about sampling, (4) compliance, and (5) therapy adequacy, a definitive RCT can be planned.

In the presence of a solid foundation of information about the diagnosis and therapy, many important questions about clinical application of the therapy for various complaints may have been generated during the execution of intermediate trials. The questions for which a practitioner needs answers to practice evidence-based medicine may have been answered before an RCT was conducted, much less an RCT using a sham procedure.[30]

23. Do clinical research designs other than RCTs, systematic reviews, or meta-analyses provide useful data?

Although a hierarchy of research designs is generally accepted, many of the serious methodologic flaws in published RCTs stem from the fact that early, preliminary investigations were not done before a rigorous RCT design was attempted. Early studies, which admittedly are at the lower end of the research hierarchy, are necessary to determine where bias may be introduced into any design using the therapy of interest and sources of bias.[20] In addition, unless the therapy has a long history of safety, even if little information about efficacy is available, toxicologic data using animal models should be considered as a first step. For example, in developing a research track for several ayurvedic herbs, the authors conducted a thorough review of the literature, performed a descriptive case study and prospective experimental case study, followed by an outcome study, before initiating an RCT.

24. How important is randomization?

The notion that randomizing patients completely eliminates bias in a clinical design is not accurate. Many RCTs, particularly when funding is limited, use a small sample size.[31] The smaller the sample size of groups in a clinical trial, the less likely randomization will equally distribute participant characteristics across the groups. In addition, use of randomization does not insulate trial participants from factors that occur during the trial and may influence outcomes. Intervening variables, such as media campaigns, may create bias.

In addition, an RCT in which the treatment modality is "inadequate" can be disastrous—for example, if one expects a few yoga sessions to reverse years of chronic back pain or uses inadequate doses of echinacea in a trial of colds. If the treatment is not sufficient to produce change in patient status, the study may be reported as a negative trial. As a result, the intervention is perceived as not useful when it was simply not delivered properly or in sufficient strength to produce change. Keep in mind that the design should match the questions being asked and that designs other than an RCT may indeed be more appropriate.[32,33]

25. What about systematic reviews for CAM?

Systematic reviews (SRs) are a qualitative method to evaluate a group of RCTs dealing with a similar therapy or diagnosis.[34] Currently very few RCTs in CAM can be included in SRs. In the first place, not enough CAM RCTs have been published. Moreover, current SRs in CAM are affected by the heterogeneity of RCTs available for review, design flaws, and changing expectations for rigor of CAM research over the past 10 years. Even using pooled data, many SRs include small numbers of RCTs. Therefore, other levels of data analysis continue to be important in clinical decision-making.

26. What is the value of meta-analyses for CAM?

Meta-analysis in CAM is extremely difficult at this point.[35] Search strategies are similar to those for SRs; however, the analysis is quantitative rather than qualitative. An attempt is made to collect data from authors of RCTs, to normalize the scores across all of the trials included, and to determine the usefulness of a particular therapy. Meta-analyses also have been attempted to extrapolate systematic quantitative data from published reports. This approach is more problematic in terms of accuracy of analysis than receiving raw data from investigators. However, the research modality is designed to offer quantitative information about the success of a therapeutic option. This method is a shift from SRs, in which a large proportion of the emphasis is on qualitative evaluation of included trials.

27. Can homeopathy be researched using established scientific parameters?

Homeopathy is a complex and holistic system of medicine. It is an unconventional Western system developed in Germany and based on the principle that "like cures like" (i.e., the same substance that in large doses produces the symptoms of an illness in minute doses cures it). Homeopathy believes that even dilute remedies have great potency, provided that they are precisely selected based on detailed evaluations of symptoms to determine the patient's sensitivity. Therefore, homeopaths use small doses of specially prepared plant extracts and minerals to stimulate the body's defense mechanisms and healing processes in order to treat illness. The use of small doses of substances to promote significant biologic or chemical activity is not new to science or medicine (see Chapter 13).

Although it is considered difficult to design a clinical trial in classic homeopathy because the prescriptions are based on criteria such as pattern of symptoms as well as the diagnosis,[36] many studies have been published in medical journals and other scientific publications. For example, a systematic review of 89 double-blind or randomized placebo-controlled trials concluded that the clinical effects of homeopathic medicines are not simply the results of placebo. In fact, the authors found that homeopathic medicines had a 2.45 times greater effect than placebo.[37,38] Another survey[39] indicated that 107 controlled clinical trials have been conducted, 81 of which show beneficial effects of homeopathic medicines. A review of RCTs reporting homeopathic safety has recently been completed. Attempts are ongoing to evaluate both efficacy and safety of homeopathic therapy.

28. Is there any other mechanism to review the quality of published articles in CAM?

Scientific critiques of already published articles can analyze the various aspects of the study, such as sample size or poor design. Two journals (*FACT* and *Evidence-based Medicine*) deal exclusively with scientific critiques of CAM research, but most CAM journals frequently include critical reviews of already published articles. In *Medical Herbalism*, Hoppe and Bergner criticize a recent publication about SJW in the *Journal of the American Medical Association*, in which the authors claim that SJW is ineffective in major depression and discredit previous SJW studies. Hoppe and Bergner explain how the bias of the statistical analysis masks possible efficacy. They also challenge criticisms such as systematic biases in evaluation or reporting, nonstandard diagnostic practices, failure to use standardized symptom-rating instruments (i.e., Hamilton Depression Scale [HAMD]), short study duration, and low depression severity (< 18 on the HAMD).[40]

29. List sources for information about current research trials in CAM.

The Internet is the biggest and easiest tool to access various sources. Some of these resources, which are both popular and vigorous in selection criteria, are listed below:
- CAM on Pubmed
  http://www.ncbi.nlm.nih.gov/entrez/query.fcgi?db=PubMed&orig_db=PubMed&cmd_current=Limits&pmfilter_Subsets=Complementary+Medicine
  The National Center for Complementary and Alternative Medicine (NCCAM) and the National Library of Medicine (NLM) have launched CAM on PubMed—a new subset of PubMed—to provide free, web-based access to sources of information about CAM.
- Combined Health Information Database (CHID)
  http://chid.nih.gov
  CHID Online is a reference tool that leads health professionals, patients, and the general public to thousands of journal articles and educational materials that contain information about different health topics.
- International Bibliographic Information on Dietary Supplements (IBIDS)
  http://dietary-supplements.info.nih.gov/databases/ibids.html
  IBIDS is a database of published international, scientific literature about dietary supplements, including vitamins, minerals, and botanicals.
- National Institutes of Health Computer Retrieval of Information on Scientific Projects (NIH CRISP) Database
  http://www.crisp.cit.nih.gov/
  CRISP is a searchable database of federally funded biomedical research projects conducted at universities, hospitals, and other research institutions.
- Cochrane Collaboration
  http://www.cochrane.org
  Cochrane Collaboration is a searchable database available directly or through OVID. It is updated periodically and has the latest information about CAM research.
- Evidence-based Medicine (EBM)
  http://cebm.jr2.ox.ac.uk/
  The Center for Evidence-based Medicine maintains a database of the studies conducted with scientific methods.

- National Center for Complementary and Alternative Medicine (NCCAM) at the National Institutes of Health (NIH)
  http://nccam.nih.gov
- Alternative Therapies in Health and Medicine
  http://www.alternative-therapies.com
  The website of the leading peer-reviewed journal in CAM indexes all articles, features and abstracts, some of which are not captured in MedLine.
- NAtural PRoducts ALERT
  http://www.ag.uiuc.edu/~ffh/napra.html
  The brainchild of pharmacognosist Norman Farnsworth, the NAtural PRoducts ALERT is the largest relational database of world literature describing the ethnomedical or traditional uses, chemistry, and pharmacology of plant, microbial, and animal (primarily marine) extracts.

A larger compendium of CAM databases and online access can be found at http://cpmcnet. columbia.edu/dept/rosenthal/Databases.html. Specific websites related to CAM, such as holistic-online and acupuncture.com, give information about research in their respective fields.

... science's potential as an instrument for identifying the cultural constraints [imposed] upon it cannot be fully realized until scientists give up the twin myths of objectivity and inexorable march toward truth."

Stephen Jay Gould, *The Mismeasure of Man*

ACKNOWLEDGMENT

The authors thank Bhaswati Bhattacharya for her aid with the data sources.

REFERENCES

1. Eisenberg DM, Davis RB, Ettner SL, et al: Trends in CAM use in the United States 1990–1997: Results of a follow-up national survey. JAMA 280:1569–1575, 1998.
2. Eisenberg DM, Kessler RC, Foster C, et al: Unconventional medicine in the United States: Prevalence, costs, and patterns of use. N Engl J Med 328:246–252, 1993.
3. Berman BM, Singh BK, Lao L, et al: Physician's attitudes toward complementary/alternative medicine: A regional survey. J Am Board Fam Pract 8:361–366, 1995.
4. Berman B, Singh BB, Hartnoll S, et al: Primary care physicians and alternative/complementary medicine: knowledge, attitudes, and usage. J Am Board Fam Pract 11(4):272–281, 1998.
5. Eisenberg DM, Kessler RC, Van Rompay MI, et al: Perceptions about complementary therapies relative to conventional therapies among adults who use both: results from a national survey. Ann Intern Med 135(5):344–351, 2001.
6. Hammerly M: Integrative medicine—Who gives a CAM? Wellness eJournal, 2000. Accessed on 09/27/01.
7. Linde K, Jonas WB: Evaluating complementary and alternative medicine: The balance of rigor and relevance. In James WB, Levin JS (eds): Essentials of Complementary and Alternative Medicine. Philadelphia, Lippincott Williams & Wilkins, 1999, p 57.
8. Singh BB: Anecdote to RCT: Botanicals and the Regulatory Process.Washington, DC, DIA, 1997.
9. Sackett DL, Rosenberg WMC, Gray JAM, et al: Evidence-based medicine: What it is and what it isn't. Br Med J 312:71–72, 1996.
10. Evidence-based medicine, in its place [editorial]. Lancet 346:785, 1995.
11. Kaptchuk TJ: The double-blind, randomized, placebo-controlled trial: Gold standard or golden calf? J Clin Epidemiol 54:541–549, 2001.
12. Imrie R: The evidence for evidence based medicine. Complement Ther Med 8:123–126, 2002.
13. White A, Ernst E: The case for uncontrolled clinical trials: A starting point for the evidence base for CAM. Complement Ther Med 9(2):111-116, 2001.
14. Meenan R: Developing appropriate measures of the benefits of complementary and alternative medicine. J Health Serv Res Pol 6(1):38–43, 2001.
15. SCUHS, 16200 E. Amber Valley Drive, Whittier CA, 90604, 1997.
16. SCUHS, 16200 E. Amber Valley Drive, Whittier CA, 90604, 2001.
17. Boline P, Kassak K, Bronfort G, et al: Spinal manipulation vs. amiltriptyline for the treatment for the treatment of chronic tension-type headaches: A randomized clinical trial. J Manip Physiol Ther 18(3):148–154, 1995.

18. Hurwitz EL, Aker PD, Adams AH, et al: Manipulation and mobilization of the cervical spine: A systematic review of the literature. Spine 21:1746–1760, 1996.

19. Kjellman GV, Skagren EI, Oberg BE: A critical analysis of randomised clinical trials on neck pain and treatment efficacy: A review of the literature. Scand J Rehabil Med 31:139–152, 1999.

20. Singh BB, Berman BM: Research issues for clinical designs. Compl Ther Med 5:3–7, 1997.

21. Berman BM, Swyers JP, Hartnoll SM, et al: The public demand over alternative medicine: The importance of finding a middle ground. Altern Ther 6(1):98–101, 2000.

22. Lee N: Principles of Statistics. New York, Wiley, 1960.

23. Kraemer H: Coping strategies in psychiatric clinical research. J. Consult Clin Psychol 49:309–319, 1981.

24. Pocock SJ, Simon R: Sequential treatment assignment with balancing for prognostic factors in the controlled clinical trial. Biometrics 31(1):103-115, 1975.

25. Research Policies and Research Applications in CAM. Available at www.nccam.nih.gov. Accessed on 10/03/01.

26. Haslam R: A comparison of the acupuncture with advice and exercises on the symptomatic treatment of osteoarthritis of the hip: A randomised control trial. Acupunture Med 19(1):19–26, 2001.

27. Hrobjartsson A, Gotzsche PC: Is the placebo powerless? An analysis of clinical trials comparing placebo with no treatment. N Engl J Med 344(21):1594–1602, 2001.

28. Kaptchuk T: Subjectivity and the placebo effect in medicine. Altern Ther 7(5):101–108, 2001.

29. Talbot M: The placebo prescription. New York Times Magazine, January 9, 2000

30. Singh BB, Berman B, Hadazhy V, Bareta J: Clinical decisions in the use of acupuncture as an adjunct therapy for osteoarthritis (OA) of the knee in the elderly. Altern Ther Health Med 7(4):58–65, 2001.

31. Berman B, Leino V, Singh B: Ongoing investigation of sample size insufficiency in RCTs. Cited in Singh BB: A fully dressed outcome study vs a naked clinical trial. Presented at the Methodological Conference: What Can Be Done If Randomization Is Not Possible, Munich, October 1996.

32. Jadad AR, Rennie D: The randomized controlled trial gets a middle aged check up. JAMA 279:319–320, 1998.

33. Jadad AR, Moore RA, Carroll D, et al: Assessing the quality of randomized clinical trials: Is blinding necessary? Control Clin Trials 17:1–12, 1996.

34. Chalmers I, Haynes : Systematic reviews: Reporting, updating, and correcting systematic reviews of the effects of health care. Br Med J 309: 862–865, 1994.

35. Shapiro DA, Shapiro D: Comparative therapy outcome research:Methodological implications of meta-analysis. J Consult Clin Psychol 51:42–53, 1989.

36. Fisher P, Greenwood A,Huskisson EC, et al: Effect of homoeopathic treatment on fibrositis (primary fibromyalgia). Br Med J; 299:365–366, 1989.

37. Linde K, Clausius N, Ramirez G, et al: Are the clinical effects of homoeopathy placebo effects? A meta-analysis of placebo-controlled trials. Lancet 350:834–843, 1997.

38. Reilly D, Taylor MA, Beattie NGM, et al: Is the evidence for homoeopathy reproducible? Lancet 344:1601–1606, 1994.

39. Kleijnen J, Knipschild P, ter Riet G: Clinical trials of homoeopathy. Br Med J 302:316–332, 1991.

40. Hoppe J, Bergner P: St. John's wort and major depression: A critique of the JAMA trial. Med Herb 12(2):18–21, 2002.

3. THE INTEGRATIVE MEDICINE APPROACH

Wendy Kohatsu, M.D.

1. Define health and healing.

Health is defined by the World Health Organization as "a state of complete physical, mental and social well-being and not merely the absence of disease or infirmity."[1] **Healing** is the inherent quality of humans to make themselves whole. It is a dynamic process, calling into play the intricate interactions of mind, body, and spirit to bring about an internal sense of balance. Healing is distinct from curing. Curing implies finite resolution of the problem. Unfortunately, too often in Western medicine, a "curing" mentality is applied to all illnesses, and patients are seen as problems to be solved, not as people to be healed. Healing in the broader sense may be deeply connecting with one's inner self, spirituality, community, and environment. An integrative view acknowledges that healing comes from within the person and that all external methods simply activate the healing process. An expanded definition of health comes from Patch Adams, M.D.: "Health is an exuberant, joyful existence every single day of your life; anything less is a certain amount of disease."

2. What is integrative medicine?

The increasing percentage of the population using CAM confirms that people adopt multiple healing practices even when conventional biomedicine is available.[2] Various terms have arisen to describe the phenomenon of seeking health care outside allopathic medicine, including unconventional, unorthodox, alternative, holistic, complementary, and New Age medicine. Although the term complementary and alternative medicine (CAM) is commonly recognized, accepted, and easy to use, CAM is only a part of integrative medicine.

Integrative medicine is a healing-oriented approach that draws upon all therapeutic systems to form a comprehensive approach to the art and science of medicine. Despite its title, this book promotes a distinctly integrative approach, putting CAM in perspective as the authors do in their everyday practice of medicine and healing. Integrative medicine is not the domain of any particular subspecialty; surgeons and ophthalmologists can practice integrative medicine as well as primary care physicians and nurses. An integrative approach focuses on how medicine is practiced—not what particular discipline is used. It neither rejects conventional medicine nor uncritically accepts alternative medicine. It also represents a unified view of medicine and healing. As Andrew Weil of the University of Arizona Program in Integrative Medicine states, "Hopefully in the future, there will be no distinction between conventional, alternative, integrative medicine... it will simply be 'good medicine.'"

3. What are the principal tenets of integrative medicine?

1. **Provide patient-centered care.** Integrative medicine is relationship-based. It establishes a partnership between patient and practitioner in the healing process and considers all factors that influence health, wellness, and disease, including mind, spirit, and community as well as body.

2. **Foster healing; do not just address disease.** The central belief of integrative medicine is that the body has ability to heal itself. Natural, less invasive interventions are recommended whenever possible ("first do no harm"). The focus is on treating the root cause of disease rather than just symptoms.

3. **Support a dynamic model of health.** Health is a dynamic equilibrium, not a single endpoint. It is a constantly evolving view of the person over time.

4. **Maintain open-minded skepticism.** An integrative approach includes awareness of what the patient is doing and the intelligent synthesis of research and education. It recognizes that good medicine should be based in good science and open to new paradigms.

5. **Synthesize the best of allopathic medicine and other systems of medicine.** Synthesis fosters the appropriate use of both conventional and alternative methods, taking advantage of the best of evidence-based medicine with an appreciation of the complexity of the individual patient.

6. **Make a commitment to self-care and self-development.** Integrative medicine also acknowledges that the well-being of its practitioners plays a vital role in fostering healthy change in medicine. Understanding and enrichment of our own lives increases the quality of our relationships with patients and peers.

4. Why do patients seek integrative medicine?

A study in 1998 showed that people interested in alternative therapies have a greater belief in the healing power of the mind and spirit, had a "transformative experience" that changed their world view, and/or were looking for a more holistic orientation to health. Of interest, most people reported that their primary reason for using CAM services was not dissatisfaction with conventional care but rather a need to participate to a greater extent in their own health care by using more natural means.[3] Jonas and Levin also suggest that, in addition to holism and desire for lifestyle enhancement, patients are motivated by pragmatic reasons (e.g., allopathic medicine proved ineffective for their condition, especially chronic illnesses; adverse effects of conventional medicine; increasing costs), declining faith in the personal relevance of scientific breakthroughs, and social factors such as the increased access of health information to the public via media and the Internet (the so-called "democratization of medicine").[4] A study at the University of Arizona showed that patients with cancer chose integrative medicine because they saw the combination of CAM with allopathic medicine as superior to either alone.

A striking feature of allopathic biomedicine is the "sick role."[5] While assuming this role, the patient receives care, follows doctor's orders, and has permission to suspend his or her ordinary responsibilities of life. Unfortunately, this viewpoint fosters dependency rather than self-efficacy. For patients to take a more active role in their healing process, both empowerment and education are necessary ingredients. As Lown observes in *The Lost Art of Healing*:

> A doctor must rely on the art of human understanding to amplify the insights provided by science. A patient likewise must cultivate a special art, that of dealing with a physician. Whereas the medical transaction is largely concerned with curing a disease, the patient craves to be healed. . . . To heal requires a relationship marked by equality—a key element in a sound doctor-patient relationship—and reciprocal respect. This is not automatically granted by either; it needs to be earned.[6]

5. What is the role of self-care in integrative medicine?

Another key aspect to integrative medicine is commitment to self-care, self-development, and reflection. Chronic stress, heavy responsibility, demanding work pace, mastery of an ever-changing field, rapidly progressing technology, and the politics and changes in the financing of medicine add up to a prescription for dissatisfaction, burnout, and even illness. The allopathic training system is abusive, and little if any time is spent on quiet contemplation and personal reflection. Ideally, physician/healers should serve as role models of wellness. Because our lives do not stop the moment we enter the clinic, feeling secure, happy, satisfied, and fulfilled in our own lives translates into a more balanced work life and mindset. Healing is about making a life—not just a living.

Many physicians today feel that they would not choose their profession again, and many are clinically depressed. Rachel Naomi Remen, M.D., describes this "crisis of meaning" as unprecedented in the history of medicine:

> [B]ecause meaning is the antecedent to commitment, there's a growing interest in enabling physicians to reclaim the meaning of their work. . . . We may need to learn to pursue meaning in the same way that we now pursue expertise and knowledge, to recognize it for the resource that it is, and to protect it against the erosion of time. The meaning of medicine is not science, but service. . . . Service is a human relationship. It is the most powerful antidote to cynicism, depression, and burnout which are so widespread in our profession today.[7]

6. How does intuition fit into integrative medicine?

Intuition has been defined as the ability to have a "distinctive feel for what's important" or to follow a hunch and 'know' something without being able to offer a conscious reason.[8] Intuition is not the same as making an emotional decision based on avoiding an unpleasant outcome that we previously encountered.

Integrative medicine acknowledges there are different ways of knowing. Use of rational thinking is imperative in allopathic medicine, but time and time again doctors will tell one another about an incident that was guided by intuition or a "gut" feeling rather than reason. We routinely rely on our five senses to give us information, yet we are limited by our ability to perceive. We may trust logic, but it is important to recognize that medicine will never be free from value judgments and personal/cultural interpretations. Physicians are trained to collect and process objective data, but experience is a non-linear process and can guide us into tuning into what is most important at any given time. However, intuitive ways of thinking are not only discouraged, but often actively suppressed in medical training. It is important to rely on good judgement, but also to be open to other ways of knowing that may provide equally valid information.

7. What other tools does an integrative provider use?

Probably the single most powerful tool of any physician is the ability to listen. It is important to hear the "story" behind the chief complaint. Patients who feel that their doctors do not spend enough time listening or answering their questions report that this feeling promotes a lack of trust. This problem is also the primary reason that patients in the U.S.consider changing doctors.[9] Unspoken communication flows between the physician and patient at every intervention. Some suggest that in up to 75% of clinic visits, patients have an unvoiced agenda.[10] Greater awareness of this phenomenon and learning to bring out any suppressed concerns can help to foster more authentic relationships with patients. Learning to pick up such clues makes us not only better listeners but also better informed physicians. Empathic listening is time-efficient: "The effectiveness of empathy promotes diagnostic accuracy, therapeutic adherence, patient satisfaction while remaining time-efficient."[11]

The other major tool is talking. There is great power in words and language. *How* we communicate information may be more important than the actual content. Rushed words of advice, no matter how well-intended, may go unheard. Learning to be present and conscious in our communications helps to ensure that the message actually gets heard. Being mindful of how we come across to others is a valuable feedback tool and is a skill that can be mastered with disciplined practice.

8. How important is the factor of time in integrative medicine?

Doctors and patients cite the lack of time as major reason for dissatisfaction. Time may be the most precious of all health care resources. Family practitioners see patients every 20 minutes; general internists, every 26 minutes.[12] Our British counterparts spend even less time (7–9 minutes) per patient. The erosion of time for health care encounter exacts a heavy toll on both physicians and patients.

One expert analyst finds that "short-visit treatment promotes reactive medicine and pharmaceutical approaches. Harmed is the healing connection in the physician-patient relationship." The system has no financial incentives to change this approach, however, because superficial care pays better. Seeing three patients for 15 minutes each is 31% more profitable that seeing one patient for 45 minutes.[13] Speed and volume are rewarded, not quality of care. However, other studies show that more patient problems were discovered during the longer visits. In our haste, we may miss legitimate concerns that need attention. Osler's admonishment that it is "far better to know the patient that has a disease...than the disease that has a patient" rings true. Even if the only goal achieved by integrative medicine is to create more time for getting to know each patient, this goal will go a long way to fostering breakthroughs in healing.

9. What is psychoneuroimmunology?

An understanding of psychoneuroimmunology is important in integrative medicine. Candice Pert, Ph.D., has shown that a systemic flow to information directly links emotions and thoughts to our bodies. Receptors for neuropeptides are found not only in the brain but also in the entire GI tract, endocrine, cardiovascular, and immune systems: "Thus, neuropeptides can act at great distances with linear connections to their cellular targets; it is the specificity of the receptors that allows for such far-flung bodymind communication."[14] Greater understanding of the interconnectedness of our bodies is the crucial to integrative medicine. Recognition and appreciation of the relationship of stress to the immune and endocrine systems have increased significantly. It is well-established that stress affects physiology and that the relaxation response enhances healing mechanisms. A drug, herb, massage treatment, or prayer has the ability to affect health on multiple levels despite its initial mode of action. Greater understanding of psychoneuroimmunology may help us to use the inter-linked mechanisms within to foster greater healing.

10. What advice can we give to patients seeking CAM therapies?

Because it is unlikely that any single integrative practitioner will be fully versed in all of allo-pathic medicine and CAM, many integrative practitioners collaborate or make referrals to CAM practitioners who offer the specific expertise that patients need. It is advisable to check the creden-tials of all providers and even to receive a treatment to appreciate what the patient may experience. Identifying suitable licensed providers is important. Other advice includes discussing why patients desire a particular therapy (was it because Aunt Martha had impressive results using homeopathy or because of the latest enticement over the web?), inquiring about costs, and having patients keep a symptom diary. Shared responsibility should be encouraged. Whenever possible, review safety and efficacy data, but realize that a Medline search may be inadequate to obtain pertinent information for decision-making. Follow up, either in person or by phone to assess the adequacy of the CAM treat-ment and ask whether it interferes or interacts with other treatments. For example, if a patient takes supplements that lower blood sugar, diabetic medications may need to be adjusted. Requesting records from the CAM provider may allow one to see directly what took place during the appoint-ment and fosters more open communication.[15]

11. Where can one learn more about integrative medicine?

- The University of Arizona has both a 2-year residential fellowship in integrative medicine de-signed to create leaders in the field and an associate fellowship, which is a 2-year, web-based interactive curriculum in which participants study at home and receive 3 weeks of on-site training for certification in the field (see http://integrativemedicine.arizona.edu).
- The American Board of Holistic Medicine (ABHM) offers 5-day educational seminars with a formal examination based on a peer-developed standard of achievement. Students completing the course successfully receive diplomate status as a specialist in holistic medicine. The ABHM is not yet accredited but intends to apply for status in the American Board of Medical Specialties (see www.amerboardholisticmedicine.org).
- The Consortium of Academic Health Centers for Integrative Medicine is a think-tank group composed of 11 major universities with programs in integrative medicine, including Harvard, University of Massachusetts, University of Minnesota, Duke University, University of Arizona, Stanford, and University of California at San Francisco. At present, the consortium does not set formal policy but collaborates to implement change in medical education.

12. How can I make all of this information practical?

Don't just take SOAP (subjective, objective, assessment, and plan) notes; take SOAP-EE notes. Add the two Es:

1. **Education.** It is not enough to formulate a one-sided assessment and plan. A patient-centered approach also focuses on educating the patient. A visit is an opportunity to educate, remembering that "doctor" comes from the Latin *docere*, to teach. Asking what diabetic patients understand about their disease and overcoming barriers in knowledge may set the foundations for greater treatment adher-ence. Education may take the form of counseling about nutrition (e.g., switching to olive oil for cook-ing), demonstrating a simple relaxation technique to help alleviate anxiety, or simply explaining how drugs work in the body. Communicating in a way that the patient understands is critically important.

2. **Empowerment.** The job of the healer/physician is to bear witness, listen, support, offer nec-essary monitoring and therapeutics (both allopathic and CAM), and enable patients to evolve from passive victims into masters of their own health. The psychology of the "sick role" perpetuates the pathology. Healing the patient's perception of himself or herself may be the first step in breaking this cycle. Conventional medicine and even certain forms of CAM tend to foster dependency—on drugs, repeat appointments, or the physician as keeper of knowledge. Discussing with patients their level of

comfort in assuming the role of equal partner in the patient-provider relationship is the first step. Some patients may have been acculturated to feel that only the "doctor knows best" instead of learning to tune in and trust themselves. Each clinic visit can lead to further growth, movement along a dynamic continuum between disease and wellness. For example, patients with hypertension can learn to monitor their blood pressure and to incorporate healthy eating, exercise, and stress reduction techniques as tools to handle their disease. Empowerment moves people to take control of their own state of health.

13. What is the direction of the future of integrative medicine?

Some experts and philosophers of science view the current era as the emergence of a new era of postmodern medicine.[16] Different perspectives will clash with old perspectives—much as Galileo was ridiculed for proposing a heliotropic view of the galaxy, or as Pasteur struggled to convince the medical authorities of his day of the existence of microbes. The innovator becomes an outcast because he or she runs counter to the dominant paradigm/world view that defines the culture, including the culture of medicine. Whereas discovering the molecular properties of herbs meshes well with our current belief system in biomedicine, the effects of energy medicine or intentional prayer remain beyond our ken. The seeming incongruities in CAM/integrative medicine may be due to differences in perspective and not to any inherent weakness in its basic premises. Application of evidence-based approaches and rigorously controlled clinical trials to "prove" CAM may be motivated more by a desire to fit CAM into a familiar schema than of scientific necessity.[17] Modern science may be inadequate in a postmodern system to capture, measure, or quantify healing—the healing that may mean the most to patients.

On a practical level, there are two training possibilities for integrative medicine:[18] (1) seamless integration into medical school curricula or (2) development of integrative medicine as a separate medical specialty The first tries to foster change from within the system using a bottom-up approach; the second uses a top-down approach. Each possibility has its own strengths and weaknesses. Because they are distinct movements occurring independently, in the future a golden spike may be placed at the junction.

The future of integrative medicine depends on developing critical thinkers "fluent" in CAM—not just in how to dissect articles on acupuncture. It also depends on training (and retraining) compassion and humanism in medicine. Like health, the practice of medicine is a dynamic balancing act. The success of biomedicine of the past century shifted the burden of illness from acute infectious disease to more chronic, degenerative diseases, largely secondary to personal attitudes and lifestyles. We need to heartily acknowledge the technologic advances of the past century as well as embrace the new era of postmodern medicine. Integrative medicine represents the balance of the art and science of medicine, the balance between caring and knowing and the synthesis of high tech with high touch.

REFERENCES

1. World Health Organization: Preamble to the Constitution of the World Health Organization. WHO Basic Documents, 26th ed. Geneva, World Health Organization, 1976.
2. Kaptchuk TJ, Eisenberg DM: Varieties of healing. 1: Medical pluralism in the United States. Ann Intern Med 135(3):189–204, 2001.]
3. Astin JA: Why patients use alternative medicine: Results of a national study. JAMA 279:1548–1553, 1998.
4. Jonas W, Levin JS: Introduction: Models of medicine and healing. In Jonas W, Levin JS, (eds): Essentials of Complementary and Alternative Medicine. Philadelphia, Lippincott Williams & Wilkins, 1999 pp 4–6
5. Krippner S: Introduction: Common aspects of traditional healing systems across cultures.. In Jonas W, Levin JS (eds): Essentials of Complementary and Alternative Medicine. Philadelphia, Lippincott Williams & Wilkins, 1999, p 196.
6. Lown B: The Lost Art of Healing. New York, Houghton Mifflin, 1996.
7. Remen RN: Crisis of meaning [editorial]. Fam Pract News Jan 15, 2002, p 10.
8. Philipp R, Phillip E, Thorne P: The importance of intuition in the occupational medicine clinical consultation. Occup Med 49:37–41, 1999.
9. Keating NL: How are patients' specific ambulatory care experiences related to trust, satisfaction and considering changing physicians? J Gen Intern Med 17(1):29–39, 2002.

10. Lang F, Floyd M, Beine K: Clues to patients' expectations and concerns about their illnesses. Arch Fam Med 9:222–227, 2000.
11. Coulehan JL, et al: "Let me see if I have this right…": Words that help to build empathy. Ann Intern Med 135:221–227, 2001.
12. Davidoff F: Time. Ann Intern Med 127:483–485, 1997.
13. Weeks J: Coding time and complexities in health creation. Integr Med Consult Vol 4(1), Jan. 2002.]
14. Pert CB, Dreher HE, Ruff MR: The psychosomatic network: foundation of mind-body medicine. Altern Ther Health Med 4(4):30–41, 1998.
15. Eisenberg DM: Advising patients who seek alternative medicine therapies. Ann Intern Med 127:61–69, 1997.
16. Dacher E: The development of an integrated medical model: Toward a postmodern medicine. In Micozzi MS (ed): Fundamentals of Complementary and Alternative Medicine. New York, Churchill Livingstone, 2001, pp 57–71.
17. Tonelli MR, Callahan TC: Why alternative medicine cannot be evidence-based. Acad Med 76:1213–1220, 2001.
18. Weeks J: The Integrative MD: Giving shape to an informal, fragmented entity. Integr Med Consult. Nov:102, 2001.

II. Therapeutic Modalities

4. PLACEBO

Opher Caspi, M.D., M.A.

1. Define placebo.

A placebo can be described as a form of therapy without its content.[1] In other words, it is a biologically inert therapy designed to look like a real therapy. In Latin the word *placebo* means *I shall please*.[2] Placebos come in many forms: medications (e.g., sugar pill, normal saline injection), medical procedures (e.g., sham acupuncture, sham surgery), psychological interventions (e.g., attention-placebo treatments), and as part of the nonspecific components of treatment that may affect outcome (e.g., patient-doctor relationship).

2. How do we know that something is a placebo?

It is often difficult to tell. As medical knowledge changes, what may be regarded as an effective treatment at one point may become regarded as a placebo at a later time. Internal mammary artery ligation is a good example. A popular surgery in the 1950s to relieve angina, it is now known to be devoid of specific merit; any subjective improvement in symptoms should be attributed to the placebo effect rather than to the artery ligation itself. As a matter of fact, because of the many examples of failed therapies that worked, some believe that the history of medicine is the history of placebos. Thus, the labeling of an intervention as a placebo depends to a significant degree on the current state of medical knowledge about the proposed mechanism of action.

3. Define the placebo effect.

There is no universal definition of the placebo effect. Examples include the following:
- The psychological or psychophysiologic effect produced by placebo[3]
- A change in an illness attributable to the symbolic import of a treatment rather than a specific pharmacologic or physiologic property[4]
- A positive healing effect resulting from the use of any healing intervention that is presumed to be mediated by the symbolic effect of the intervention on the patient[5]
- A change in the body (or the body-mind unit) that results from the symbolic significance that one attributes to an event or object in the healing environment[6]
- The difference in outcome between a placebo-treated group and an untreated control group in an unbiased experiment[7]

For practical purposes, the two terms *placebo effect* and *placebo response* are synonyms. Yet some authors regard the placebo effect as the part of the therapeutic outcome that can be attributed directly to the administration of placebos, whereas the placebo response refers to the totality of the outcome.

4. True or false: The placebo response is about 30%.

The 30% figure often quoted as the average magnitude of the placebo effect is a myth. It is based on an article published in 1955 by Beecher, who summarized the results of several studies across conditions. His study, however, was methodologically flawed.[4] Placebo response rates vary enormously from study to study and may range from 0% to 100% without any scientific meaning attached to its average. This variability is not altogether surprising if one considers that the apparent benefits of treatment for any complex condition depend on both the targeted symptoms and the method of measuring symptoms. Each of these factors may vary from study to study, as may the overall context in which the study is carried out. For example, specialized placebo studies, in which the primary focus is the placebo effect itself, often yield high response rates, as do studies in which the main target symptom is psychological.

5. Is the placebo effect distinct from healing?

Both placebo effect and healing are inferential concepts; neither can be observed directly but only inferred. We observe specific phenomena that we attribute to healing (e.g., wound healing, DNA repair) but which may be manifestations of something else. Likewise, positive outcomes in the placebo arm of a study are attributed to placebo effect, but this conclusion is inferred—we do not know the exact mechanism by which positive outcomes occur. Misattribution of cause and effect, especially when placebos are involved, poses an important methodologic challenge that requires great attention and critical thinking. It is entirely possible that the same biologic events are labeled by different observers as spontaneous remission, spontaneous healing, or placebo effect, depending on their perspective, belief system, and/or context.

That said, the placebo effect is believed to promote health and healing. The power of placebo draws on the innate ability of the body to heal itself spontaneously. This innate capacity is best represented in the fundamental biologic principle of homeostasis, which is believed to exist in all living beings. Evidence indicates that self-repair occurs at all levels of physiology and anatomy.

6. Are all placebos known to be biologically inert considered equal?

No. It is generally accepted that the strength of a drug's placebo response is related to its route of administration. An intravenous injection, for example, is thought to be more effective than oral administration of the same placebo medication.[9] It is further believed that surgery and other medical devices, including those used in complementary/alternative medicine (CAM) such as acupuncture needles, may have an enhanced or mega-placebo effect.

7. What if we simply do not know the precise mechanism of action?

This difficult question is often raised in the context of CAM. The best approach is comparison of the intervention with a well-matched placebo in a well-designed clinical trial (other factors being equal). If the outcome in both arms is the same, the mechanism of action is most likely the placebo effect, and the intervention is classified as a placebo. If the intervention arm shows a superior outcome but the specific mechanism of action is unknown, some authors still hesitate to regard the intervention as real. At this point the author's worldview comes into play. An excellent example is the debate about homeopathy.[10] Some studies show that homeopathy has therapeutic effects greater than placebo, but the mechanism of homeopathy is not precisely known or even considered ludicrous. For some authors, a statistically significant difference is acceptable without full understanding of mechanisms, but for others the lack of a scientifically verifiable mechanism precludes acceptance of any data pertaining to homeopathy.

8. What is an active placebo?

Used mainly in research, an active placebo is typically an ineffective drug or a drug used at an ineffective dose that is administered to mimic the potential side effects of the intervention under study without having any direct influence on the condition itself. Although the placebo in this case is not biologically inert, its chemical properties are not relevant to the condition under consideration. Examples of active placebos include caffeine for the study of stimulants, atropine (which causes dry mouth) for the study of tricyclic antidepressants, and various sedatives for the study of the anxiolytic properties of benzodiazepines. An example of active placebos in CAM is the needling of real yet irrelevant acupoints (rather than sham acupuncture) in the study of the specificity of acupuncture for various conditions. Generally, in clinical trials that include active placebos as controls, the intervention under study shows decreased efficacy compared to trials that use truly inert placebos as controls.

9. Describe the nocebo effect.

The nocebo effect is the causation of a negative effect, sickness, or even death by expectations of sickness or death and associated emotional states. There are two forms of the nocebo effect.[11] In the generic form, subjects have vague negative expectations. For example, they are diffusely pessimistic and do not expect to get well; their expectations are realized in terms of symptoms, sickness, or death, none of which were specifically expected. In the specific form, the subject expects a particular negative outcome, which subsequently occurs (e.g., voodoo death). On the whole, physicians try to avoid the nocebo effect. However, a nocebo effect may occur when practitioners unintentionally convey negative messages related to prognosis or response to therapy (e.g., "you have 12 months to live").

10. Is the nocebo effect the same as placebo side effect?

No. Placebo side effects occur when expectations of healing produce sickness, however minor, or when a positive expectation has a negative outcome. For example, a rash may occur after administration of a placebo. Placebo side effects can be numerous. The nocebo effect, on the other hand, requires both negative expectations and negative outcome. To make matters more complicated, nocebos also may have side effects; that is, negative expectations produce positive outcomes or outcomes other than those expected.[11]

11. Are placebo effects and nonspecific effects the same?

The terms *placebo effect* and *nonspecific effect* of therapy often are used interchangeably, reflecting some confusion about their meaning. The popular definition of placebo as nonspecific treatment is not entirely accurate, because placebo effects tend to be highly specific. For example, subjects given placebo are known to report the same type of effect (e.g., pain reduction, healing of a peptic ulcer, bronchodilation in asthmatics) that is experienced by subjects given an active treatment.[12]

Nonspecific effects, on the other hand, refer to the common features of *all* therapeutic interventions, regardless of theoretical orientation, that are not measured and often ignored, such as the quality of the patient-physician relationship, potential healing ambiance of the clinical setting, extra time and attention spent on the study patient, and the patient's expectations.[13]

12. How can we estimate the magnitude of the placebo effect?

It is important to distinguish between the perceived and the true placebo effect. We often wrongly equate the response seen in the placebo arm of a clinical trial with only the placebo effect. To obtain the true placebo effect, other nonspecific effects need to be identified by including an untreated control group in clinical trials. The magnitude of the placebo effect is then the difference in outcome between a placebo-treated group and an untreated group in an unbiased experiment.[14]

13. What can we learn from the placebo arm of randomized, controlled trials? What can we not learn?

Unfortunately, there is still confusion between research methods that test efficacy and research methods that shed light on mechanisms of action. For some researchers, placebo control conditions are a means of setting a minimal standard of effectiveness for treatments. However, the mechanism of action is being evaluated rather than the effectiveness of the treatment. In the evaluation of medications, the assumption of the model being tested is that the effect of a medication consists of two components: a specific physiologic component and a nonspecific psychological component. The effect of a placebo, however, consists only of the nonspecific psychological component. Thus, total effectiveness is not being evaluated, but rather the extent to which the physiologic component adds significantly to the psychological component.[12]

14. Why is double-blinding important in randomized trials?

The concept of the double blind is fundamental to clinical research. It is considered a cornerstone of clinical trials evaluating the efficacy and often even the effectiveness of interventions. A true double blind study requires that both parties—subjects and caregivers—be ignorant of the true intervention. Blindness is used in clinical studies to control for potential external or nonspecific influences such as beliefs and expectations as well as to maintain as much objectivity as possible on the part of the researchers. The most common use of the double-blind method is within the context of double-blind, placebo-controlled, randomized trials, often considered by clinicians and researchers as the gold standard for clinical studies.

15. Are there any limitations to the placebo effect?

No. The belief that the placebo effect is limited to mild cases that would resolve with or without the placebo is not supported by the literature—nor is the belief that the placebo effect does not last as long as the effect elicited by real medications. Ample data show that a medication effect is, in fact, indistinguishable from a placebo effect.[15] Pharmacologically, placebos behave just like drugs: they elicit dose- and time-dependent effect and can have cumulative effects just like real drugs. Placebo effects play a role in the recovery from self-limited disease as well as from life-threatening conditions.

16. Is the placebo effect all in the mind?

No. The somewhat popular view that the placebo effect is psychological (thus not-so-real), whereas drug effects are physiologic (thus real), is a sad reflection of the Cartesian mind-body dichotomy. Plenty of evidence supports the bidirectional communication of mind and body under all circumstances, whether real medications or placebos are introduced. Placebo effects are manifested physiologically (as explained above), and the mechanisms involved are well specified (e.g., classic conditioning).[16]

17. Can the placebo effect be viewed as simply a nuisance artifact that occurs in randomized, controlled trials?

No. The placebo effect is real and occurs in all domains of health care. As a matter of fact, a maximally effective treatment can be expected to maximize the placebo effect. Recognizing that a treatment has a powerful placebo effect does not imply that it is entirely psychologically mediated. Two common examples illustrate the complexity of attributing cause and effect in medicine.

1. A patient is evaluated for a sore throat. Pending the results of a throat culture, a course of antibiotics is prescribed. The patient improves within a short period, even though the culture turned out to be negative. Clearly the antibiotics did nothing, and the improvement resulted either from the natural history of the disease or from the placebo effect (i.e., the belief in the medication itself triggered healing).

2. The same patient is evaluated for yet another episode of sore throat 1 year later. Again a throat culture is taken and a course of antibiotics is recommended. Again the patient improves within a short period, but this time the culture is positive for streptococci A. To what can we attribute the patient's recovery? Did the antibiotics trigger the cure, or was it possibly the natural history of the disease? Or is it once again a classic example of the placebo effect, in which he belief in the medication triggered healing?

In both cases any one of the above mechanisms—or any interaction among them—may have helped the patient recover. But we cannot be 100% certain that the cause of recovery was one or the other(s).

18. Is the placebo powerless?

In 1955 Beecher's seminal article, *The Powerful Placebo*, concluded that the magnitude of the placebo effect is about 30%.[17] On the other hand, a meta-analysis published in 2001 denounced the placebo as powerless.[18] Which study is right? Probably neither.[19] The only way to assess the power of placebos is to conduct a set of prospective, rigorous clinical trials during which the strength of placebo interventions is intentionally manipulated, and neither of these studies did so. Furthermore, as emphasized above, there is real doubt about the extent to which we can extrapolate from clinical trial findings to clinical practice guidelines. Estimating the magnitude of placebo effects in clinical trials, at best, may educate researchers (e.g., when they calculate the number of subjects needed in a study to show an effect, i.e., the study's power), but it has little relevance to clinical practice. Outside the realm of double-blind, randomized clinical trials, ample evidence supports the contention that the capacity to elicit placebo effects is inherent in each of us. Thus, the question is not whether placebos work but rather how we can maximize their effects in clinical practice.

19. Can improved patient outcome be misattributed to the placebo effect?

Yes. Some effects attributed to placebos are, in fact, methodologic artifacts. An evaluation of placebos and their mechanisms requires attention to the research literature in which placebo effects have been found. Such literature is of variable quality, and not all effects claimed to be placebo effects can be attributed to placebos. Among the most important alternative explanations are the following:

1. **Natural history of the disorder**. Many disorders are cyclical or improve spontaneously. An important reason for including no-treatment control groups in the evaluation of treatment effects is to

rule out natural history as an explanation of the observed improvement. For example, if a study explores the use of an herb as a novel treatment for multiple sclerosis and shows significant improvement after 1 month, it is difficult to determine whether the improvements were due to the herb or the cyclic nature of multiple sclerosis.

2. **Reactivity of measurement and patient biases.** This explanation refers to the extent to which patients are aware that they are being assessed. In clinical trials, typically all measures are reactive. The patient is assessed before and after treatment and knows that the assessments are an evaluation of the effectiveness of the interventions. Because the patient is aware of the assessment, incentives for biasing the response may play a role. For example, at the beginning of the study, patients may bias their responses to indicate increased severity so that they qualify for treatment. At the end of the study, patients may bias responses toward improvement as a means of being a good patient and as a means to end therapy. This pattern, often called a "hello-goodbye effect," results in demonstrating or exaggerating improvement even when little or no improvement has occurred.

3. **Regression to the mean.** This explanation refers to a statistical phenomenon that occurs when measurements are subject to error or vary randomly within patients. Individual scores that are high or low on one measurement occasion are likely to be closer to the mean of all scores on the second measurement occasion. The degree to which regression to the mean occurs in a study depends on the reliability of the measurement and the extent to which patients are selected for a study on the basis of extreme measurements. Patients may show improvement, both in the clinic and in research studies, even in the absence of treatment effects because of the variability of the intensity of symptoms over time (an effect of natural history) or because of the random error in the measurements being used (regression to the mean). On subsequent occasions, then, improvement is likely to be demonstrated even if the treatment or placebo had no effect. A no-treatment control group is essential to rule out regression to the mean as an explanation for the improvement of placebo interventions.

20. Is the placebo effect limited to certain types of patient personalities?

Several recent studies across different medical conditions and cultures reexamined the potential personality dimension of the placebo response. A review of the research concluded that personality traits found in one study differ from those reported in other studies. Contradictory findings can result from differences in clinical conditions, patient populations, research procedures, and settings. No data consistently relate either personality variables or demographic variables (e.g., age, sex, intelligence, race, social class, ethnicity, religiosity, religious background) to placebo reaction.[12]

The capacity to elicit the placebo reaction is probably inherent in everyone. The placebo effect seems to be contextual, situational phenomenon more than an enduring personality trait.

21. Can expectations trigger a placebo effect?

Yes. In fact, there are three different types of expectations[20]:

1. **Outcome expectations** refer to consequences that follow actions (e.g., taking a pain killer and immediately feeling much better).

2. **Self-efficacy expectations** are beliefs that one can successfully perform the actions required to achieve valued outcomes (e.g., I believe I can do it).

3. **Response expectations** are held by the person about his or her own emotional and physiologic responses, such as anxiety, pain, and mood. The person does not consider these responses to be volitional. Some authors have proposed that response expectations are the major determinant of placebo effects.

Expectations may be altered by even small variations in instructions and experimental designs in clinical research. For example, it has been shown that differences between double-blind and deceptive administration of placebos can produce different outcomes. In one study of response expectations about coffee,[21] all subjects were given decaffeinated coffee after being told either that (1) they may receive either caffeinated or decaffeinated coffee (similar to a double-blind setting) or (2) they would receive caffeinated coffee (deceptive administration). Results confirmed that the different protocols produced different results and that the subjects' expectations about the effect of caffeine were correlated significantly with performance across both experimental conditions.

22. Is the placebo effect a conditioned response?

Most early observers of the placebo effect attributed it to human suggestibility. Others, however, suggested that pavlovian conditioning of drug effects provided an alternative explanation. Many demonstrations indicate that inactive substances, after being paired with drugs, elicit pharmacologic responses. Such conditioned responses can be demonstrated with animals as well as humans. They may manifest as a new response to a previously neutral substance or as a modulation of the drug's effect. A few examples are caffeine, nicotine, cyclophosphamide, and nitroglycerin. Substantial evidence suggests that some placebo effects are best conceptualized as pavlovian conditioned responses, whereas others are not. Probably there are several placebo effects, each mediated by a different process.[22]

23. Discuss the role of culture in the placebo effect.

Cultural differences play a role in the response to placebos. For example, in a sample of 117 studies of treatment for peptic ulcer disease, the placebo healing rate was 7% in Brazil vs. 36% in the rest of the world. The placebo effects for the treatment of peptic ulcer disease were significantly higher in Germany than elsewhere in the world. A study of Czech patients with a variety of somatic and psychological problems showed that capsules with warm colors induced sympathicotonic symptoms, extending to aggressiveness with explosive manifestations, whereas cold colors evoked vagotonic sedative symptoms, extending to collapse. A Dutch survey found that stimulant medications tend to be marketed as red, yellow, or orange tablets, whereas depressants tend to be marketed as blue, green, or purple tablets. In Italy, on the other hand, blue medications are associated with arousal among men.[23]

24. How is placebo analgesia mediated?

In placebo analgesia, the administration of a substance known to be nonanalgesic (e.g., saline injection) produces an analgesic response when the subject is told that it is a pain killer. Several theories attempt to explain this effect by means of anxiety mechanisms, cognitive process, and classic conditioning. The neurobiology of the placebo was born when it was discovered that placebo analgesia is mediated by endogenous opioids. In addition, the opioid antagonist naloxone can reverse placebo analgesia, and the blockade of the receptors for the neuropeptide cholecystokinin potentiates the placebo analgesic response. One intriguing study demonstrated that placebo as well as a true analgesic increased blood flow to specific opioid parts of the brain, as seen on positron emission tomography. Thus, it seems that the endogenous pain-killing system can be activated by placebo analgesia, which somehow taps into the specific neuropeptide pathways.[24]

25. Define the Hawthorne effect.

Named after a social experiment done in 1927 in a factory called Hawthorne Works, the Hawthorne effect refers to the positive effects associated with the mere enrollment in a study. It is the tendency of people to improve in behavior and functioning simply because they are being observed or monitored. The Hawthorne effect can be controlled in clinical research by the administration of treatment to all subjects under equal conditions. The Hawthorne effect contributes to the placebo effect, but the two terms are not synonymous.[25]

26. To what extent is it ethical to use placebos as controls in research?

This topic is highly controversial. On one hand, the Declaration of Helsinki, based on the principle that in human research the interest of science and society should not take precedence over considerations related to the well-being of the subject, explicitly forbids the use of placebo groups *if* an accepted treatment exists. Proponents of this view contend that under these guidelines placebo comparisons are unethical if any treatment is demonstrably effective and hence should not be used at the researcher's discretion. On the other hand, federal regulatory authorities, such as the Food and Drug Administration, contend that a placebo group is needed to provide the benchmark from which the effect of a new treatment should be measured. Proponents of this view fear that comparing new drugs with approved drugs without using a placebo anchor point can lead to approval of ineffective drugs.[26]

27. Is it ethical to use placebos in clinical practice?

This question is by no means easy to answer. For most practitioners, giving a product with no known activity represents deception and betrayal of a patient's trust. However, we probably unwittingly contribute to the placebo effect all of the time via nonspecific effects. For example, what are the legitimate indications, if any, for which placebo prescription is at all justified? Are practitioners always obliged to tell the truth, the whole truth, and nothing but the truth to their patients—even if they believe that a placebo in fact may help the patient? Are practitioners allowed to deceive patients? For example, can they deliberately exaggerate the potential benefit of a medication because optimism and positive expectations are associated with improved outcome? When the efficacy of an intervention is not evidence-based (as is the case with most interventions in medicine, including CAM), should practitioners disclose this fact to their patients? What is the fine balance between the practitioner's obligation to maximize the placebo effect and his or her obligation to respect the patient's autonomy to make informed decisions? To what extent may discussion of rare side effects potential a nocebo response? The answers to these and many other related questions are by no means black and white.

28. What wisdom can be gained about people who demonstrate a strong placebo response?

In nearly every published clinical trial, a certain subset of patients in the placebo arm experiences exactly the same therapeutic effects and adverse effects as the treatment group. Is belief the mechanism of action? Do these subjects falsely believe that they are receiving active treatment, and is this belief strong enough to mimic the exact positive effects of the active treatment? The surest testimony to the power of the placebo response occurs when a supposedly inert substance creates objective findings similar to those of the active treatment without administration of the active substance. Such placebo responders somehow have triggered a healing response from within or by the power of belief, since it cannot be attributed to the drug itself. Rather than just a technical nuisance, placebo can be regarded as the greatest gift to self-healing. It would be a grand experiment to explore how placebo responders in randomized, controlled trials manage to accomplish self-healing.

29. Can the placebo effect be called into play purposefully?

Optimal care of patients requires maximization of the placebo effect. The placebo effect is more likely to occur in the clinic when the patient regards the clinician as experienced, competent, and optimistic and when the clinician expects the treatment to help. One study suggests that the placebo effect occurs only when patient and physician are of like mind.[28] According to this supposition, both need to share positive beliefs and expectations as well as a good relationship. A study of the impact of the physician's positive attitude on patient outcomes found that the physician's advice was a more effective placebo intervention than the administration of a placebo prescription. The placebo effect thus depends on the interaction among the clinician, the treatment process, and the patient. The patient's perception of that interaction often ignites the healing/placebo process.[29] The premise is simple: the clinician is a therapeutic agent, and the medical encounter is its playing field. As one writer observed, the physician is a vastly more important institution than the drug store.

REFERENCES

1. Ernst E: Make believe medicine: The amazing powers of placebos. Eur J Med Rehabil 6:124–125, 1996.
2. Aronson J: When I use a word . . . . Please, please me. Br Med J 318:716, 1999.
3. Shapiro AK: Factors contributing to the placebo effect. Am J Psychother 18:73–88, 1964.
4. Brody H: Placebos and the Philosophy of Medicine: Clinical, Conceptual, and Ethical Issues. Chicago, University of Chicago Press, 1980.
5. National Institutes of Health, OAM sponsors placebo and nocebo conference. CAM Newsletter 1997.
6. Brody H: The Placebo Response: How You Can Release the Body's Inner Pharmacy for Better Health. New York, Harper Collins, 2000.
7. Götzsche PC: Is there logic in the placebo? Lancet 344:926–926, 1994.
8. Kienle GS, Kiene H: Placebo effect and placebo concept: A critical methodological and conceptual analysis of reports on the magnitude of the placebo effect. Altern Ther Health Med 2:39–54, 1996.
9. Kaptchuk TJ, et al: Do medical devices have enhanced placebo effects: J Clin Epidemiol 53:786–792, 2000.
10. Linde K, Clausius N, Ramirez G, et al: Are the clinical effects of homeopathy placebo effects? A meta-

      analysis of placebo-controlled trials. Lancet 350:834–843, 1997.
11. Hahn RA: The nocebo phenomenon: Concept, evidence, and implications for public health. Prevent Med
      26(5 Pt 1):607–611, 1997.
12. Bootzin RR, Caspi O: Explanatory mechanisms for placebo effects. In Guess HA, et al (eds): The Science of
      the Placebo: Toward an Interdisciplinary Research Agenda. London, BMJ Books, 2002.
13. Grencavage L, Bootzin RR, Shoham V: Specific and nonspecific effects in psychological treatments. In
      Costello CG (ed): Basic Issues in Psychopathology. New York, Guilford Press, pp 359–376.
14. Ernst E, Resch KL: Concept of true and perceived placebo effects. Br Med J 311:551–553, 1995.
15. Kirsch I, Sapirstein G: Listening to Prozac but hearing placebo: A meta-analysis of antidepressant medica-
      tion. Prevent Treat 1, 2000.
16. Ader R: The placebo effect: If it's all in your head, does that mean you only think you feel better? Adv Mind-
      Body Med 16:7–11, 2000.
17. Beecher HK: The powerful placebo. JAMA 159:1602–1606, 1955.
18. Bjartsson HR, Götzsche PC: Is the placebo powerless? An analysis of clinical trials comparing placebo with
      no treatment. N Engl J Med 344:1594–1602, 2001.
19. Greene PJ, Wayne PM, Kerr CE, et al: The powerful placebo: Doubting the doubters. Adv Mind-Body Med
      17:298–307, 2001.
20. Kirsch I, Sapirstein G: Automaticity in clinical psychology. Am Psychol 54:504–515, 1999.
21. Kirsch I, Weixel LJ: Double-blind versus deceptive administration of a placebo. Behav Neurosci 102:319–
      323, 1999.
22. Siegal S: Explanatory mechanisms of the placebo effect: Pavlovian conditioning. In Guess HA, et al (eds):
      The Science of the Placebo: Toward an Interdisciplinary Research Agenda. London, BMJ Books, 2002.
23. Moerman DE: Cultural variations in the placebo effect: Ulcers, anxiety, and blood pressure. Med Anthropol
      Q 14:51–72, 2000.
24. Price DD, Soerensen LV: Endogenous opioid and non-opioid pathways as mediators of placebo analgesia. In
      Guess HA, et al (eds): The Science of the Placebo: Toward an Interdisciplinary Research Agenda.
      London, BMJ Books, 2002.
25. Bailar JC III: The powerful placebo and the Wizard of Oz. N Engl J Med 344:1630–1632, 2001.
26. Temple R, Ellenberg SS: Placebo-controlled trials and active-control trials in the evaluation of new treat-
      ments. Part I: Ethical and scientific issues. Ann Intern Med 133:455–463, 2000.
27. Levine RJ: Placebo controls in clinical trials of new therapies for which there are no known effective treat-
      ments. In Guess HA, et al (eds): The Science of the Placebo: Toward an Interdisciplinary Research
      Agenda. London, BMJ Books, 2002.
28. Benson H, Epstein MD: The placebo effect: A neglected asset in the care of patients. JAMA 232:1255–1227,
      1975.
29. Di Blasi Z, et al: Influence of context effects on health outcomes: A systematic review. Lancet 357:757–762,
      2001.

5. CREATIVE ARTS THERAPY

Pali Delevitt and Aga Lewelt

1. What are the creative art therapies?

The most commonly used modes of creative art therapy include music, art, dance or movement, journaling, and poetry. As the name implies, all of these interventions use creative expression to offer therapeutic benefit— including improvement in quality of life, expression of unspoken and often unconscious concerns about illness, increased self-awareness, and coming to terms with emotional conflicts. Music therapy and journaling have been the most extensively studied.

2. Why is it important to consider the use of creative arts in healing?

Creative expression can be used to cope with life challenges or as a means of transcending. It offers the opportunity for each of us to tap into parts of ourselves that often have been neglected or left unexpressed. One could simply acknowledge that it is good therapy to express the unconscious self and that humans are inherently creative in their life force. When the life force has been shut down or limited, disease may be a natural result. A logical antidote to encourage people to begin to express themselves freely in whatever medium they may feel most comfortable.

The rational mind may limit perceptions through the use of internal censors. Creative expression, like dreaming, often gives rise to insight and information that is not accessible through intellectual means. Cognitive therapy may not create as much of a breakthrough as the freedom to express the self through the powerful nonverbal medium of crayons or the heartfelt flow of a poem. We may not always be able to measure the healing response in terms of numbers or data, but we can experience it in our patients' response to disease, treatment, and the world around them.

If healing is about becoming whole, creative expression can help us to heal the grief that comes from loss to our bodies and psyche through the course of illness or loss of a loved one in death. There is no more powerful healing instrument than the gift of heartfelt expression for what we have lost. When we allow our hearts to speak through the medium of our creative spirit, we find release and perhaps a reframing of the experience into one of personal power and triumph. Furthermore, all of these interventions carry a highly reasonable risk-to-benefit ratio and are usually not costly. They are often excellent complements to conventional treatments.

I am no longer afraid of mirrors
Where I see the sign of the Amazon
The one who shoots arrows.
There was a fine red line across my chest
    where a knife entered.
But now a branch winds around the scar
And travels from arm to heart.
Green leaves cover the branch, grapes hang there,
    and a bird appears.
What grows in me now is vital
    and does not cause me harm.

I think the bird is singing.
I have relinquished some of the scars.
I have designed my chest with the care
    given an illumined manuscript.
I am no longer ashamed to make love.
Love is a battle I can win.
I have the body of a warrior
    who does not kill or wound.
On the book of my body
I have permanently inscribed
    a tree of life.

        —Deena Metzger

From *Tree: Essays and Pieces.* Berkeley, CA, North Atlantic Books, 1997; "Warrior Poster," distributed by Donnelly/Colt, Hampton, CT. With permission.

3. What are the general functions of the creative arts therapies? Which specific populations have used them?

All creative arts therapies afford an opportunity to use our "artistic side." Several authors have written about the value of using the creative side to learn new tasks and experience a new way of viewing the world. In *Drawing on the Right Side of the Brain: A Course in Enhancing Creativity and Artistic Confidence*,[1] Betty Edwards outlines a method to see the world with our artistic right brain instead of using the mechanistic left brain. Left-brain activities, such as mathematical and technical reasoning, are believed to be more prevalent in Western culture. Seeing the world in a different light and learning to utilize the other 50% of the brain may be therapeutic. Case reports have been published for patients with a wide range of disease types, and studies have shown positive physiologic effects in normal volunteers.

4. Are we prewired to pursue pleasure and play?

One need only look at the normal routine of most young children to recognize the benefits of play— as both learning tool and therapy. Evidence indicates that our brains are preprogrammed to encourage experiences of play and pleasure through the release of certain neuropeptides. Pessimism, depression, anxiety, social isolation, and hostility have been linked to greater mortality and morbidity. Pleasurable activities, such as watching fish swim in a tank, hearing the sounds of nature, and eating delicious food, enliven our senses and allow us to enjoy fuller lives. Laughter has been shown to have significant neurohormonal effects, including drops in epinephrine and cortisol. Humor has the power to dispel hostile and resentful feelings and to bind people together. For a review of the medical benefits of pleasure, read *Healthy Pleasures* by Ornstein and Sobel.[2]

5. Is laughter really the best medicine?

Humor therapy involves the use of humor as a relief of physical and emotional difficulties. One of the most famous instances of this approach was documented in Norman Cousins in *Anatomy of an Illness, As Perceived by the Patient*. Cousins recovered from ankylosing spondylitis by using humor therapy as a significant part of his self-designed regimen, which included watching Marx Brothers videos from his hospital bed. Significant neuroendocrine changes take place in the body during laughter, and these hormonal changes certainly may account for a physiologic healing response. Some literature documents the physiology and neuropsychologic benefits of mirthful laughter. For information from one of the leaders in the field, see www.patchadams.org.

6. Give examples of ways in which music has been used in healing throughout history.

Music was almost certainly the first art form to be used to treat illness.[3] In the Bible David plays his harp for King Saul to ease his melancholy. Ancient Egyptians believed that music bestowed fertility. Ancient Greeks used music as medicine to mend the body by way of the soul. Greek physicians used music to move patients form their original emotional condition into an intense orgiastic state that they considered to be cathartic as well as essential in guiding the patient toward a healthy emotional balance. More than 1000 years ago, Arab and Judaic healers used music to help patients with psychiatric disorders. The effects of music on specific physiologic processes, such as cardiac output, respiratory rate, pulse rate, and blood pressure, were originally reported in the late 1800s.[4]

Music also has been used to help people in the transition between life and death. In Medieval times, beautiful music was played in hospices for the dying. This tradition is carried forward by Theresa Shroeder-Shaker in *The Chalice of Repose*. In the Buddhist tradition, the dying person is chanted over for the hours before and after death to ease the transition. Music therapist Deforia Lane, herself a cancer survivor, has designed and implemented an outstanding music therapy program at the Ireland Cancer Center, part of the University Hospitals of Cleveland. This program has brought the experience of both listening to and creating music to pediatric patients and their families. Lane views music from a spiritual perspective; it has transcendent powers to heal and to touch people at a deep and personal level.

Music affects our moods, emotions, and performance. One study found that, depending on the type of music to which they listened, participants reported noticeable changes in either negative feelings, such as hostility, sadness, tension, and fatigue, or positive feelings, such as caring, relaxation, mental clarity, and vigor.[5]

7. **Summarize the beginning of music therapy in the United States.**

The use of recorded music as therapy began after World War I with the accumulation of research that tested the morale-boosting effects of music during the war. The music therapy movement developed into a profession and in the 1940s established its first formal four-year training program. The National Association of Music Therapy (NAMT) was formed as a forum for research and development of music therapy.6 Currently there are over 5000 registered music therapists (RMTs) and certified music therapists (CMTs) in the United States.

8. **What are the theoretical mechanisms for the effects of music?**

Singing and chanting are a part of many traditions, and we are just beginning to understand the potential physiologic implications. Tibetan monks use chanting and other toning devices to help "tune" the physical body to a more balanced resonance that may aid the healing process. The physical body may resonate to different notes or sounds, and when these sounds are played, the body becomes "in tune" or harmonized. Scientist Hans Jenny's experiments reveal that sound causes random particles to assume orderly geometric patterns. Mathematical patterning of certain music has an effect on brain-wave patterns. Baroque music improves the brain's ability to study and assimilate information.

We do not know the exact mechanism responsible for the observed effects of music in our bodies. However, researchers in neuroanatomy have proposed two main theories. One postulates that music acts as a nonverbal medium that can move through the auditory cortex directly to the limbic system to affect brain function. Secondly, music may stimulate release of endorphins, which in turn act on specific receptors to affect brain function.[5]

9. **What does research reveal about the physiologic effects of music?**

Music has been shown to have an effect on physiologic parameters such as galvanic skin response, vasoconstriction, muscle tension, immune system function, respiration rate, heart rate variability, pulse rate, and blood pressure. Data show that listening to different types of music can lower levels of the stress hormones coritsol, adrenaline, and noradrenaline and increase levels of atrial natriuretic peptide, a potent antihypertensive produced by the atria of the heart.[5]

Music has been successfully used to reduce drug use and length of labor in obstetric patients; to reduce anxiety in preoperative pediatric patients; to reduce pain reactions in postoperative obstetric/gynecologic patients; to decrease the occurrence of myocardial infarctions and mortality in intensive care units; to reduce total time to reach weight criterion for discharge of premature infants in neonate nurseries; and to reduce fear, anxiety, and distress in hospitalized pediatric patients and their families.[4] Furthermore, music has numerous uses in nursing homes, burn units, pain clinics, and rehabilitation settings.

For example, when patients admitted to the cardiac unit with a presumptive diagnosis of acute myocardial infarction listened to music through earphones for three sessions over two days, their apical heart rates were more effectively lowered, and their peripheral temperatures were more effectively raised than in a control group. Moreover, heart rates were lowered significantly more after the third session than after the first two sessions, showing a cumulative effect. The incidence of cardiac complications in the group receiving music therapy was lower than in the control group.[7]

10. **Explain the "Mozart effect."**

The Mozart effect is an inclusive term signifying the transformational powers of music in health, education, and general well-being. Specifically, it uses the music of Mozart to improve memory, awareness, relaxation, and integration of learning styles. French physician Alfred Tomatis noted that sounds distracted many people and spent years researching many different styles of music. He found that Wolfgang Amadeus Mozart 200 years earlier had composed music that could stimulate the brain, yet relax the body. Composer Don Campbell has carried on this work.[8] Some preliminary studies show that certain Mozart pieces may stimulate brain areas involved in spatial- temporal reasoning. The take-home message is that music can have an effect on the functional capacity of the brain and may ultimately be a useful adjunct to learning and development.

11. Should surgeons listen to music in the operating room?

A study examined the effects of surgeon-selected and experimenter-selected music on perfor-mance and autonomic responses of surgeons during a standard laboratory psychological stressor.[9] The results showed that music had beneficial effects both autonomically and behaviorally. The bene-ficial autonomic effects were observed as reduced cardiovascular reactivity during task performance. As we know, cardiovascular reactivity contributes to cardiovascular disease, such as coronary artery disease and hypertension. The behavioral effects of music were demonstrated by improved task per-formance. Of note, no specific category of surgeon-selected music had better physiologic responses or task performance. The surgeons gained the most benefit by listening to the music that they per-sonally chose. This finding supports the belief that it is not the type of music that matters, but the participant's individual taste.

12. How has art been used in healing throughout history?

The connection between art and mental health was recognized in the late 1800s. *Artistry of the Mentally Ill*, published in 1922, sparked interest in the value of art for rehabilitation. In the 1940s, prominent psychologists included the interpretation of art and symbols in psychoanalysis. Carl Jung defined certain symbols as archetypes—universally held pictures from the collective unconscious mind that may be used to help solve life problems. In 1969, the American Art Therapy association was established and now has over 4,000 members. The Art Therapy Credentials Board sets standards for art therapists and provides public education.

In ancient times the healer/shaman used a combination of music, chanting, dancing, and paint-ing to invoke the spirits or to tap into the unconscious of the person in need of healing, but only in the past 30 years has art therapy become a specialty complete with degrees and accreditation. Some institutions may have an art therapist on staff or hire an art therapist for consultations, but it is not necessary to have a specialized therapist to use creative arts with patients.

13. How does art therapy work? What effects does it have and why?

No one knows exactly how art therapy works, but it is theorized that the act of creating influ-ences brain-wave patterns and chemicals released by the brain. Numerous case studies have reported benefits in eating disorders, cancer or other terminal illnesses, burn recovery, chemical addiction, grief, sexual abuse, and emotional impairment. Art therapy works for both children and adults. Through the act of drawing, parts of our personality or psyche may be revealed in ways that other-wise would not be apparent. Forms of art therapy range from crayon drawing and making sculpture to viewing masterpieces of art and discussing the feelings that they evoke.

14. Why is art therapy beneficial to hospitalized children?

Art provides a therapeutic outlet for the many psychosocial needs of young patients and their families. The hospital, with all its strange people, procedures, rules, routines, and machines, is ex-tremely stressful to children. An inpatient experience can lead a child to become withdrawn and angry and can even halt development and cause regression.

Because most decisions in the hospital are made without the child's input, the arts offer an op-portunity for children to make their own choices, including what materials to use, what to draw, and how much paint to use. Secondly, the arts provide an experience in which the child can have an active role instead of a passive role. The arts also allow children to communicate their true feelings and provide a safe setting in which fears can be addressed. To children who are temporarily or per-manently physically impaired, the arts offer the opportunity to focus on and nourish abilities. The children may also use their imagination to experience activities that they are unable to experience physically. The joy associated with creating and participating in an art project may be the only time that a child feels the powerful and healing sense of hope. Finally, by using the arts children may demonstrate whether they understand their condition and treatment.[10]

15. What is therapeutic writing? What effects does it have on health?

In therapeutic writing, people write about the innermost thoughts and feelings related to an im-portant emotional issue that has affected their life. Confronting deeply personal issues and conflicts via creative self-expression promotes physical health, subjective well-being, and selected adaptive behavior. Specifically, patients writing or talking about emotional experiences in comparison with a writing control group assigned a superficial topic showed significant decreases in physician visits, enhancement of immune function, and long-term improvement in mood. Such a disclosure paradigm has equal benefit for a wide range of people, independent of education level, personality, age, ethnicity, or native language.[11] A recent randomized trial showed that writing about previous stressful and traumatic events relieved symptoms of both asthma and rheumatoid arthritis.[12]

16. Explain the therapeutic use of journaling and story-telling.

Journaling and storytelling are two powerful mediums through which a person may express inner dialogues and emotions in a safe yet significant manner. Encouraging patients to keep a journal that chronicles their feelings, thoughts, dreams, and personal reflections deepens the dialogue with health care providers and encourages optimal healing in various ways. Having a child tell a story or a fable may invite symbols and metaphors that speak to their hopes and fears and the anticipated outcome of their illness. It allows them to tell their own story in a language of the heart, not the mind.

The process of taking experiences and structuring them into stories is called story-ing, and it provides a means of thinking about and giving meaning to our lives. Story-telling gives us a chance to express fears, hopes, and dreams and requires a willingness to be vulnerable and share our deepest feelings. Mutual story-telling between patient and practitioner has numerous potential benefits. For example, story-telling can assist in establishing a more intimate patient-doctor relationship that allows exploration of often neglected issues, such as death, dying, and disability.[13]

17. Poetry on rounds? How was the idea born, played out, and received by participants?

A physician noticed that, although medical schools have begun to incorporate the teaching of humanities, there was no model for teaching humanistic values in residency programs. Therefore, he chose rounds, a time when attendings, residents, and students meet to influence each other and patient care, as an opportunity to read and discuss poems brought in by team members. Most of the poems were about illness and the nature of being a physician; surprisingly, many were written by team members or one of their friends or family members.[14] The openness of the discussions was remarkable. It allowed participants to integrate arts and humanities with medicine; to explore feelings about medical care, diagnosis, and treatment; and to set aside many of the hierarchical distinctions that usually exist during traditional rounds. Poetry on rounds was received favorably as a reminder of humanization, an opportunity for exploration of feelings, and a change from the routine.

18. In what other ways can physicians tap into their creativity and humanism using the arts?

An increasing number of academic journals, professional organizations, and national conventions are dedicating space, activities, contests, and topics to the discovery and nurturing of the artists within physicians. Monthly features of the *Journal of the American Medical Association* include poetry, a story-telling column called "A Piece of My Mind," and great works of art on the cover. Exploration of our creative side may help to open new avenues of patient-doctor communication and deepen appreciation for our humanity.

19. What are the physiologic effects of dance therapy?

There have been few scientific studies of dance therapy, but clinical reports suggest that dance and movement therapy may be beneficial in improving self-esteem, reducing stress, and maintaining mobility. Many of the physiologic benefits of dance therapy may be similar to those obtained through exercise. We know that exercise releases powerful neurotransmitters (endorphins) in the brain that enhance the sense of well being. These physical benefits, in combination with the self-expressive aspects of movement, may be synergistic in promoting health and healing.

20. What resources are available for more information?
- Furth GM: The Secret World of Drawings: Healing through Art. Boston, Sigo Press, 1988.
- Bach S: Life Paints Its Own Span: On the Significance of Spontaneous Pictures by Severely Ill Children. Einsiedeln, Switzerland, Diamon Verlag, 1990.

• Jenny H: Cymatics: Wave Phenomena, Vibrational Effects, Harmonic Oscillations with Their Structure, Kinetics and Dynamics, vol. 2. Switzerland, Basilius Presse, 1972.
• Lippin RA: Expressive and creative arts therapies. In Micozzi MS (ed): Fundamentals of Complementary and Alternative Medicine, 2nd ed. New York, Churchill Livingstone, 2001, pp 257–275.

REFERENCES

1. Edwards B:Drawing on the Right Side of the Brain: A Course in Enhancing Creativity and Artistic Confidence. New York, G. Putman's Sons, 1989.
2. Ornstein R, Sobel D: Healthy Pleasures. Reading, MA, Addison Wesley, 1989.
3. Lockmer K: The healing arts: Sometimes a song is the best medicine. Free Spirit Mag Oct-Nov:39–41, 1997.
4. Stadley JM: Music research in medical/dental treatment: Meta-analysis and clinical applications. J Music Ther 23:56–122, 1986.
5. McCraty R, Barrios-Choplin B, Atkinson M, Tomasino D: The effects of different types of music on mood, tension, and mental clarity. Altern Ther 4:75–84, 1998.
6. Schiedermayer D: Music yherapy for the relief of postoperative pain. Altern Med Alert 2(8):89–91, 1999.
7. Guzzetta CE: Effects of relaxation and music therapy on patients in a coronary care unit with presumptive acute myocardial infarction. Heart Lung 18:609–616, 1989.
8. Campbell DG: The Mozart Effect. New York, Avon Books, 1997.
9. Allen K, Blascovich, J: Effects of music on cardiovascular reactivity among surgeons. JAMA 272:882–884, 1994.
10. Rollins JH: The arts: Helping children cope with hospitalization. Imprint 37:79–83, 1990.
11. Pennebaker JW: The effects of traumatic disclosure on physical and mental health: The values of writing and talking about upsetting events. Int J Emerg Mental Health 1:9–18, 1999.
12. Smyth JM, et al: Effects of writing about stressful experiences on symptom control in patients with asthma or rheumatoid arthritis: a randomized trial. JAMA 281(14) 1304-09, 1999.
13. Banks-Wallace J: Storytelling as a tool for providing holistic care to women. In Integrated Women's Health: Holistic Approaches for Comprehensive Care. Gaithersburg, MD, Aspen Publishers, 2000.
14. Horowitz HW: Poetry on rounds: A model for the integration of humanities into residency training. Lancet 347:447–449, 1996.

6. HYPNOSIS AND IMAGERY

Sherry L. Robbins, M.D., and Michael R. Floyd, Ed.D.

1. What is hypnosis?

Hypnosis is an altered state of consciousness, characterized by a narrowing of one's concentration to a more limited but heightened focus.[1] Hypnosis is a relaxed state of mind and body, in which one tends to be more responsive to suggestion; it is a pervasive phenomenon that everyone has experienced at some point. There are two popular misconceptions about hypnosis:

1. Hypnosis is a state of sleep. In fact, trance experience is highly individualized, but hypnosis is best considered as a state of heightened concentration with a narrowed scope.

2. Hypnosis occurs only after formal induction by a hypnotist. In fact, there are many forms of trance. "Highway hypnosis" is but one of many examples: Behind the wheel of a car on a familiar road we may not consciously negotiate every turn or be aware of precisely how much time has passed, but we abruptly "wake up" as we reach our destination.

2. What is guided imagery?

Imagery is a mental process produced by the action of the imagination. A common example is daydreaming: The person gives attention to the part of the brain that thinks in images. The images are usually visual or pictorial images, but other senses may be incorporated. Imagery is classified by its primary sensory content: visual, verbal, auditory, olfactory, tactile, gustatory, or kinesthetic. A talented speaker may captivate an audience by evoking images or by drawing on collected memories. Guided imagery involves the use of focused concentration of formed mental images and has been found to be an effective intervention for increasing comfort when cure may not be possible.[2] Guided imagery is also used clinically in psychotherapy and plays an important role in hypnosis, autogenic training, relaxation techniques, and behavior therapy.

Although hypnosis has been described as "controlled imagination," the two terms are not interchangeable.[3] Mental imagery is an aspect of self-hypnosis and is a skill that can be used to promote relaxation, an important component of health and well-being. One can experience imagery without hypnosis and vice versa. Common uses of imagery in the waking state include imaging an improvement in performance of a task and rehearsing a future event. In hypnosis, suggestions given during the trance tend to evoke imagery, which can be quite vivid. Personal images created by the subject are generally more powerful than those suggested by the hypnotist. For example, when imagery is used in hypnotherapy to control pain, the therapist may ask subjects to visualize their pain as an object with a distinct shape or color. Then, the suggestion is given that the mind has control over the pain, just as the mind has been able to visualize it. With practice, this skill becomes more powerful.

3. Summarize the history of hypnosis as a therapeutic modality.

Hypnosis is as old as history itself. The Celts and Druids, as well as the ancient Egyptian, used it. There are references to hypnosis in the Bible. James Braid, an English physician, was the first to coin the word *hypnosis*, which was derived from the Greek word *hypnos* (sleep). He later realized that suggestion, rather than sleep, was the main factor responsible for hypnotic phenomena.[3a] Franz Mesmer is credited with inventing the modern techniques of hypnosis and was the first physician known to use hypnosis as a medicinal tool. A commission appointed by the King of France and headed by Benjamin Franklin investigated Mesmer's claims of "animal magnetism" and reached the conclusion that any reported effects were due to imagination. Thomas Jefferson, in France at the time, described Mesmer's ideas as "an imputation of so grave a nature as would bear an action of law in America." Ironically, it was a Frenchman, Lafayette, who brought the practice to America in 1774. He was a close associate of both Mesmer and George Washington.[4]

Mesmeric societies persisted in America in the early and mid-nineteenth century. By the 1880s hospital hypnosis became more credible, first in France with Burnheim and Charcot. Through the influence of Sigmund Freud, Clark Hull, and Milton Erickson, hypnosis was brought into the modern era, and it was accepted by the British Society of Medicine in 1955 and by the American Medical Association in 1958.

4. How are hypnosis and imagery related to health?

Hypnosis and guided imagery have been shown to enhance a wide variety of physical functions, ranging from athletic performance to the facilitation of mind and body healing. Much of this work has involved pain treatment, especially for cancer and surgery.[5,6] Other applications have involved migraine[7] and muscle tension[8] headaches, as well as other chronic health conditions.[9] However, these methods have been shown to be particularly effective with psychological aspects of health, such as anxiety and hopelessness.[10]

5. Give examples of the use of hypnosis or imagery for improved athletic performance.

Visualization and imagery have become an important feature in developing athletic performance. These methods have been used to improve self-concept, concentration, and rapid relaxation and to effect positive mental states. Unlike running or musical performance, which involve slowly increasing speed or tempo to achieve full performance, certain athletic activities (e.g., basketball, skiing, gymnastics[11]) involve more complex actions that cannot be learned in slow motion. Through imagery, the mind imagines athletic performance, often in "slow motion," rehearsing, practicing and perfecting complex neuromuscular movements,while reducing both external and internal distractions.

6. What is the role of the hypnotist or therapist during a session?

The hypnotist or therapist serves as facilitator. It is the patient who determines his or her response to the suggestions made by the facilitator. The patient always has an "interested observer" within him- or herself that rejects any unacceptable suggestion. Trust between therapist and patient is conducive to a productive hypnotic session.

7. What are the basic components of a hypnotic session?

1. **Introduction.** The therapist explains the techniques to be used and solicits information from the patient about the problem or diagnosis. The therapist also should seek information about past experiences that may be useful during the trance session.

2. **Induction** is the process by which the patient enters the hypnotic state. The scope of his or her focus becomes more narrowed and intensified.

3. **Deepening** refers to continued narrowing of focus and intensification of attention, as the patient relaxes more deeply.

4. **Suggestion.** Once the subject has achieved an appropriate depth of trance, suggestions are made by the facilitator pursuant to the therapeutic plan.

5. **Awakening** refers to returning the patient to the fully alert state.

6. **Debriefing.** During discussion at the end of the session, the therapist elicits feedback from the patient about the experience

8. Describe the process of trance induction.

During the induction phase of hypnosis, attention is fixated and the field of awareness becomes narrowed. The therapist may ask the patient to fix his or her gaze on a particular object or spot. Usually, the patient becomes progressively more relaxed and begins to reduce voluntary movements. As trance progresses, ideas become more focused and concentration becomes directed on suggestions offered by the therapist. The trance state is usually produced by repetition of visual, auditory, and/or tactile stimuli in a rhythmical, even monotonous manner.

Although most therapeutic interventions occur with patients in a light-to-medium stage of trance, many believe that suggestions given in deeper hypnotic stages may be more beneficial. Suggestions are often woven into the trance through inflections in speech or stories or through deepening techniques involving imagery or direct suggestions indicative of greater relaxation. For example, the therapist may suggest that the patient sink "deeper and deeper" into a chair or imagine walking down a flight of stairs to a deeper level of trance.[12]

9. What responses in the patient confirm an appropriate trance state?

Mild trance state is characterized by slow breathing, feelings of lethargy, inhibition of voluntary movements, relaxation, and eyelid and limb catalepsy.

Moderate trance is characterized by glove anesthesia, partial posthypnotic anesthesia, age regression, time distortion, and positive mental imagery.

Deep trance is characterized by more complete age regression, both positive and negative hallucinations, extensive anesthesia and amnesia, and marked decrease in mental activity.[12a]

10. How are suggestions given during the hypnotic trance?

Typically, suggestions are positive, rather than negative. For example, a suggestion that the patient's breath will come more easily after quitting smoking seems to be more effective than suggesting that the patient concentrate specifically on not smoking. Suggestions also seem to be most beneficial when they are individualized, presented in a simple form that makes use of the patient's own language, and stated in the present tense. Pertinent points need to be reinforced throughout the session. Suggestions to be internalized generally should be given during inhalation, whereas suggestions to release should coincide with exhalation. The patient also should be encouraged and should be allowed as much time as he or she needs to respond. The patient also should try to define everything in experiential terms.

11. What subjects or situations are not appropriate for hypnosis?

Although experts debate the assertion that "not everyone can be hypnotized," some people are more difficult to hypnotize than others. In general, however, everyone has the potential to enter some degree of trance. Some precautions should be observed:

1. The therapist should not attempt to treat any condition with hypnosis that he or she is not qualified to treat by other means (a cardinal rule of hypnosis). For example, a dentist may appropriately use hypnosis to decrease pain from a procedure but should not hypnotize patients to treat asthma.

2. Stage hypnosis or party hypnosis (i.e., hypnosis performed for entertainment purposes in which the hypnotist has no therapeutic relationship with the subject) is not appropriate and carries some potential dangers. Although the "interested observer" of the subject can reject unacceptable suggestions, the chance of an adverse reaction is increased in the absence of an established professional relationship between facilitator and subject, and the appropriate history-taking and rapport-building steps are ignored. (See question 15.)

3. Hypnosis should not be attempted in a subject who does not wish to be hypnotized.

4. Caution subjects who may consider taking legal action against a third party for alleged abuse. Recollections that either surface during or are enhanced by hypnosis are often inadmissible in court; therefore, undergoing hypnosis may potentially eliminate the ability to seek legal action. Therapists can be held liable if they do not caution the subjects before the session about this possibility.

5. Depressed subjects are potentially in danger of developing increased suicidality in some hypnotherapeutic situations (particularly when they are directly told to give up a particular habit or symptom, which may be serving as a coping mechanism).

12. What medical conditions have been demonstrated to derive benefit from hypnosis?

One of the best examples is cancer.[13,14] Various problems in patients with cancer can be minimized by hypnosis. For example, cancer pain can be attenuated by several means. Time distortion can be suggested to decrease the duration of a painful episode; amnesia can be induced so that the patient does not dread a future episode; the pain can be diminished in severity or replaced by an alternative sensation such as numbness; or the pain can be moved to a less sensitive area of the body. Similarly, a patient with cancer may be able to develop amnesia for chemotherapy-associated nausea and vomiting; alternatively, the appetite can be stimulated; or the symptom may be minimized directly.[15] In addition, hypnosis and imagery can effect immunomodulation. Data support the mind-body connection for immune system function, as well as improvement of immune system function with the use of imagery/hypnosis. One of the most intriguing potential benefits of hypnosis in patients with cancer is in treating fear of death. Certain patients who fear death can benefit from undergoing a "hypnotic death rehearsal," in which hypnotic techniques allow the patient to envision the death process in a nonthreatening and supportive manner.

Another medical condition known to respond positively to hypnosis is thermal injury.[16] A hypnosis session should be performed as soon as possible (at least within the first 12 hours of injury) for optimal results. The therapist gives suggestions to make the affected area "cool and comfortable." This intervention has been shown to limit the depth of the wound. Extremely painful debridement procedures are often required in the treatment of extensive burns, and pain control can be enhanced by methods similar to those described above for cancer. By making suggestions during trance to enhance blood flow to the affected areas on the day after injury, healing may be hastened by several days. For patients with extensive thermal injuries, good nutrition is essential for healing and is often a challenge to achieve. Hypnosis can help by increasing the appetite. For patients with disfiguring injuries, ego strengthening during trance can be of potential benefit by enhancing self-image.

13. What problems are involved in reviewing the literature for proof of the efficacy of hypnosis?

Definitively determining the utility of hypnosis and imagery based on current literature is often made difficult by the diversity of variables in published studies. For example, many distinctly different treatment protocols have been labeled as "hypnosis." At other times the hypnosis element of the study was only part of the interventional treatment, and many studies are limited by small sample size. If we limit the search to conditions that have been studied a sound, objective manner, we can affirm that the following medical conditions can be positively affected by hypnosis: irritable bowel syndrome, some cases of asthma, hemophilia, chemotherapy-associated nausea and vomiting, dermatological disorders, and preoperative preparation for surgery.

14. What are some of the myths surrounding hypnosis?

1. The hypnotist has absolute power and can make the person in trance do whatever the hypnotist commands. This myth is simply false.

2. The hypnotized subject becomes a "zombie." In fact, participants are usually aware of the suggestions being given, and in "alert hypnosis" they are able to walk, talk, and open their eyes. They do not get "stuck" in a trance accidentally.

3. One session of hypnosis can cure any problem. In fact, hypnosis is most often an additional treatment—not the sole treatment. Rarely is one session curative.

4. A subject cannot lie under hypnosis. Evidence clearly indicates that subjects have successfully lied while under hypnosis.

5. Whatever information is recalled in trance must be accurate. Hypnosis has been helpful in some forensic cases. Because the participant's mind may unintentionally embellish some recollections, information obtained must be taken with some skepticism. Without corroborating evidence, accuracy cannot be assumed.

15. What are the potential side effects and complications of hypnosis?

As clinicians we hold tightly to the admonition, "above all, do no harm." Mild side effects may occur in about 1% of inductions, but more serious adverse reactions are possible. Therefore, the hypnotic therapist must be skilled and experienced in addressing a wide range of emotional expression and licensed within a health profession.

The broad spectrum of potentially undesirable hypnotic experiences ranges from more common, mild, transient side effects to rare, acute emotional or psychological events. Examples of mild side effects include sleepiness, cognitive distortions, and headaches. Examples of acute psychological events include suicidality, panic, psychosis, or regression to a past traumatic experience. As with medications, not all side effects are "bad," and some may be "reframed" as progress toward a goal. Participants are at greater risk of complications when hypnosis is used in an inappropriate setting or performed by someone untrained to treat a particular condition or when an inappropriate suggestion is given.

16. What is the role of self-hypnosis?

It has been said that "all hypnosis is self-hypnosis." Therefore, even without a hypnotherapist as facilitator, patients may have the ability to enter trance on their own. Self-hypnosis can be used to accomplish a relaxed state. It is also a valuable technique for reinforcing the therapeutic process initiated by a hypnotherapist. For successful outcomes in some cases, self-hypnosis practice sessions are essential for reinforcement (e.g., for control of pain during labor and delivery).

17. How can I learn more about hypnosis?

The **Society for Clinical and Experimental Hypnosis** (SCEH), which was founded in 1949 and now has approximately 1,000 members, may be contacted at SCEH Central Office, Washington State University, P.O. Box 642114, Pullman, WA 99164-2114; fax: (509) 335-2097; e-mail: sceh@pullman.com.

The **American Society of Clinical Hypnosis** (ASCH), which was founded in 1957 and now has approximately 3,000 members, sponsors training workshops, a journal, and a library of resource materials. The society may be contacted at 2250 East Devon Avenue, Suite 336, Des Plaines, Illinois 60018 or at http://asch.net.

American Psychological Association, Division 30, Psychological Hypnosis, has approximately 1,700 members.

Informative books and articles include the following:

- Hammond DC (ed): Hypnotic Induction and Suggestion. Chicago, ASCH Press, 1990.
- Pratt GJ, et al: A Clinical Hypnosis Primer. San Diego, Psychiatric Consulting Association Press, 1984, pp 118–143.
- Hammond DC: Clinical Hypnosis and Memory: Guidelines for Clinicians for Forensic Hypnosis. Seattle, WA, ASCH, Committee on Hypnosis and Memory, 1995.
- Hammond DC (ed): Handbook of Hypnotic Suggestions and Metaphors. New York, W. W. Norton, 1990.
- Pinnell CM, Covino NA: Empirical findings on the use of hypnosis in medicine: A critical review. Int J Clin Hypnosis 48(2):170–194, 2000.

18. How do I find a reputable hypnotherapist and what credentials should he/she have?

The ASCH may be able to identify members in your area. Not all reputable hypnotherapists have chosen to undergo the certification process by the American Board of Clinical Hypnosis, but those who have done so have undergone at least three training workshops and passed a certification exam in hypnosis. A reputable hypnotherapist will spend time during the initial visit getting to know you and your particular problem and will tailor your sessions to individual needs, explaining in advance what you are to expect from each session. Finally, no professionals should attempt to treat a condition by hypnosis techniques that they would not be competent to treat within the bounds of their profession by other means. Hypnotherapy is an adjunctive technique only.[18]

REFERENCES

1. Edmonson WE: The Induction of Hypnosis. New York, John Wiley, 1991, pp 300–313.
2. Kolcaba K, Fox C: The effects of guided imagery on comfort of women with early stage breast cancer undergoing radiation therapy. Onocol Nurs Forum 26:67–72, 1999.
3. Gravitz M: Early theories of hypnosis: A clinical perspective. In Lynn S, Rhu J (eds): Theories of Hypnosis: Current Models and Perspectives. New York, Guilford Press, 1991, pp 19–42, 1991.
3a. Rossi and Cheek: Mind-Body Therapy. Ideodynamic Healing and Hypnosis. New York, W.W. Norton, 1988.
4. Gravitz M: Early American Mesmeric Societies: A historical perspective. Am J Clin Hypnosis 37(1):41–48, 1994.
5. Steggles S, Maxwell J, Lightfoot NE, et al: Hypnosis and cancer: An annotated bibliography 1985–1995. AmJ Clin Hypnosis 39(3):187–200, 1997.
6. Spiegel D, Moore R: Imagery and hypnosis in the treatment of cancer patents. Onocology 11:1179–1189, 1997.
7. Ilacquoa GE: Migraine headaches: Coping efficacy of guided imagery training. Headache 34:99–102, 1994.

8. Mannix LK, et al: Effect of guided imagery on quality of life for patients with chronic tension-type headache. Headache 39:326–334, 1999.
9. Maguire BL: The effects of imagery on attitudes and moods in multiple sclerosis patients. Altern Ther Health Med 2(5):75–79,1996.
10. Royle JA, et al: The research utilization process: The use of guided imagery to reduce anxiety. Can Onocol Nurs J 6:20–25, 1996.
11. Liggett DR, Hamada S: Enhancing the visualization of gymnastics. Am J Clin Hypnosis 35(3):190–197,1993.
12. Hammond DC (ed): Handbook of Hypnotic Suggestions and Metaphors. New York, W. W. Norton, 1990.
12a. Hammond DC (ed): Hypnotic Induction and Suggestion. Chicago, ASCH Press, 1990.
13. Levitan AA: The use of hypnosis with cancer patients. Psychiatr Med 10(1):119–129, 2000.
14. Ernst E: Complementary therapies in palliative cancer care. Cancer 91:2181–2185, 2001.
15. Marchioro G, Azzarello G, et al: HyOpnosis in the treatment of anticipatory nausea and vomiting in patients receiving cancer chemotherapy. Oncology 59(2):100–104, 2000.
16. Peebles-Kleiger MJ: The use of hypnosis in emergency medicine. Emerg Med Clin North Am 18:327–336, 2000.
17. Pinnell CM, Covino NA: Empirical findings on the use of hypnosis in medicine: A critical review. Int J Clin Hypnosis:170–194, 2000.
18. Dowd ET: Cognitive Hypnotherapy. Livingston, NJ, Jason Aronson., 2000.

7. MEDITATION

Shauna L. Shapiro, Ph.D.

1. Define meditation.

Various methods whose background and techniques are quite different are placed collectively under the umbrella term *meditation*. To enhance clarity and avoid misunderstanding, it is important to have a clear definition of meditation. In its simplest form, meditation can be defined as an attempt to regulate attention consciously.

This definition has three important components. First, it uses the word *conscious* to introduce the importance of intention: the *intention* to focus attention. Second, it is a definition independent of any religious framework or orientation (although meditation can occur within a religious framework). Finally, the word *attempt* places an emphasis on the process of meditation, as opposed to the specific goals or results.

2. What is the relationship between meditation and Buddhism?

Meditation was originally conceived within the religious/philosophical context of Eastern spiritual disciplines, including Buddhism. However, meditation has been an essential element in nearly all religious and spiritual traditions, including Judaism, Christianity, and Islam.[1] You do *not* have to be Buddhist to meditate because the essence of meditation, "intentionally paying attention," has universal applications. When applied as a health care intervention, mediation can be used effectively regardless of a patient's cultural or religious background.

3. How can meditation affect physical and mental health?

Research has examined primarily the effects of meditation as a strategy for stress management and symptom reduction. Over the past three decades, considerable research has examined the psychological and physiologic effects of meditation,[2] and meditative practices are now used in a variety of health care settings. The research demonstrates that meditation is an effective intervention for a variety of physical and psychological disorders :
- Cardiovascular disease[3,4]
- Chronic pain[5]
- Substance abuse[6]
- Dermatologic disorders[7]
- Anxiety and panic disorder[8–10]
- Reduction of depressive symptoms[11,12]

4. What are the positive psychological benefits of meditation?

Research[2,13] demonstrates positive psychological and behavioral benefits, including improvements in the following:
- Self-actualization
- Empathy
- Sense of coherence and stress-hardiness
- Increased autonomy and independence
- Positive sense of control
- Moral maturity
- Heightened perception
- Improvements in reaction time and responsive motor skill, increased field independence (correlated with independent judgment and strong sense of body and self)
- Increased concentration and attention
- Deepening sense of spirituality[11,12]

The literature[2] also includes positive psychological and behavioral changes identified by subjective report. Examples include improved perception of internal and external events; greater equanimity, pleasure, bliss, and ecstasy; increased energy, and excitement; unusual dreams and dream recall; and greater acceptance of self.

5. Are there any negative consequences of meditation?

Meditation appears to be a safe practice for most people. However, case reports and descriptive studies document some adverse effects. Some practitioners report initial increases in stress, anxiety and depression (although these reactions can represent normal emotional mood states).[14] Furthermore, for people who are at high risk for emotional flooding or uncovering of repressed material, such as those with posttraumatic stress disorder or suicidal ideation, concurrent psychotherapy may be necessary. Finally, it has been suggested that meditation may be contraindicated for people with psychotic or borderline personality disorders.

6. What is the difference between formal and informal meditation practice?

Formal meditation refers to the practice of meditation in a disciplined fashion during specific times of day, in a specified place, and usually in a specific posture.[15] The formal practice is the typical image that most Westerners have of meditation: a meditator sits in lotus style, eyes closed, deeply focused and paying attention.

However, the **informal practice** is equally as important, although less typically associated with the Western concept of meditation. The informal meditation can be practiced throughout the day; it involves an attempt to be conscious of everything one does, feels, and experiences without judging or evaluating. Common activities can become an informal practice—all that is required is a shift in consciousness from the automatic pilot mode to being fully present. For example, if you are eating, try paying attention to one bite, then the next, then the next. The informal practice becomes simply the experience of eating—not eating while watching television, reading the newspaper, or talking on the phone. Complete awareness is brought to the process of eating. Informal practices include driving, washing dishes, making love—in fact, *anything* can become an informal practice, depending on the person's ability to pay attention.

Western researchers have focused primarily on formal practice. However, the goal of meditation is not simply to focus attention during formal sittings but to maintain and generalize conscious awareness to all parts of life (informal practice). Therefore, both formal and informal meditation practice are essential. The formal practice of meditation strengthens the informal practice, planting the seeds and the skills to eventually bring awareness to each moment of our lives.

7. What are the major types of formal meditation?

The family of meditation techniques traditionally has been divided into two basic groups: concentrative meditation and mindfulness meditation.[15] All types of **concentrative meditation** attempt to restrict awareness by focusing attention on a single object. Examples of the object of meditation include the breath, the body, a mantra, a single word (for example, one), or specific sounds.

In **mindfulness meditation**, one attempts to pay attention nonjudgmentally to all stimuli in the internal and external environment, but not to become fixated (ruminate) on any particular stimulus. Through the process of mindfulness, one becomes aware of unconscious and automatic thoughts, behaviors, and emotions, which often are driven by deep-seated fear and anxiety. Through the process of paying attention in the present moment to whatever arises, mindfulness meditation cultivates insight into how to lead happier, more adaptive lives.

A third category, **contemplative meditation**, has recently been introduced.[16] Contemplative meditation involves opening and surrendering to a larger Self (e.g., God, benevolent other). From this receptive place one may ask questions and address unresolved issues. Kabat-Zinn proposes contemplation of larger questions—for example, "What is my Way?"—during meditation practice while remaining open to *not knowing*.[17] He suggests that inquiry of this kind leads to openings and new understandings, visions, and actions. Examples of contemplative meditation include certain types of Jewish meditation, centering prayer, and labyrinth meditations.

8. How is meditation different from relaxation training?

Meditation training differs significantly in both practice and intentions from relaxation training.[14] First, an emphasis of meditation is the development of greater understanding through the systematic cultivation of inquiry and insight, whereas the goal of relaxation training is simply to achieve a state of low autonomic arousal, with little or no emphasis on the cultivation of insight. Relaxation often occurs during the practice of meditation, but it is not an objective of the process. Furthermore, relaxation is taught as a technique, a tool to be used during stressful or anxiety-provoking situations. Meditation, in contrast, is conceived as a "way of being," cultivated daily regardless of circumstances.[14]

9. What were the original intentions of meditation?

The intention behind meditation is to "wake up" from a suboptimal state of consciousness, and to realize our true nature. Traditions of wisdom, from which meditation stems, concur that the normal waking state is often automatic and dreamlike; in essence, people live their lives without being present, on auto-pilot. Meditation is referred to as a "consciousness discipline" because waking up, learning to live our lives mindfully instead of mindlessly, requires considerable effort and discipline.

At their core, meditative disciplines provide roadmaps to reach optimal openness, awareness, and transcendent states of consciousness.[18] Within its original spiritual/religious context, meditation is practiced as a means for developing insight and wisdom, purification (reducing greed, anger and selfishness), concentration, enhanced connection, and transcendence (including altered states of consciousness). It is a means for changing an individual's perception of the world and for developing a more accurate, unified, and accepting view of one's self, other people, nature, and the universe.

10. How do I begin a formal meditation practice?

Many steps are involved in beginning a meditation practice. Exploring different books and essays is a good first step. You can learn of the many different traditions and techniques and choose one that speaks most to you and your current belief system. It also may be helpful to seek out a meditation community and teacher in your area through searching the worldwide web or the local phone book. Once you have chosen a specific type of meditation, three steps are involved in beginning a formal practice.

Step 1. First, it is essential to form an *intention* for your practice. You may ask yourself, "Why am I meditating? What do I hope to gain?" There is no right answer to these questions. Some people begin meditation as a form of stress management, others to reduce physical or mental discomfort, and still others to cultivate greater insight and compassion. Regardless of your intention, it is important to remind yourself of it before you sit down to practice meditation. Your intention may (and probably will) change and evolve over time; continue to explore it consciously before each meditation practice.

Step 2. The second step in developing a practice is to find a place to meditate. It is often difficult to find a safe and quiet place where you will not be interrupted. Some meditators set aside a specific room in their house, others find a special place outdoors, still others meditate in their office with the door closed. It is essential that you that feel this place is special and your own.

Step 3. The third step in developing a practice is to establish a routine. It is valuable to find a time of day or night that feels right to you. In beginning a meditation practice people often play around with different times, such as first thing in the morning, at lunch break, when they get home from work, or immediately before bed. To date, research has not demonstrated any specific time as superior. What is most important is that you feel that the time is right; in this way you will be more likely to continue the practice.

11. What should the length of my formal meditations be? And how often should I meditate?

There is no gold standard for length of meditation practice. In the beginning it may be helpful to start with 15 minutes once or twice a day. As your practice deepens, you can gradually increase the amount of time. A well-established meditation program, which demonstrates significant physical and psychological improvements in its participants, suggests 45 minutes a day, 6-days a week. However, other studies demonstrate benefits with less practice.

Research has not yet determined whether it is more important to meditate every day for a brief period or to meditate only a few times a week for longer sittings. The most widely held theory is that frequency is more important than duration, which suggests that it is more important for meditation to become a part of your daily life as opposed to sporadic practice for longer periods. This approach is similar to exercise, it is better to do a little bit of exercise each day than to do one huge workout once a week.

12. Can anyone learn to meditate?

Yes. In fact it is impossible to "fail" as long as you are consciously attempting to bring attention into the present moment. However, meditation is called a consciousness **discipline** because it requires discipline! Beginning a meditation practice is an arduous challenge. It is important to have a strong commitment and intention, but it is equally important to stay gentle and kindly with yourself as you proceed. This attitude can be referred to as compassionate discipline. Lastly it is helpful to remember a wise saying from Ram Das when you are feeling particularly discouraged.: "You fall off the path a thousand times; the trick is to get back on a thousand and one."

REFERENCES

1. Goleman D: The Meditation Mind. Los Angels, Tarcher, 1998.
2. Murphy M, Donovan S, Taylor E: The Physical and Psychological Effects of Meditation: A Review of Contemporary Research with a Comprehensive Bibliography. Sausalito, CA, Institute of Noetic Sciences, 1997.
3. Zamarra JW, Schnieder RH, Besseghini I, et al: Usefulness of the transcendental meditation program in the treatment of patients with coronary artery disease. Am J Cardiol 77:867–870, 1996.
4. Castillo-Richmond A, Schneider RH, Alexander CN, et al: Effects of stress reduction on carotid atherosclerosis in hypertensive African Americans. Stroke 31:568–573, 2000.
5. Kaba-Zinn J: An outpatient program in behavioral medicine for chronic pain patients based on the practice of mindfulness meditation: Theoretical considerations and preliminary results. Gen Hosp Psychiatry 4:33–47, 1982.
6. Gelderloos P, Walton K, Orme-Johnson D, Alexander C: Effectiveness of the transcendental meditation program in preventing and treating substance misuse: A review. Int J Addict 26:293–325, 1991.
7. Kabat-Zinn J, Wheeler E, Light T, et al: Influence of mindfulness meditation-based stress reduction intervention on rate of skin clearing in patients with moderate to severe psoriasis undergoing phototherapy (UVB) and photochemotherapy (PUVA). Psychosom Med 60:625–632, 1998.
8. Edwards DL: A meta-analysis of the effects of meditation and hypnosis on measures of anxiety. Dissert Abstr Int 52 (2-B):1039–1040, 1991.
9. Miller F, Fletcher D, Kabat-Zinn J: Three year follow-up and clinical implications of a mindfulness-based intervention in the treatment of anxiety disorders. Gen Hosp Psychiatry 17:192–200,1995.
10. Kabat-Azinn J, Massion AO, Kristeller J, et al: Effectiveness of a meditation based stress reduction program in the treatment of anxiety disorders. Am J Psychiatry 149:936–943, 1997.
11. Astin JA: Stress reduction through mindfulness meditation: Effects on psychological symptomatology, sense of control, and spiritual experiences. Psychother Psychosoms 66:97–106,1997.
12. Shapiro SL, Schwartz GER, Bonner G: The effects of mindfulness-based stress reduction on medical and pre-medical students. J Behav Med 21:581–599, 1998.
13. Shapiro DH, Walsh RN (eds): Meditation: Classic and Contemporary Perspectives. New York, Aldine, 1984.
14. Kabat-Zinn J: Mindfulness meditation: What it is, what it isn't, and its role in health care and medicine. In Haruki Y, Suzuki M (eds): Comparative and Psychological Study on Meditation. Netherlands, Eburon Press, 1996, pp 161–170.
15. Shapiro DH: Meditation: Self-regulation Strategy and Altered State of Consciousness. New York, Aldine, 1980.
16. Shapiro SL, Schwartz GE, Santerre C: Positive Psychology and Meditation [in press].
17. Kabat-Zinn J: 1994. Wherever You Go, There You Are. New York, Hyperion, 1994.
18. Walsh R: The transpersonal movement: A history and state of the art. J Transpers Psychol 25 (2):123–139, 1993.

8. SPIRITUALITY

Ken Olive, M.D.

1. Why has spirituality been largely ignored in contemporary medicine?

Historically, spirituality and medicine were tightly intertwined. In indigenous cultures, the shaman was the source of healing knowledge and access to the spirits. In medieval Europe the first hospitals were run in monasteries. With the advent of the scientific era, a schism developed between religion and medicine in western societies because of restraints placed on scientific inquiry by established religious organizations. Despite noteworthy exceptions (e.g., William Osler, Carl Jung), most academicians avoided the intermingling of religion and medicine. Throughout this time, however, a medical missionary movement remained active. The schism between religion and medicine persisted largely until the late 20th century. Most physicians in practice today received no formal training in the role of spirituality, the meaning of the illness experience, or how to address spirituality in the clinical setting. Although physicians in practice usually come to realize that spirituality plays a significant role in the lives of their patients, many choose not to address it. Instead they typically retreat to the realm of the familiar and comfortable—the biomedical and technical realms.

2. How common are spiritual and religious beliefs in the U.S. population?

The U.S. population is a highly religious group. The Gallup Poll has surveyed Americans several times during the last four decades and has consistently found that 95% believe in God or a higher power.[1] In various surveys, 70–75% indicate that their religious beliefs are the most important influence in their lives. Over 40% attend religious services on a weekly basis, and over 50% pray on a daily basis. Although some people identify strongly with an organized religion, others recognize their spirituality as a personal relationship to their life force, higher power, or source. If the concept of spirituality is considered to be that which gives meaning and purpose to life, virtually everyone possesses some form of spirituality.

3. Do patients want their doctors to address spiritual and religious issues with them?

Many patients want doctors to address their beliefs—in some cases, because the beliefs directly affect clinical decisions. Noteworthy examples include Jehovah's Witnesses who choose not to receive blood products and Christian Scientists who eschew traditional medical therapy. In other cases, the illness experience challenges patients' concepts of wholeness and produces spiritual angst as they address questions such as "How can I be of value to my family in this broken state?" Acknowledgment by the physician that these concerns are valid reassures the patient. Knowing that the physician empathizes can assuage some of the sense of loneliness. In some cases, simply the knowledge that the physician recognizes a higher power is reassuring to the patient. Patients who are actively involved in religious activities have a greater desire for physicians to address spiritual issues, as do patients who are facing life-threatening or end-of-life issues. In one study, 75% of patients indicated that physician inquiry about beliefs that may affect end-of-life medical decisions would increase the patient's trust in the physician.[2]

4. How do physicians address spiritual and religious issues with patients?

The approach varies widely from physicians who do not address spiritual issues at all to those who address them in depth with all patients. Most physicians address beliefs in a limited number of patients when they deem it appropriate. Although this approach is the norm, its main disadvantage is that it is based on the physician's subjective assessment of when it is appropriate to address beliefs. Many experienced clinicians indicate that they have been surprised at times to find spiritual issues operative in patients in whom they were unexpected. Based on such experiences, it is a wise practice to open the door for spiritual discussion with all new patients, with patients experiencing emotional distress, and with all patients facing life-threatening and end-of-life issues.

5. Is it ethical for doctors to address spirituality and religion with patient?

An equally appropriate question is "Is it ethical for doctors *not* to address spirituality and religion with patients?" Given that most patients have some religious beliefs, that all have some basic form of spirituality, that patients often depend on these beliefs for coping with illness, and that those who effectively use their personal spiritual resources often do better, there appears to be no ethical problem with addressing spiritual issues with patients. If, however, a physician approaches this issue from the perspective of trying to achieve a personal religious outcome as opposed to what is in the best interest of the patient, such actions may not be ethical.

6. Does the medical literature suggest that religious belief or behavior is associated with health benefits?

Yes. Multiple studies examining a variety of health outcomes suggest that religious beliefs and behavior are associated with benefits. Patients who attend religious services weekly or more have lower total mortality rates, lower rates of substance abuse, and are less likely to have elevated levels of interleukin 6, one of the inflammatory cytokines. Higher levels are associated with a variety of diseases.[3-5] HIV-infected patients who are actively involved in religious practices have higher CD 4 counts.[6] Elderly women with hip fractures who have high levels of religiosity ambulate further and have less depression after surgery.[7] Elderly patients undergoing elective heart surgery who derive strength and comfort from their religious beliefs have a lower 6-month mortality rate than those who do not.[8] Heart transplant recipients with higher levels of religiosity are more compliant with complex drug regimens.[9] Hypertensive patients who attend religious services regularly tend to have lower blood pressure.[10] Patients with rheumatoid arthritis who received an active prayer intervention, in which the prayers involved physically touching the patient, demonstrated objective improvement compared with preintervention symptoms and control patients.[11]

7. Do religious beliefs affect wellness behaviors?

A variety of wellness behaviors are beneficially influenced by religious beliefs. Many religions discourage a variety of behaviors, which may negatively impact health, such as alcohol use, illicit drug use, and sexual promiscuity. Multiple studies have shown that religious service attendance is a potent factor in preventing substance abuse in adolescents.[4] College students who hold their religious beliefs to be important are less likely to be sexually active or to abuse substances and more likely to use safety belts and to exercise.[12] Many Buddhists regularly engage in meditation, which not only instills deeper meaning to their lives but has also been shown in studies to be beneficial for reducing anxiety, cardiovascular disease, and pain (see Chapter 7).

8. How do patients use spirituality or religious beliefs to cope with illness?

Patients rely on spirituality to cope with illness in three general ways: (1) to search for an explanation for suffering, (2) to derive strength for dealing with suffering, and (3) to receive support from other members of their spiritual community. As they work through the illness experience, patients commonly ask such questions as "Why is this happening to me?" and "What did I do to deserve this?" Answers to such questions are not typically found in medicine but are based on a patient's belief system. Although it is not primarily the job of the physician to answer such questions, it is essential to recognize their importance and to facilitate patients' engagement of the questions by encouraging the use of their own spiritual resources.

Numerous studies of chronic illness indicate that patients rely on religious and spiritual resources. Elderly patients with serious medical problems most commonly report that God helps them through their illness and suffering. HIV-infected patients with stronger religious coping have lower levels of depression. Patients with cancer consistently define God as their most important strength of comfort, commonly followed by family and friends. Support from spiritual communities can take many forms, ranging from emotional and spiritual support to tangible material and physical support. Emotional support can include physical presence, phone calls, cards, and letters as well as prayers. More tangible support can include transportation, household cleaning, and cooking meals.

9. Is prayer an effective therapy?

This question is highly controversial in research. Both advocates and skeptics have expressed concern about studies that examine the effectiveness of prayer. Those who believe that prayer can invoke a supernatural response from God frequently argue that an all-knowing and all-powerful God cannot be expected to conform to certain rules of behavior regarding actions in particular situations. Their faith is not likely to be shaken by negative prayer studies. Others argue that testing God contradicts the teachings of their faith. The skeptic argues that to use empirical methods to explain non-empirical phenomena is inherently unscientific and that any results of such work are dubious.

That being said, a few brave (or foolish, depending on one's perspective) researchers have ventured into this minefield, and their results have been mixed. One of the earliest to examine this question was the nineteenth century British researcher Francis Galton, who conducted a crude epidemiologic study.[13] He believed that of all people, monarchs were the most prayed for. Thus, from his perspective, if prayers were effective, their longevity should exceed that of the general population. Finding that in actuality monarchs had shorter life spans, he concluded that prayer must not be effective.

10. What studies have examined the effectiveness of prayer?

Current studies of prayer have shown improvement in methods since Galton's time. A randomized trial of children with leukemia assigned them to receive standard antileukemic therapy with or without intercessory prayer.[14] Children who were prayed for had a much lower mortality rate. However, the study design did not provide enough patients to demonstrate a significant difference. A randomized controlled trial of intercessory prayer for patients admitted to a critical care unit showed reduced rates of congestive heart failure, pneumonia and cardiopulmonary arrest among patients who were prayed for.[15] In addition, their overall hospital course was better. However, there was no difference in other important outcomes, such as mortality, occurrence of ventricular fibrillation, or length of stay. A more recent study attempted to confirm this trial and demonstrated some, but not all, of the same findings.[16]

In another study, healers from a variety of faiths (Christian, Jewish, Buddhist, Native American, shamanic traditions, and secular schools of healing) prayed for patients with advanced AIDS.[17] Each study patient received prayer from a distance (healers and patients never met) from 10 different healers on a rotating basis. Significant improvements compared with controls included lower incidence and severity of illness, fewer hospital stays and doctor visits, and improvement in mood—all without significant changes in the CD4 levels.

In summary, limited literature with some methodologic limitations suggests that prayer may be associated with beneficial health outcomes. Regardless of proven affects on physical health outcomes, most patients pray in times of illness. Many find it to be a source of strength and comfort.

11. Is religion ever harmful to health?

Overviews of the varied literature examining religion and health generally show that about 75% of the studies indicate a beneficial relationship between religion and medicine. The remainder is divided roughly evenly between studies indicating a neutral relationship and those indicating an adverse relationship. Obvious anecdotal examples include religious cults, which have advocated mass suicides for religious gains. The most recent of these sensational events in the United States involved members of the Heaven's Gate Cult. Many committed suicide by poisoning to free their souls to join a waiting space ship, which they believed would take them to a higher level of existence.

The best examples provided in the medical literature involve medical neglect based on religious reasons. The Faith Assembly declines acceptance of prenatal and obstetrical care. In one study in Indiana, maternal and perinatal mortality were 10- to 100-fold higher among Faith Assembly members than among other patients.[18] A study of over 172 pediatric deaths involving religiously motivated neglect suggested that many of the children may have had an excellent outcome with standard medical care.[19] Examples included untreated cases of appendicitis, pneumonia, and diabetes mellitus type I. Clearly not all religion is associated with beneficial health outcomes.

12. How do you take a medically relevant spiritual history?

A medically relevant spiritual history should open the door for discussion, communicate that the clinician realizes the potential importance of the topic, and determine whether the patient has particular beliefs or practices relevant to health care. Three recent publications[20-22] provide different mnemonics for taking a spiritual history; an example of the **SPIRIT** questionnaire[20] is included below. There is much overlap between these approaches, and they can be modified to fit the physician's personal style of questioning.

S : Spiritual belief system
  • What is your formal religious affiliation?
  • Name or describe your spiritual belief system.

P: Personal spirituality
  • Describe the beliefs and practices of your religion or spirituality system that you personally accept or do not accept.

I: Integration with a spiritual community
  • Do you belong to any spiritual or religious group or community?
  • What importance does this group have to you?
  • Is it a source of support? In what ways?

R: Ritualized practices and restrictions
  • Are there specific practices that you carry out as a part of your religion/spirituality (e.g., prayer or meditation)?
  • Are there certain lifestyle activities or practices that your religion/spirituality encourages or forbids? Do you comply?
  • Are there specific elements of medical care that you forbid on the basis of religious/spiritual grounds?

I: Implications for medical care
  • What aspects of your religion/spirituality would you like me to keep in mind as I care for you?

T: Terminal events planning
  • As we plan for your care near the end of life, how does your faith affect your decisions?
  • Are there particular aspects of care that you wish to forgo or have withheld because of your faith?

Maugans TA: The SPIRITual history. Arch Fam Med 5:11–16, 1996.

13. What is spiritual care in the clinical context?

Spiritual care begins with obtaining the spiritual history. Basic spiritual care of the patient involves compassion, presence, listening, and encouragement of realistic hope. Any caring physician can provide this level of care. A visit from a hospital chaplain or community religious leader is often welcomed by the patient and may be especially helpful if medical issues concerning specific theologic beliefs or conflicts are involved.

14. Is it appropriate for doctors to pray with patients?

Opinions vary widely on the propriety of physicians praying with patients. Many physicians do so. Others strongly believe that this practice crosses professional boundaries. The guiding principle is that physician-patient interactions should not be perceived as coercive by the patient.

For: Many patients want it. Praying with patients can strengthen the doctor-patient relationship, especially when doctor and patient have the same or similar religious backgrounds. The literature suggests that prayer is an effective coping mechanism for dealing with the stress associated with illness.

Against: Praying with patients may contribute to the patient's belief that the physician has greater power than he or she would have without prayer. Praying with patients may represent religious coercion in which patients do not feel the freedom to decline.

Patient-initiated requests to pray avoid concerns about coercion and privacy. Whether a physician prays with the patient depends on the physician's own comfort. Nonreligious physicians or physicians of a different faith may listen respectfully as the patient prays.

15. How should doctors respond when patients ask about the doctor's beliefs?

If a patient inquires into a physician's spiritual beliefs, it may be an indirect way of trying to address other issues. Thus, it is helpful to understand patients' motivation for asking and what they are truly interested in knowing. Some may be interested in knowing whether the physician is open to spiritual issues and willing to incorporate patients' beliefs and desires into their care. When confronted with such a situation, it is reasonable to ask patients why this issue is important to them. Then the physician is better equipped to address patients' concerns.

It is appropriate to share beliefs with the patient in such a situation if both you and the patient are comfortable. This issue has been addressed in guidelines formulated by Foster[23]:

1. Religious dialogue may take place but does not have to take place.
2. Religious dialogue must be invited by the patient, not imposed by the physician.
3. Physicians must be open, nonjudgmental, and honest. They may share their own religious beliefs as personally valuable and helpful but must not insist that those beliefs be considered ultimate truth by the patient with whom they are shared.

Whatever its nature, the purpose of religious dialogue should be to lift or share burdens—not to produce them.

16. Should physicians address the issue of miracles with patients?

Some patients raise the question of miracles with the physician. Although uncommon, such questions tend to arise either when the patient is doing poorly or (less likely) when the patient has done much better than expected. In responding to such questions, the physician must find the balance between avoiding inappropriate false hope and taking away all hope. The physician can respond in a supportive way, regardless of personal belief in miracles as supernatural phenomena. When a patient appears to have no hope of recovery, it is important to restate the known facts and expected or likely outcome. Then one can make a qualifying statement: although this is the expected outcome, it cannot be known with certainty whether it will apply a specific patient, because at times unexpected and unexplainable outcomes occur. If the physician believes in miracles, it is reasonable to state this belief as long as it is placed in a realistic context for patient or family. Even in the most dire of circumstances the physician should not take away all hope.

Some physicians have described events that they believe to be miracles in the supernatural sense of the word. Examples include patients who met all criteria for brain death but awoke shortly before termination of life support. Others have described less dramatic events in which a clearly unexpected outcome occurred.

17. If a patient's beliefs interfere with appropriate medical care, is it appropriate to attempt to change the patient's belief?

Adults have the right to believe what they choose. They also have the right to decline medical interventions, even if an adverse outcome is expected as a result. Physicians have a professional obligation to explain the expected medical consequences of a faith-based decision to forego treatment or choose an alternate treatment of uncertain empirical value (informed consent). With the patient's permission, physicians may share personal beliefs about the issue in question, including their personal wish that the patient accept the proposed medical intervention. However, it is considered unethical to make a patient's care conditional on accepting the physician's beliefs.

18. What is an appropriate response when a patient requests an intervention that would cause the physician to violate his or her own moral code?

At some time in the physicians' career, a patient may make a request that would require the physician to violate a deeply held moral code. Examples include assisting with abortion, performing euthanasia, or assisting with suicide. Even if they are legal, it is widely accepted that physicians are not required to engage in such practices. In such situations physicians should be honest and straightforward about their position, yet respectful of the patient's perspective. It is critical that the physician not behave in a way that may be construed as abandonment. The physician may not withdraw from care of the patient until alternative care is arranged. If an intervention of which the physician does not approve could be potentially life-saving, the physician must arrange for its provision by another physician.

19. Which specific beliefs may affect the medical care of Jewish patients?

Issues of particular importance for observant Jewish patients may include the need for kosher foods and recognition of the importance of the Sabbath or Jewish festivals. The need to consult with a religious advisor may arise if medical interventions create religious questions. The belief that only God gives life and that only God may take it away may raise significant concerns for patients facing end-of-life issues.[24]

20. How do the beliefs of Native Americans affect medical care?

The use of native healers remains a rich part of many Native American cultures. Each of the approximately 500 nations in North America may have its own unique traditions of healing, although beliefs in healthy living and spiritual principles that restore balance are shared by many.[25] A recent study among Navajo patients attending a rural Indian Health Service clinic found that one-third used native healers on a regular basis and that two-thirds have used native healers at some point.[26] Age, education, income, and fluency in English did not distinguish users of native healers from those who did not. Native healers were consulted for problems such as arthritis, depression, and diabetes mellitus. Conflict between the advice of native healers and medical providers was rare.

A separate study involving Midwestern Native Americans (primarily Ojibwa, Oneida, Chippewa, and Menominee) found that 38% see a native healer.[27] Types of native healers included herbalists, spiritual healers, and medicine men. The most common treatments included sweat lodge ceremonies, spiritual healing, and herbal remedies. In contrast to the previous study, more than one-third received different advice from native healers and physicians; they rated the healer's advice higher than the physician's advice in almost two-thirds of cases. These studies illustrate the high value that Native American populations may place on the use of native healers and suggest that physicians should be open to address these issues with patients.

21. Which specific Islamic beliefs may affect health care?

Islam considers life as sacred and belonging to Allah.[28,29] In general Muslims are supportive of preventive health care and contemporary medical care for illness. Preserving life and avoiding suicide are high priorities. On the other hand, Islamic ethical authorities do not require futile therapy. For the Western health care practitioner, gender issues may be the most obvious difference in caring for Muslim patients. Islamic doctrine mandates same-sex providers, if possible; in some cases, the Muslim patient will wish to be cared for only by a provider of the same gender. This requirement is voided in cases of medical emergency or when expert care is needed.

Two specific Muslim ritual practices have health care implications. The Hajj (pilgrimage to Mecca) can be physically demanding for devotees making the 4-day trip across the desert. In addition, because millions of people participating in the Hajj are in close proximity, the Centers for Disease Control and Prevention operates an office in Mecca to help the Saudi government prevent outbreaks of infectious illnesses, including meningococcal infection. Ramadan is a month of spiritual consciousness during which Muslims fast from dawn to dusk. Fasting during Ramadan involves total abstention from eating, drinking any fluids, and sexual relations. Physicians can be sensitive to observant Muslims' needs by modifying their medication dosing schedule during Ramadan and realizing the psychosocial implications for Muslim patients, who may be unable to fast for medical reasons during Ramadan.[30]

22. What sources are available for further information?

- King DE: Faith, Spirituality, and Medicine: Toward the Making of the Healing Practitioner. Binghamton, NY, Haworth Press, 2000.
- Koenig HG: The Healing Power of Faith: Science Explores Medicine's Last Great Frontier. New York, Simon & Schuster, 1999.
- Larson DB, Larson SS, Puchalski CM, Koenig HG: Patient spirituality in clinical care: Parts I and II. Primary Care Rep 6:165–180, 2000.
- Matthews DA: The Faith Factor: Proof of the Healing Power of Prayer. New York, Viking, 1998.

REFERENCES

1. Gallup G: Religion in America—50 years, 1935–1985. The Gallup Report. Princeton, NJ, Princeton Religion Research Center, 1989.
2. Ehman JW, Ott BB, Short TH, et al: Do patients want physicians to inquire about their spiritual or religious neliefs if they become gravely ill? Arch Intern Med 159:1803–1806, 1999.
3. Strawbridge WJ, Cohen RD, Shema SJ, Kaplan GA: Frequent attendance at religious services and mortality over 28 years. Am J Public Health 87:957–961, 1997.
4. Guinn R: Characteristics of drug use among Mexican-American students. J Drug Educ 5:235–241, 1975.
5. Koenig HG, Cohen HJ, George LK, et al: Attendance at religious services, interleukin-6, and other biological parameters of immune function in older adults. Int J Psychiatry Med 27:233–250, 1997.
6. Woods TE, Antoni MH, Ironson GH, Kling DW: Religiosity is associated with affective and immune status in symptomatic HIV-infected gay men. J Psychosom Res 46:165–176, 1999.
7. Pressman P, Lyons JS, Larson DB, Strain JJ: Religious belief, sepression, and ambulation status in elderly women with broken hips. Am J Psychiatry 147:758–760, 1990.
8. Oxman TE, Freeman DH, Manheimer ED: Lack of social participation or religious strength and comfort as risk factors for death after cardiac surgery in the elderly. Psychosom Med 57:5–15, 1995.
9. Harris RC, Dew MA, Lee A, et al: The role of religion in heart-transplant recipients' long-term health and well-being. J Religion Health 34:17–32, 1995.
10. Larson DB, Koenig HG, Kaplan BH, et al: The impact of religion on men's blood pressure. J Religion and Health 28:265–278, 1989.
11. Matthews DA, Marlowe SM, and MacNutt FS: Effects of Intercessory Prayer on Patients With Rheumatoid Arthritis. Southern Medical Journal 93:1177-1186, 2000.
12. Oleckno WA, Blacconiere MJ: Relationship of religiosity to wellness and other health-related behaviors and outcomes. Psychol Rep 68:819–826, 1991.
13. Galton F: Statistical inquiries into the efficacy of prayer. Fortnight Rev 12(new series):125–135, 1872.
14. Collipp PJ: The efficacy of prayer: A triple-blind study. Med Times 97(5):201–204, 1969.
15. Byrd RC: Positive therapeutic effects of intercessory prayer in a coronary care unit population. South Med J 81:826–829, 1988.
16. Harris WS, Gowda M, Kolb JW, et al: A randomized, controlled trial of the effects of remote, intercessory prayer on outcomes in patients admitted to the coronary care unit. Arch Intern Med 159:2273–2278, 1999.
17. Sicher F, Targ E, Moore D II, Smith HS: A randomized double-blind study of the effect of distant healing in a population with advanced AIDS. West J Med 169(6):356–363, 1998.
18. Spence C, Danielson TS, Kaunitz AM: The Faith Assembly: A study of perinatal and maternal mortality. Ind Med March:180–183, 1984.
19. Asser SM, Swan R: Child fatalities from religion-motivated medical neglect. Pediatrics 101:625–629, 1998.
20. Maugans TA: The SPIRITual history. Arch Fam Med 5:11–16, 1996.
21. Anandarajah G, Hight E: Spirituality and medical practice: Using the HOPE questions as a practical tool for spiritual assessment. Am Fam Physician 63:81–88, 2001.
22. Puchalski C and Romer AL: Taking a spiritual history allows clinicians to understand patients more fully. J Palliat Care 3(1):129–137, 2000.
23. Foster DW: Religion and medicine: The physician's perspective. In Marty ME, Vaux KI (eds): Health/Medicine and the Faith Traditions. Philadelphia, Fortress Press, 1982, pp 245–270.
24. Rosner F: Principles of practice concerning the Jewish patient. J Gen Intern Med 11:486–489, 1996.
25. Cohen K: Native American medicine. Alt ern Ther 4(6):45–57, 1998.
26. Kim C, Kwok YS: Navajo use of native healers. Arch Intern Med 158:2245–2249, 1998.
27. Marbella AM, Harris MC, Diehr S, et al: Use of Native American healers among Native American patients in an urban Native American health center. Arch Fam Med 7:182–185, 1998.
28. Sarhill N, LeGrand S, Islambouli R, et al: The terminally ill Muslim: Death and dying from the Muslim perspective. Am J Hosp Palliat Care 18(4):251–255, 2001.
29. Daar AS, al Khitamy AB: Bioethics for clinicians. 21: Islamic bioethics. Can Med Assoc J 164:60–63, 2001.
30. www.islamcity.org [accessed December 13, 2001].

9. YOGA

Russell H. Greenfield, M.D.

1. What is yoga?

The discipline of yoga can be traced back 4,000 years to the Indus Valley. It is an essential component of ayurveda, one of the oldest complete medical systems in the world. The word *yoga* is derived from a Sanskrit root (*yuj*) meaning to unite or yoke. Traditionally, regular yoga practice is believed to unite body, mind, and spirit, thereby enhancing health and quality of life. First introduced to the United States at the 1893 Chicago World's Fair,[1] yoga is now practiced regularly by over 12 million Americans. Far from indicating a fad, these numbers reflect the growing awareness that yoga offers an intimate sense of involvement in health care and wellness.

Although many view yoga as an activity for relaxation or stretching, it is more a discipline in the art of living, complete with physical, mental, spiritual, and community practices.

2. Is yoga a religious practice?

Yoga is a discipline of conscious living that encourages, but does not mandate, spiritual reflection. It can complement any religious practice or be practiced completely apart from one.

3. Is yoga appropriate only for the relatively healthy and flexible?

People of any fitness level or age can practice yoga, whether as a regular practice to help quiet the mind (and thereby manage stress), as a means of becoming more aware of the body, as an intense work-out for competitive athletes, or as the first step on the path toward a regular exercise program.

It has been said that only in the United States is yoga a competitive sport. The object of practice should be to take the body and mind from a place of discomfort to a place of comfort. Yoga is to be enjoyed, not suffered through. Rather than "no pain, no gain," the principle behind yoga is stated more correctly as" no pain, no pain."

4. Describe the types of yoga practice.

The various schools of yoga encompass all styles, from those requiring a high degree of fitness and emphasizing physical exertion to those promoting the meditative aspects of practice. All offer a path by which people may attain balance in their lives, greater self-awareness, and improved health by paying attention to mind, body, and spirit. Yoga is not simply about physical postures; it is a full lifestyle discipline. The major branches of yoga include, among others, **bhakti** (the path of devotion and love), **hatha** (the forceful path), **jnana** (the path of wisdom and knowledge [study]), **karma** (the path of service and action), and **raja** (the path of meditation and spirituality).[1,2]

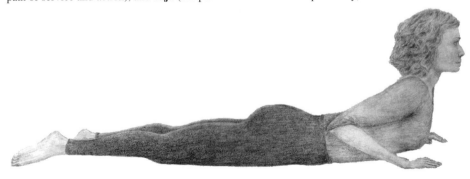

The cobra pose is a classic example of the physical postures adopted in yoga. (Drawing by Matthew Flesch.)

5. Describe the different styles of hatha yoga.

Hatha yoga is the most popular form in the US, focusing significant attention on the physical postures (asanas), breath work, and meditation. Some of the most commonly practiced yoga styles come under the umbrella heading of hatha yoga:

Ashtanga: a form that emphasizes physical exertion and stamina and considers the creation of internal body heat to be an essential component of practice, along with a challenging sequence of postures. It is sometimes referred to as "power yoga."

Bikram: performed in a heated room to promote the removal of toxins and increased flexibility, this style emphasizes physical exertion during the performance of asana sequences.

Integral: a meditative form of yoga that includes gentle postures and breathing exercises.

Iyengar: emphasizes attention to detail with regard to proper alignment in the performance of postures. Restorative yoga, a gentle therapeutic technique emphasizing stretching, movement, and breath work, is derived mainly from this style of yoga.

Kripalu: emphasizes the way the postures feel (body awareness), deep breathing exercises, and the spiritual nature of yoga.

Viniyoga: promotes the union and coordination of breath and sequential movements. This gentle style form can offer a good introduction to the therapeutic benefits of yoga practice for the elderly, those in acute or chronic discomfort, or any beginning student.

6. Describe a typical yoga session.

Because of the variety of styles, there is no such thing as a "typical" yoga session. That said, the majority of yoga classes in the United States last an average of 45–60 minutes. Participants often engage in the performance of postures called asanas. Thousands of asanas have been described, but most practitioners use only a few dozen on a regular basis. Some people most enjoy the physical aspects of assuming the postures, which enhance flexibility and relaxation for tired muscles. Others, however, find that regular practice provides an opportunity for mental relaxation, stress reduction, and self-discovery. Classes commonly end with students in a fully relaxed position, followed by appropriately inspiring comments of closure.

7. What is pranayama?

For people in search of a deeper practice, the asanas are done not as ends unto themselves but in preparation for breath work (pranayama), performed both alone and together with the various postures. The breath, when tied to the postures, helps participants experience greater awareness of how they feel in each pose, providing a greater sense of each individual's body. Breath work is done in preparation for meditation, and meditation prepares participants for the real work of yoga—finding greater connection with oneself and the community at large.

8. Can yoga be adapted for people with limitations in mobility?

Yoga therapists, who have experience with or receive additional training in applying yoga to specific maladies, use carefully chosen, gentle postures in association with breath work to create a healing opportunity for people with various illnesses. Often the instructor recommends the use of various props, such as blocks or chairs, to enable participants to perform asanas without having to invite discomfort (see figure at top of following page).

9. Identify a representative research study that supports a therapeutic role for yoga.

One of the more widely recognized studies focused on yoga and carpal tunnel syndrome.[3] Forty-two people with carpal tunnel syndrome were enrolled in an 8-week, single-blind, randomized controlled study. Control subjects were offered a wrist splint in addition to regular therapy, whereas participants assigned to the yoga group used postures designed to enhance upper body joint health and also practiced relaxation therapy. At the end of the study, participants in the yoga group showed significant improvement in grip strength and had reduced pain compared with the control group. Yoga is helpful not only for musculoskeletal problems; it has a broad range of benefits.

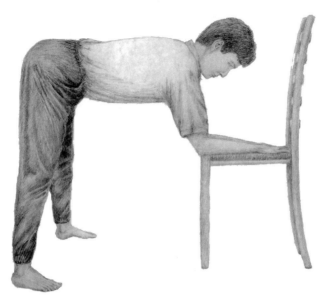

The use of a chair enables participants with limitations in mobility to perform asanas without having to invite discomfort. (Drawing by Matthew Flesch.)

10. What health benefits are associated with yoga?

Most participants agree that a regular yoga practice enhances flexibility (both physical and mental), improves posture, and increases strength and balance. A regular practice also provides an enjoyable means of managing stress and offers a sense of personal involvement, even control, in maintaining or improving health. Although poses have been used in association with specific maladies for millennia, yoga therapy has not generally been considered disease-specific. A regular yoga practice can benefit people with a variety of health problems, including:

Asthma[4–9]	Headaches
Chronic pain[10]	Hypertension[15–17]
Depression and anxiety[11–14]	Insomnia
Dysmenorrhea	Irritable bowel syndrome
Fatigue	Lower back and other musculoskeletal problems
Fibromyalgia	(e.g., osteoarthritis, carpal tunnel syndrome)[3,18,19]

Yoga may not offer participants a cure for their ailments, but practice can help people create balance in their lives and enhance quality of life.

11. Summarize the research studies related to yoga.

The majority of studies addressing the therapeutic potential of yoga suffer from serious methodologic flaws. Many designs include only a small number of subjects, are uncontrolled, include numerous confounding factors, and use various "cleansing procedures" that make interpretation difficult at best. Only a few articles have focused on any negative effects related to the practice of yoga. This may be due to a relative lack of such effects or to publication bias. Still, yoga has been studied in association with the majority of conditions listed above, and the results suggest that regular practice can benefit certain people.

12. How does yoga work?

The precise mechanisms behind yoga's therapeutic benefits have not been conclusively identified. One of the most commonly posited explanations is stress reduction and systemic relaxation. Yoga practice may calm the autonomic nervous system, thereby eliciting the physiologic changes associated with deep relaxation. Such changes include reduced muscle tension, decreased oxygen consumption, overall calming of vascular tone, and improvement in the mechanical aspects of breathing (improved flexibility of thoracic musculature, increased tidal volumes, and decreased bronchial reactivity).[20] Regardless of the exact mechanisms, yoga appears to encourage health and healing.

13. How safe is the practice of yoga?

Yoga is safe as long as participants do not push themselves beyond a point of mild tension. A sense of competition (with others or oneself) often leads to straining in an attempt to attain or maintain a pose, and injury may follow.

There are rare reports of disability related to the practice of yoga, including vertebral artery dissection,[21–24] persistent out-of-body experiences,[25] and development of orbital varices.[26] Patients with known cerebrovascular insufficiency should be cautioned against prolonged head turning during yoga practice. Common sense should always prevail. Inverted poses should be avoided during menses, and pregnancy mandates a gentle practice performed under the guidance of an instructor well-versed in yoga for expectant mothers.

14. Give some suggestions for finding a yoga teacher.

Yoga books and tapes can be found at any large bookstore, but the best way to be safely introduced to yoga is by taking a class. First ask around for a yoga studio with a good reputation, and check into the instructor's credentials. No national standard exists for teacher certification, and the range of credentials varies widely from a few days of intensive training to decades of immersion in study. Look for an instructor with at least 4 years of teaching experience who has worked with people with chronic illness or disability. It is worthwhile to watch a few classes, especially with differing styles, before deciding which class to join. People may ask for one or two private lessons so that an individualized practice plan can be devised, taking into account any limitations that may be present. Ultimately, one can develop a daily practice to be done at home as well as in the studio.

15. List sources of further information.

Austin M: *Yoga for Wimps.* New York, Sterling Publishing, 2000.

Devi N: *The Healing Path of Yoga: Time-Honored Wisdom and Scientifically Proven Methods That Alleviate Stress, Open Your Heart, and Enrich Your Life.* Three Rivers, 2000.

Farhi D: *Yoga Mind, Body and Spirit : A Return to Wholeness.* Henry Holt, 2000.

Iyengar BKS: *Light on Yoga: Yoga Dipika.* Schocken Books, 1995.

Kraftsow G: *Yoga for Wellness: Healing with the Timeless Teachings of Viniyoga.* New York, Penguin Books, 1999.

Lasater J: *Relax and Renew: Restful Yoga for Stressful Times.* Rodmell Press, 1995.

REFERENCES

1. Knaster M: Discovering the Body's Wisdom. New York, Bantam Books, 1996.
2. Budilovsky J, Adamson E: The Complete Idiot's Guide to Yoga. New York, Alpha Books, 1998.
3. Garfinkel MS, Singhal A, Katz WA, et al: Yoga-based intervention for carpal tunnel syndrome: A randomized trial. JAMA 280:1601–1603, 1998.
4. Nagarantha R, Nagendra HR: Yoga for bronchial asthma: A controlled study. Br Med J 291:1077–1079, 1985.
5. Khanam AA, Sachdeva U, Guleria R, et al: Study of pulmonary and autonomic functions of asthma patients after yoga training. Indian J Physiol Pharmacol 40:318–324, 1996.
6. Nagendra HR, Nagarantha R: An integrated approach of yoga therapy for bronchial asthma: A 3–54 month prospective study. J Asthma 23(3):123–137, 1986.
7. Singh V, Wisniewski A, Britton J, et al: Effect of yoga breathing exercises (pranayama) on airway reactivity in subjects with asthma. Lancet 335:1381–1383, 1990.
8. Singh V: Effect of respiratory exercises on asthma. The Pink City lung exerciser. J Asthma 24(6):355–359, 1987.
9. Birkel DA, Edgren L: Hatha yoga: Improved vital capacity of college students. Altern Ther Health Med 6(6):55–63, 2000.
10. Nespor K: Pain management and yoga. Int J Psychosom 38(1–4):76–81, 1991.

11. Ray US, Mukhopadhyaya S, Purkayastha SS, et al: Effect of yogic exercises on physical and mental health of young fellowship course trainees. Ind J Physiol Pharmacol 45:37–53, 2001.

12. Janakiramaiah N, Gangadhar BN, Naga Venkatesha Murthy PJ, et al: Antidepressant efficacy of Sudarshan Kriya Yoga (SKY) in melancholia: A randomized comparison with electroconvulsive therapy (ECT) and imipramine. J Affect Disord 57(1–3):225–229, 2000.

13. Era TK, Gore MM, Oak JP: Recovery from stress in two different postures and in Shavasana: A yogic relaxation posture. Ind J Physiol Pharmacol 42:473–478, 1998.

14. Kamei T, Toriumi Y, Kimura H, et al: Decrease in serum cortisol during yoga exercise is correlated with alpha wave activation. Percept Mot Skills 90(3 Pt 1):1027–1032, 2000.

15. Brownstein AH, Dembert ML: Treatment of essential hypertension with yoga relaxation therapy in a USAF aviator: A case report. Aviat Space Environ Med 60:684–687, 1989.

16. Sundar S, Agrawal SK, Singh VP, et al: Role of yoga in management of essential hypertension. Acta Cardiol 39(3):203–208, 1984.

17. Murugesan R, Govindarajulu N, Bera TK: Effect of selected yogic practices on the management of hypertension. Ind J Physiol Pharmacol 44:207–210, 2000.

18. Garfinkel MS, Schumacher HR Jr, Husain A, et al: Evaluation of a yoga based regimen for treatment of osteoarthritis of the hands. J Rheumatol 21:2341–2343, 1994.

19. Garfinkel M, Schumacher HR: Yoga. Rheum Dis Clin North Am 26:125–132, 2000.

20. Benson H, Lehmann JW, Malhotra MS, et al: Body temperature changes during the practices of g Tum-mo yoga. Nature 295:234–236, 1982.

21. Pryse-Phillips W: Infarction of the medulla and cervical cord after fitness exercises. Stroke 20:292–294, 1989.

22. Nagler W: Vertebral artery obstruction by hyperextension of the neck. Arch Phys Med Rehabil 54:237–240, 1973.

23. Russell WR: Yoga and the vertebral arteries. Br Med J 1:685, 1972.

24. Hanus SH, Homer TD, Harter DH: Vertebral artery occlusion complicating yoga exercises. Arch Neurol 34:574–575, 1977.

25. Kennedy RB: Self-induced depersonalization syndrome. Am J Psychiatry 133:1326–1328, 1976.

26. Cohen JA, Char DH: Bilateral orbital varices associated with habitual bending. Arch Ophthalmol 113:1360–1361, 1995.

10. AYURVEDA

Robert E. Svoboda, BAMS, and Bhaswati Bhattacharya, M.P.H., M.D.

1. What is ayurveda?

Ayurveda, the classical system of healing and health enhancement that arose in the Indian sub-continent at least 5000 years ago, takes as its subject every aspect of embodied life, from before conception until after death. Traditional ayurveda is, simultaneously, a body of therapies, a constellation of health-enhancement practices, a way of life, and a philosophy of living. The word *ayurveda* can be translated as "the knowledge of life," "the art of living," or "the science of longevity," but its true thrust is "life-adaptability." According to ayurvedic philosophy, all embodied organisms must acclimate accurately to every environmental shift; the more appropriate and effortless the adjustment, the better the health. Disease states characteristically result when adaptation fails.

Although ayurveda's original therapies most likely focused on eclectic shamanic practices, for the past 3000 years or more it has widened its approach to include dietary regulation, exercise, yoga, massage, herbs, minerals, cathartic purification, surgery, psychological counseling, psychodrama, and other empirical methods both conventional and unconventional. There are also applications to veterinary medicine.

2. Is ayurveda the only traditional medicine practiced in India today?

No. Ayurveda is one of the six systems of medicine officially recognized, licensed, and supported by the government of India. India currently boasts more than 100 colleges of ayurveda, with a similar number of hospitals, both public and private, that identify themselves as ayurvedic. Ayurvedic wards are found in many hospitals otherwise devoted to other medical systems.

3. What is the original source of ayurveda? When did it originate?

Ayurveda originated from the Vedas, the ancient books of wisdom and sacrificial ritual that form the basis of classical Indian civilization. A lack of unambiguous documentation has prevented scholars from agreeing on when precisely the Vedas appeared or whether the Indus Valley civilization, the earliest Indian culture about which we any useful data, followed the Vedic religion. Some substances that have ayurvedic medicinal uses have been located in Indus Valley remains, which cover roughly the period from 3000 to 1500 BC, but no firm evidence supports the idea that ayurveda as such was practiced in the Indus Valley at that time.

The Vedic religion was clearly active during at least the second millenium BC, however, and classical ayurveda appeared no later than 1000 B.C. Until about 1000 A.D., ayurveda appears to have been India's dominant medical system, practiced by Vedics, Buddhists, and Jains alike. Thereafter it has competed with, and been influenced by, Greco-Arab medicine and biomedical principles and practices.

4. What are the most important texts of ayurveda?

The textbooks of ayurveda derive from the oral hymn traditions of Vedic ritual, compiled into collections called "samhitas." The most important of these samhitas were the Four Vedas: Rg, Yajur, Sama, and Atharva, which were put in written form around 1500 BC. From them were derived the *Charaka Samhita*, a treatise on internal medicine that is the first and still most important of all ayurvedic texts. Ayurveda's most famous surgical text is the *Sushruta Samhita*. Both books were originally compiled during the latter part of the first millennium B.C. and took on their current form during the early centuries of the first millennium A.D.

During the 7th or 8th centuries A.D., *Ashtanga Sangraha* and *Ashtanga Hrdaya* appeared, two famous ayurvedic treatises that are condensations of the earlier works, with some updating. *Madhava Nidana*, *Sharngadhara Samhita*, and *Bhavaprakasha* are renowned later texts, each adding new diseases and therapies. *Bhavaprakasha*, for instance, first described syphilis, calling it "the foreigners' disease" in honor of the Portuguese, who introduced it.

Modern instruction in ayurveda uses these texts primarily, with some adapted texts combining traditional ayurvedic and biomedical understanding of pharmacology, anatomy, or physiology and texts from other traditional medical systems, such as unani or siddha, to adapt ayurveda into modern practice.

5. What are the major branches or specialties of ayurveda?

As taught in the two chief texts, the *Charaka Samhita* and the *Sushruta Samhita*, Ayurveda consists of eight major branches, with knowledge organized by clinical symptoms or organ dysfunctions:

1. Internal medicine (kayachikitsa)
2. Surgery (shalya tantra)
3. Eye, ear, nose, and throat (shalakya tantra)
4. Gynecology, obstetrics, and pediatrics (kaumara bhritya)
5. Toxicology (visha tantra)
6. Psychiatry/psychology (bhuta vidya)
7. Rejuvenation (rasayana)
8. Virilization (vajikarana)

Both texts also contain detailed sections on various preclinical sciences:

- Basic concepts and terminology
- Anatomy and physiology
- Pharmacy and pharmacology (including the use of minerals and metals)
- Preventive and social medicine
- Pathology and diagnosis of disease

Some of these specialties may seem rather alien to the modern scientist, and even ones that seem familiar are not necessarily so. For example, psychology (bhutavidya) focuses chiefly on states of possession. However, other ayurvedic principles and practices are more familiar, such as the operation for repair of damaged noses and ears, whose details nineteenth century German scholars translated from the *Sushruta Samhita*. This operation inaugurated plastic surgery, making *Sushruta* the father of that specialty.

6. How does ayurveda define health and disease?

One of the words for "healthy" in Sanksrit is *svastha*, which literally means "established in oneself." According to one ayurvedic definition of svastha, the body and its physiologic processes are balanced and harmonious (sama), and the mind, senses, and spirit are "pleased" (prasanna). Disease develops when a devitalized body-mind fails to respond properly to a challenge (from within or without) and thus loses its equilibrium. Physical manifestations of illness may manifest from physiologic causes, and pathologies of the psyche can result from physiologic imbalances. Misalignment is the cause of disease, and good alignment is the cause of health. Thus, realignment of body and mind is the chief goal of ayurvedic intervention.

7. What are the three doshas?

After long observation, India's physicians of old found that organisms display certain patterns of abnormal activity when they fail to adapt well to changing conditions.[1] In Sanskrit, these patterns are referred to as doshas. Most vaidyas (ayurvedic doctors) recognize three doshas: **vata** (a pattern of unfocused overactivity, often leading to depletion), **pitta** (a pattern of focused overactivity creating abnormal heat), and **kapha** (a pattern of accumulation and stagnation). Wind, bile, phlegm, and other bodily constituents are the vehicles of the three doshas; they are the substances that carry these patterns and through which these patterns act. As long as the doshas remain in balance with one another, they keep the organism healthy; when they go out of balance, they cause disease. The vata pattern governs all motion of every kind in the mind and body; the pitta pattern is in charge of all transformation; and the kapha pattern, which lubricates, maintains, and contains, is the living being's stabilizing influence. All people are composites, and there are elements of each dosha in each person.

8. What are the characteristics of people dominated by the vata pattern?

They are typically thin with dry skin, quick-minded, alert, active, flexible, and creative. When unbalanced, they become fearful, nervous, and anxious. They are more susceptible to diseases involving the air principle (see question 11) such as emphysema, pneumonia, and arthritis. Other common vata disorders include flatulence, tics, twitches, aching joints, dry skin and hair, nerve disorders, constipation, and mental confusion.

9. Describe people dominated by the pitta pattern.

They are of medium build with ruddy skin and have warm bodies, penetrating ideas, and sharp intelligence. Unbalanced, they are easily agitated and aggressive and tend toward hate, anger, and jealousy. They tend to have diseases involving the fire principle (see question 11), such as fevers, inflammatory diseases, and jaundice. Common symptoms include skin rashes, burning sensation, ulceration, fever, inflammations or irritations (e.g., conjunctivitis), colitis, and sore throats.

10. Describe people dominated by the kapha pattern.

They have thick skin, and their bodies and muscles are well developed. They tend to be calm, tolerant, and forgiving and have strength and endurance. Unbalanced, they become lethargic and tend to experience greed, envy, attachment, and possessiveness. They are likely to have diseases associated with the water principle (see question 11), such as flu and sinus congestion.

11. How do the doshas relate to the five elements?

The three doshas are said to derive from the five great elements that make up the physical universe: space, air, fire, water, and earth. These "elements" are actually states of matter, with earth representing the solid state, water the liquid state, and air the gaseous state. Fire is the power of transmutation, which can change the state of any substance; space is the field that is simultaneously the source of all matter and the locale in which all matter exists.

The *Charaka Samhita* defines a human as the assemblage of these five elements plus the "indwelling spirit." Matter in all of its forms is derived from consciousness. Every substance with which we come in contact also is made up of these five elements and their attendant attributes. Each substance, when consumed, will influence the balance of these elements—and thus the doshas—in the organism's body and mind alike. For example, vata, which is associated with space and air, can be aggravated by gas-producing foods, such as beans, and pacified by foods cooked with water and butter. Pitta, which is associated with fire, is aggravated by hot spices and pacified by coconut and milk. Kapha, which is associated with water and earth, is aggravated by dairy products and pacified by ginger and garlic.

12. What is the role of yoga in ayurveda?

The word *yoga*, which means "union" and traditionally indicated practices intended to forge a union of body with mind, suggests to most people one version of the systematized practices of bodily postures (and sometimes breathing exercises) that have become widely popular in the West. In India, however, the generic term *yoga* represents a wide range of methods that seek to create "one-pointedness" (ekagrata) of mind and purpose. One of the most popular of these methods is the ashtanga ("eight-limbed") yoga of Patanjali, which details an eight-step formula for "one-pointing" the individual. Ayurvedic physicians were once expected to practice some form of yoga for self-cultivation, and yoga appears in the curriculum of the current ayurvedic course of study. Ayurvedists who espouse yoga may use the techniques of Patanjali's yoga, particularly asana (postures) and pranayama (breath control), for therapeutic purposes.

13. What is the relationship between Tibetan medicine and ayurveda?

Commonly accepted as the fusion of several medical systems adapted to the Tibetan environment and way of life, Tibetan medicine originated around the seventh century A.D. A medical conference is thought to have taken place between 755 and 797 A.D. at Samye in Central Tibet, where renowned philosophers and physicians gathered from Persia, Greece, India, China, Afghanistan, Nepal, East Turkestan, and Kashmir.

The *yGyud-bzhi*, meaning four roots and pronounced gyu-shi, are the current standard Tibetan texts, with most elements adapted from Greek (unani) medicine, traditional Chinese medicine, Indian Buddhist philosophy, and ayurvedic medicine. Significant ayurvedic influences on Tibetan medicine include the practice of seasonal food adjustments, prescribing diet according to taste, the use of food as medicine, the philosophy of karma in healing, and the use of mind-body therapies.

14. What kinds of diseases are treated by ayurveda?

Grouped differently from biomedical pathology textbooks, diseases in ayurveda are interpreted as dysfunctions with physiologic more than with anatomic correlates.[2] For example, diseases of the liver and cardiovascular system are discussed together. Blood production, cirrhosis, jaundice, anemia, leukemia, hemorrhage, hypertension, and low blood pressure are discussed in the same chapter. Although such grouping may seem superficially disparate, in fact clotting factors, blood components, and detoxification of blood occur in the liver to produce healthy cardiovascular function.

Although ayurveda can be quite effective in treating both acute and chronic diseases, its most conventional use within biomedically dominated societies is in the realm of preventive health. Conditions such as obesity, poor physical conditioning, indigestion, fatigue, and other disease states that are not considered life-threatening in biomedicine are treated with a blend of exercise, massage, herbs, yoga, detoxification, and rejuvenation in ayurveda to prevent more serious disorders from developing.

Acute diseases are effectively treated by ayurvedic formulations. Viral infections of the skin and mucosa are treated with herbal formulations that have been shown to contain potent antiviral compounds such as curcumin. Joint diseases, such as osteoarthritis, are treated with ayurvedic massage and anti-inflammatory herbal preparations. Neurologic conditions, especially those with toxic origins, are treated with oil detoxification using panchakarma. One particularly effective application of ayurvedic surgery is kshara sutra therapy,[3] which is used for anorectal disorders, particularly fistula-in-ano. A kshara sutra is a thread that has been soaked in herbal alkalis and dried. The dried threads are passed into the fistula's tract and tied off, whereupon the alkalis efficiently cauterize the tract from within. This procedure represents one of the most advanced ancient understandings of surgery and rivals current biomedical procedures.

15. What lifestyle factors are most crucial to developing and preserving health in ayurvedic medicine?

Ayurveda's hallmark is preventive medicine, and its health maintenance cornerstones are regular exercise and toning of the body; cultivation of deep, abdominal breathing; body-appropriate diet in harmony with the environment; proper sleep; and regular bowel habits. Ayurveda's emphasis on diet, exercise, and hygiene far exceeds that of allopathic medicine, and most ayurvedic practitioners emphasize these factors more regularly during visits with patients than do biomedical physicians.

Specific dietary modifications as well as regular exercise may be suggested to balance the doshas. A vaidya may recommend the use of massage and deep meditation breathing to assist in smoking cessation, using the ayurvedic principles of detoxification. Supervised fasting, rejuvenating herbs, and hypoglycemic preparations are often used in detoxification programs for diabetic patients, who often see both weight loss and better sugar control after such programs.

16. Describe ayurvedic pathology.

Detecting disease even before it organizes into clinical pathology is a strong point of ayurveda. Ayurvedic medicine pays great attention to clinical symptoms because they create imbalances in the patient's daily life and health. Symptoms that are significant or persistent are pursued with urine diagnosis, pulse diagnosis, tongue diagnosis, or more detailed history and addressed with lifestyle-rebalancing techniques before overt pathology manifests.

The six stages of disease development begin with the accumulation of the doshas and proceed first to their aggravation and then to their extension into parts of the system where they do not belong. Doshas are active. When the doshas encounter a particularly devitalized region of the body-mind, they localize, manifest into perceptible disease patterns, and finally erupt into clinical disease. These stages, which are gauged through detailed history and meticulous observation of the eyes, skin, voice, and gait, can be correlated with what scientists know about spread of disease and progression of pathology on a cellular level. For example, when the pitta is high, skin is yellow, and heat in the body and mind increases. Changes in bile, sweat, endocrine glands, and color occur. One of the conditions associated with exacerbated pitta is hepatitis. Another is cholecystitis. In each, subtle changes of the external body can signal early changes in the internal body, and action can be taken to correct excessive pitta before overt disease erupts.

17. How does diagnosis in ayurveda differ from diagnosis in allopathic medicine?
Ayurvedic diagnosis entails two avenues of investigation: what is balanced with the patient and what is imbalanced. What is "balanced" involves an assessment of the patient's overall level of health and resilience, including an estimation of which organs and tissues are particularly vital, well formed, and well functioning. A "wellness" evaluation also inspects the condition of the patient's more subtle aspects, including mental status and state of the life force (prana).

Diagnosis of disease involves appraisal of weaknesses, innate and acquired, in body and mind; measurement of dosha levels (searching primarily for relative increase); and identification of specific disorder(s). In practice it is not always necessary (or realistic) to make a precise diagnosis of a specific disorder. A specific diagnosis, however, helps tailor treatment and can increase the patient's confidence in a potentially positive outcome, whereas the lumping together of conditions that are related but not identical heightens the risk of delivering inadequate or improper treatment.

18. Are modern diagnostics and therapeutics used in ayurveda?
Ayurvedic practitioners, especially those trained in the past 30 years after medical curricula became more cosmopolitan and integrated, commonly use laboratory blood tests, histopathology, x-rays, scans, and stethoscopes to aid diagnosis. The diagnosis is usually framed in the mind-body-spirit context of the disease, although biomedical terms such as cancer and tic disorder are retained. If an ayurvedic term for the biomedical syndrome exists, it is used, such as prameha for diabetes in general and madhumeha for diabetes mellitus. Although a small cohort of ayurveda's conservative practitioners insist on administering only treatments mentioned in the ancient texts, many others use a combination of ayurvedic techniques, pharmacology, and biomedical principles Despite this attitude of "curative inclusiveness," however, it remains "un-ayurvedic" to use surgery or any other similarly intensive intervention as a first line of defense.

19. What are the different styles of ayurveda in India?
In the many areas where ayurveda has long been practiced continuously, localized methods and formulations have developed in response to local environments and diseases. Classic rivalries among the ayurvedists of these regions still persist. In addition to northern (Varanasi) and southern (Kerala) styles, the states of Maharashtra and Gujarat in western India have a style of their own, as does eastern India. As practitioners take ayurveda to other countries (e.g., Switzerland, Australia, United States, Britain) and adapt their interpretation of the Vedas to new environments, ambiguity over whose practice ist "authentic" has flourished. There is no overall arbiter to determine which of these systems is "valid" or "most valid."

20. What are the different styles of ayurveda in the West?
A few well-known ayurvedic authorities are now based in the West. Vasant Lad, one of the best known of the group of ayurvedic physicians who were trained in India and came to the U.S. to propound traditional principles, is the founder of the Ayurvedic Institute in New Mexico. (http://www.ayurveda.com)

Maharishi Mahesh Yogi, who introduced transcendental meditation in the 1970s, claims to have rescued ayurveda by reformulating it for the modern world through extolling the benefits of regular and sacred meditation. His university, the Maharishi Ayurved University in Fairfield, Iowa, has actively recruited M.D.s interested in lifestyle approaches to health, and a community of followers is dedicated to his diet, lifestyle, and philosophy of health. (http://www.mum.edu/CMVM/index.html)

In the early 1980s Deepak Chopra was an active speaker and proponent of the Maharishi philosophy. Later he branched off into this own philosophy of life and healing. He first espoused this philosophy in *Quantum Healing*, which combines elements of modern physics with principles of healing on the subcellular level in ways that resonate with the body-mind philosophies of classic ayurveda. Using his training as a practicing biomedical physician and his upbringing in ayurvedic philosophy, Chopra has authored popular works for Western readers (http://www.chopra.com/).

More recently, as yoga centers and institutes initiate courses in ayurveda, a new style has developed that centers on yogic health with a reduced emphasis on medical intervention.

21. What are the major treatment modalities of ayurveda?

In preventive care, lifestyle approaches such as balanced diet, exercise, therapeutic work, support systems, and abstinence from toxic habits are emphasized. For acute care conditions, herbal formulations, surgery (especially reconstructive), aromatherapy, massage, and counseling are used. For rejuvenation, massage, detoxification, and internal purification through enemas and supervised fasting, yoga, and meditation are the main elements.

Panchakarma, which means "five actions," is a unique system of rejuvenation based on therapeutic emesis, purgation, evacuative enema, nasal cleansing, and blood-letting to purge the body of toxins. Within this process, each cycle of which can last 21–30 days, is a cycle of fasting, sweating, oil massage, and exercise along with regular meditation and regulated nutrition.

22. Describe a typical ayurvedic treatment plan, particularly in the context of terminal illness.

The art of ayurvedic practice consists of knowing how best to adapt ayurveda's axioms to any situation at any time or place. Except in the most acute cases, the initial emphasis is placed firmly on accomplishing the simplest tasks: rebalancing the doshas, removing toxins, enhancing the digestive fire, and inculcating good health habits. The method works when physician and patient are willing to examine dietary habits, physical activity, substance use and abuse, relationship and support issues, degree of significant life stresses, and available coping mechanisms, in addition to the significance derived from symptoms.

Ayurveda seeks the highest quality of life for all patients, particularly in preparing for death, which, though inevitable, is the life event for which most people least prepare themselves. Death is often a positive outcome, particularly when all effective management options have been exhausted, and assisting a person to depart from this world with grace and composure is one of an ayurvedic physician's most important tasks.

23. How important to ayurvedic treatment is diet?

"You are what you eat" is ayurveda's watchword. Some sources maintain that dietary impropriety is responsible, directly or indirectly, for 90% of all disease states. Whether or not this estimate is accurate, it is a strong statement of the crucial role that ayurveda assigns to diet. Ayurveda recommends fresh food, freshly prepared and consumed in moderate amounts, without between-meal snacks, for those who value their health. Organic food is preferred.

Highly processed food, food that is highly preserved (or even worse, spoiled), fast food, and junk food are strongly discouraged because of their minimal nutritional value and substantial propensity to disturb homeostasis and promote food intolerance. Alhough evidence in the literature supporting associations between food intolerance and specific pathologies is still limited, many practitioners and patients report improvement in symptoms after dietary change.

Timing of meals is also important. Ayurveda proposes that the gastrointestinal system works best when the main work of eating is confined to the period that begins just before midday and ends just after dark (roughly 11 AM to 7 PM, depending on locality). This time frame provides the body a full 8 hours (roughly from 7 PM to 3 AM) in which to assimilate , followed by 8 hours (roughly 3 AM to 11AM) for elimination .

24. What is the significance of the six tastes (rasas) in ayurvedic diet?

The six tastes in ayurveda are sweet, sour, salty, pungent, bitter, and astringent. The tastes are associated with the three doshas. Sweet, sour, and salty foods increase kapha; sour, salty, and pungent foods increase pitta; and pungent, bitter, and astringent foods increase vata. Dosha aggravations may be balanced by foods associated with the complementary doshas—for example, vata with kapha. However, including each of these tastes in every meal is part of a balanced diet, because each taste signals the digestive system to trigger a different set of enzymes and digestive juices. In addition, balances of taste also ensure satiation and inclusion of a wider variety of nutrients.

25. List some of the well-known plants used in ayurveda.[4,5]

COMMON NAME	BOTANICAL NAME	CLINICAL USE
Tulsi	*Ocimum sanctum*	Antiviral
Neem	*Azadirachta indica*	Dental caries, antimicrobial
Ashwagandha[6]	*Withania somnifera*	Immunostimulant
Bitter melon	*Momordica charantia*	Hypoglycemic, antidiabetic
Turmeric[7]	*Curcuma longa*	Antiviral, dermatologic agent
Guggul[8]	*Commiphora mukul*	Cholesterol-lowering agent
Fenugreek	*Trigonella foenum-graecum*	Hypoglycemic, antidiabetic

26. What scientific studies of ayurveda are available?

In the past decade, the number of clinical studies in ayurveda has dramatically increased in the West. Fueled by the export of ayurvedic herbs into other markets and the increasing popularity of indigenous medicines in the West, companies that seek to market and license such products have engaged in studies, sometimes using the pharmaceutical model of research and development.

The National Institutes of Health (NIH) has funded several scientific studies in ayurveda, one of which is the NIH CAM Specialty Center for Research in Natural Medicine and Prevention. At the Maharishi Ayurved University, clinical trials in dardiovascular disease and aging in elderly, high-risk African Americans are under way. The subjects of the trials include the effects of meditation on atherosclerosis and the effects of ayurvedic herbal preparations on carotid atherosclerosis and oxidative stress. To learn more about ongoing studies, go to http://nccam.nih.gov/fi/research/desc.html#cnma.

Hari Sharma's text on research in maharishi ayurveda is another resource for clinical and basic scientific studies of ayurvedic treatments.[9]

Several human studies have been completed by Bala Manyam[10] and colleagues in the use of *Mucuna pruriens* (atmagupta in Sanskrit) for Parkinson's disease. Found to be a safe and less toxic alternative to levodopa pharmaceuticals, atmagupta contains natural levodopa and related pre- and postcursor compounds. *M. pruriens* is used traditionally with other natural antiparkinson agents found in plants, such as the anticholinergics in *Datura stramonium*, levodopa in *Vicia faba*, and dopaminergic *Claviceps purpura*.

Studies of guggul and guggulipids have demonstrated potent effects in lowering cholesterol comparedwith statin drugs and validated use in other inflammatory diseases (e.g., osteoarthritis).[11]

Studies of ayurveda, many of which are unavailable through mainstream American sources and databases, have been collected at the Ayurvedic Institute in Santa Fe, New Mexico. For more information, visit www.ayurveda.com. A recent study released by the U.S. Public Health Service's Agency for Healthcare Research and Quality (AHRQ Publication No. 01-E040) in September 2001 examines the current literature and basis for ayurvedic medicine in diabetes mellitus. It is titled, *Ayurvedic Interventions for Diabetes Mellitus: A Systematic Review*[12] and reviews herbal treatments for diabetes but finds no English evidence-based trials of other ayurvedic approaches. It is useful for its many references and summary of botanical literature.

27. What types of certification, registration, and licensing are currently available for ayurvedic practitioners?

In the United States, there is no official licensing process for ayurvedic doctors. Certificate programs have been initiated and approved by ayurvedic organizations, but there is no national approval for licensure. Regulation of health practitioners who are not conventionally licensed varies widely from state to state.

No certification boards yet exist for developing national standards for licensure of ayurvedic practitioners. A few physician groups, such as the American Academy of Ayurvedic Medicine

(AAAM) and the American Association of Physicians of Indian Origin (AAPI), have projects in their infancy to examine collaborations with doctors who observe biomedical standards but practice with ayurvedic doctors in the plurimedical system used in India. The government of India recently established funding through the Department of Indian Systems of Medicine and Homoeopathy for creating continuing medical education programs for U.S .doctors interested in receiving lectures provided by traditional ayurvedic scholars.

In addition, practitioners trained in India have opened schools in America; the Ayurvedic Institute in New Mexico is perhaps the leading example. Others include the Chopra Center for Well-Being,and the California College of Ayurveda. Several organizations also offer preliminary courses in ayurveda, designed more for scholars than for aspiring practitioners.

The most authentic method of obtaining training for an M.D. is a certification course of study in India.Well-reputed institutions include the Arya Vaidya Sala in Kottakal, Kerala; the Benaras Hindu University in Varanasi,Uttar Pradesh; the University of Poona, in Pune, Maharashtra; and the Gujarat Ayurved University, in Jamnagar, Gujarat.

To find a complete listing of courses at the 196 ayurvedic colleges in India, visit http://indian-medicine.nic.in/html/edu/augpg.htm. The official government site for locating ayurvedic training programs in India is http://indianmedicine.nic.in/html/edu/aemain.htm.

28. What resources are available for additional information?
- Priya Vrat Sharma: Sodasangahrdayam: Essentials of Ayurveda. New Delhi, Motilal Banarsidass Publishers, 1993.
- Vaidyaratnam PS Varier: Chikitsa Samgraham, 4th ed. Kottakkal, The Arya Vaidya Sala, 1999.
- Vasant Lad: Ayurveda: The Science of Self-healing. Santa Fe, Lotus Press, 1984.
- Robert Svoboda: Ayurveda: Life, Health, and Longevity. New York, Penguin Books, 1992.
- Government of India, Department of Indian System of Medicine and Homoeopathy: The Ayurvedic Pharmacopoeia of India. New Delhi, National Institute of Science Communication, 1999.

REFERENCES

1. Lad V: Ayurveda: The Science of Self-Healing. Santa Fe, NM, Lotus Press, 1984.
2. Murthy NA, Pandey DP: Ayurvedic Cure for Common Diseases, 5th ed. New Delhi, Orient Paperbacks, 1995.
3. Sharma SK, Sharma KR, Singh K: Kshara Sutra Therapy in Fistula-in-Ano and other Ano-Rectal Disorders. New Delhi, Rashtriya Ayurveda Vidyapeeth Publications, 1994.
4. Sharma H, Clark C: Contemporary Ayurveda: Medicine and Research in Maharishi Ayur-Veda. New York, Churchill Livingstone, 1998.
5. LaValle JB, Krinsky DL, Hawkins EB, et al: Natural Therapeutics Pocket Guide, 2000-2001. Hudson, OH, Lexi-Comp, 2000.
6. Ziauddin M, Phansalkar N, Patki P, et al: Studies on the immunomodulatory effects of Ashwagandha, J Ethnopharmacol 50(2):69–76,1996.
7. Szapary PO, Cirigliano MD: Turmeric in the treatment of dyspepsia. Altern Med Alert 3(5):49–53, 2000.
8. Singh RB, Niaz MA, Ghosh S: Hypolipidemic and antioxidant effects of *Commiphora mukul* as an adjunct to dietary therapy in patients with hypercholesterolemia. Cardiovasc Drug Ther 8:659–664, 1994.
9. Sharma H, Clark C: Contemporary Ayurveda: Medicine and Research in Maharishi Ayur-Veda. New York, Churchill Livingstone, 1998.
10. Manyam B: HP-200 in Parkinson's Disease Study Group. An alternative medicine treatment for Parkinson's disease: Results of a multicenter clinical trial. J Altern Compl Med 1(3):249–155, 1995.
11. Singh BB, Mishra L, Aquilina N, Kohlbeck F: Usefulness of guggul (*Commiphora mukul*) for osteoarthritis of the knee: An experimental case study. Altern Ther Health Med 7(2):112–124, 2001.
12. Hardy M, Coulter I, Venuturupalli S, et al: Ayurvedic Interventions for Diabetes Mellitus: A Systematic Review. Evidence Report/Technology Assessment No. 41 (Prepared by Southern California Evidence-based Practice Center/RAND under Contract No. 290-97-0001). AHRQ Publication No. 01-E040, 2001. Available at http://www.ahcpr.gov/clinical/ayurvinv.htm.

11. TRADITIONAL CHINESE MEDICINE

Julia Thie, L.Ac.

1. What modalities are used in traditional Chinese medicine (TCM)

All methods of TCM are based on holism; living in harmony with nature, ourselves, and others is seen as the foundation of good health. Between 200 B.C. and 100 A.D., the fundamentals of Chinese medicine were compiled in the oldest known text, *Huang Di Nei Jing (The Yellow Emperor's Inner Classic)*. The text states that the more out of balance one is with nature, the more invasive the type of medicine that is necessary. TCM has progressed with time, and many texts have expounded on the historical concepts.

The methods chosen for treatment may be as simple as a lifestyle or attitude change or as complex as herbal therapy or acupuncture (see Chapter 12). Other modalities include heat therapy (moxibustion), medicinal nutrition, forms of bodywork known as tui-na and shiatsu, and energy work called qi-gong. Different modalities are chosen for case-specific efficacy. All are based on a philosophy that expands into many aspects of Chinese culture.

2. How does the theory of yin and yang apply to this medicine?

Yin and yang are relative concepts based in ancient Taoism. They represent the nature of opposites: yin is dark and inward moving, whereas yang is bright and outward moving. The dynamic nature of yin and yang is within all things. Nothing is purely yin or purely yang. Because they are in constant transformation from one to the other, there is always some yang within yin and some yin within yang. The opposition and transformation of yin and yang are considered the spark of life.

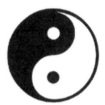

The tai-ji symbol shows a spot of white on the black and a spot of black on the white, symbolizing the concept that nothing is purely yin or purely yang.

Yin and yang also describe the nature of illness and predict what will happen if the illness is unheeded. For example, if a person with a hyperthyroid condition (yang in nature) goes untreated, the condition may eventually collapse into hypothyroidism (yin in nature). The same person left untreated may then develop an inflammatory disorder, cycling back into excess (yang), although with less strength. The circle of change continues with pathologic force unless some intervention occurs. The goal is to create a closer state of balance between the patient's yin and yang natures so that a check-and-balance system between the two allows neither to become too dominant.

3. What is qi?

Qi is one of the "three treasures" in Chinese medical philosophy. It is best explained as the vital energy that moves through and sustains all life. Normal flow of qi in the body creates and maintains health, whereas blockage of qi can lead to disease. Qi is subcategorized into different types that perform particular functions. For example, wei-qi describes the defensive energy of the immune system, based primarily on lung function, and gu-qi is the energy of the stomach and spleen that digests food. The other two "treasures" are essence (jing) and spirit (shen).

4. How is a diagnosis obtained in TCM?

To understand diagnostic terminology in TCM, a philosophical language barrier must be overcome. The actual diagnosis is not a name of a disease but rather a systematic description of disharmonies using terms that are synonymous with elements in nature or terms that describe energetic functions. Wind, damp, dry, cold, and heat are descriptions of pathogenic elements that can afflict a person either externally or internally. For example, a person may develop a cough after exposure to an external dry wind; a rash may break out in response to heat in the blood; or diarrhea may result from excessive internal damp heat. TCM does not simply treat the cold, rash, or diarrhea; it finds ways to balance the underlying disharmony so that the body can eliminate its manifestations. Other common terms that are described in relative excess or deficiency include qi, blood, body fluids, and yin and yang. For example, a deficiency of qi within the digestive systems creates an inability to digest foods properly. A bruise is considered a localized stagnation of excessive blood.

Many paradigms govern Chinese medicine. A few methods of classifying pathology include the eight principles, five elements, zhang-fu theory, four levels, and six stages. All are philosophies designed to obtain a TCM diagnosis and treatment plan.

5. Explain tongue and pulse diagnosis.

Tongue diagnosis is unique to TCM. The tongue's shape, motility, color, coating, and moisture are signs that help shape a diagnosis. The figure below shows the geographic locations that correspond to internal organs. The presence of color changes, coatings, or cracks in these areas indicate disharmonies within the corresponding organ system For example, a thick yellow coating is an indication that the body is not processing foods well and that dampness has accumulated.

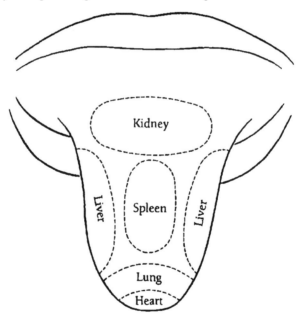

Zones of the tongue that correspond to internal organs. (From Between Heaven and Earth by Harriet Beinfield and Efrem Korngold, copyright © 1991 by Harriet Beinfield and Efrem Korngold. Used by permission of Ballantine Books, a division of Random House, Inc.)

Pulse diagnosis is a highly-refined art form included in the earliest texts of oriental medicine. The most commonly used pulse location is the radial artery. There are three pulse positions at this location (see figure on following page). Each position has three depths that indicate the status and location of the patient's energy and fluids. There are many ways of describing the qualities of the pulse (e.g., wiry, slippery, superficial). Each indicates a condition that helps to shape the diagnosis.

Both tongue and pulse are subjective tools that may be altered by exterior factors. Part of the intake should verify whether the tongue or pulse has been influenced by medications or other substances.

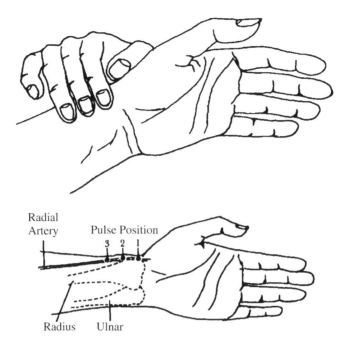

Radial
Artery   Pulse Position
                3 2 1

Radius   Ulnar

Pulse taking, Chinese style. (From Kaptchuck T: The Web That Has No Weaver. Congdon & Weed Inc., Chicago,IL, 1983, with permission.)

6. What are the eight principles?

Yang	Excess	Hot	External
Yin	Deficient	Cold	Internal

The eight principles offer a starting point in diagnosis that determines the type of treatment necessary to resolve the disharmony. For example, symptoms of the common cold may be categorized as a yang/excess/hot/external condition. Treatment consists of expelling heat from the exterior. Edema, on the other hand, may be categorized as a yin/excess/cold/internal condition. Treatment consists of draining excessive yin and warming the interior. The eight principles provide a method of categorizing the location and nature of the patient's condition.

7. Explain the five element theory.

The five element theory, also known as the five phase theory, is another paradigm in Chinese medical diagnosis and practice. The relationships among these elements explain the interconnectedness of all of the body's systems, which are represented as fire, earth, metal, water, and wood. These terms correspond to signs and symptoms that determine the focus of treatment. For example, the coloring of a person's skin can point to an elemental disharmony. Jaundice, which is typically yellowish-green, classically affects the wood and earth elements.

Five Element Sample Correspondences

	FIRE	EARTH	METAL	WATER	WOOD
Yin organ (zhang)	Heart	Spleen	Lung	Kidney	Liver
Yang organ (fu)	Small intestine	Stomach	Large intestine	Urinary bladder	Gallbladder
Color	Red	Yellow	White	Black	Green
Emotion	Joy	Worry	Grief	Fear	Anger
Tissue	Vessels	Muscles	Skin	Bones	Sinews
Sense organ	Tongue	Mouth	Nose	Ears	Eyes

As seen in the chart, the colors associated with wood and earth are green and yellow. The involved organs are the liver and spleen, which would be addressed in the treatment of most cases of jaundice. Furthermore, the nature of the person with jaundice may be classified as a wood type. This "type" is determined by personality and history of symptoms. Knowing a patient's elemental type can help in counseling against behavioral extremes that negatively affect health.

8. What is five element acupuncture?

The use of acupuncture in five element treatment requires an understanding of the cycles and relationships among the five elements.

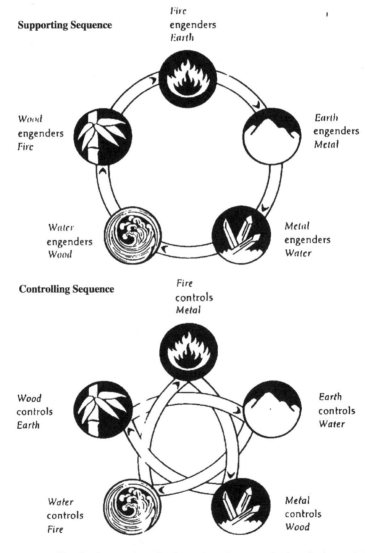

Top, Supporting sequence. The five lements in a circular order—the generation/ mothering cycle in which each generates the next. *Bottom,* Controlling sequence, also known as cross-effecting. For example, the wood element "nourishes" fire, whereas water "controls" fire. Each element has corresponding organs, one solid and one hollow. (From Beinfeld H, Korngold E: Between Heaven and Earth. New York, Ballantine Books, 1991, with permission.)

After determining elemental excesses or deficiencies that affect the health of a patient, the acupuncture points are selected by their ability either to tonify or to sedate the proper elements. For example, a person with deficiency in the metal element may have symptoms of shortness of breath or wheezing, indicating imbalance in lung functions, and an allopathic diagnosis of asthma. Points are chosen to correct these imbalances, either by nourishing the earth element (support), which helps transform phlegm, or by sedating the wood element (control) ,which helps in cases of allergy-induced asthma.

9. How does TCM approach the person with depression?

The following cases of depression are quite different when viewed within the framework of TCM diagnosis. Both have a disturbance of shen (spirit), yet from different causes. Keep in mind that the organs listed need not be the anatomic organ but rather a system of functions.

1. A woman has depressive symptoms. Her concurrent symptoms are premenstrual cramping and low self-esteem. Her stools are loose, and she frequently has indigestion. Her pulse is wiry and slippery; her tongue is pale and swollen. She shows signs of liver qi stagnation and spleen qi deficiency. Her depression is categorized as yin/excess/cold/internal, or as wood overcontrolling earth. The treatment is to nourish spleen qi and move liver qi. In the five element treatment paradigm, wood is sedated and earth tonified. These goals can be achieved internally with herbs and nutrition; externally with massage, acupuncture, moxibustion, and qi-gong exercises.)

2. A man has depressive symptoms. He also has bouts of anger that are expressed in a passive-aggressive manner. He complains of heartburn, flank pain, and temporal headaches. His pulse is wiry and rapid, and his tongue is red. This case is categorized as yang/excess/hot/internal. He shows signs of liver qi stagnation with heat. The treatment is to move liver qi and clear heat. This condition may be resolved with acupuncture, vigorous exercise, and herbs as well as other methods.

Both patients would benefit from a referral to a qualified psychological therapist in conjunction with treatment. Antidepression medication may not be necessary. These examples show how a TCM practitioner may evaluate disease. Although the two people carry the same allopathic diagnosis of depression, they are conceptualized differently and thus treated differently. Matching the appropriate treatment principle to the correct TCM diagnosis is the key to achieving the desired results.

10. What is unique about the selection and use of herbs in oriental medicine?

Records of Chinese herbal therapy have been traced back to the third century B.C.[1] Each herb has a temperature, also called its nature (hot, warm, neutral, cool, or cold), a taste (bitter, sweet, pungent, sour, or salty and bland), a corresponding meridian, and certain actions. An herb is not used primarily because it treats an ailment but rather because its nature addresses the pattern shown by the patient. Herbal formulation is a key concept in TCM. Rarely are herbs used singly, and each herb has a specific role within a formula. A substance may be used as the chief herb addressing the imbalance or as a guide herb that helps to direct the formula to a certain area of the body; other roles are also possible roles. The herbs may be chosen in pairs because their synergistic effect has a specific function. The art of combining Chinese herbal formulas is known as feng ji.

11. Are Chinese herbs safe?

The question of safety lies less in the herbs themselves and more in their proper use and the quality of the herbal products used. There are different categories of herbs. Tonic herbs have a good safety profile and can be taken for long periods . Medicinal herbs are used in times of illness and should be taken only for short periods. Many herbs are specifically processed to remove toxicity or are neutralized by combination with other herbs within a formula. Herbs are used with dose specificity and are appropriate and safe when used properly.

Product validity and quality are important issues for herbal practitioners. Unfortunately, some Chinese-made formulas, also known as "patents," are adulterated with pharmaceuticals such as non-steroidal anti-inflammatory drugs, steroids, and narcotics,[1] which raises justified suspicion for herbal products imported from countries without adequate quality controls. Chinese labeling laws allow these ingredients to be listed merely as "other." To ensure quality control, many practitioners use American-made products that name both the genus and species of the herbs used and are backed by adequate laboratory testing. Practitioners may also directly compound the bulk herb ingredients in their office to ensure quality. Chinese herbs have a long history of traditional use. Serious problems exist in some commercial formulations, but when used responsibly, herbs are an asset to patient care.

12. What is qi-gong?

Qi-gong translates as energy (qi) and cultivation (gong); hence, the term refers to energy cultivation. It is the practice of moving one's own or another person's energy with intent. Qi-gong is practiced both internally and externally in many styles and forms. For more information, see www.acupuncture.com.

Many styles use stillness or simple body movements in conjunction with visualization. It is best to seek out guidance when learning to practice qi-gong techniques. Practitioners who perform qi-gong on a patient or teach others how to cultivate energy usually have worked many years on cultivating their own energy. Most are taught in an apprentice format, and schooling is not usually institutionalized. In China, retreat centers focus on this work. Qi-gong is also used in hospital settings, where it is both taught to and performed on patients. Research in this field is growing rapidly.

The benefits of qi-gong range from simple well-being to reversal of serious illnesses. The sensation of moving energy can be tangible and highly rewarding. One review of the medical benefits of qi-gong documents improvements in a wide variety of conditions, including hypertension, bone density (in men), reduced medication doses in stroke patients, improved weight gain and strength in patients with advanced cancers, and functional improvement in senile patients.[3]

13. What are the barriers to research in TCM?

TCM has been successfully practiced for more than 5000 years. Most of the clinical acupuncture research has been done in the United States since approximately the 1970s, when TCM was introduced. Much of the research previously done in China is empirical and case-based. Although the previous research was promising, no controls or scientific testing methods were used. Control groups were considered unethical because they deny treatment to those who may need it. It is a challenge to design clinical trials while preserving the diagnostic and treatment principles unique to the tradition of Chinese medicine. Some of the challenges in TCM research include creating believable placebos for acupuncture, doubling-blinding the practitioner to the unique one-on-one treatment plan designed for each patient, and heterogeneity of techniques and training of various practitioners.

Some successful methods include the use of previously proven treatments as a comparison. "Sham points" or non-acupoints are sometimes needled in lieu of a no-treatment placebo. Needling "nontreatment" points, however, introduces a confounding factor, because these points elicit some response of their own, although not as much as the true acupoints. Qi-gong studies are now gaining some popularity, and herbal research has also been noted, although acupuncture has received the most attention. *Acupuncture Efficacy* by Birch and Hammerschlag provides seventy valid studies focusing on chronic pain, emesis (nausea and vomiting), stroke, respiratory disease, and substance abuse.[4]

14. Discuss recent research studies in TCM.

Two good clinical studies have used moxibustion (see Chapter 12) for correction of breech presentation.[5,6] In a 1998 study, 260 healthy primagravidas with a breech presentation in their 33rd week of gestation were randomized to either moxibustion for up to 2 weeks or no intervention. Results showed that at 35 weeks the rate of cephalic presentation was 75% vs. 48% in the control group (p <. 0.001). Only one woman in the moxa group required external version compared with 24 in the control group.

Other studies[7,8] have shown that acupuncture and electroacupuncture are as effective as amitriptyline in the treatment of mental depression. The results indicate that acupuncture is a viable treatment option for depression, especially when antidepressive medication is contraindicated. No studies have yet compared acupuncture with newer agents.

15. How do I find a qualified practitioner of TCM?

Each state in the U.S. regulates acupuncture licensure independently. Most states recognize national certification by the National Certification Commission for Acupuncture and Oriental

Medicine (NCCAOM). Other states have self-governed licensing exams and regulatory boards (see www.acupuncture.com for listing). Oriental herbalists and bodyworkers are also certified by the NCCAOM, although certification usually is not required by law. Qi-gong practitioners are independently credited. Many instructors are proud of their lineage of instruction and style. In looking for a qualified practitioner, it is best to interview the teacher and ask for background information and references. Growing organizations provide information to the public (see www.qigonginstitute.org).

16. Are there any allopathic diagnoses that seem to respond well to TCM?

Many illnesses respond well to the application of TCM, which in the West often is viewed as an alternative when allopathic treatment fails, especially for medical problems that are more chronic in nature or elude easy treatment. In China and other parts of Asia, however, TCM is an established medical system often practiced side by side with the "newer" Western forms of medicine. Specifically for acupuncture, the National Institutes of Health[9] has listed conditions for which adequate studies have documented benefit (see Chapter 12).

The main goal of TCM is the prevention of illness. According to an old saying, "Do not wait until you are thirsty to begin to dig a well; do not wait until you are at war to make your arrows." The lifestyle practices of TCM are designed to keep a person healthy and to avoid the necessity of invasive methods.

17. What resources are available for additional information?

Websites
- www.nccaom.org
- www.acupuncture.com
- www.nccam.com
- www.qigonginstitute.org

Books
- Beinfeld H, Korngold E: Between Heaven and Earth. New York., Ballantine Books, 1991.
- Maciocia G: The Foundations of Chinese Medicine. New York, Churchill Livingstone, 1989.
- Tierra L: The Herbs of Life. Freedom, CA, Crossing Press, 1992.
- Ni M (translator): Huang Di Nei Jing (The Yellow Emperor's Classic of Chinese Medicine). Boston, Shambala Publications, 1995.
- Kaptchuk T: The Web That Has No Weaver. Chicago, Congdon & Weed, 1983.
- Reichstein G: Wood Becomes Water: Chinese Medicine in Everyday Life. New York, Kodansha America, 1998.

REFERENCES

1. Bensky D, Gamble A: Materia Medica. Seattle, WA, Eastland Press, 1993.
2. Huang WF, Wen KC, Hsiao ML: Adulteration by synthetic therapeutic substances of traditional Chinese medicines in Taiwan. J Clin Pharmacol 37:344–350, 1997.
3. Saucier KM: Medical applications of qigong. Altern Ther 2:40–46, 1996.
4. Birch S, Hammerschlag R: Acupuncture Efficacy. Tarrytown, NY, National Academy of Acupuncture and Oriental Medicine, 1996.
5. Cardini F, Weixin H: Moxibustion for correction of breech presentation: A randomized controlled trial. JAMA 280:1580–1584, 1998.
6. Cardini F, Marcolongo A: Moxibustion for correction of breech presentation: A clinical study with retrospective control. Am J Chin Med 21:133–138, 1993.
7. Huo H, Jia Y, Shan L: Electro-acupuncture vs. amitriptyline in the treatment of depressive states. J Trad Chin Med 5:308, 1985.
8. Tang X, Liu X, Luo H, et al: Clinical observation on needling extrachannel points in treating mental depression. J Trad Chin Med 14:14–18, 1994.
9. http://odp.od.nih.gov/consensus/cons/107/107_intro.htm.

12. ACUPUNCTURE

Julia Thie, L.Ac

1. What is the basic concept of acupuncture?

The basic concept of acupuncture is to foster health via the correction of imbalances of internal energy flow. The insertion of fine needles into specific points on the body elicits the production of various chemicals, which in turn contribute to a healing response. The acupuncture points are mostly located along pathways of concentrated bioelectric energy called qi. These pathways are called meridians or channels. Many of the meridians are named after and correspond to internal organs.

Qi is the energetic substance in all things. Although invisible, it is a tangible force when one is trained to perceive it. There are many kinds of qi. The type manipulated by acupuncturists is called yuan qi. Acupuncture moves this energy by techniques of ascending or descending, reinforcing, reducing, warming, and clearing.[1] The selection of technique is based on a Chinese medical diagnosis. The goal is to move qi in the appropriate direction to create the desired physical and emotional response.

2. What is the significance of meridians?

Meridians are often mistakenly conceptualized as nerves. They usually parallel major blood vessels and nerves, sometimes flowing with them and, in other areas, apart from them. There are twelve main and eight extra meridians, fifteen collaterals, and twelve divergent meridians. There is also a complex series of "submeridians," called luo vessels, that connect the organs to the meridians. Each main meridian, which is the focus of this basic overview, has an internal pathway as well as an external pathway. The figure to the right shows the gallbladder main meridian, with both internal (dotted lines) and external pathways (solid lines).

The meridians are used as a diagnostic tool by palpation, signs and symptoms associated within an area, and associated organ function. When points are needled, quite often a sensation traverses the meridian on which the point is located.[2] The concept of meridians gives an understanding of the flow of energy in the human body and its relationship to the environment as viewed from an Asian medical perspective.

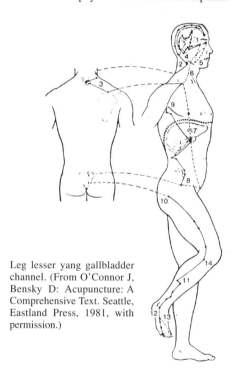

Leg lesser yang gallbladder channel. (From O'Connor J, Bensky D: Acupuncture: A Comprehensive Text. Seattle, Eastland Press, 1981, with permission.)

3. What types of needles are used? How?

In 1996, the Food and Drug Administration changed the status of the acupuncture needle from experimental device to medical device. Most acupuncturists use disposable needles rather than resterilize used needles. The solid filiform needles are made mostly from stainless steel, although some practitioners prefer gold or silver needles for certain conditions; 4,000 years ago they were made of stone.

The length of filiform needles varies from 5 to 60 mm. Other types include intradermal and cutaneous needles and lancets. Filiform needles are inserted perpendicularly, obliquely, or horizontally, depending on the underlying structures and the technique used for a particular response. Needles are usually retained for 20–60 minutes. In some cases, the needles are immediately removed; in other cases, auricular tacks are applied superficially to acupoints on the outer ears and are retained for up to 2 days.

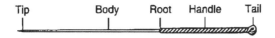

The structure of hte filiform needle. (From Qiu ML: Chinese acupuncture and moxibustion. Edinburgh, Churchill Livingstone, 1995, p 186, with permission.)

4. Does acupuncture hurt?

The style of acupuncture determines the amount of discomfort in needling. Korean style acupuncture is quite aggressive, whereas the Japanese style penetrates more superficially and is not as intense. The form most commonly used in the United States is a modified Chinese style that is relatively painless, mainly because Americans do not comply well with painful methods. The most commonly used needles are very sharp and very thin. They break through the skin quickly without much sensation. Some practitioners use guide tubes to assist insertion.

A sensation that most practitioners will try to elicit is called "da qi", or the arrival of qi. It is felt after the needle is inserted and the qi at the point is stimulated. It is not pain; usually it is described as a surge or pressure around the area of the point or traversing along the meridian. Once the needles are inserted, the patient usually has a sensation of relaxation and well-being. Patients may even fall asleep.

5. Describe the neurologic response to needle insertion.

Neurologic response to acupuncture needle insertion is believed to be a pain-blocking mechanism. According to the gate theory, acupuncture stimulates A-beta fast-twitch nerve fibers, blocking the slower A-delta fibers and thus inhibiting the substantia gelatinosa in the spine. This process blocks the pain signal to the brain[3,4] and is, in a sense, a volume control for pain signals. Acetylcholine concentration in the brain is increased in animals after 20-minute retention of needles.[5]

Acupuncture is believed to stimulate endogenous production of serotonin and opiates. Experimental blockage of serotonin synthesis reduces effectiveness of acupuncture, whereas synthesis of serotonin potentiates its effect.[6] Use of the morphine antagonist naloxone blocks the increased pain threshold obtained by acupuncture, implying the presence of at least two hormonally induced systems.[7] In animal studies, nonresponders to acupuncture tend also to be nonresponders to morphine.[8]

6. Describe the systemic response to needle insertion.

Acupuncture not only decreases pain but also can play a role in immune enhancement and many other regulating functions[9]:

- Lysis of foreign bacteria and cells
- Increased vascular permeability
- Smooth muscle contraction
- Mast cell degranulation
- Oponisation of bacteria (labeling as foreign),
- Stimulation of phagocytic activity of immune cells
- Chemotaxis (attracting immune cells to site of injury)
- Enhanced coagulation to prevent severe blood loss in the presence of vascular damage

7. Is acupuncture safe?

Blood contamination from acupuncture needles is very unlikely. All licensed acupuncturists must successfully perform the clean needle technique established by national acupuncture certifying boards and based on standards developed by the Occupational Safety and Health Administration and Centers for Disease Control and Prevention. In the hands of a trained practitioner, acupuncture has shown evidence of being safe.[10] The risks involved are bruising, fainting, vomiting, and local bleeding from acupuncture sites. More serious risks include nerve damage and pneumothorax. The incidence of these events is significantly low,[11] and acupuncture is considered one of the safer forms of medical intervention.[12]

8. What recent scientific studies support the use of acupuncture?

Two recent studies,[13,14] using magnetic resonance readings, demonstrate the effect of laser acupuncture on brain function. A specific point (urinary bladder 67) on the lateral side of the fifth toe, which is used classically to improve vision, was stimulated. The unactivated laser was used as the placebo. In allopathic medicine, there is obviously no correlation between vision, the bladder, and the fifth toe, but the results showed a significant difference between the two groups in regard to activation of the corresponding brain visual cortex. These studies help to confirm some of the "unexplainable" energetic phenomena that underlie the principles of acupuncture.

9. How are acupuncture points chosen?

Chapter 11 gives a more detailed explanation of this complicated question. A treatment plan, which includes point selection, is based on the parameters of the diagnosis. A traditional Chinese medicine diagnosis is not a disease per se but a description of a pattern. For example, if the pattern of a patient is generally "excessive heat," symptoms may include high fever, loud voice, and odorous secretions. Points are chosen that clear the excess from either the affected system or the "level" at which the excess is located. Depending on signs and symptoms, the points are chosen to reduce the heat in the body, possibly by diaphoresing, stimulating bowel movement or urination, or decreasing an inflammatory response. This view of point selection is more clinical. Bear in mind that many successful treatment plans are selected for reasons that do not conform to a scientific model but instead reflect a long history of traditional clinical and esoteric practices.

10. What other therapies are used with acupuncture?

Electroacupuncture is a modern technique of running a low-voltage electric current though needles placed in the points singly or in a circuit. It strengthens and lengthens the acupuncture response. Because of its enhanced effect, it is not appropriate in all cases.

Moxibustion is a warming technique that applies heat by burning certain herbal preparations on acupuncture points. It can be applied directly on the skin, at the end of a needle, or as a stick burned close to the skin. The most common moxa substance is *Artemesia vulgaris* (mugwort). The herb is dried and the fibrous material removed. It is used loosely or rolled into a cigar-shaped stick. When an open flame is not applicable, a spray form of the moxa extract is used in conjunction with a heat lamp.

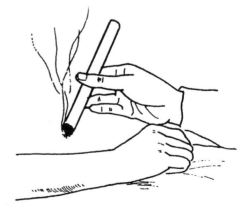

Moxibustion with cigar-shaped stick. (From Xinnong C: Chinese Acupuncture and Moxibustion. Beijing, Foreign Language Press, 1993, with permission.)

Cupping. A specially made glass cup is attached by suction to the skin surface. A flame is placed in the cup and quickly removed, creating a vacuum necessary to attach it to the skin. This method is used mostly in cases of pain and swelling and respiratory disorders. Cupping leaves a mark for a day or two and should not be misinterpreted as an injury. This technique increases blood flow to an area. In the language of traditional Chinese medicine, cupping releases heat from the muscle layer out to the surface.

11. What types of ailments does acupuncture treat?

Traditionally, acupuncture does not treat disease but rather patterns of disharmony. These patterns often correspond to known disease patterns. Below is a list of conditions for which acupuncture may be used, according to the World Health Organization:

Digestive disorders
Abdominal pain
Constipation
Diarrhea
Hyperactivity
Indigestion

Emotional disorders
Anxiety
Depression
Insomnia
Nervousness
Neurosis

Eye, ear, and oral disorders
Cataracts
Gingivitis
Poor vision
Tinnitus
Toothache

Gynecologic disorders
Infertility
Menopausal syndrome
Premenstrual syndrome

Musculoskeletal disorders
Arthritis
Back pain
Muscle cramping
Pain/weakness
Neck pain
Sciatica

Neurologic disorders
Headaches
Migraines
Bladder dysfunction
Parkinson's disease
Postoperative pain
Stroke

Respiratory disorders
Asthma
Bronchitis
Common cold
Sinusitis
Smoking cessation
Tonsillitis

Miscellaneous disorders

Addiction control
Athletic performance
Blood pressure regulation

Chronic fatigue
Immune system tonification
Stress reduction

In addition, a consensus panel formed in 1997 by the National Institutes of Health[15] concluded that many conditions are appropriate for acupuncture therapy. The complete report is available at http://odp.od.nih.gov/consensus/cons/107/107_intro.htm.

12. How many treatments are necessary to obtain the desired results?

The old saying, "Long time cause, long time cure", usually rings true. It takes longer to see lasting results for a chronic degenerative disorder than for an acute symptom. An acute symptom may need only 2–4 treatments. For chronic cases, approximately 12 visits within 8–10 weeks is a general estimate. Some patients may need a longer course of treatment. Success also hinges on the patient's compliance with suggested lifestyle and dietary changes. Regular visits about once per month may be used as a preventative measure and are suggested to decrease stress and boost immune function.

13. What are the licensing or certification requirements for practicing acupuncture?

- A licensed acupuncturist (L.Ac.) holds a license in one or more states.
- A person certified by the National Certification Commission for Acupuncture and Oriental Medicine (NCCAOM) is called a diplomate of acupuncture (Dipl.Ac.).
- An oriental medicine doctor (O.M.D.) has obtained advanced training in acupuncture.

Schools of oriental medicine are accredited by the Accreditation Commission for Acupuncture and Oriental Medicine (ACAOM). Most commonly they are based in traditional Chinese medicine. Most schools require a minimum of an associate's degree for admission and offer a 3- to 4-year program. On completion of the program, the student becomes a master of traditional oriental medicine. Some programs offer a master's degree.

Each state independently regulates acupuncture licensure. Most states recognize national certification by the NCCAOM (www.nccaom.org). Other states have self-governed licensing exams and regulatory boards (see www.acupuncture.com for listings). Medical doctors are also legally eligible to perform acupuncture, although acupuncture alone is usually not the extent of training in traditional Chinese medicine. It is suggested that they be certified by the Academy of Medical Acupuncture in Los Angeles (www.medicalacupuncture.org.).

Addiction withdrawal treatment may be performed by an acupuncture detox specialist (ADS), who learn a specific protocol separate from the practice of oriental medicine. Five specific points are pierced bilaterally in each ear for 45 minutes/day during active treatment. ADSs are certified by the National Acupuncture Detox Association (NADA) and practice in the context of a substance abuse treatment program (www.acudetox.com).

14. What resources are available for additional information?

Websites

- www.acupuncture.com
- www.nccam.com

Organizations

- Accreditation Commission for Acupuncture and Oriental Medicine, Silver Springs, MD
- National Acupuncture Foundation, Washington, DC
- Society for Acupuncture Research, Bethesda MD

Books

- Birch S, Hammerschlag R: Acupuncture Efficacy. New York, National Academy of Acupuncture and Oriental Medicine, 1996 (a helpful compendium of controlled studies in acupuncture, categorized by condition).
- Beinfeld H, Korngold K: Between Heaven and Earth. New York Balantine Books, 1991 (excellent, readable guide with good discussion of philosophy of traditional Chinese medicine).
- Maciocia G: The Foundations of Chinese Medicine. New York, Churchill Livingstone, 1989 (textbook with in-depth explanations of theory, pathology, diagnosis, and point functions).
- Kapchuck T: The Web That Has No Weaver. Congdon & Weed, Chicago, 1983 (classic book that was the first to break down barriers to understanding the basics of traditional Chinese medicine fort Western readers).
- Reichstein G: Wood Becomes Water: Chinese Medicine in Everyday Life. New York, Kodansha America, 1998 (good, easy-to-read overview, well-illustrated with excellent clinical examples for the beginner).

REFERENCES

1. Xinnong C: Chinese Acupuncture and Moxibustion. Beijing, Foreign Language Press, 1993.
2. Lazorthes Y: Acupuncture meridians and radiotracers. Pain 40:109–112, 1990.
3. Melzack R, Wall P: Science 150:971–979, 1965.
4. Melzack R, Dennis P: Psychology of Pain. New York, Raven Press,1978.
5. Developments in Acupuncture Research. Beijing, TCM Research Institute, 1981.
6. Han JS, Terenius L: Neurochemical basis of acupuncture analgesia. Annu Rev Pharmacol Toxicol 22: 193–220, 1982
7. Cheng R, Pomeranz B: Pain relieving mechanisms of acupuncture. Life Sci 25:1957–1962, 1979.
8. Han JS: Neurochemical Basis of Pain Relief by Acupuncture. Beijing, Beijing Medical University, 1988.
9. Kendall DE: A scientific model for acupuncture. Am J Acup 17:257–258, 1989.
10. Rampes H, James R: Complications of acupuncture. Acup Med 345:1576, 1995.
11. White AR, Hayoe S, Ernst E: Survey of adverse events following acupuncture. Acup Med 15:67–70, 1997.
12. McPherson J, et al: The York acupuncture safety study: Prospective survey of 34,000 treatments by traditional acupuncturists. Br Med J 323:485–486, 2001.
13. Cho ZH, et al: New findings of the correlation between acupoints and corresponding brain cortices using functionl MRI. Proc Natl Acad Sci USA 95:2670–2673, 1998.
14. Golaszewski S, et al: Effects of laser acupuncture on activation within the visual cortex: A functional MRI study. Available at http://www.academicpress.com/www/journal/hbm2001/11314.html. Accessed 7/16/01.
15. NIH Consensus statement on acupuncture. JAMA 280:1518–1524, 1998.

13. HOMEOPATHY

Malcolm Riley, B.D.S.

1. Define homeopathy.

Homeopathy is a therapeutic modality based on the principle of similars. The word *homeopathy* comes from the Greek words *homoios*, meaning similar or like, and *pathos*, meaning suffering. Therapeutically, homeopaths use remedies that are dilute preparations of many different substances.

2. Describe the origin of homeopathy.

Samuel Hahnemann, M.D. (1755–1843), a distinguished German physician, discovered the principles of homeopathy in the second half of the 18th century. Unhappy with the conventional treatments of his time, which included blood-letting and purging, he actively sought a more humane system of medicine. Homeopathy is now practiced all over the world, particularly in Germany, France, England, and India.

3. What is meant by the the principle of similars?

The principle of similars can be explained by the phrase, "like cures like." Disease can be treated with substances that, when given to healthy persons, elicit the *same* symptoms as the disease. The substances do not cause the disease but trigger a response in the body that can mimic the symptoms. An example of similars in conventional medicine is vaccinations, which use minute quantities of pathogens to induce a healing reaction in the body. The result of vaccination, an antibody response, is different, however, from the response to a homeopathic remedy.

An example of the principle of similars in homeopathy is the use of coffea cruda (homeopathically prepared coffee). The symptoms produced by drinking coffee can include restlessness, sleeplessness, and an overactive mind. Homeopathic coffea may be prescribed to treat conditions such as sleeplessness due to an overactive mind and/or anxiety accompanied by restlessness, even though the symptoms may not be caused by coffee.

4. How was the principle of similars discovered?

Hahnemann was translating Cullen's *Materia Medica* from English into German and came across a treatment for swamp fever using cinchona bark (quinine). Cullen, a professor at the University of Edinburgh, postulated that the effect was due to the astringent action on the stomach. Hahnemann thought this an unlikely explanation and, in the true manner of a pioneer, decided to take quinine himself to observe its action.

To Hahnemann's surprise, as he took the quinine he began to experience the exact symptoms of swamp fever, except for the pyrexia. He had discovered a strange phenomenon—a substance used to treat an illness was also capable of causing the symptoms of the same disease. Hahnemann spent the remainder of his life identifying more **similia** (i.e., more substances that produced the same symptoms as diseases).

5. What is the homeopathic *Materia Medica*?

As Hahnemann and his followers took the various substances, the thousands of symptoms that they caused were systematically recorded in a text called the *Homeopathic Materia Medica*. This is the basic tool from which homeopaths prescribe. Today many materia medica exist, some still in 18th and 19th century language, although some have been brought up to date with modern terminology.

6. What is a homeopathic remedy?

Homeopaths refer to the substances that they use as "remedies" rather than medicines or drugs to separate the more gentle homeopathic remedies from the toxic drugs that were used at the time and also to stress the different philosophical basis of homeopathy. Virtually anything can be prepared homeopathically. The three main groups are animal, vegetable, and mineral. Remedies also have been prepared from x-rays and other forms of radiation. A special group of remedies prepared from diseased tissue are called **nosodes**.

7. How is a homeopathic remedy prepared?

Hahnemann was concerned with the toxicity of many of the substances and experimented with finding the minimal dose to get a healing effect. He began by diluting the remedies and shaking them vigorously between dilutions. The folk tale is that Hahnemann made house calls and used a wooden cart to transport his remedies. The cart used to vibrate the remedies as it traveled over the rough streets, and Hahnemann thought that this vibration explained why patients treated as the end of the day did better than those treated earlier in the day.

Dilution and shaking were standardized to the current process and are termed **serial dilution and succusion** (vigorous shaking). Dilutions of 1:10 (decimal) or 1:100 (centesimal) are the most commonly used. The combination of the dilution and the number of times that dilution and succusion are repeated determine the potency of the remedy. For example 6x (6d in German products) is a remedy that has been diluted 1:10 six times. 30c refers to the potency of a remedy that has been serially diluted 1:100 thirty times.

8. If these substances are so dilute, how can they work?

There is no accepted scientific answer. Homeopathic remedies greater than 24x or 12c contain virtually none of the original substance; thus, conventional physics and chemistry cannot explain their action.

Homeopathic principles are completely counterintuitive to allopathic medicine, yet studies show effects greater than placebo.[1] The facts that infinitesimal amounts of substance are used as therapy and that the strength of a homeopathic remedy is inversely proportional to its physical amount are ludicrous to the thinker rooted in scientific reason. Because it does no make sense on a molecular basis, there must be another explanation. Homeopathy is considered an energy-based therapeutic system, and there is yet much to be discovered about the mechanisms of homeopathic treatments in the human body.

Considerable research is being done into the structure of water and how the substance and its subsequent dilution and succusion may be affected. Pischinger postulates that homeopathy may act through regulation of connective tissue.[2] Shui-Yin Lo[3] recently identified rigid stable structures in water called I_E structures; I_E stands for ice formed under an electric field. These structures appear to be highly stable and offer at least a mechanism for water to hold "memory" of a homeopathic remedy.

9. What forms of homeopathic remedies are available?

The most common form is the compressed lactose tablet, but sucrose pills and pillules, alcohol-based drops, injectable saline ampules, and topical preparations are available.

10. Describe the typical history taken by a homeopathic practitioner.

The homeopathic approach has much in common with the conventional approach: a good history of the chief complaint and the associated symptoms are recorded. The homeopathic history varies in the scope and focus of the questions. A homeopath wants to know all about the patient, not just the symptoms of disease. Information as specific as fear of dogs, feeling cold in the afternoon, nasal-sounding voice, and food preferences may be important during a homeopathic history. The intent is to find the similium—that is, the remedy that matches as close as possible to the patient, not to his or her disease(s). This is the basis for the individualized remedy and a source of considerable confusion to conventional physicians.

It is highly probable that patients presenting with the same diagnosis—for example, rheumatoid arthritis—will be given different remedies because the homeopath prescribes for the patient, not the disease. This principle is seen clearly in traditional Chinese medicine and ayurveda, which also individualize treatments based on the energetics of the patient (see Chapters 10 and 11).

11. Describe the different schools of homeopathic practice.

The various schools of homeopathic practice are based on the same principles of the similium and the minimal effective dose. In the U.S. the most prevalent school is **classic homeopathy**, which emphasizes finding a single best remedy for all symptoms with which a patient presents. On the other hand, European homeopaths (particularly French and German) may use multiple homeopathic remedies, each aimed at treating specific conditions or illnesses.

12. How is the homeopathic remedy selected?

The patient's symptoms are matched to a remedy that has the same characteristics as recorded in the *Materia Medica*. There are many thousands of remedies, and the characteristics of many are several pages long; memorizing all of them is almost impossible.

The traditional way to aid the practitioner in the selection of remedies is the process of reporatization. A **reporatory** is a list of all symptoms and characteristics that are associated with a particular remedy. For example, symptoms of vertigo may point to a whole list of possible homeopathic remedies (e.g., cocculus, gelsemium, sepia), each with defining characteristics (e.g., vertigo when riding, vertigo starting from the occiput, vertigo with rolling sensation). Other symptoms from the patient, such as craving for sweets, emotional factors, and side of body most affected, also are reporatized. Each time a remedy comes up, it is assigned a value; after all of the symptoms are reporatized, usually there are a few remedies with a high score. Each of these remedies is then compared with the patient's symptom picture and the closest match is the correct remedy. This process is time-consuming and often computerized.

13. How are the remedies prescribed?

There is no clear agreement. A **constitutional homeopath** usually prescribes a single remedy selected to treat the majority of a patient's symptoms and waits for up to 2 or 3 months to assess the action of the remedy before selecting another. European homeopaths often use a mixture of remedies; many of these mixtures are available in health food stores in the U.S.

Homeopathic remedies for acute conditions are usually prescribed only for symptoms of the acute complaint rather than for the symptoms of the whole patient. Arnica for trauma and bruises, hypericum for nerve pain, and oscillococcinum for flu are common examples.

14. Describe the doses, frequency, and duration of homeopathic treatment.

Lower potencies (6x, 12c) are often repeated 3–4 times/day, whereas middle potencies (30c) may be given once a day and higher potencies (200c and above) usually are given as a single, one-time dose. Potency and frequency vary considerably among homeopathic practitioners. In fact, the different groups often refer to each other as high or low prescribers.

One key and rather unusual aspect of homeopathic prescribing is that the remedy is given until some improvement is noted; then it is stopped. It is prescribed again only if the improvement does not continue. The rationale is that homeopathy stimulates the healing process; once the healing has begun, the body should then be left to heal itself.

15. What are the side effects and complications of homeopathic treatment?

There are two areas of concern with homeopathic remedies: direct and indirect effects. **Direct effects** are rare, and the few reported cases involved misuse of remedies. For example, low potencies still contain small amounts of the original substance. There was one report of a child taking an overdose of homeopathic mercury.[4]

Indirect effects are more insidious and result mainly from the withholding of appropriate medical care while homeopathic remedies are taken. Usually they are associated with self-prescribing, but there have been instances of physician homeopaths using only homeopathic medicine when conventional treatment was indicated.

16. What is homeopathic aggravation?

Homeopathic aggravation is often misinterpreted as a side effect of treatment. Aggravation is the temporary worsening of symptoms, and to a homeopath it is a good sign, indicating that the patient's healing ability is intact and has been stimulated by the remedy. Aggravation occasionally causes some alarm, and if patients seeing a homeopath report worsening of symptoms, check with the homeopath. It can be difficult to distinguish between an aggravation and actual worsening of the symptoms. An aggravation is identified as an initial worsening, which gradually begins to improve; in contrast, a progression of disease continues to worsen with no improvement.

17. What special precautions are appropriate with homeopathic remedies?
Electromagnetic radiation and volatile oils such as camphor and mint may interfere with the action of homeopathic remedies. Remedies should be kept away from airport security scanners, computers, and other electrical equipment. Coffee and garlic should be avoided during homeopathic treatment and the remedies should be taken at least 15 minutes before or after food or teeth cleaning.

18. What evidence indicates that homeopathy works?
Considerable use of homeopathy by veterinarians probably eliminates the question of placebo response. Merck[5] successfully used homeopathy in the treatment of acute mastitis in cattle. In vitro studies by Belon[6] demonstrated that highly diluted doses of histamine inhibit degranulation in basophils.

Over 100 double-blinded studies have evaluated the use of homeopathy in humans. A Cochrane review concluded that the homeopathic remedy oscillococcinum does not prevent flu, but taking it once the flu has developed probably can shorten the illness.[7] Two recent meta-analyses[8,9] concluded that homeopathy was more effective than placebo, but both commented on the suboptimal methodology of many of the trials.

Despite the lack of definitive scientific data, clinical success is often reported by patients empirically. Because substances are so dilute, risk is minimal when high-quality remedies are used; thus, the benefit-to-risk ratio of homeopathic treatment usually remains quite high.

19. For which conditions has homeopathy been proved effective?
The homeopathic literature has numerous case studies of the success of individual homeopathic treatments. Historically, homeopathy was successful in the cholera epidemics in Europe in the 18th century. In the conventional literature, two studies stand out. In a study of allergic bronchial asthma, lung function parameters improved in 77% of patients treated with homeopathics compared with 36% taking placebo.[10] In another trial, acutely ill Nicaraguan children receiving a homeopathic remedy had significantly shorter duration of diarrhea compared with their placebo counterparts.[11] Otitis media and rheumatoid arthritis also have responded to homeopathic treatment.

Another study showed that a topical homeopathic gel (containing *Symphytum officinale, Rhus toxicodendron,* and *Ledum palustre*) was as effective as topical piroxicam gel in the reduction of pain in patients with osteoarthritis of the knee.[12] More studies need to be done to evaluate the efficacy of homeopathic treatments.

20. What is the legal status of the practice of homeopathy in the U.S.?
It is legal for medical doctors to practice homeopathy anywhere in the U.S. At present, three states—Connecticut, Nevada, and Arizona—have homeopathic medical boards that license medical doctors who practice homeopathy. Homeopathy also is practiced by other licensed practitioners, such as dentists, podiatrists, veterinarians, naturopaths, chiropractors, acupuncturists, physician assistants, nurse practitioners, and nurses, depending on scope of practice.

Numerous training programs and correspondence courses in homeopathy are offered for lay practitioners. These courses offer certification, although certification does not necessarily grant licensure to practice. Lay homeopaths are not allowed to diagnose or treat disease, but conventional diagnosis is not necessary for the practice of classic homeopathy.

21. What does homeopathy not treat?
Homeopathy works better with functional conditions (e.g., headache, allergies, psychological complaints) and is generally less successful with overt pathology (e.g., diabetes, stroke). Homeopathic remedies, however, often relieve the severity of overt illnesses. For example, the deformities of

rheumatoid arthritis are unlikely to be helped by homeopathy, but the pain and limitation of movement can be improved.

22. Why do homeopaths prefer that their patients not take other medications?

Homeopaths want to see the patient's exact symptom picture, which often is obscured by concomitant medication use. This preference is obviously problematic with illnesses that require medication, such as diabetes and uncontrolled hypertension. In such instances, the homeopath attempts to obtain a history of symptoms before the medication was begun. Homeopaths do not withhold essential medication.

23. How are homeopaths credentialed?

Some states license only M.D.s or lay practitioners working with M.D.s, whereas other states have no licensing requirements. Because credentialing for homeopathy varies widely by state, it is advisable to contact each state board directly. Other credentialing bodies include:
- American Board of Homeotherapeutics, which certifies M.D.s and D.O.s and awards them a D.Ht. (http://www.homeopathyusa.org/home/).
- Council for Homeopathic Certification, which provides certification to licensed and unlicensed practitioners (http://www.homeopathicdirectory.com/old/).
- North America Society of Homeopaths (http://www.homeopathy.org/).

24. Where do I find further information about homeopathy?

Homeopathic Education Services (http://www.homeopathic.com/) has a considerable number of books, remedies, and other information about homeopathy. For an interesting narrative account of homeopathy, read the first few chapters in *Health and Healing* by Andrew Weil, M.D. Other resources:
- Dana Ullman: *Consumer's Guide to Homeopathy: The Definitive Resource for Understanding Homeopathic Medicine and Making It Work for You.* New York, Jeremy P. Tarcher/Putnam, 1996.
- Thomas Kruzel: *Homeopathic Emergency Guide: A Quick Reference Handbook to Effective Homeopathic Care.* Berkeley, CA, North Atlantic Books, 1992.

REFERENCES

1. Linde K, Clausius N, Ramimez G, et al: Are the clinical effects of homeopathy placebo effects? A meta-analysis of placebo-controlled trials. Lancet 350:834–843, 1997.
2. Pischinger A: Matrix and Matrix Regulation: Basis for a Holistic Theory in Medicine. Haug Verlag, Heidelberg, 1991.
3. Shui-Yin L: Physical properties of water with I_E structures. Mod Phys Lett 10:921–930, 1996.
4. Montoya-Cabrera M, Rubio-Rodriguez A, Velazquez-Gonzalez S, et al: Mercury poisoning caused by a homeopathic drug. Gac Med Mex 127:267–270, 1991.
5. Merck C, Sonnenwald C, Rollwage B, Berl H: The administration of homeopathic drugs for the treatment of acute mastitis in cattle. Munch Tierarztl Wochenschr 102:266–272, 1989.
6. Belon P, Cumps J, Ennis M, et al: Inhibition of human basophil degranulation by successive histamine dilutions: Results of a European multi-centre trial. Inflamm Res 48(Suppl 1):S17–S18, 1999.
7. Vickers AJ, Smith C: Homoeopathic oscillococcinum for preventing and treating influenza and influenza-like syndromes. Cochrane Database Syst Rev 2001.
8. Cucherat M, Haugh MC, Gooch M, Boissel JP, for the Homeopathic Medicines Research Advisory Group: Evidence of clinical efficacy of homeopathy: A meta-analysis of clinical trials. Eur J Clin Pharmacol 56:27–33, 2000
9. Linde K, Melchart D, Altern J: Randomized controlled trials of individualized homeopathy: A state-of-the-art review. Complement Med 4:371–388, 1998.
10. Reilly D, Taylor MA, Beattie NG, et al: Is evidence for homeopathy reproducible? Lancet 344:1601–1066, 1994.
11. Jacobs J, Jimenez LM, Gloyd SS, et al: Treatment of acute childhood diarrhea with homeopathic medicine: A randomized clinical trial in Nicaragua. Pediatrics 93:719–725, 1994.
12. Van Haselen RA, Fisher PAG: A randomized controlled trial comparing topical piroxicam gel with a homeopathic get in osteoarthiritis of the knee. Rheumatology 39:714–719, 2000.

14. ALLOPATHIC MEDICINE

Reid Blackwelder, M.D.

1. Define allopathic medicine.

The origin of the term *allopathic* is one of the most unusual as well as ironic in the history of Western medicine. Samuel Hahnemann, M.D., a renowned German physician of the eighteenth century, is credited with coining the term. Hahnemann became dissatisfied with the orthodox medicine of his day, in which the most common treatments were aggressive bleeding and purging. He pursued another approach to medicine that he called the law of similars, which states that "like cures like." He called this practice "homeopathy," which in Greek means "like the disease." Hahnemann also coined the term *allopathy,* which in Greek means"other than the disease," referring to the heroic practices of the day that, in his opinion, had no logical relationship to symptoms.[1] Thus, the term that we routinely use to describe our system of medicine was created by a doctor dissatisfied with its practice.

Other commonly used terms include Western medicine, biomedicine, conventional medicine, and traditional medicine. The last term is an interesting word choice. According to the World Health Organization, 80% of the world population seeks health care from "traditional" and cultural healers in systems that are not allopathic medicine. By this definition, one may question what is truly traditional.

2. Discuss the roots of allopathic medicine.

Hippocrates is often called the father of modern medicine, and allopathic physicians routinely graduate from medical school with some version of the Hippocratic oath. The contributions of Galen to anatomy, Harvey to the understanding of circulatory medicine, and William Osler are frequently mentioned. Louis Pasteur (1822–1895) was also a seminal figure in allopathic medicine. His support of the germ theory created a powerful foundation for our approach to the practice of medicine. In his perspective, the environment was hostile; bacteria invaded the body and caused disease. The role of physicians was to utilize all medicines to kill bacteria. The body had a limited influence in this process. This reductionist perspective forms the basis of western biomedicine.

Of interest, allopathic medical training does not emphasize much of its history. Key points in how medicine redirected itself from other healing traditions are not explored. In particular, missteps of Western medicine are rarely discussed. We do not often remember that modern physicians routinely recommended radiation treatment of children's thymus glands, gave vaccines with toxic mercury loads to newborns, and almost excluded osteopathic physicians from specialty membership. Most allopathic physicians are not aware of the relationships to other healing systems, such as homeopathy, chiropractic, and midwifery. Allopathic history is full of powerful and disturbing examples of antagonism toward these groups, as outlined by John Robbins in *Reclaiming Our Health: Exploding the Medical Myth and Embracing the Source of True Healing.*[2]

3. How is allopathic medicine different in other cultures?

Allopathic medicine is practiced all over the world. Medical training in different specialties is in fact quite similar, regardless of the culture involved. How allopathic medicine is practiced, however, differs dramatically from place to place. As Lynn Payer states in *Medicine and Culture*[3]:

> Some of the most common prescribed drugs in France, drugs to dilate the cerebral blood vessels, are considered ineffective in England and America; an obligatory immunization against tuberculosis in France, BCG, is almost impossible to obtain in the United States. German doctors prescribe from six to seven times the amount of digitalis-like drugs as their colleagues in France and England, but they prescribe fewer antibiotics. . . . French people have seven times the chance of getting drugs in suppository form as do Americans. In the late 1960s American surgery rates were twice those in of England; and the intervening years have seen this surgery gap widen, not close.

These differences result from the prevailing culture of medicine rather than any difference in competence or training. Take, for example, the differences in allopathic medicine in four scientific Western cultures. A patient with vague but mild symptoms of malaise may be diagnosed with a viral illness in the U.S., "liver crisis" in France, hertzinsufficie (low blood pressure) in Germany, and "catching a chill" in England. Patients with the same objective findings received a different diagnosis in different allopathic settings, depending on the cultural view of illness. Cultural context certainly colors how we practice medicine.

4. How did the Flexner report affect allopathic medicine?

The Flexner report is discussed elsewhere in this book, but its impact warrants further review. Abraham Flexner was an instrumental figure in the dramatic change that occurred in the training of American medicine in the early 1900s. Previously a number of different healing systems existed, some familiar and some not: schools of homeopathy, osteopathy, and Thomsonian herbalism; medical schools for minorities and women; and chiropractic schools. Unfortunately, much of the education available in most of these systems was not standardized. Flexner was hired to investigate and report on the state of medical education to help philanthropists determine the best areas in which to invest.

The fledgling American Medical Association was also invested in the outcome of this study. The recommendations of the report had far-reaching consequences. Ultimately, most of the other healing systems and their training programs were closed, and select allopathic schools, particularly in larger cities, were supported politically as well as practically with large financial grants. Unfortunately, the distinctions of which schools were worthy were not based on outcomes measurement of the different healing systems or approaches. The ultimate decisions were much more political.

Certainly the Flexner report had many positive outcomes. Many practitioners of all kinds of medicine were questionable at best. The American people deserved more consistent training as well as care. Moreover, the rapidly growing areas of science and technology could be more easily evaluated and implemented in a standardized system.

5. What is the basis of the national discussion about generalist vs. specialist physicians?

This question relates to general information about the physician workforce. After the Flexner report, a standard medical education and training process were created. A physician had to complete medical school and one year of postgraduate training, called an internship, before practicing medicine freely. In early 1900s most graduates of medical schools became general practitioners, because little formal specialty training was available. As the basic sciences exploded with new information and new technology became available, the trend toward mastering a more narrowed field of medicine increased. Accordingly, specialties and subspecialties began to formalize their training. Today almost all physicians practicing allopathic medicine complete additional training after internship, called a residency.

Residency matching data (www.NRMP.org) reveal that in 2001 15% of positions were in family medicine, 10.5% in pediatrics, and 23% in internal medicine. Historically, generalists and family physicians are more likely than subspecialists to practice in rural or underserved areas. The needs of underserved parts of the country or populations play a key role in the political discussions of how doctors are trained and where they should practice.

6. Describe the strengths of allopathic medicine.

The science and technology revolution, development of molecular pharmacology, imaging techniques, and standardization of medical care have contributed to making biomedicine a highly appropriate and successful approach to acute illness and trauma. Above all, allopathic medicine is a tremendous antidisease system. In addition, surgical techniques have improved so that almost miraculous treatments and approaches have become routine and their risks have decreased. Recent advances in medical management have led to greatly improved outcomes for such acute and life-threatening problems as heart attacks and strokes. Trauma care, transplant procedures, genetic research, and artificial limbs and organs are highlights of allopathic medicine.

In addition, medicine is beginning to look at its critical thinking processes. More and more emphasis is being placed on making decisions based on outcomes. This approach will dramatically alter what we consider medical standards of care. For example, placement of a Swan-Ganz catheter was long believed to be a critical step in managing patients in the intensive care unit, whereas recent studies have shown that it actually causes more harm than benefit. This procedure is now used with much less frequency. Similar evaluations are placing emphasis on preventive services and screening tests. The U.S. Preventive Health Services Task Force is doing groundbreaking work to explore the evidence supporting many of the diagnostic and treatment approaches that have long been considered standards of care. All in all, allopathic medicine is working to improve how it is practiced in many ways.

7. What areas are not well addressed by allopathic medicine?

The benefits of allopathic medicine are often unavailable or unaffordable to many people in the U.S. In 1999, 15.5% of the population was uninsured and unable to obtain diagnostic or therapeutic technologies and medications.[4] Medicare, developed in 1965 to secure the health coverage for retirees, does not cover prescription drugs, preventive services, or long-term care for the elderly. This problem will continue to grow as the baby boomers reach retirement age. The average person over age 65 spends 2% of his or her income on health care, and 79% of people over age 65 have incomes less than $25,000.[5] Despite the glut of physicians in many urban centers, other areas of the country continue to be underserved. Even for patients with insurance, some doctors and practices limit the number of patients with government-supported health insurance (Medicaid and state agencies), thus creating further access barriers. Not surprisingly, many uninsured and underinsured populations have poorer health outcomes.

As one examines these concerns and remembers the legacy of Pasteur, allopathic medicine does not seem to fit the criteria for a "health care" system. It has a strong focus on disease diagnosis and management but lacks training in health, healing, and optimizing wellness. Although new therapies continue to be developed, the prevalence of chronic illnesses such as diabetes, hypertension, obesity, and autoimmune diseases remains essentially unchanged—or even higher than before.

8. How does allopathic medicine address preventive medicine?

Physicians routinely state that diet, exercise, and lifestyle choices are important in managing medical problems; medical students, however, are not trained to provide in-depth dietary or exercise counseling and, once in practice, are given neither time nor reimbursement to do so. In fact, health maintenance visits or preventive services may be restricted by insurance companies. Medicare, for example, allows only one "well" visit per year.

More and more studies support the critical roles of diet, exercise, and lifestyle in supporting health and fighting illness. Studies such as the Life Style Heart Trial[6] and the Lyon Diet Heart Study[7] emphasize the critical role of diet and behavioral choices in the development or reversal of heart disease. Sadly, it seems much easier to prescribe a pill, for both physician and patient. Thus, prevention, and lifestyle modification are more preached than practiced.

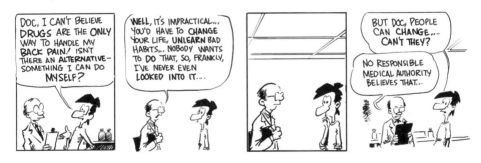

From Sinclair P: Alex's Restaurant: The Cartoon of Mind, Body, and Planet! With permission.

The reports of the U.S. Preventive Health Services Task Force will challenge this transition further. The yearly complete physical is no longer supported as an appropriate means to provide routine preventive care. Instead, age-specific health maintenance evaluations (HMEs) will receive increasing emphasis.

The task force continues to publish information indicating that education and counseling about preventive issues have a much greater impact on health than any aspect of the physical exam or specific lab tests. This changing emphasis will mark a paradigm shift for the coming generation of physicians.

9. Why are so many physicians seemingly unhappy with their chosen career?

Recent job satisfaction surveys have suggested that as many as 50% of physicians across the board question whether they would repeat their decision to go into medicine. The allopathic "health care" system has failed not only patients but also healers. Physicians have higher-than-normal rates of depression, suicide, drug and alcohol abuse, and divorce. These extremely concerning numbers suggest a strong need to recreate ourselves.[8] Factors contributing to physician "burnout" probably begin in medical school, and continue through residency.

Residency work hours have been debated for years. Concerns were made public by a New York journalist, whose daughter received care from resident physicians and died after a mistake was overlooked.[9] The question was raised whether overworked and sleep-deprived residents should be providing any medical care at all. Almost all medical students start with strong altruistic feelings. Somewhere along the line, however, many physicians become what they most wanted to avoid. They lose their idealism and are frustrated rather than nurtured by their patients and careers.

10. What else in the allopathic model contributes to burnout?

Both subtle and overt pressures contribute to job dissatisfaction. Information technology, which has exploded to the point of overload, contributes to feelings of frustration simply with keeping current. The separation of the first two years of medical school from clinical experience begins the process of objectifying patients into anatomic parts, diseases, and biochemical pathways. This process continues in the clinical years through the tendency to refer to patients as diagnoses,or unnamed lists of signs and symptoms (e.g.,"the appy [appendectomy] in room 207," "the train wreck with the GI bleed"). Time pressures, real and imagined, have challenged physicians' innate desire to get to know their patients. Inefficient systems cause patients to use emergency departments as ambulatory clinics, and insurance regulation of physician assignment disrupts continuity of care.

Even the language we use contributes to an attitude of "us" against "them." "Noncompliance" means that patients are not doing what the doctor told them to do without taking into consideration factors such as access, cost, literacy, and support systems. A "poor historian" is often simply not giving the history that the physician wanted or expected or took too long for the limited time available. The patient with the "laundry list" of problems may feel pressured to get his or her issues into the open before the doctor takes control of the interview and directs which problem is addressed. Calling patients "trolls," "gomers," or "drug-seekers" only creates negative images and expectations, often before personal introductions occur. Such emotions make it difficult to remember the idealistic altruism that led physicians to medicine.

11. What is allopathic medicine doing to address the problem of burnout?

A number of medical schools have recognized how critical communication is to the practice of medicine. In fact, more and more research confirms the beneficial health effects of a patient-centered interview.[10] Further investigation has clarified some of the foundation skills that can be helpful. Exciting research is under way to document positive patient outcomes as well as improved efficiency in the physician/patient interaction. These foundation skills include:

- Rapport building
- Agenda setting
- Identifying cues and clues
- Recognizing and responding to emotions and feelings
- Use of summary
- Negotiaton of common ground

These techniques are invaluable and relatively easy to learn. Through their use, patients have more than seventeen to nineteen seconds of uninterrupted time to set their agenda early in the interview, and the provider gains a deeper understanding of the patient.

12. Is evidence-based medicine the current standard of practice?

Surprisingly, much of what is taught in medical school and implemented in practice is based on theoretical possibilities rather than evidence-based review. Several recent articles have documented that commonly held medical beliefs are not, in fact, supported by published evidence. Examples include the beliefs that pernicious anemia must be treated with intramuscular rather than oral replacement of vitamin B_{12}; that corneal abrasions heal more quickly with patching; and that patients with diabetes should not be given a beta blocker because it will hinder their ability to recognize hypoglycemia.[11] In fact, these and other examples are actually medical myths; they are not supported by the best available evidence.

One of the dangers of not practicing evidence-based medicine is that tests replace clinical thought and abnormal numbers are treated instead of patients. This approach creates cascades of tests and procedures. If 20 lab tests are done in a completely healthy person, the chance that at least one test will have an abnormal result is 20% on the basis of statistic probability alone. Thus, a "simple" screening test can lead to more and more expensive and potentially dangerous diagnostic tests and procedures.

The *Journal of Family Practice* provides one of the best and most readily available approaches to beginning the transition from the practice of disease-oriented evidence (DOE) to the practice of patient-oriented evidence that matters (POEM). This approach is outlined at the following website: http://www.medicalinforetriever.com/index.cfm.

13. How can experiential information become part of evidence-based medicine?

Randomized, double-blinded, controlled (RDBC) studies are considered the gold standard of research. Physicians often assume that a medical standard is supported by an RDBC trial when in fact it is not. During a 1976 review of medical practices, the Office of Technology Assessment estimated that less than 20% of standards were supported by controlled trials. As evidence-based medicine becomes more commonly practiced, that number is likely to increase, although no similar review explores current evidence for global standards.[12] In addition, unawareness of research does not equate with lack of available research. Unfortunately, approaches are often disregarded because of ignorance of available research. This position will become harder and harder to support in the era of rapid information accessibility.

One of the biggest challenges for allopathic medicine is deciding how to balance different ways of knowing. An important part of knowledge comes from anecdotal or experiential sources, which are perfectly legitimate bases for making medical decisions, especially since evidence-based medicine is neither universally available nor universally applicable.

14. How do experience and chance factor into evidence-based medicine?

Much of medical education emphasizes the acquisition and regurgitation of facts, and the information explosion makes this approach even more likely during medical school, residency training, and rounds—even in board certification exams. Physicians readily admit that "Patients and diseases do not read textbooks"; in other words, textbook presentations differ from real-life scenarios. Moreover, doctors at times rely on intuition to guide diagnostic and therapeutic decisions. They need to learn to be comfortable with a certain level of uncertainty and chance in their decision-making process.

Current teaching and testing structures suggest a linear process to medical decision-making, when in actuality it is quite free-form. Physicians learn this more practical method of clinical thinking from their mentors. They also make daily use of certain aspects of gaming theory and probabilities, although courses in these subjects are not part of medical school curricula. For example, it is wasteful to order an MRI to rule out brain tumor in every patient complaining of a mild headache on the basis of probability alone. The art of medicine is truly about knowing the patient, applying astute clinical skills, learning odds tables and probabilities, and perceiving a balance between more and less likely events.[13]

15. Even with good information, why do discrepancies exist in medical care?

More and more evidence indicates that much of how medicine is practiced in the U.S. is driven by the preferences of physicians rather than by evidence-based medicine. Some of the initial work in this area was done in the 1960s by John Wennberg,[14] who was recruited to analyze practice patterns of hospitals in Vermont. The data demonstrated that, regardless of biomedical research, the rates of appendectomies, prostatectomies, herniorrhaphies, tonsillectomies, and so on varied tremendously even in the same state. In an attempt to understand these trends, a single university hospital was studied, anticipating that more consistent practice patterns would emerge. What emerged instead was a clear indication that the determining factor was the preferences and tendencies of individual physicians and hospitals rather than the disease itself.

Even today, with information available in the form of sound studies, best evidence practices, and organized educational processes, habits of practicing physicians do not necessarily change. Proven therapies go unused, and old familiar practices persist.

16. Discuss the relationship of allopathic medicine to the pharmaceutical industry.

Pharmaceutical companies have become an increasingly important part of medical education at every level. Although strict guidelines are being developed and implemented, a number of gray areas still exist. More and more research is sponsored by pharmaceutical companies. Many pharmaceutical companies have included clauses to reserve the right not to publish data that does not support the anticipated outcome. Thus, some of the information that seems like good evidence may be based on skewed data. Concerns have been raised about selective publication or biased interpretations of results in manufacturer-supported trials.[15] Moreover, the cost of advertising to students, residents, and physicians is staggering and contributes directly to the cost of medications for patients. The papers, pens, toys, and lunches are designed to enhance product recognition. They have nothing to do with whether a medication is appropriate for a particular patient.[16]

17. How has managed care affected the way in which allopathic medicine is practiced?

This area has undergone a dramatic change in recent years. Under managed care, selecting a personal physician is largely driven by who is covered rather than free choice. As people make life transitions and change jobs or location, often their insurance coverage also changes (sometimes every 2–3 years), and continuity of care suffers. Gone are the days when the family doctor would provide care for life. Providers suffer, too. Many physicians feel less in control of their practice and more like workers in a corporate enterprise in which performance is judged by numbers, profitability is the bottom line, and freedom, pride, and personal fulfillment are lost.

Such changes have generated an entirely new need for educating physicians about how to document and code. Physicians now devote significant time and resources to paperwork for fear of submitting fraudulent claims. The cost of overhead to support this level of administration and oversight continues to increase. It is common to have staff dedicated solely to billing.[17,18] Chart audits by third-party payers are routine and are done by nonclinicians, who are interested primarily in billable components rather than quality of care.

18. How has managed care affected physician reimbursement?

Reimbursement issues affect medical decision-making and even specialty choice. For many years, specialties with a procedural emphasis (e.g., surgical subspecialties) have had higher reimbursement rates from insurances companies and third-party payers than specialties with more cognitive approaches (e.g., general internal medicine, psychiatry). This bias means, for example, that ophthalmologists make more for cataract surgery than an internist who spends several hours talking with a suicidal patient and arranges for in-patient stay, potentially saving the patient's life. These discrepancies are currently the subject of significant analysis and legal processing. In addition, the decisions as to which doctors can perform and charge for certain procedures has become highly political and is driven primarily by economics. Such "turf battles" ignore the capacity for competent training in the same procedure in different specialties. Insurance companies also play a role in determining which physician specialty is reimbursed for what procedure.

In addition, the flexibility that old-style physicians may have had in terms of patients' bills is coming under increasing scrutiny by third-party payers. Medicare, in particular, is working to ensure that everyone is treated equally with respect to how bills are generated and submitted. Bartering, professional courtesy, and even "down-coding" a visit because someone is in tight financial circumstances are illegal options under Medicare guidelines.

19. Discuss examples of complementary/alternative medicine (CAM) techniques that have become part of mainstream allopathic medicine.

The following statement by Marsha Angell, former editor of *The New England Journal of Medicine,* has been widely quoted : "There cannot be two kinds of medicine—conventional and alternative. There is one medicine that has been adequately tested, and medicine that has not, medicine that works and medicine that may, or may not work. Once a treatment has been tested rigorously, it no longer matters if it was consider alternative at the outset."[19] This perspective of exploring scientifically proven and evidence-supported medicine is instrumental in the changes facing current students and residents. Techniques and practices evolve from being labeled as quackery or questionable to becoming mainstream. Although it may be confusing, this blurring is entirely appropriate and should be embraced.

Techniques such as hypnosis and acupuncture have now become acceptable; in fact, many physicians seek to use them in their practice. As support for prevention and positive behavioral choices increases, nutrition becomes an even more appropriate aspect of medical care. Botanical medicine is undergoing a dramatic transition. Numerous botanicals have been standardized, researched, and validated and are becoming essentially newer prescription drugs. In addition, 25% of all pharmaceuticals are botanically derived, and antitumor and antimicrobial drugs are even more likely to be derived from plants.[20]

20. Is allopathic medicine embracing proven CAM techniques?

A disturbing aspect about some of these changes, however, is that CAM techniques are not becoming truly integrated or no longer exist in their original form. Instead, they essentially are becoming westernized, especially with respect to philosophy. For example, acupuncture is only one part of a thoroughly integrated approach to medicine in China and other Asian countries. These approaches involve diet, nutrition, family, philosophy, and spirituality. Western medicine has taken it out of its original context and essentially changed it into an invasive procedure. Similarly, when Western physicians prescribe botanicals, they are not practicing herbal medicine. Western physicians are pleased that popular botanicals are becoming easier to prescribe and that their effects and drug interactions are better documented. To an herbalist, on the other hand, the whole plant is the drug. The Western approach of identifying single active ingredients has great benefits, but it also is fraught with danger (see Chapters18 and 61).

21. What rituals underlie allopathic medicine?

Ritual and ceremony are key parts of other healing systems. Compared with the ceremony of a Native American shaman, for example, we may not think that ritual is pertinent to the practice of allopathic medicine. But consider some of the trappings of its culture. The selection process to become a healer is not open to everyone, and many who are selected make great sacrifices to attend medical school. An arcane language is taught, mysteries of the human body are revealed, and a new alphabet is learned. Altered states caused by heightened expectations, sleeplessness, intense study, and strange diet contribute to a powerful rite of passage. At each stage, a white robe of differing lengths is used to identify the initiate's level of training. Sacred instruments and tools are used and carried on the healer's body or in the pockets of the healer's robes. When patients come to the hospital for treatment, they are subjected to ritualized actions, a controlled environment, and often a gathering of many practitioners in their room.

The bottom line is that all healers, regardless of culture and process, can tap into ritual as part of their power. Certainly they should have at their disposal all of the knowledge and tools of their training. But rituals serve to initiate, familiarize, bond, and mark rites of passage; like the shaman, we can learn to maximize this experience for the recipient.

22. What is the Planetree system?

One of the most dramatic and potentially rejuvenating effects on how health care is practiced in the hospital system may come out of the Planetree system,which was begun by a patient and nurses in California. Planetree is another name for the sycamore tree under which Hippocrates shared his wisdom with students. The essence of Planetree is a complete philosophical shift to create a more nurturing and healing environment in the hospital setting. This shift involves aesthetic changes such as hanging pictures or photographs in the halls. It involves making the family a more active part of patients' health care. It may include open charts, unrestricted visiting hours, healing pet therapy, music therapy, and massage. Through this nurturing process, the way that western medicine is practiced, at least in hospitals, may undergo a much needed and exciting change. More information is available at the following website: http://www.planetree.org.

23. How can I practice evidence-based, time-efficient, prevention-oriented care and still have satisfied patients, enjoy my job, and get paid?

The key steps in this dance relate to communication. The core communication skills discussed above are invaluable for improving time efficiency. When used properly, they decrease the "Oh, by the way, doctor" comment that often frustrates many physicians at the end of an encounter. Patients can get what they need in the average 20 minutes allotted to them and can feel that much more time was actually spent with their concerns. In this fashion, physicians can create a collaborative rather than antagonistic relationship with their patients.

Comfort with how they handle information overload is another important step for physicians. Emphasis on patient-oriented outcome studies can increase the quality of care. At the same time physicians need to find ways to value the intuitive side of medicine. A key part of this approach is openness to perspectives other than their own. Moreover, willingness to change their perspective as information becomes available allows physicians to take advantage of the best evidence and to create the most appropriate and individualized treatment approaches for their patients.

Physicians need to become more and more comfortable in collaborating with patients, nurses, and other practitioners. Allopathic medicine has emphasized thinking over doing throughout the training period. One way in which physicians can open their horizons to new perspectives is to experience personally different approaches to health and healing and to pursue individual interests. Physicians should strive to become positive role models for medical students as they begin to create their own path in the profession. Core communication skills should be used not only in patients' rooms but throughout life as physicians learn to listen for everyone's stories. This technique is invaluable in the physician's as well as the patient's family and support system. The goal is to live passionately as well as experientially.

REFERENCES

1. Weil A: Health and healing. Boston, Houghton Miffin, 1998.
2. Robbins J: Reclaiming Our Health: Exploding the Medical Myth and Embracing the Source of True Healing. Tiburon, CA, H.J. Kramer, 1996.
3. Payer L: Medicine and Culture. Varieties of Treatment in the United States, England, West Germany, and France. New York, Henry Holt & Company, 1996.
4. Grumbach K: Insuring the uninsured: Time to end the aura of invisibility. JAMA 284:2114–2116, 2000.
5. Bodenheimer T: Questions and answers about Medicare. Intl J Health Serv 29:519–523, 1999.
6. Ornish D, et al: Can lifestyle changes reverse coronary heart disease?: The Lifestyle Heart Trial. Lancet 336:129–133, 1990.
7. De Lorgeril M, et al: Mediterranean diet, traditional risk factors, and the rate of cardiovascular complications after myocardial infarction: Final report of the Lyon Diet Heart Study. Circulation 99:779–785,1999.
8. Shearer S, Toedt M: Family physicians' observations of their practice, well being, and health care in the United States. J Fam Practice 50:751–756, 2001.
9. Underwood W: Residents and fellow work hours reform 2001. AMA Resident and Fellow Section Report: F(A-01), 2001.
10. Stewart M, et al: Patient-centered Medicine: Transforming the Clinical Method. Thousand Oaks, CA, Sage Publications, 1995.
11. Paauw DS: Did we learn evidence-based medicine in medical school? Some common medical mythology. JABFP 12:143–149,1999.
12. Imrie R, Ramey DW: The evidence for evidence-based medicine. Compl Ther Med 8:123–126, 2000.
13. Bravata DM: Making medical decisions under uncertainty. Semin Med Pract 3(2):6–13, 2000.
14. Millenson ML: Demanding Medical Excellence: Doctors and Accountability in the Information Age. Chicago, University of Chicago Press, 1999.
15. Rochon PA, et al: A study of manufacturer-supported trials of nonsteroidal anti-inflammatory drugs in the treatment of arthritis. Arch Intern Med 154:157–163, 1994.
16. Coyle SL: Physician-industry relations. Part 1: Individual physicians. Ann Intern Med 139:396–402, 2002.
17. Bodenheimer T: Physicians and the changing medical marketplace. N Engl J Med 338:584–588, 1999.
18. Bodenheimer T: The movement for improved quality in health care. N Engl J Med 338:488–492, 1999.
19. Angell M, Kassirer JP: Alternative medicine: The risk of untested and unregulated remedies. N Engl J Med 339:839–841, 1998.
20. Calixto JB: Efficacy, safety, quality control, marketing and regulatory guidelines for herbal medicine (phytotherapeutic agents). Braz L Med Biol Res 33:179–189, 2000.

15. OSTEOPATHIC MEDICINE

David N. Grimshaw, D.O.

1. What is osteopathic medicine?

Osteopathic medicine is a branch of medicine whose philosophy embraces the concept of the unity of the living organism's structure (anatomy) and function (physiology). Osteopathy was founded by Andrew Taylor Still, M.D. in 1892. The term "osteopathy" was chosen by Still, because "we start with the bones." He stated that the Greek stem *osteo* includes the idea of "causation" as well as "bone" and that *pathos* means "suffering." A critical juncture in his life occurred when he lost two members of his family to meningitis. Unable to help them, he resolved to change the course of how medicine was practiced. The key paradigm shift was a change from treating disease to treating the host and assisting the host's capacity to overcome disease. Because the established medical profession largely rejected his ideas, he declared a "new" profession to allow him to apply the principles that he believed were operative in caring for patients. The first school, called the American School of Osteopathy, was located in Kirksville, MO, where the Kirksville College of Osteopathic Medicine stands today.

2. List the basic tenants of osteopathic philosophy.

- A person is the product of a dynamic interaction among body, mind, and spirit.
- An inherent property of this dynamic interaction is the person's capacity to maintain health and recover from disease.
- Many forces, both intrinsic and extrinsic, can challenge this inherent capacity and contribute to the onset of illness.
- The musculoskeletal system significantly influences the person's ability to restore this inherent capacity and therefore to resist disease processes.

3. What principles guide osteopathic approaches to patient care?

- The patient is the focus for health care delivery.
- The patient has the primary responsibility for his or her health.
- The role of the physician is to facilitate the healing process within the patient.
- The patient is treated in the context of the disease process that he or or she is experiencing.

Through many changes in science, technology, and society, the essential aspects of this philosophy have remained a constant. The uniqueness of osteopathy is not the principles on which its philosophy is based but the systematic manner in which they are applied in the care of patients. As Still observed, "To find health should be the object of the doctor. Anyone can find disease."

4. What factors have influenced the growth of osteopathy?

From its beginnings in Kirksville, MO to its present status with 19 colleges and approximately 49,000 practicing doctors of osteopathy (DOs) in the United States, osteopathic medicine has largely been a profession defined by the forces influencing its development. The struggle with regulatory agencies and traditional physicians to attain equal practice rights and licensure required the great majority of the profession's resolve and resources for the first 70 years of its existence. The denial of privileges to practice in traditional hospitals prompted DOs to form their own hospitals, which were private community hospitals financed by the physicians themselves. The success of these hospitals facilitated the growth of the profession. Denial of the right to practice in the military during World War II also led to rapid growth, because the DOs who stayed home took care of civilians left without a doctor.

The first school to be affiliated with a major university was the Michigan State University College of Osteopathic Medicine, founded in 1969. This was a landmark event, because all previous schools had been private. The trend of affiliation with universities has continued in the newer schools and has given the profession its first real opportunity to develop a culture of research and association with teaching hospitals.

In the 1960s, DOs in California were offered MD degrees, in what many view as an attempt to "buy out" the osteopathic profession. One of the largest medical schools at that time was originally an osteopathic institution. Many beleaguered DOs, tired of the battle for acceptance, took the M.D. degree, but a committed handful persisted in keeping osteopathic medicine as a distinct healing profession. The percentage required to declare the entire profession legally "converted" was never achieved; thus osteopathy kept its unique identity.

5. Describe the difference in how DOs and MDs make a diagnosis.

The osteopathic physician sees disease and health as states that exist along a continuum for each person. Disease can be seen and felt as a loss of connection within the person from inherent intrapersonal and interpersonal rhythms. The diagnosis of the patient usually includes two components: the aspect that relates to a disorder of a given tissue or organ, typically a medical diagnosis (e.g., gastroesophageal reflux disease [GERD]), and then the associated functional aspect of that disorder, such as somatic dysfunction in the mid-thoracic spine and rib cage. The functional aspect gives a sense of how ill the patient is, a quantitative measure of well-being, a context in which the GERD takes place.

As for the use of the hands in making a diagnosis, the DO looks for structural findings that correlate with the patient's complaints, such as abnormal posture, loss of range of motion in a particular region, and altered patterns of movement that may suggest a functional component to the problem. The DO listens to the patient's body with his or her hands, taking a measure of the feel of the tissues. Treatment is directed toward both components of the diagnosis. In the example of GERD , a medication may be prescribed initially. Then osteopathic manipulative medicine (OMM) can be applied to maximize the function of the thoracic spine and rib cage, facilitating the ability of the body to heal itself, enhancing the delivery of the medication to the affected area, and perhaps changing the underlying patterns that led to the development of the illness in the first place.

6. How does the more inclusive diagnostic paradigm translate into treatment?

The issue of cause and effect is more directly addressed with osteopathic philosophy. Why did the patient develop this problem? What underlying factors need to be addressed to change this pattern and prevent the problem from recurring? Rather than just treating the effect with medication, the cause is sought. Early osteopathic writings implied a bias toward thinking that most disease began as an alteration in function within the musculoskeletal system. This bias is no longer taught; rather, one looks for associations between the structural and functional aspects of the disease process. There is a similarity between osteopathic thought and traditional Chinese medicine in the awareness that cause is a susceptibility of the host to outside influences, whereas the more Western disease-oriented model focuses on a more external locus of control. Thus, nutrition, lifestyle choices, body habitus, and patterns of behavior are considered contributing factors in the development of an illness. Changing these patterns , therefore, can alter the course of the illness toward health.

7. What are the most common types of osteopathic manipulation?

The most commonly used methods among osteopathic practitioners are the muscle energy technique (MET); high-velocity, low-amplitude thrust (HVLA); strain-counterstrain; functional techniques, facilitated positional release; myofascial release techniques; and cranial osteopathy. The reader is referred to comprehensive texts for greater detail (see question 31).

8. Explain the muscle energy technique.

MET, which, was first developed in the 1950s by Mitchell, uses the patient's intrinsic activating force of muscle contraction. The operator positions the patient at the edge of a barrier to normal motion, then asks the patient to contract the hypertonic muscles, and resists the effort for 3–5 seconds, allowing no movement to occur. The result is an isometric contraction. Next one can advance the segment further to a new barrier, which is closer to normal range. A series of contractions followed by relaxation and repositioning of the segment is used, and then the segment is retested to see if motion has been restored.

9. What principles underlie the high-velocity, low-amplitude thrust?

HVLA or mobilization with impulse is the technique most frequently associated with the word "manipulation." It requires a precise localization of forces and is also usually applied at the barrier to motion in all three planes. A quick, short movement is used (about an eighth of an inch) in the direction of motion that the operator wishes to increase. The force in this case is supplied by the operator. This technique is most useful when the restriction is caused by a joint and tends to work best for chronic restrictions. It is often reserved for the fibrotic type of restrictions, when other, gentler methods fail.

10. How is the strain-counterstrain technique applied?

Strain-counterstrain, developed by Jones, is a gentle, indirect technique in which the operator positions the body in a specific manner to produce relaxation in a particular muscle. This position is held for approximately 90 seconds, and then the body is slowly returned to normal. The technique works extremely well for acute injuries, when muscles are still quite irritable and shortened. Jones developed a mapping of tender points related to involved muscles and positions in which to hold the patient for the alleviation of pain at the points.

11. Explain functional techniques and facilitated positional release.

The techniques in this category were developed simultaneously but independently by different groups during the 1940s and 1950s. The concept is often described as finding the region within the body that is "out of step"with the structures around it and bringing it back into harmony with its environs. Functional techniques are usually indirect, meaning that one finds the position of ease for the affected segment in all planes to facilitate dissipation of tissue tension. When the tension dissipates, the structure is returned to its normal position and retested. This gentle and subtle method relies heavily on the ability to palpate tissue and test for ease and fluidity of motion. It works well for both chronic and acute problems.

12. What are myofascial release techniques?

Myofascial release techniques, developed by Ward, focus on restrictions found within the soft tissues. Typically, the myofascial release technique is used directly, taking up the range of movement of the soft tissues in three planes. The tissues are then loaded, taking them into the direction of restriction and thus increasing tissue tension. The patient then can be asked to perform enhancing maneuvers, such as taking a deep breath, which increases tension further, or reaching upward with the arms to load the tissues further. The tension in the tissues builds and then gives way, usually after 15–30 seconds, and a release phenomenon occurs. The tissue elongates, softens, often flushes, and gives off heat as the stored energy within it is released. This method is effective in acute and chronic conditions and requires fairly significant upper body strength on the part of the operator.

13. How does cranial osteopathy work?

This method of osteopathic manual medicine was first described in the 1940s by Sutherland, who was struck by the idea that the anatomy of the bones of the skull, which are beveled like the gills of a fish, suggested that they were built for motion. He coined the term *primary respiratory mechanism* to describe an inherent motion that he felt within the body and on the cranium. This motion, which was rhythmic and independent of breathing and pulse, occurred between 8 and 14 times per minute.

Sutherland described five components of the primary respiratory mechanism, which included articular, fluid, membranous, and inherent motility of the brain and spinal cord as well as the sacrum below. He developed techniques for assessing the motion and treating restrictions within the mechanism. Subsequent research has shown that his novel ideas were indeed correct. This technique is subtle but powerful and is useful in treating children with recurrent infections, some types of headaches, late effects of traumatic brain injuries, and temporal mandibular joint disorders (usually in conjunction with a dentist). It also helps to alleviate the effects of trauma.

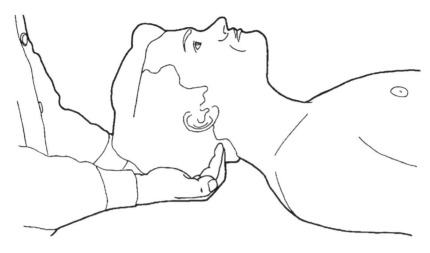

Release of the cranial base.

14. How is a DO different from an MD?

The paradigm used to train DOs is a holistic model of health and disease. The primary difference is in the way a DO thinks about illness and perceives the patient. A DO takes into account factors such as lifestyle, nutrition, and the context in which the illness occurred when considering the problem with which the patient presents. DOs tend to be open-minded about using a wider variety of treatment options to deal with a given problem, including the use of manual medicine. This philosophical bias translates into the type of specialties that DOs choose. Compared with MDs, a higher percentage of DOs are primary care physicians; 60% of all DOs are in general practice, family practice, internal medicine, pediatrics, and obstetrics/gynecology compared with 35% of all MDs. Approximately 5% of all physicians in the United States are DOs, but DOs constitute 20% of general/family practitioners.[1]

Secondly, a basic curriculum in the use of osteopathic manipulative diagnosis and treatment is taught to all DOs in medical school. Whether or not it is used for patient care, this training allows the DO to perform a more detailed examination of the neuromusculoskeletal system and to appreciate the role that it may play in the genesis and perpetuation of disease processes. This additional tool allows the DO both to diagnose more accurately and to treat more effectively a broad array of illnesses. For instance, manual medicine can be used to enhance recovery from an illness such as an upper respiratory infection. Using the hands to improve lymphatic drainage from the head and neck helps maximize the patient's inner resources (circulatory and immune system function).

15. Is osteopathy like chiropractic?

Not in the United States. Both professions began in the late 1800s, both incorporated the use of manual procedures in treatment, and both were influenced by bone setters from England and France. However, several differences have existed from the beginning. Unlike osteopathy, chiropractic at first did not claim to be a complete school of medicine. The most obvious difference between the professions is their scope of practice. DOs have unlimited medical licenses in all 50 states, effectively giving them equality with MDs in terms of access, rights, and responsibilities. Chiropractors have only recently sought to broaden their scope of practice and never claimed to be a total school of medicine.

Chiropractic approaches to manipulation vary widely (see Chapter 16). There are some similarities in manipulation techniques in the two professions. In medical and chiropractic literature, the term *manipulation* usually implies the quick high-velocity, low-amplitude thrust method of joint mobilization. However, many manual medicine procedures do not use a thrusting type impulse. DOs tend to use a broad spectrum of manual methods, not just the thrusting type, and all are included under the umbrella term o*steopathic manipulative treatment* (OMT). Chiropractors use the term *subluxation* to describe the entity treated with manipulation, whereas osteopaths use the term *somatic dysfunction*.

16. Define somatic dysfunction.

Somatic dysfunction is defined as impaired or altered function of related components of the somatic (body framework) system, including skeletal, arthrodial, and myofascial structures and their related vascular, lymphatic, and neural elements. The all-inclusive nature of the definition suggests an understanding of the interrelatedness of structure and function and places the emphasis on function. This definition implies that the corrective measure used for treatment should restore function, allowing patients to use their own set of internal self-regulatory mechanisms to stay well.

The diagnosis of somatic dysfunction requires the doctor to observe and palpate the structure in question throughout its range of motion. Objective findings of asymmetry, altered range of motion, and tissue texture changes are necessary for the diagnosis. Such a diagnosis cannot be based on a static view on x-ray or physical examination. Somatic dysfunction also has recognized region-specific ICD-9 codes (somatic dysfunction, ICD-9 CM #739.1–739.9).

17. How is osteopathic manipulative medicine (OMM) used?

OMM is used within the context of total patient care and can be of value in diagnosis, treatment, and assessment of therapeutic response. For example, it can be used in diagnosis to identify a somatic component of visceral disease. Most allopaths are unaware of structural (musculoskeletal) components of visceral diseases.

One area in which this approach has been explored is the correlation of physical findings in the structural exam with coronary artery disease (CAD). The most common structural findings associated with documented CAD were chronic tissue texture abnormalities and persistent somatic dysfunction at the T3 and T4 level on the left side in the paravertebral musculature just lateral to the spinous processes.[2] The neuroanatomic rationale[3] for these associations is the convergence of visceral and somatic afferents within the spinal cord at the T3–T4 level. The often seen changes in tissue texture may be caused by an elevated sympathetic efferent output from that level of the cord in response to the increased visceral afferent input into the nervous system. These somatic markers for visceral disease processes are part of the osteopathic tradition and represent an area that deserves further research and exploration.

18. For what types of conditions is OMM helpful?

Treatment using OMM can be curative for a number of disorders, helpful in management of several chronic conditions, and palliative in still others. OMM can be applied over a broad range of situations. One of the most common applications is in the treatment of back and neck pain, particularly when it is related to mechanical restrictions and injuries (see figure on following page). As another example, OMM management of patients with chronic obstructive pulmonary disease includes maximizing the function of the thoracic spine, rib cage, and diaphragm. Whereas the medications for COPD are designed primarily to facilitate function of the gas exchange mechanism, OMM can be used in conjunction with pulmonary rehabilitation to facilitate function of the mechanical pump aspect of the problem.

19. For what specific diagnoses has manual medicine been proven beneficial?

This is one of the most commonly asked questions about OMM. Osteopathic literature is not referenced by disease. Review of the medical and chiropractic literature for controlled trials reveals that the following problems can be improved by using manipulative approaches: low back pain, headache (migraine, muscle tension, and cervicogenic are the most commonly studied),[4,5] neck pain, dizziness,[6] carpal tunnel syndrome, pancreatitis, postoperative pain and pulmonary dysfunction, gait disturbance in Parkinson's patients,[7] and pneumonia in elderly patients.[8] In infants, torticollis, GERD, and colic have been found to improve with manual procedures. Several case studies have been published suggesting positive effects on sucking dysfunction in infants,[9] chest wall and rib pain after thoracic surgery, thoracic outlet syndrome, sciatica, spinal stenosis, traumatic brain injury, low back pain of pregnancy, postural imbalances, and several other conditions.

Osteopathic medicine originated with and still maintains a philosophy of treating the patient rather than the disease. A large percentage of the osteopathic literature consists of case reports. As the trend of affiliation with universities continues, clinical trials in osteopathy are expected to become more common.

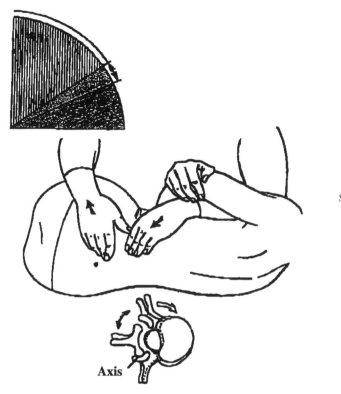

Side posture mobilization.

Axis

20. What is treated with manual medicine?

The patient. The manipulable lesion is somatic dysfunction, found on examination as a combination of three factors: altered tissue texture, decreased range of motion, and asymmetry of form and function. It can be and usually is a component of an additional problem, such as osteoarthritis or emphysema. The somatic dysfunction is treated with the intention of improving the patient's capacity to recover from disease and achieve a greater measure of health. Manipulation affects disease processes by enhancing the capacity of the host to respond to the disease process. Hagopian explains the process as follows: "We work with relationships of structure and function, body to mind, parts to whole, past to present, individual to environment . . . . How and where to treat will be dictated by the body's own purposeful changes in the direction of its inherent perfect design."[10]

21. What mechanisms are thought to be operative in manual medicine?

For the most part, the mechanisms are theoretical. Research is needed to elucidate what actually happens with hands-on therapies. One fairly well understood mechanism is the postisometric relaxation phase of a muscle contraction. MET uses this phenomenon to change the resting length of a hypertonic muscle. Once the shortened muscle is identified, the patient is positioned in such a way as to control the muscle so that the patient contracts it and the operator applies an equal and opposite counterforce to prevent it from shortening. This technique is referred to as an isometric contraction. Shortly after the patient relaxes the muscle as completely as possible, the operator can stretch it to a new length. This maneuver can be repeated several times to reset the resting tone of the muscle, allowing the joint to achieve an increase in its range of motion.

Technologies such as magnetic resonance imaging, positron emission tomography, electromyography, and three-dimensional computed tomography coupled with functional measures commonly used in research will allow investigators to observe and document the effects of manual therapies in the years to come.

22. How is OMM used as a palliative treatment?

OMM can be a powerful tool at end of life for pain management, comfort, and assisting the patient and family with the process of dying. Several forms of manual medicine are extremely gentle and can be used even in patients with metastatic disease, osteoporosis, and end-stage pulmonary and cardiovascular disease. Osteopathic manipulative treatments given twice weekly over the last few months of a person's life can afford a great deal of relief from pain and allow more restful sleep.

23. What training do DOs receive in manual medicine?

OMM as taught in U.S. schools is evaluated by the National Osteopathic Board of Medical Examiners (http://www.nbome.org). This organization provides the testing for licensure of osteopathic physicians in the U.S. All U.S.-trained DOs are expected to have a basic understanding of and rudimentary skills in OMM at graduation from medical school. DO medical students receive approximately 200 hours of formal education in OMM during their first two years. Exposure in the third and fourth years of medical school varies considerably; not all schools require a rotation in OMM specifically.

Approximately 50% of DOs do their internship and residency in MD programs, which rarely include training in any type of manual medicine. Many osteopathic postgraduate programs also lack training in OMM, particularly specialties that do not typically incorporate manual medicine (e.g., surgical specialties, pathology, ophthalmology). Hence, many DOs have not been exposed to OMM since their early years in medical school. In a survey of osteopathic practitioners, Fry[5] found that the primary predictor for the use of OMM was learning a new OMM format since graduation from medical school. The second predictor was an interest in OMM during internship, which often is a DO's last exposure to osteopathic manual medicine training before going into a residency.

24. Do all DOs use manipulative treatment in their practice?

No. In a study of randomly selected Osteopathic physicians,[11] Johnson et al. reported the use of OMM by osteopathic physicians. Only 6% of more than 1000 respondents stated that they treated more than half of their patients with OMM, and nearly one-third used OMM on less than 5% of their patients. Two factors were cited as the most common explanations: (1) barriers (time, finances) to its use and (2) OMM protocol. Another study[12] using a mailed survey found that 71% of 100 practicing osteopathic physicians use OMM, but only 14% used it on more than half of their patients. Only 1% of D.O.'s specialize in OMM.

25. In which specialties is OMM most often used?

The most common specialties that use manipulation are family practice, osteopathic manipulative medicine, physical medicine and rehabilitation, sports medicine, internal medicine, and obstetrics and gynecology. A few DOs occasionally use OMM in subspecialties, such as cardiology (for musculoskeletal chest wall pain), pulmonology (to enhance rib cage and diaphragmatic function), surgery (to enhance postoperative outcomes), and emergency medicine (primarily for musculoskeletal complaints). Of interest, in the U.S. orthopedic medicine is so strongly identified as a surgical specialty that, despite frequent opportunities for its application, DO orthopedic physicians rarely use OMM in their care of patients.

Another specialty with an enormous potential for the use of OMM is pediatrics, particularly for treatment of otitis media.[13] Again, very few pediatricians use manual medicine, perhaps because the types of manual medicine most useful in the care of infants, children, and even adolescents are cranial, myofascial release, and functional techniques. These techniques are more difficult to learn, require a higher level of skill, and are seldom mastered by the typical primary care DO.

26. Describe the process for certification and demonstration of expertise in OMM.

Certification in OMM is overseen by the American Osteopathic Board of Neuromusculoskeletal Medicine (known until 2000 as the American Osteopathic Board of Special Proficiency in Osteopathic Manipulative Medicine). The American Academy of Osteopathy (AAO) is the primary professional society within the American Osteopathic Association that includes members who devote a significant percentage of their time to manipulative medicine. In Pennsylvania and California, rudimentary knowledge and ability to perform OMM are part of the licensing procedure. Board certification in osteopathic family medicine also requires demonstration of the ability to evaluate and treat a given problem with OMM methods.

Fewer than 500 DOs in the U.S. are board-certified in neuromusculoskeletal medicine, and membership in the Fellows of the Academy (FAAO), the highest recognition that can be attained by a U.S.-trained D.O. in the field of manipulative medicine, is limited to just over 100. To find a DO who does manipulative medicine, contact the AAO in Indianapolis at http://www.academyofosteopathy.org.

27. How is osteopathy practiced in the United States compared with other countries?

Only DOs trained in the United States are allowed to practice an unlimited scope of medicine and surgery. This training gives them the opportunity to offer their skills in the context of total patient care. Osteopaths in other countries do not have the same training; their practice, therefore, is limited to manual therapies.

28. How are osteopathic principles applied in pediatrics?

Pediatrics is a particularly potent area for the use of osteopathic techniques. Because children are growing, one has the opportunity to assist with maximizing their ability to adapt and develop. A few of the common problems for which children are seen for osteopathic manual treatment are plagicephaly (abnormally shaped head after delivery), torticollis, recurrent ear and sinus infections, frequent respiratory infections, and developmental delays. The principles are the same as with adults, but children respond much more readily. The methods most commonly used in children are cranial, functional, and muscle energy. Of note, a trial sponsored by the National Institutes of Health was begun in 1999 at the University of Arizona to explore use of OMT for recurrent pediatric otitis media.

29. What are the risks of manipulation?

The most frequently cited severe complication of manipulation is vertebral artery syndrome.[14] The mechanism of injury is a tear of the intimal lining of the vertebral artery caused by a sudden thrust that combines rotation and extension of the cervical spine or prolonged positioning in an extended and rotated position. This mechanism results in formation of a thrombus, which extends upward into the posterior circulation of the brain and lodges most frequently in the distribution of the posterior inferior cerebellar artery. No reliable tests can predict who is at greater risk for this complication. The average age of persons affected is 38 years. The frequency of this complication is estimated to be about one in one-million manipulations of the high-velocity, low-amplitude type.[15] It has not been reported using muscle energy procedures, which avoid the forceful maneuver and the position of hyperextension combined with rotation. Other possibilities include minor treatment reactions, such as dizziness, muscular soreness for 1–2 days after a treatment, and aggravation of underlying problems.

According to persons with extensive experience in reviewing cases with negative outcomes in both the osteopathic and chiropractic professions, the most common mistake that has resulted in complications is misdiagnosis. In other words, manual procedures were used inappropriately because the practitioner did not make the correct diagnosis. For example, utilization of high-velocity techniques in people with metastatic disease, osteoporosis, or an unstable vertebral motion segment secondary to injury, disk disease, or ligamentous laxity is clearly inappropriate. One should use manual medicine procedures to treat hypomobility or somatic dysfunction. It is the responsibility of the practitioner to make an accurate diagnosis and to apply these methods correctly for the correct reasons.

30. Discuss the contraindications to manipulation.

There are very few **absolute contraindications**, given the fact manual techniques can be applied in so many different ways. The first contraindication is hypermobility. For instance, patients with advanced rheumatoid arthritis and patients with Down syndrome develop ligamentous laxity in the joints of the upper cervical spine, which should not be treated with any type of manipulation. Other obvious contraindications include fractures and septic joints, central nervous system infections, acute bleeding, and abnormal intracranial pressure. However, even in acutely ill patients, some forms of manual medicine can be useful in conjunction with standard medical care. A prime example is gentle soft tissue techniques to the thoracic spine, rib cage, and diaphragm in the days after coronary artery bypass grafting to reduce pain in the chest, to decrease the need for medication, to enhance the patients' ability to take a deep breath, and to reduce the risk of postoperative complications such as atelectasis and pneumonia.

Relative contraindications include vigorous articulation applied to actively inflamed joints. Knowledge that the patient has metastatic disease to bones, joints, or areas of soft tissue needs to direct the approach. It is not necessary to avoid touch in such patients. In fact, touch used in palliative care of the dying can be profoundly comforting. However, the methods must be gentle and not place strain on the injured tissues. In instances of acutely injured spinal disks, caution must be exercised. Typically the injured segment is not treated, but the joints above, below, and around the injured area often are affected in predictable patterns. Treatment of the surrounding regions can facilitate recovery, reduce pain and edema, and allow more rapid healing. One treats the whole patient, not the disease.

31. What resources are available for additional information?
- Butler DS: Mobilisation of the Nervous System. Melbourne, Churchill Livingstone, 1991.
- Chaitow L: Cranial Manipulation Theory and Practice: Osseous and Soft Tissue Approaches, Edinburgh, Churchill Livingstone 1999.
- Gallagher RM, Humphrey, FJ II (eds): Osteopathic Medicine: A Reformation in Progress. New York, Churchill Livingstone, 2001.
- Gevitz N: The D.O.'s: Osteopathic Medicine in America. Baltimore, Johns Hopkins University Press, 1982 (the best historical book about the profession).
- Greenman PE: Principles of Manual Medicine, 2nd ed. Baltimore, Williams & Wilkins, 1996.
- Isaacs EI, Bookhout MR: Bourdillon's Spinal Manipulation, 6th ed. Butterworth Heinemann, Boston, 2002 (recent and well-referenced).
- Kuchera M, Kuchera WA: Osteopathic Considerations in Systemic Dysfunction, 2nd ed. Kirksville, MO, KCOM Press, 1992 (the best book about use of OMM outside neuromusculoskeletal medicine).
- Ward RC (ed): Foundations for Osteopathic Medicine. Baltimore, Williams & Wilkins, 1997 (the best compilation to date; referenced, multiauthored text).

REFERENCES

1. Ross-Lee B: Primary care medicine. In Gallagher H (ed): Osteopathic Medicne: A Reformation in Progress. New York, Churchill-Livingstone, 2001, pp 65–67.
2. Barnes MW: Academy of Applied Osteopathy 1965 Yearbook of Selected Osteopathic Papers, Vol. 1. Carmel, CA, Academy of Applied Osteopathy, 1965.
3. Korr IM: The Collected Papers of Irvin M. Korr, Vols. 1 & 2. Indianapolis, IN, American Academy of Osteopathy Year Book, 1997.
4. Vernon H, McDermaid CS, Hagino C: Systematic review of randomized clinical trials of complementary/alternative therapies in the treatment of tension-type and cervicogenic headache. Complement Ther Med 7(3):142–155, 1999.
5. Nilsson N: A randomized controlled trial of the effect of spinal manipulation in the treatment of cervicogenic headache. J Manipul Physiol Ther 18(7):435–440, 1995.
6. Heikkila H, Johansson M, Wenngren BI: Effects of acupuncture, cervical manipulation and NSAID therapy on dizziness and impaired head repositioning of suspected cervical origin: A pilot study. Manipul Ther 5(3):151–157, 2000.
7. Wells MR, Giantinoto S, D'Agate D, et al: Standard osteopathic manipulative treatment acutely improves gait performance in patients with Parkinson's disease. J Am Osteopath Assoc 99(2):92–98, 1999.
8. Noll DR, Shores, JH, Gamber, GR, et al: Benefits of osteopathic manipulative treatment for hospitalized elderly patients with pneumonia. J Am Osteopath Assoc 100(12):776–782, 2000.
9. Holtrop DP: Resolution of suckling intolerance in a 6-month old chiropractic patient. J Manipul Physiol Ther 23(9):615–618, 2000.
10. Hagopian S: On Becoming an Osteopath [interview]. Altern Ther 7:85–91, 2001.
11. Johnson SM, Kurtz ME, Kurtz JC: Variables influencing the use of osteopathic manipulative treatment in family practice. J Am Osteopath Assoc 97(2):80–87, 1997.
12. Fry LJ: Preliminary findings on the use of osteopathic manipulative treatment by osteopathic physicians. J Am Osteopath Assoc 96(2): 91–96, 1996.
13. Pratt-Harrington D: Galbreath technique: A manipulative treatment for otitis media revisited. J Am Osteopath Assoc 100(10):635–639, 2000.
14. Di Fabio RP: Manipulation of the cervical spine: Risks and benefits. Phys Ther 79:50–65, 1999.
15. Klougart N, Leboeuf-Yde C, Rasmussen LR: Safety in chiropractic practice. Part II: Treatment to the upper neck and the rate of cerebrovascular incidents. J Manipul Physiol Ther 19:563–569, 1996.

16. CHIROPRACTIC

Robert D. Mootz, D.C., and Ian Coulter, Ph.D.

1. Define chiropractic.

Chiropractic is a health care profession, not a procedure, although spinal adjusting or manipulation procedures are frequently associated with or mistaken for "chiropractic." The word was coined near the turn of the 20th Century from the Greek word meaning "done by hand." Today the chiropractic profession is licensed or recognized as a distinct health care profession in all U.S. states and jurisdictions as well as over 75 countries around the world. Chiropractic has its own professional associations and educational institutions and is typically recognized and regulated through separate legislative acts.

2. How did chiropractic originate?

The profession of chiropractic began in the 1890s in the Midwestern United States. A Canadian immigrant named Daniel Palmer was a self-taught naturalist healer who observed that spinal manipulation seemed to help a variety of ailments and reasoned that the function of the nervous system was affected. He began teaching his principles to others and eventually founded the Palmer School of Chiropractic in Davenport, Iowa, which graduated its first class in 1898. Early students were mostly medical physicians, but eventually the field took on a life of its own.[1] Although chiropractic is now practiced throughout the world, its origin and early development took place in North America.

3. What education do chiropractors receive?

A chiropractic education in many ways resembles that of the other health sciences. For all chiropractic colleges a minimum of two years university education in the biologic sciences with some courses in the social sciences and humanities is required for entry (although some colleges now require the completion of an undergraduate degree). Over half of all doctors of chiropractic (DCs) now have a bachelors' degree in addition to a doctor of chiropractic degree. The chiropractic program consists of 4 years with an average of 4826 contact hours (compared with an average of 4667 contact hours for medical schools).[2] About 30% of the time is devoted to basic sciences and 70% to clinical sciences. An additional 1,405 hours are spent in a clinical clerkship.

For the first two years of the program the emphasis is on the basic biologic sciences and is relatively similar to medical education (e.g., anatomy, biochemistry, microbiology, physiology, pathology, neurology, physics). Chiropractors spend less time on public health but more time on such issues as radiology, nutrition, biomechanics, physical therapies, and manipulation. Medical students complete considerably longer clinical practice internships (over twice the amount). In addition, chiropractic resembles dentistry in that no residency is required for a license after completion of the degree.

4. Describe the subspecialty and postgraduate education programs in chiropractic.

Nearly all jurisdictions mandate continuing education requirements for relicensure. Over 96% of U.S. practitioners attend postgraduate conferences and seminars. Beyond minimal continuing education requirements, several part-time and full-time postgraduate diplomate or fellowship programs are offered by chiropractic schools. Extended part-time postgraduate programs are available in family practice, applied chiropractic sciences, clinical neurology, chiropractic orthopedics, sports injuries, pediatric nutrition, rehabilitation, and industrial consulting. Less than 10% of practitioners obtain certification.[3] Full time 1- to 3-year chiropractic residency programs are also offered in radiology, orthopedics, and clinical sciences. Both residency and postgraduate programs lead to eligibility for competency examinations administered by specialty boards recognized by the American Chiropractic Association or International Chiropractors Association. The specialty boards typically confer diplomate status for successful completion of the training/residency programs and competency examination.

5. What kinds of clinical evaluation do chiropractors perform?

Chiropractors approach clinical diagnosis in a similar fashion to that of all health care practitioners. History, physical examination, regional examination, special studies, and specialty-specific evaluation procedures are routinely incorporated. Case history, physical examination, and neuromusculoskeletal examination are routinely performed and rated of high importance by chiropractors. Standard history and physical examination methods are basic chiropractic clinical competencies. and clinical differential diagnosis is routinely used. Chiropractic also emphasizes biopsychosocial considerations in patient care.[4] A history is similar to any medical history. A chiropractic physical examination differs somewhat in that chiropractors have refined and developed many of their own methods for evaluating articular function. Some of the mechanical assessment strategies are common to physical medicine procedures, whereas others are unique to chiropractic.[5]

The table below lists many commonly used mechanical assessment procedures. Osterbauer[6] reviewed the evidence for reliability and utility of several chiropractic mechanical assessment procedures for detection of joint dysfunction or "vertebral subluxation," a term often preferred by chiropractors. Procedures with reasonable (fair to good) reliability included assessments of osseous and soft tissue pain or tenderness. To date, procedures for determining mobility, cutaneous temperature differences, and joint position have not fared as well in reliability studies. This problem is not unique to chiropractic methods; many commonly used orthopedic and physical examination procedures in all clinical fields have similar problems.

Commonly Used Chiropractic Mechanical Assessment Procedures

Pain provocation	Dynamic spinal loading
Static palpation	Tissue compliance
Motion palpation	Reactive leg-length discrepancy
Range-of-motion measurement	Gait analysis
Postural symmetry	Functional capacity and physical performance evaluation

6. Discuss the role of lab studies and radiographic imaging in chiropractic.

Chiropractic training includes the use of standard clinical laboratory studies, but they are used less frequently than in typical medical practice, probably because of the nature of presenting conditions frequently seen by chiropractors. Radiology and imaging are used with far greater frequency than other special studies; plain radiographs are the most common choice. Computed tomography (CT) and magnetic resonance imaging (MRI) are used much less frequently. Other special studies sometimes used or ordered by chiropractors include nerve conduction studies, bone scans, and electromyography. Chiropractors obtain x-rays for approximately one-half of new patients and far less frequently with established patients.[3,7] Appropriateness criteria for chiropractic radiography have been developed and implemented, and effective quality improvement efforts have been in place in colleges and private practices for more than a decade.[8,9]

7. What interventions do chiropractors use?[3,7]

Spinal manipulation is the therapeutic procedure most closely associated with chiropractic, but patient management often includes lifestyle counseling, nutritional management, rehabilitation, various physiotherapeutic modalities (e.g., ultrasound, electrical muscle stimulation), and a variety of other interventions such as mobilization, exercise, relaxation, electrical stimulation, traction, heat, acupuncture, and manual therapy (deep tissue massage, trigger point therapy). Chiropractors report that they "routinely" perform chiropractic adjustive techniques. Nearly all chiropractors recommend corrective or therapeutic exercise. In addition, most chiropractors recommend nutritional counseling, supportive techniques, or supplements but only on a "sometimes" basis.

For example, one large study showed that 84% of patients who presented with low back pain received spinal manipulation (or adjustment); 79% received non-thrust manual therapies (e.g., mobilization, massage, heat packs); 31% received education; and 5% received other forms of therapy such as acupuncture.

8. **Summarize the use of spinal and extremity manipulation.**

Chiropractors generally prefer the term *adjustment* over the term *manipulation* because it is believed to imply a more specific or precise maneuver and distinguishes it from other forms of manipulation. There are at least 100 distinct chiropractic, osteopathic, and physical therapy manipulation techniques, a large array of highly specialized adjusting tables and equipment, and a great deal of variation in the specific techniques used by individual practitioners.

9. **How important are exercise and rehabilitation?**

Ninety-eight percent of chiropractors reported that they use corrective and therapeutic exercises. Chiropractors have incorporated patient activation and exercise into their management strategies since at least the 1930s. Evidence-based guidelines published by the Agency for Health Care Policy nd Research (AHCPR) stress the importance of early activation of patients with acute low back pain to optimize recovery. Chiropractors are involved in the treatment of professional and amateur athletes and have been included by many countries as Olympic team physicians. A clinical journal is devoted to sports chiropractic and rehabilitation has been published for the better part of a decade. Chiropractic authors frequently address rehabilitation and activation strategies.

10. **What ancillary and complementary procedures may be used?**

Chiropractors may incorporate a variety of complementary and ancillary procedures, including cryotherapy, trigger point therapy, nutritional counseling, and bracing. The majority of practitioners also use massage, heat, traction, and electrical muscle stimulation modalities. Acupressure and meridian therapy are used by about 66% of practitioners; less than 10% report the use of acupuncture.

11. **How do chiropractors address issues of lifestyle and activities of daily living?**

Promotion of wellness and lifestyle strategies is also a significant, if underexplored, aspect of chiropractic management. More than two-thirds of chiropractors report using nutritional counseling, and chiropractic college curricula include courses on the subject. Health promotion strategies for chiropractors can be found in the literature.

12. **Define the following terms commonly used in chiropractic manipulation.**

Mobilization: passive movement within physiologic joint range of motion (the range typically performed by intrinsic musculature).

Manipulation: passive movement into paraphysiologic range (the range that typically requires application of external force) but not beyond anatomic range of motion.

Spinal manipulative therapy: generic umbrella term used for various procedures that may include any or all of the other terms.

Chiropractic adjustment: term typically favored by DCs to characterize neurologic and segmental specificity in application (as opposed to mechanical and directional articular specificity typical of manipulation descriptions).

Manipulable spinal lesion models
- *Generic:* biomechanical, neurophysiologic, trophic, psychosocial, combination models.
- *Profession-derived:* chiropractic vertebral subluxation, osteopathic somatic dysfunction, manual medicine joint block or fixation.

Active care: manual movement performed by patients themselves.

Passive care: manual movement performed by or with assistance from a clinician.

Manipulation technique categories
- *Generic:* mechanical/clinical descriptions (e.g., specific contact thrust) or manual force mechanically assisted.
- *Developer-named* (e.g., Gonstead, Cox technique)
- *Diversified, Logan-basic, craniosacral*

From Mootz RD, Meeker W: An evidence-based update on spinal manipulation with considerations for an aging population. 19th Annual Geriatric Research Education and Clinical Center (GRECC) Symposium, St. Louis University School of Medicine and Logan College of Chiropractic, St. Louis, MO, 2000, with permission of authors.

13. What is the difference between joint mobilization, manipulation, and adjusting?

Mobilization involves passive movement (applied by the clinician) within a joint's physiologic range of motion (see question 12) This is the maximal range of motion that typically can be achieved by voluntary movement of the patient's intrinsic musculature. Mobilization is performed within this usual range of motion but often under gentle joint distraction (opening up or stretching the joint) while the patient voluntarily relaxes muscles associated with the joint.

Manipulation is defined as passive movement (performed by the clinician) into the paraphysiologic range of motion. This range of motion is the range in which a joint can be moved with the application of external force but not exceeding the anatomic limitation of the joint's intrinsic connective tissue (e.g., ligaments, joint capsule, tendons, musculature).

Chiropractic adjustment is the phrase typically favored by DCs to characterize specificity in segmental and neurologic terms as opposed to manipulation to reduce simple joint restriction. In great measure, these traditional distinctions are academic because thrust applied for the purpose of influencing joint movement may affect proprioceptive and other reflex activities and vice versa.

14. What conditions respond to chiropractic interventions?

Acute, subacute, and chronic low back pain as well as neck pain and certain types of head pain are favorably influenced by spinal manipulation.[10,11] Chiropractors report that they often diagnose and manage joint dysfunction, headaches, degenerative joint disease, muscular strains, spinal disc problems, myofascitis, radiculopathies, spinal curvatures, tendinitis/tenosynovitis, and peripheral neuralgias. They also report that patients with tumors, infectious disease, hereditary disease, and other systemic disorders are never or rarely evaluated and managed in their practices. About two-thirds of diagnoses recorded in DCs' practices are for musculoskeletal problems.[7]

15. What are the benefits of spinal manipulation?

Chiropractic services are the most frequently used of the complementary and alternative medicine approaches.[12] Among outcomes assessed in manipulation studies, pain level, physical function, and patient satisfaction have rated highly. Actuarial reviews have consistently indicated that chiropractic care is somewhat less expensive or similar to medical care for treatment of injury-related conditions.[13] However, the sophistication of research design in much of the literature to date cannot definitively distinguish which effects may be directly attributed to spinal manipulation vs. other concurrent management strategies used by chiropractors.

16. What is the "pop" that one often hears when a joint is manipulated?

When a synovial joint is moved from its physiological joint range into its paraphysiologic joint range, a negative pressure develops within the joint. In many instances, this negative pressure can create a cavitation where gaseous molecules (most likely CO_2) temporarily come out of solution in synovial fluid. This can be associated with a an audible "pop" sound (what is experienced when one "cracks" one's knuckles for example). Studies have verified radiographically that an intra-articular gas bubble develops and remains visible for 15-20 minutes. During this "refractory" period the joint will not cavitate again, and after cavitation, an increased range of motion has been documented. This range of motion increase appears to persist beyond the refractory period.[14]

17. What are the potential complications of manipulation?

Manipulation can have side effects, but serious complications are extremely rare. In more than 50 randomized clinical trials of manipulation, including about 2500 subjects, no serious complication has been reported.[11] A literature review performed by RAND (a health care think-tank) identified 118 cases of serious complications from cervical spinal manipulation reported in the English literature, including 21 fatalities and 51 major impairments. The other 42 reported serious complications resolved favorably.[7] Complications from lumbar manipulation are much rarer, with only 29 cases reported since 1911. Serious complications include vertebrobasilar and cerebral reactions, disc herniation, and cauda equina syndrome. Half of the cases of cauda equine reported in the literature resulted from lumbar manipulation under anesthesia, which is rarely performed and usually not by chiropractors.[15]

RAND estimated the rates of serious complications as 5–10 in 10 million manipulations for vertebrobasilar reactions, 3–6 in 10 million for major impairment, < 3 fatalities per 10 million manipulations, and about 1 per 100 million complications involving the cauda equina.[10] At the high end, occurrences have been estimated to be 1 in 400,000–500,000. Other estimates indicate 1 per 1.3–2 million manipulations.[16] Strategies to minimize risk have been developed in chiropractic and are standard within the profession, including the identification of appropriate clinical indications, appropriate patient selection and appropriate expertise. To help put the issue in perspective, the most common comparable medical treatment for routine musculoskeletal conditions typically seen by chiropractors is the prescription of nonsteroidal anti-inflammatory drugs (NSAIDs). Complications from NSAIDs have been documented at 0.04% fatality rate (accounting for 3200 deaths annually)[17] and a 2.74% rate of serious gastrointestinal events.[18] These complications account for 20,000 hospitalizations annually.

18. Does manipulation have any side effects?

Nearly half of all patients who experience side effects usually have local discomfort, headache, or tiredness with onset within 4 hours of the procedure. Some 15% describe effects as "severe" in intensity, but most disappear within 24 hours. Side effects do not appear to have an age-dependency, although a slightly higher incidence may exist among women.[19]

19. Is chiropractic covered by insurance?

Insurance covers at least a portion of chiropractic costs for most Americans (see table below). Chiropractic services are covered by most employer-sponsored health plans, and many states have passed regulations governing insurance equality for services of chiropractors. Although insurance plans may not be required to cover chiropractic, most employer-sponsored plans still do, with the exception of health maintenance organizations. Some plans cover radiology services, some limit total visits to 12 or 20 per year, and some require referral from a medical physician gatekeeper. Medicare first incorporated a chiropractic benefit in 1972. Chiropractic physicians are explicitly recognized by regulation or statute as "attending providers" (i.e., providers whom workers may access directly and who can oversee management of the case) in the workers compensation systems of 39 states and the District of Columbia.[16]

Payment for Chiropractic Services by Source

PAYMENT SOURCE	ACA (1996) SURVEY[1] (% INCOME)	RAND (1998) STUDY[2] (% PATIENTS)	NBCE (2000) SURVEY[3] (% PATIENTS)
Direct payments from patients (cash)	27.7	20.9	24.1
Private insurance (indemnity)	28.6	41.8	23.1
Auto insurance	14.5	9.8	16.7
Workers' compensation	10.8	10.4	9.6
Medicare	8.4	7.3	10.7
Prepaid/managed care	8.6	3.7	14.0
Medicaid	1.2	1.5	1.8
Other	0.9	2.3	0.0

[1] Goertz C: Summary of 1995 ACA annual statistical survey on chiropractic practice. J Am Chiropr Assoc 33(6):35-41, 1996.
[2] Hurwitz EL, Coulter ID, Adams AH, et al: Utilization of chiropractic services in the United States and Canada: 1985-1991. Am J Publ Health 88:771-776, 1998.
[3] Christensen MG, Kerkhoff D, Kollasch MW (eds): Job Analysis of Chiropractic: A Project Report, Survey Analysis and Summary of the Practice of Chiropractic in the United States. Greeley, CO, National Board of Chiropractic Examiners, 2000.

20. What distinguishes chiropractic methods from other manual medicine approaches?

Mobilization and manipulation are approaches sometimes used by other practitioners, including physical therapists and osteopathic physicians and some medical physicians. However, well over

90% of spinal manipulation care in the U.S. is provided by chiropractors. Key differences may exist in techniques and how manipulation is incorporated into overall patient management. Typically, manual medicine and physical therapy approaches to manipulation focus predominantly on joint pain and restriction findings. In contrast, chiropractors may factor more global clinical presentations and reflex effects into overall management strategies.[1] Although specific joint signs and symptoms may factor into how manipulative thrust is applied in chiropractic settings, other factors may be more prominent in determining where to apply manipulation as well as the frequency and duration of interventions.

For example, regardless of how restricted an individual joint might be, the decision as to which segment or region should be manipulated may be based on pain radiation patterns, tautness of paraspinal muscle regions and how they are enervated, biomechanical function of affected joints compared with adjacent areas, and mechanics involved in initial onset. Thus, the regions manipulated by chiropractors may not directly correspond to the symptomatic region or to the area that a nonchiropractor may feel is the site of the manipulable lesion. In addition, many unique features are associated with chiropractic techniques, including how patients are positioned, the kinds of equipment used (e.g., specialized adjusting table and instruments that administer thrust), and characteristics of prestressing joints and thrust.

21. Why do procedures vary among different chiropractors?

Chiropractic treatments may vary somewhat by geographic region because of differences in state or provincial laws as well as individual practice preferences. Despite this variation, chiropractors report substantial consistency in the procedures that they use. More than 90% of 4000 chiropractors from a random national sample indicated that they use standard high-velocity manipulation procedures (e.g,. diversified technique) for spinal and extremity joints. Two-thirds indicated that they use some kind of a mechanically assisted technique (e.g,. special instruments or tables that assist with patient positioning and/or administration of manipulative procedures). Eighty to 90% also report inclusion of therapeutic exercise and rehabilitation methods, thermal therapy, myofascial work, nutritional counseling, activities of daily living counseling, and bracing and supporting.[3] Variation in chiropractic practice results from numerous factors, including patient preferences and tolerances, nature and severity of conditions, practitioner training, and frequency and duration of care.

22. What research has been done on chiropractic methods?

Spinal manipulation is a well-studied intervention. Its evidence base includes long-term clinical experience, observational studies, randomized clinical trials, meta-analyses and systematic literature reviews, formal expert consensus panels, and government reports and guidelines. Manipulation has been compared with placebos, exercise and advice, no treatment (natural progression), back school, analgesics and NSAIDs, infrared, shortwave diathermy, ultrasound, flexion exercises, massage, electrical stimulation, and various combinations of these. In general, some 39 randomized clinical trials have evaluated spinal manipulation for low back pain. At least 26 favored manipulation (including 8 of the 10 best designed studies), and 13 found outcomes from manipulation comparable to other treatments. There have been at least 18 randomized trials for manipulation with head and neck pain complaints. Nine favored manipulation, and eight found manipulation equal to other treatments.[11]

Most trials and reviews conducted to date favored manipulation; no studies report that any comparable treatments work better than manipulation.[11,20] Far fewer studies have considered manipulation for nonmusculoskeletal disorders, but among the few available studies evidence favoring benefit has been much less robust. Among the better-designed studies are comparisons of manipulation with usual care for primary dysmenorrhea, chronic pelvic pain, childhood asthma, and hypertension.[21,22] The primary outcomes of all studies have been essentially equivocal in terms of nontreatment or random treatment groups. Some benefit with reduced medication use was reported in the asthma study.

23. Can children benefit from chiropractic care?

Despite some controversy, chiropractors have long been involved in pediatric care, and some practitioners emphasize pediatric care as a specialty. Chiropractic literature and training emphasize the special needs of children. However, effectiveness studies of manipulation interventions in pediatric populations are uncommon as in other biomedical research settings. For the most part, case studies and case series reports predominate.[23] Otitis media is an example of a common pediatric condition addressed by chiropractors. Practitioners have frequently encouraged conservative management strategies over routine use of antibiotics, suggesting that manual manipulation and soft tissue procedures in the cervical spine region may help facilitate drainage through the eustachian tube. Observational studies and expert panels have resulted in guidelines for chiropractic conservative care and monitoring.

24. Can the elderly benefit from chiropractic care?

Older patients may make up approximately 15% of chiropractic patient populations. Of patients between 65 and 75 years of age, 14% report using chiropractic services, but the percentage declines to 6% among those over the age of 75. However, access issues may account for the decline. Regional variation is significant, and one study examining two rural Midwestern communities found that two-thirds of people over the age of 65 used chiropractic care.[24] That number increases substantially among men over 70 years old. Overall, chiropractic utilization by the elderly mirrors that of the general population. Those that use chiropractic services tend to be in good health and less likely to use nursing home or hospital services; they use fewer prescription drugs but more over-the-counter medications.[25]

Research specifically in elderly populations has not been conducted, and care in extrapolation of results in younger populations is warranted. However, considerations about elderly patients that are relevant to all providers apply to chiropractic settings as well. For example, multiple medications can be a source of masked treatment effects, healing times prolong with age, and access to care locations may be challenging. In one study[25] involving a small group of self-selected chiropractic patients within a large trial of a comprehensive home-based geriatric assessment, follow-up, and health promotion program, the chiropractic group was less likely to be hospitalized, to have used a nursing home, or to use prescription drugs but more likely to report better health status, to exercise vigorously, and to be more mobile in the community.

Manipulation techniques can be modified to suit the exigencies and tolerances of patients and other specific considerations. For example, lower force and soft tissue techniques may be preferable in severe osteoporosis or in acutely inflamed regions.

25. How does one find a good chiropractor?

The simplest answer is the same way one finds any good doctor. As with other health care practitioners, expertise, personality, practice style, and availability can factor into deciding how to find a chiropractor. Different patients may have different needs and preferences that affect the relative effectiveness of one practitioner compared with another. Recommendations of friends or family members are often the most ready source of information. Internal medicine specialists are one of the more common interdisciplinary referral sources reported by chiropractors. Therefore, asking internists or family practitioners for recommendations may be a good starting place.

Obtaining a list of practitioners in the community from a state licensing board is also a starting point. One can inquire about complaints or disciplinary actions. In general, in looking to establish an interreferral relationship, it may be worthwhile to meet with and interview a number of chiropractors to get a sense of their educational background and practice style. Asking questions such as "How do you determine how much care someone needs?" and "How do you work and communicate with other providers?" can provide insight into clinical styles and preferences that can be compared with your own. Will the chiropractor provide written reports and updates of findings, recommendations, and progress? In addition, asking chiropractors what they do when patient progress is slower than expected and what they do to cultivate a patient's own self-reliance may be important issues.

Last but not least, the extent to which the chiropractor takes care of his or her own health may be an important consideration. Because much of chiropractic care is about increasing the patient's knowledge and behavior modification for self-care and prevention, it seems reasonable to expect the chiropractor to live by the same standards. If the chiropractor's knowledge does not lead to appropriate personal behaviors, it seems difficult to believe that it will do so for the patient.

26. Summarize the philosophy of chiropractic.

Apart from its specialized therapies, chiropractic is distinguishable by certain philosophical positions that contrast with medicine but are in harmony with other CAM modalities. These positions affect the way in which chiropractors perceive health and health care. Traditionally chiropractic combined five dominant metaphysical positions:

1. Vitalism, which postulates that the body has inherent capacities to heal itself (which Palmer termed the body's innate intelligence).

2. Preference for "natural remedies" (e.g., the hands).

3. Holism (treatment of the whole person, not merely the symptoms)

4. Humanism (recognizing the dignity of the patient)

5. Therapeutic conservatism (belief that, because the body has a substantial capacity for self-healing, the best care may often be the least care)

6. Critical rationalism (the belief that science and scientific investigation provide the best foundation for a health practice; shared with medicine)

These principles, in turn, give rise to a philosophy of health and health care. Health is the natural state, and the tendency of the body is to restore that state. The role of the provider is to facilitate the healing process. Health is seen as the expression of the body, mind, and spirit. The role of the provider is as much about educating as it is about treating. Because health is unique for each individual, care is highly personalized. In this approach health comes from within the patient and is not given by the provider. Chiropractic makes a distinction between disease and "dis-ease" and assumes that health is not simply an absence of disease. It also postulates that treatment (focused on the condition) is not the same as care (focused on the person).

The extent to which these philosophical distinctions make a difference in outcomes is not known, but they clearly color the health encounter. Some patients select CAM therapy on the basis of philosophical positions such as postmodernist values. An increasing body of qualitative research indicates that patients view the chiropractic encounter as quite distinct from a medical encounter.[26]

REFERENCES

1. Mootz RD, Haldeman S: The evolving role of chiropractic within mainstream health care. Top Clin Chiropr 2(2):11–21, 1995.

2. Coulter I, Adams A, Coggan P, et al: A comparative study of chiropractic and medical education. Altern Ther Health Med. 4(5):64–75, 1998.

3. Christensen MG, Kerkhoff D, Kollasch MW (eds): Job Analysis of Chiropractic: A Project Report, Survey Analysis and Summary of the Practice of Chiropractic in the United States. Greeley, CO, National Board of Chiropractic Examiners, 2000.

4. Hansen DT: Psychosocial predictors in spine care. Top Clin Chiropr 6(2):38–50, 1999.

5. Souza TA: Differential Diagnosis and Management for the Chiropractor: An Algorithmic Approach, 2nd ed. Gaithersburg, MD, Aspen, 2001.

6. Osterbauer P: Technology assessment of the chiropractic subluxation. Top Clin Chiropr 3(1):1–9, 1996.

7. Hurwitz EL, Coulter ID, Adams AH, et al: Utilization of chiropractic services in the United States and Canada: 1985–1991. Am J Publ Health 88:771–776, 1998.

8. Mootz RD, Hoffman LE, Hansen DT: Optimizing clinical use of radiography and minimizing radiation exposure in chiropractic practice. Top Clin Chirop 4(1):34–44, 1997.

9. Mootz RD, Hansen DT, Souza TA, et al: Application of incremental change strategies in chiropractic and multidisciplinary clinical settings for quality improvement. Qual Manage Health Care 8(3):42–64, 2000.

10. Coulter ID, Hurwitz EL, Adams AH, et al: The Appropriateness of Manipulation and Mobilization of the Cervical Spine. Santa Monica, RAND, MR-781-CCR, 1996.

11. Meeker WC: Effectiveness and safety of spinal manipulation for low back pain, neck and head pain. In Faass N (ed): Integrating Complimentary Medicine Into Health Systems. Gaithersburg, MD, Aspen, 2001.

12. Eisenberg DM, Davis RB, Ettner SL, et al: Trends in alternative medicine use in the United States, 1990–1997: Results of a follow-up national survey. JAMA 280:1569–1575, 1998.

13. Branson R: Cost comparison of chiropractic and medical treatment of common musculoskeletal disorders: A review of literature after 1980. Top Clin Chiropr 6(2):57–68, 1999.

14. Brodeur R: The audible release associated with joint manipulation. J Manip Physiol Ther 18(3):155–164, 1995.

15. Assendelft WJ, Bouter LM, Knipschild PG: Complications of spinal manipulation: A comprehensive review of the literature. J Fam Pract 42:475–480, 1996.

16. Cherkin DC, Mootz RD (eds):Chiropractic in the United States: Training, Practice and Research. AHCPR Pub No. 98-N002. Rockville, MD, Agency for Health Care Policy and Research, Public Health Service, US. Depart,emt of Health and Human Services, 1997.

17. Fries JF: Assessing and understanding patient risk. Scand J Rheumatol Suppl 92:21–24, 1992.
18. Gabriel SE, Jaakkimainen L, Bombardier C: Risk for serious gastrointestinal complications related to use of nonsteroidal anti-inflammatory drugs: A meta-analysis. Ann Intern Med 115:787–796, 1991.
19. Senstad O, Leboeuf-Yde C, Borchgrevink C: Frequency and characteristics of side effects of spinal manipulative therapy. Spine 22:435–440,, 1997.
20. Shekelle PG, Adams AH, Chassin MR, et al: Spinal manipulation for low back pain. Ann Intern Med 81:439–442, 1992.
21. Balon J, Aker PD, Crowther ER, et al: A comparison of active and simulated chiropractic manipulation as adjunctive treatment for childhood asthma. N Engl J Med 339:1013–1320, 1998.
22. Hondras MA, Long CR, Brennan PC: Spinal manipulative therapy versus a low force mimic maneuver for women with primary dysmenorrhea: A randomized, observer-blinded, clinical trial. Pain 81(1–2):105–114, 1999.
23. Fallon JM: The role of chiropractic adjustment in the care and treatment of 332 children with otitis media. J Clin Chiropr Ped 2:167–172, 1998.
24. Lavsky-Shulan M, Wallace RB, Kohout FJ, et al: Prevalence and functional correlates of low back pain in the elderly: The Iowa 65+ Rural Health Study. J Am Geriatr Soc 33:23–28, 1985.
25. Coulter ID, Hurwitz EL, Aronow HU, et al: Chiropractic patients in a comprehensive home-based geriatric assessment, follow-up and health promotion program. Top Clin Chiropr 3(2):46–55, 1996.
26. Coulter I, Adams A, Coggan P, et al: A comparative study of chiropractic and medical education. Altern Ther Health Med 4(5):64–75, 1998.

17. MASSAGE

Seth McLaughlin

1. What is massage?

Massage is the manual manipulation of soft tissues. The target tissues and techniques used to address them vary with each of the major methods of massage. Swedish massage, however, forms the basis of modern western massage. The most common Swedish strokes are effleurage (stroking), pettrisage (kneading), and tapotement (percussion). Massage also commonly includes stretching and exercises.

2. How did massage develop?

Healing touch is one of the oldest and most instinctual methods of caring for injuries. In approximately 2600 B.C, Huang Ti discussed massage in *The Yellow Emperor's Classic of Internal Medicine*.[1] Massage has been prominently featured in China, Japan, Egypt, and Greece a well as among the ancient Mayan society in Central America and the Incas of South America.

Massage was popularized in the United States after two brothers, Charles F. Taylor and George H. Taylor, introduced the Swedish movement system in 1856. In the late 1800s, massage lost popularity, largely because of inconsistent training and overstated claims. Research in the early 1900s led to the development of many techniques still used today. From the 1960s to the present, massage has grown in popularity.[2] Acceptance of massage by the medical community has increased because of research by organizations such as the Touch Research Institute at the University of Miami.

3. How long does a massage take?

The appropriate length varies depending on the reason for the massage. A 10-minute seated massage may be used in the workplace to decrease stress and absenteeism and increase productivity. A typist, hair stylist, or other person whose work or hobby involves upper extremity motion, however, may need a full-hour massage to relieve injury from repetitive motion to the rhomboid muscles between the shoulder blades, the forearm flexors, and the forearm extensors.

4. How often should people get a massage?

Many people find monthly massage helpful for stress reduction. As with length of massage, frequency can be determined with the help of a qualified therapist. Severity of injury, financial constraints, and personal preference are among the common determinants of frequency. Most commonly, people with acute soft tissue injuries receive weekly massage until the injury resolves.

Many therapists teach clients to do self-massage or stretching. Daily self-massage may be helpful for some conditions, such as tennis elbow or carpal tunnel syndrome. For clients receiving massage, relaxation techniques, such as progressive relaxation or breath work, may be helpful.

5. Why is massage expensive?

Massage requires constant client contact. A therapist has a limited number of potential sessions each week. Because massage is highly physical work for the therapist, many therapists must further limit the number of treatments that they give. It is not uncommon for therapist's career to be limited by injury to the hands.

Massage prices vary with region, special qualifications, office location, and client load. Typically, prices range from $45–85 for a 1-hour massage. Massage tends to be more expensive at spas than with a private practitioner.

6. Is there anyone who should not have massage?

If a sponge bath is permissible, light stroking massage should not cause problems. Certainly, there are times when deep massage is contraindicated. Typically, contraindications are local. For example, massage should be avoided in cases of infectious skin disease, unhealed wounds, and blood clots; over varicose veins and directly over bruises; in acutely inflamed areas; at the sites of recent fractures; and over tumor sites. Deep work should be avoided in the proximity of an aneurysm and in the abdomen of a woman in her first trimester of pregnancy. General contraindications include conditions such as congestive heart failure with severe lymphedema, renal failure, or other organ failure.

Massage also may be contraindicated by client medications. A client who takes anticoagulants and experiences easy bruising should wait until the medication is regulated before having deep massage. Conversely, massage may alleviate the side effects of medications that stimulate sympathetic autonomic nervous system function.[2]

7. Describe the physical effects of massage.

Massage increases circulation, lymphatic flow, collagen synthesis, and digestive peristalsis. Through these effects, massage improves nutrient delivery and waste removal. Massage also may speed healing to injured tissues by increasing blood flow and collagen synthesis via deep transverse friction. By increasing peristalsis, massage can be used to improve some digestive complaints, such as constipation.

Perhaps the most common physical benefit sought by clients is interruption of the pain-spasm-pain cycle. After an injury, the splinting reflex initiates isometric contractions, which cause muscles surrounding the site to support the injured area by limiting movement. Although this reflex is helpful, if the contraction is sustained for a long period or is too strong, it may cause pain. This cycle may be especially harmful because the contraction decreases local circulation and may result in localized ischemia. The additional pain due to ischemia further reinforces the reflex to contract. Massage is effective at interrupting this cycle.[3]

8. What are the emotional benefits of massage?

Massage has been shown to reduce the levels of the stress hormone cortisol. By decreasing cortisol levels, massage may reduce the deleterious effects of stress on the body. Massage is associated with an increase in oxygen saturation of the blood. These effects combine to make massage an excellent adjunct therapy for many people who have emotional disorders.[4]

Many massage therapists have experienced a client who spontaneously bursts into either tears or laughter. If disassociation is one of the client's primary complaints, gentle nurturing massage may aid the client's reconnection with his or her body.[5]

Some methods of massage have been developed for working with clients who have emotional complaints. Examples include Rubenfield synergy, Rosen method, Phoenix Rising Yoga Therapy, integrative yoga therapy, somatosynthesis, somatoemotional release, SHEN physio-emotional release therapy, somatic experiencing, Hakomi integrative somatics, jin shin do, process scupressure, and Being In Movement.[6]

9. Is it possible to be hurt by a massage?

Yes. Little research has addressed massage-related injuries, but true injuries are usually mild and may include bruising or overstretching. More common than true injury is transient soreness on the day after a massage.

10. Should the client be sore on the day after a massage?

Soreness is common after techniques that work on fascia and other deep tissues.[7] If the client is prone to becoming sore easily, consider using heat to soften superficial layers before the massage. After a massage, ice may be used to further decrease soreness. Therapeutic bathing with Epsom salts (magnesium sulfate) also may decrease the risk of soreness after a massage through inhibition of troponin binding.[8]

The most important technique for decreasing soreness is communicating openly and clearly with the massage therapist before and during the massage. Because clients often seek out massage because of muscle tension, some discomfort is normal with most massage techniques. It should be a "this-hurts-so-good" kind of feeling. If it stops feeling good, talk to the therapist.

11. Why do massage therapists often tell clients to drink water after a massage?

When the therapist works into knotted muscles, waste products from inside the ischemic muscle knot are pushed into circulation. Lymphatic flow and venous return are increased. With these increases comes an increase in waste removal from target tissues. Extra water aids in flushing the system and may prevent a metabolic headache or soreness after the massage.

As clients relax, they tend to breathe with a larger percentage of effort from the diaphragm. This deep breathing may increase water loss from the lungs.[9] During a 1-hour massage, enough water may be lost to dehydrate the client slightly.

12. Of what are the knots in muscles composed?

Knots in muscles may be composed of a variety of substances. Some knots are trigger points, which are composed of muscles in spasm. These spasms decrease circulation to the area, leaving the area nutrient-starved and saturated in metabolic waste products. These points often refer pain to other areas when pressed. Sustained pressure often relieves the trigger point. Some physicians may also recommend trigger point injections.[10]

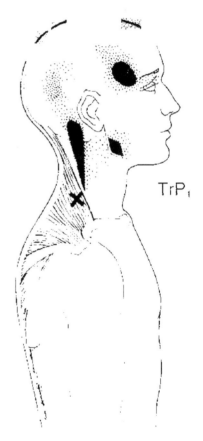

Trigger points (x) are areas of muscles in spasm and may refer to other areas (stippled/solid) when pressed. (From Simons DG, Travell JG, Simons LS: Travell and Simons' Myofascial Pain and Dysfunction: The Trigger Point Manual, Vol. 1: Upper Half of the Body. Baltimore, Williams & Wilkins, 1999, with permission.)

Fibromyalgia is associated with tender points (see diagram in Chapter 49). These points appear moth-eaten on histologic examination. Tissue breakdown is evident. Pain typically does not refer to other areas. Although trigger points are typically found in a tight band of muscle, fibromyalgia tender points tend to be in areas of decreased muscle tension. Tender points elicit diffuse localized pain, whereas trigger points elicit sharp local pain and usually refer pain to other locations in the body.[11]

A point that feels like a muscular knot also may contain calcium deposits. With damage to the periosteum, the bone may release calcium to protect the area. A common site for this type of injury is the heel. Plantar fasciitis causes increased tension on the periosteum of the calcaneus. The periosteum may release calcium, which results in a heel spur.[12]

13. What qualifications should I seek in a massage therapist?

If you are interested in massage for relaxation, the qualifications are brief. If you are in a state that requires licensure (see table at www.massagemag.com), your therapist should be licensed by the state. Usually, states allow the use of the title LMT to indicate that one has passed all of the requirements to become a licensed massage therapist. In other states, RMT refers to registered massage therapist. CMT refers to certified massage therapist; certification probably was given by the school from which the therapist graduated. In states where massage is not regulated on a statewide basis, counties or cities may have regulations of their own. In California, for example, requirements vary county by county. Whether or not your state requires a license, ask how many hours of education the potential therapist has had. If the number is less than 500 hours, the therapist does not meet the minimal number of hours suggested by the National Certification Board for Therapeutic Massage and Bodywork.

If you are interested in massage for treatment of an injury, more detailed schooling may be helpful. Numerous different advanced training programs are available for therapists. Particularly helpful are neuromuscular therapy (NMT), Rolfing, structural integration, and orthopedic massage. All of these programs prepare therapists to help with serious injuries. If your state that requires licensure, consider calling the state board of health or checking their website to verify licensure.

Membership in one of the national massage organizations may further indicate the therapist's quality. Therapists who join one of these organizations make a commitment to follow a code of ethics developed specifically for massage therapists. The three major massage organizations are the American Massage Therapy Association, Associated Bodywork and Massage Professionals, and the International Massage Association.

14. Does a massage client have to undress completely for a massage?

Seated massage is typically done with the client fully clothed. For table massage, the amount of clothing removed varies with the style of massage. Some people have their massage while still wearing underwear. However, it is rather difficult to practice Swedish massage if a client chooses to wear clothing during a massage because of limited access to the skin. That said, the client decides how much to undress, if at all. If a client is not comfortable during a massage, he or she will not be able to relax completely.

Many state laws address the issue of client modesty by requiring that massage therapists keep clients draped with a sheet, towel, or other covering. As the session progresses, the therapist uncovers the portion of the body that is to be massaged. When the therapist is finished massaging that portion, it is recovered with the drape.

15. What are the benefits of lubricants during a massage?

Lubricants allow the therapist's hands to glide smoothly over the skin or into the deep tissues instead of creating friction that may cause discomfort. Massage lubricants are typically either an oil or a cream. Both oils and creams may be effective as moisturizers for the skin. In addition, vegetable or nut oils are often high in antioxidants.

Many lubricants have additional ingredients to increase the effectiveness of the massage. Herbs such as kava kava, valerian root, St. John's wort, and calendula may be used to relax muscles and speed healing. Essential oils such as peppermint, eucalyptus, clary sage, and Roman chamomile may decrease pain. Homeopathic preparations such as *Arnica montana* may assist the therapist in treating acute conditions with swelling. Nutraceuticals such as HMB (calcium hydroxy gamma butyrate) may be used to modify catabolism and therefore decrease soreness. All of these additions to lubricants can increase benefits for the client.[13]

16. How is massage different than chiropractic therapy?

Chiropractic therapy seeks to decrease pain and improve function by improving skeletal alignment. Although schools of chiropractic therapy vary, most use quick motions to realign the spine. The effect on alignment makes chiropractic therapy a great ally of massage. Massage also improves alignment through relaxing tight muscles and thickened fascia that pull the body out of its proper position. The two techniques are complement ry. If a person receives chiropractic therapy for a problem that primarily involves soft tissues, the problem will probably reappear quickly. Conversely, if a client receives only massage but has poor skeletal alignment, soft tissue treatment may fail to provide adequate relief. Many clients find it beneficial to receive massage and chiropractic therapy on the same day fif both skeletal alignment and soft tissue discomfort are involved.

17. What are the benefits of infant massage?

Infant massage has been shown to facilitate the parent-infant bonding process in the development of warm, positive relationships; to reduce stress responses to painful procedures such as inoculations; to reduce pain associated with teething and constipation; to decrease colic; to induce sleep; to encourage weight gain; and to improve performance on developmental tasks for preterm infants.[14]

A massage therapist typically does not do infant massage. A certified infant massage instructor teaches parents to massage their child. They are often taught specific techniques for various ailments. Massage provides an especially good opportunity for parental bonding.

18. What clinical evidence supports massage for specific ailments?

The Touch Research Institute at the University of Miami has undertaken clinical studies of massage. They maintain a detailed list of abstracts at http://www.miami.edu/touch-research/.

Many of the conditions that may benefit from massage are not musculoskeletal disorders. The mood-altering effects of massage are well documented. For example, women diagnosed with anorexia nervosa were given a massage twice weekly for 5 weeks or standard treatment. The massaged women reported lower stress and anxiety levels and showed lower cortisol levels immediately after the massage. Over the 5-week treatment period, they also reported decreased body dissatisfaction on the Eating Disorder Inventory and increased levels of dopamine and norepinephrine.

Because massage affects so many body systems, it has the potential to be supportive in many disorders. Massage has been specifically studied and found to be helpful in the following situations: Alzheimer's disease-related agitation, anorexia nervosa, anxiety, asthma, attention deficit disorder, autism, back pain, breast cancer lymphedema, bulimia, cancer pain, chronic fatigue syndrome, cocaine addiction in infants, cognitive disorders, cystic fibrosis, depression, diabetes, fibromyalgia, headache, hypertension, immunology, juvenile rheumatoid arthritis, labor pain, multiple sclerosis, oxytocin production, preterm infants, psychiatric disorders, and stress.[15]

19. Why should you choose one type of massage over another?

Some clients seek a more gentle type of relaxation massage, whereas others choose deep myofascial therapy to correct a particular area of dysfunction. Culture also plays a large part in massage preference. Different styles of massage were developed in different areas. Shiatsu, Thai massage, tuina, and acupressure developed within traditional Chinese medicine. These techniques include work designed to stimulate energetic meridians. See table below for more information about different massage techniques.

Types of Massage/Bodywork

Alexander technique (technically not a massage modality): Through one-on-one lessons and postural guidance, clients learn to let go of muscle tightness, especially in the head and neck, and repattern their movements.

Craniosacral therapy (CST): Originally from osteopathy, CST is based on the craniosacral rhythm, created by the flow of cerebrospinal fluid in dura mater, which lines the inside of the cranium and vertebral column down to the sacrum. This craniosacral rhythm can be detected and gently treated by subtle movements of the 22 movable bones of the skull.

Lomilomi: This traditional Hawaiian massage uses a variety of techniques performed with hands, elbows, forearms, and feet. It also includes energy work.

Manual trigger point release: Sustained pressure is used to break the pain-spasm-pain cycle and relieve neuromuscular trigger points. After trigger point release, gentle stretching and movement help to keep trigger points from reforming. Advanced methods include Bonnie Prudden myotherapy, St. John neuromuscular therapy, or Judith (Walker) Delaney neuromuscular therapy.

Table continued on following page

Types of Massage/Bodywork (Continued)

Rolfing: This method of body work, also known as structural integration, consists of 10 basic sessions. Because Rolfing works with superficial and deep fascia, it may be uncomfortable. Because of its impressive results, it has become the foundation on which other systems have developed, such as Aston-patterning, postural integration, soma neuromuscular integration, CORE bodywork, and myofascial release.

Reflexology: Reflexology is based on the idea that the feet contain a map of the whole body. Massaging reflex points on the soles stimulates the corresponding organ and affects change throughout the body. Reflexology also may be performed on the hands or ears.

Shiatsu: Also known as acupressure, shiatsu uses the same points found in acupuncture. Instead of needles, finger pressure is applied to stimulate energy flow and healing in the meridians. Shiatsu tends to be more stimulating than relaxing.

Swedish massage: Swedish style is what most clients envision as massage. It is performed on a table, with oil applied to the body, in long, soothing strokes. It usually targets superficial tissues, promotes circulation, and tends to be relaxing.

Thai massage: This dynamic massage is performed with the client clothed. It is considered a cross between yoga and acupressure. The practitioner also performs deep stretching and manipulation. Thai massage is usually done on the floor.

Trager psychophysical integration: Trager method practitioners rhythmically rock, vibrate, and stretch the body in order to promote an effortless way of being. Clients are often taught movements to do at home to recreate the sensory state developed during work with a practitioner.

Adapted from Knaster M: Discovering the Body's Wisdom. New York, Bantam Books, 1996.

20. What is Rolfing?

Rolfing is a method of structural integration. It is a popular form of bodywork developed by Ida Rolf in the 1930s The goal of Rolfing is to organize the major segments of the body so that they are in a more vertical relationships with each other and with the field of gravity. It typically involves deep work on fascia to ensure adaptability of length elasticity and pliability of the connective tissue. Rolfers typically do not work on one specific area. They believe that work on the whole body is more effective than work on any specific portion. Rolfers work to ensure proper support. If an area is injured, they will work every area beneath it to ensure proper support. Similarly, Rolfers attempt to help their clients achieve dynamic balance. This balance occurs left to right, deep to superficial, and front to back.[16]

REFERENCES

1. Kamenetz HL: History of massage. In Rogoff JB (ed): Manipulation, Traction, and Massage, 2nd ed. Baltimore, Williams & Wilkins, 1980, pp 37–38.
2. Fritz S: Mosby's Fundamentals of Therapeutic Massage, 2nd ed. St. Louis, Mosby, 2000.
3. Juhan D: Job's Body: A Handbook for Bodywork [expanded edition]. Barrytown Ltd., Barrytown, NY, Barrytown Ltd., 1987, pp 329–334.
4. Fields T: J Bodywork Move Ther 4:31–38, 2000.
5. Nielse T: Massage Mag 60:114–117, 1996.
6. Knaster M: Discovering the Body's Wisdom. Bantam Books, New York, 1996.
7. Rolf IP: Rolfing: Reestablishing the Natural Alighnment and Structural Integration of the Human Body for Vitality and Well-Being. Rochester, VT, Healing Arts Press, 1989.
8. Fry CH, Hall SK: The role of magnesium in the regulation of muscle function. In Sigel H, Sigel A (eds): Metal Ions in Biological Systems, vol 26.. New York, Marcel Dekker: 1996 pp 464–486.
9. Tortora GJ, Grabowski SR: Principles of Anatomy and Physiology, 9th ed. New York, John Wiley & Sons, 2000, pp 775–817.
10. Finando D, Finando S: Informed Touch: A Clinician's Guide to the Evaluation and Treatment of Myofascial Disorders. Rochester, VT, Healing Arts Press, 1999, pp 25–26.
11. Smythe H. Fibrositis syndrome: A historical perspective. J Rheumatol 16(Suppl 19):2, 1989.
13. Werner R: A Massage Therapist's Guide to Pathology. Philadelphia, Lippincott Williams & Wilkins,1998.
13. Price L: Carrier Oils for Aromatherapy and Massage. New Baskerville, UK, Riverhead Publishers, 1999.
14. Field T: Massage therapy for infants and children [review].J Devel Behav Pediatr 16:105–111, 1995.
15. Field T: http://www.miami.edu/touch-research/ 2002.
16. LaRochelle C: The five principles of Rolfing. Holistic Health News, 1997.

18. BOTANICAL MEDICINE

Roberta Lee, M.D.

1. Are botanical medicines and herbal remedies new?

No. Botanical medicines and herbal remedies have been used for centuries and formed the basis for the beginnings of the pharmacologic treatment of diseases. In fact, folk healing methods of the Mediterranean region and the Orient were included in the first European herbal compendium, *De Materia Medica*, written by the Greek physician Dioscorides in the first Century A.D. In the Orient, use of numerous botanical medicines is recorded in one oldest Chinese medical text, *The Yellow Emperor's Inner Classic* (*Huang di nei jing*). This text, which was compiled by unknown authors between the years 200 B.C. and 100 A.D, sets forth the theories and philosophical foundations of traditional Chinese medicine (TCM), including the use of herbal remedies.

At present it is estimated that over 40% of prescription drugs sold in the U.S. contain at least one ingredient derived from a natural source.[1] Up to 25% of prescription drugs contain an ingredient derived from a flowering plant. Common examples include the use of the periwinkle (*Catharanthus roseus*) for chemotherapy and foxglove (*Digitalis* spp.) for production of cardiac glycosides.

2. How is the use of herbs in allopathic medicine different from traditional healing systems?

The difference is based largely in philosophy. In allopathic medicine, practitioners tend to view botanicals as "natural pharmaceuticals" or storehouses of phytochemicals. In healing traditions such as Ayurveda, TCM, and Native American herbalism, the practitioner prescribes herbs to support the systems of the body and to protect and enhance their functions. Whereas an allopathic practitioner may prescribe goldenseal to treat an infection (substituting an herb for a drug), a traditional herbalist may prescribe a combination of immune-supporting and detoxifying herbs for the same infection.

A traditional herbalist may combine many herbs in one formula, whereas the allopathic practitioner, who values specificity, usually prescribes only one herb in as concentrated and purified a form as possible. This trend is evidenced by the current movement in herbal medicines toward extraction and standardization of herbal products. This practice is helpful, perhaps even crucial, to the allopathic model of medicine. It does, however, give us a good insight into how far we have diverged from a holistic traditional view of herbal healing practices.

3. How prevalent is the use of botanical medicine?

Although a long history of botanical use has been well established, it was generally considered by most conventional health care providers to be insignificant until studies done in the 1990s revealed that approximately one of three people had used some form of alternative medical therapy (including botanical products) in the past year. In the first study by Eisenberg, botanical medicine was the sixth most common alternative therapy. By 1997, botanical medicine had become the second most common alternative.[2,3] Furthermore,6 0 million people were noted to use herbal products each year, spending over $3.4 billion.[4] It is estimated that in 2000 retail sales of herbal supplements in all channels of trade were slightly over 4 billion dollars.[5]

4. What makes the study of botanicals more complex than the study of pharmaceuticals?

Because there are often several species and families of herbs, familiarity with the specific Latin name may be helpful. For example, there are various species of ginseng: *Panax ginseng*, also known as Chinese or Korean ginseng; *Panax quinquefolius*, known as American ginseng; and several lesser known subtypes (e.g., *P. notoginseng*, *P. pseudoginseng*). Siberian ginseng, while of the same botanical family (Araliaceae) as other ginsengs, is not a true ginseng but a related plant species, *Eleutherococcus senticosus*, which is valued for its adaptogenic rather than stimulating properties.

To add to the complexity, different parts of a plant may be used for medicinal purposes.The aerial (above-ground) parts of the flowering plant *Echinacea purpurea* are often are expressed as a fresh-pressed juice, whereas the roots of *E. angustifolia* are harvested. Both are used for immunos-timulating properties. Ambient temperature, seasonal rainfall, and soil conditions may play a role in a plant's particular chemical composition. Plant harvesting and manufacturing processes may also affect herbal efficacy. For example, stinging nettles seems to work best as a freeze-dried preparation that preserves its "sting"; it is relatively ineffective as a tincture. All in all, many factors make the study of botanicals inherently different from the study of pharmaceuticals.

5. Are botanical products considered drugs?

The word "drug" comes from the Old Dutch word *drogge*, which means "to dry," because most pharmacists,and other healers dried plants for use as medicines.[6] The status of supplements and botan-ical products was unclear—at least from a legal standpoint—until 1994. In the United States, under the Dietary Supplement Health and Education Act of 1994 (DSHEA), botanical products are legally recognized as " dietary supplements," not as drugs, and thus do not fall under the scrutiny of the Food and Drug Administration (FDA). The DSHEA defines botanical products as plants "containing com-binations of many numerous naturally occurring plant chemicals; herbs generally act in a wider, more general, less specific way than most single ingredient pharmaceutical drugs. Their actions are more gentle than conventional medicine and work usually in more long-term situations."[7] With this defini-tion came the restriction that product labels can claim only general physiologic or therapeutic effects rather than efficacy for a specific disease or health-related condition. DSHEA asserted that "unlike many drugs, the role of herbal dietary supplements is to enhance the diet by adding safe and natural plants and their constituents to support and protect bodily functions and processes."

Despite this assertion, growing evidence in medical journals reveals that many plants have pow-erful pharmacologic action. But the physiologic activity of many herbals is not so simple as that of conventional pharmaceuticals. A single plant can contain hundreds of biologically active compounds that can work individually or synergistically. Furthermore, these groups of compounds create more than one physiologic effect.

6. Why are studies of herbal medications so limited?

Herbs have been traditionally used in Europe for centuries, and some governments (such as Germany) actively support herbal research. Indeed, many of the first-line "drugs" used in Europe are botanicals (e.g., ginkgo, saw palmetto, St. John's wort). In the U.S., funding for herbal studies is dif-ficult because most herbal preparations cannot be patented. Large randomized clinical trials are ex-pensive, and most herbal companies do not have the resources to fund such trials. On average, it takes about $500 million dollars to develop and patent a new drug through the FDA.[8] Pharmaceutical companies are reluctant to fund botanical trials because they cannot recover the costs with products that cannot be patented. In addition, herbal products may be perceived as competition for patented prescription medications.

7. Do botanical medicines interact with prescription medications?

Yes. Some herbal compounds are known to interact with prescription medications. For example, in 2001 an article in the *Journal of the American Medical Association* noted that St. John's wort and other medications metabolized by a particular liver enzyme (cytochrome P450) affect levels of some HIV medications (indinavir), immune suppressants (cyclosporine), and estrogens (esthinyl estra-diol).[9] The dilemma for health care professionals and people using botanical products is access to accurate information—especially because few professionals receive training in the use of botanical products. (See Chapter 61.)

8. What is the difference in quality between botanical products and prescription medications?

At present, adherence to "good manufacturing practices" (GMPs) by supplement manufacturers is not mandated by any governmental body or supervisory third party; it is the responsibility of the man-ufacturers themselves. A GMP herbal product contains only the ingredients identified on the label (not adulterated), and if an active ingredient is identified, the product contains the specific amount that it claims. In addition, the herbal product should contain the correct plant parts, appropriately harvested at the correct time and processed in the manner necessary to sustain efficacy.[10] Companies with limited funds may curtail some aspects of quality production to save money. Let the buyer beware! Furthermore, standardized regulations for testing pesticides or heavy metals is lacking. Random testing has revealed that these issues are more common than one would like to think. The largest study to date showed that 24% of approximately 2600 samples collected in Taiwan contained at least one adulterant, including caffeine, indomethacin, hydrochlorothiazide, theophylline and steroids.[11]

9. In what forms are botanical products available?

Herbs or botanical products can be prepared as tinctures, liquid or solid extracts, capsules, tablets, lozenges, teas, decoctions, vapor treatments, poultices, compresses, or bath products. Others can be rubbed into the skin as salves, creams, or oils.

Tinctures. An herb placed in alcohol or glycerin is a tincture or liquid extract. The alcohol is used to draw out the plant's active properties (both lipophilic and otherwise), helping to concentrate and preserve the contents. A tincture has more alcohol than an extract. Liquid extracts are more concentrated and therefore more cost-effective. Both may be taken as drops in tea or diluted in warm water. If the mixture is left to stand for 5 minutes, a substantial amount of alcohol will evaporate.

Glycerites. An alternative to an alcohol extract is a liquid glycerin extract called glycerite. This form may be preferable for people who need to avoid even minute amounts of alcohol. The glycerin is processed by the body as fat, not sugar.[12] In general, glycerin products have a shorter shelf life than alcohol-based products (2 years or less). Ingestion of more than 1 ounce (30 ml) of glycerin can have a laxative effect. In general, glycerin extracts should contain 60% glycerin with 40% water to ensure preservation. Some plants that contain resins or gums may not do well in a glycerin extraction and may be isolated more efficiently in alcohol.

Solid extracts. Solid extracts are derived from concentrated liquid extracts from which the alcohol or water has been removed. Capsules and tablets contain the ground or powdered herb. These preparations may have a large amount of filler, such as soy or millet powder. Fillers may be included to add bulk, to ensure disbursement, or to stabilize the active constituents. Tablets may also contain a binder such as magnesium stearate or dicalcium phosphate. Binders increase water absorption and facilitate breakdown in the body. One of the disadvantages of capsules and tablets is that fillers can make the identification an herb difficult by masking its true color or odor.

Teas. Teas are used for a wide range of purposes. Teas come in two forms: decoctions and infusions. To make a decoction, the herb is placed in boiling water and cooked for 10–15 minutes. This method is preferred for denser plant materials such as roots, barks, or berries. To make an infusion, the dried herb is added to hot water and allowed to steep for 3–5 minutes. Brewing a cup of chamomile tea is an example of making an infusion. A general rule for using fresh vs. dried plant material is that three parts of fresh herb are equivalent to one part of dried herbs.

Poultices and compresses. Poultices are produced from crushed herbs that have been made into a paste. The poultice is usually applied directly to the affected area, and cloth or gauze is used to keep the mixture on the skin. Compresses are also made for direct application on the skin. Making a compress involves soaking a cloth in a strong tea, tincture, glycerite, or oil. Potentially toxic in their concentrated form, essential oils must be diluted before use on the skin.

10. What is a standardized extract?

A standardized extract is a botanical preparation that has been concentrated through the use of a solvent and then either dried (solid extract) or reconstituted by the addition of glycerin or alcohol (liquid extract). In either case, a particular constituent(s) in the plant has been measured, and the extract has been tested chemically and is guaranteed to contain the stated amount(s) of each constituent. In addition, if the activity of the preparation is not high enough, concentrated amounts of the constituents are added to guarantee appropriate activity.

On the positive side, the consumer can feel confident that the product has the desired amount of compounds known to be active in the herb. On the negative side, because the pharmacologic activity of most plants is complex and involves a variety of different compounds and even different families of compounds, altering the native ratio of the constituents may alter the natural activity of the plant. In addition, it may not be known for sure that the "active ingredients" concentrated and/or standardized are in fact the ingredients responsible for the herb's efficacy. Some plants have been found in subsequent studies to be standardized to a compound no longer believed to be the strongest active ingredient (e.g.. hyperforin vs. hypericum in St. John's wort).[13] As another example, the active ingredient(s) in saw palmetto is still not known; thus, saw palmetto is standardized simply to contain 80–90% fatty sterols.

11. What are the major criticisms of standardized extracts?

Some botanical experts believe that inclusion of all compounds in the plant (called a whole-plant product) represents the optimal proportions that nature intended for medicinal use. In other words, concentrating the plant and increasing one or two compounds may disrupt or deter the effectiveness of the herb. In a less technological era, guaranteeing that the extract was standardized involved strict attention to the timing of harvesting as well as use of the proper plant parts and their processing. When these products were made by herbalists, the quality was judged by smell, taste, and effect. Today, because much of the plant cultivation is mechanized and industrialized, the timing of harvesting and processing may be altered in such a way that some of the quality is lost.

What is the best way to achieve the most from both worlds? In addition to seeking standardized products, read about the companies that manufacture the products. Know the actions of the botanical products that you use, and learn which specific plants are used (the Latin name or Latin binomial) and which parts create the desired effect. Buy organic herbs, if possible. Consider looking for companies that employ a knowledgeable herbalist or botanist in the manufacturing process.

12. When is it appropriate to use an herbal product instead of a pharmaceutical product?

In general, an integrative approach recommends initial use of treatments that are less invasive and have fewer side effects. For example, herbal anti-inflammatories may be recommended before nonsteroidal anti-inflammatory drugs for chronic joint pain. Because of the time required for most botanical products to become effective, it is best not to use herbs for conditions that require urgent management. Furthermore, for serious health conditions, it is a good idea to consult with a health care provider—especially because herbs may take a longer time to show effects (up to 2 months). Otherwise, herbal products can be useful for many symptoms and conditions, such as gastroesophageal disease, depression, and hepatitis (see chapters about specific diagnoses).

Side effects can be seen with herbal products just as with medicines and common foods. Common side effects include allergic reactions (hives, scratchy throat, headaches), throat irritation (*Echinacea augustifolia*), upset stomach (especially cayenne pepper and garlic), and headaches (valerian). In most cases, stopping the herb for a few days until the symptoms clear and trying a lower dose will identify true allergies. In other cases, it may take several weeks or months of use to develop an allergy.

13. Do botanical products cross-react with drugs?

Most herbal preparations are gentle, but they do have pharmacologic effects. In general, it is advisable to watch the timing of the intake of spicy herbs such as ginger or cayenne if the patient is taking prescription medications. These herbs can dilate blood vessels and thus increase absorption.[14] Patients taking digoxin or other heart medications should avoid herbal tonics such as hawthorn unless they are taken under the supervision of a qualified health care provider.[15] Patients taking heart medications or antidepressants such as fluoxetine, sertraline, or paroxetine should be careful with caffeine-containing herbs (e.g., guarana, green tea, maté tea, kola nut) or stimulating herbs such as damiana or ephedra (ma huang). Patients with hypertension should avoid licorice and Asian ginseng, which can elevate blood pressure.[16] For more possible side effects, please consult a credible source with updated drug-herb interactions (see question 21). One disadvantage of these publications is that they frequently list theoretical, unproved interactions and therefore may less useful for clinical applications. For example, echinacea has known immune-boosting properties but is commonly listed as contraindicated in systemic lupus erythematosus because of theoretical concerns that it may exacerbate autoimmune disorders, even though this effect is not seen clinically.

14. Are herbs safe because they are natural?

In general, herbs are safer because they are less concentrated, but not all herbs are safe. Three of the best known problem herbs are comfrey, chaparral, and ephedra. Comfrey has been shown to have alkaloid compounds that, when ingested, cause liver damage.[17] The herb also has been implicated as a cause of liver and bladder cancer. However, it is highly effective as a topical remedy for wound healing. Chaparral is a desert shrub used as a cold and flu remedy. From the late 1950s to the 1970s it was used in the fight against cancer, but later it was linked to serious liver damage requiring liver transplantation.[18]

Ephedra, or ma huang, popular as a decongestant and used in TCM formulas, contains a potent alkaloid called ephedrine. It has the ability to give an extra jolt of energy and for this reason is included in many natural botanical products for weight loss and energy boosting. Sensitive people may experience heart palpitations, nervousness, anxiety, and disturbed sleep. Of 140 reports of adverse effects of over-the-counter ephedra products studied by the FDA, half of the cases involved cardiovascular symptoms, about 20% involved central nervous system symptoms, and 10 cases resulted in death.[19]

As is often the case with pharmaceutical medications, overuse, abuse, and misuse of botanical products can lead to harmful effects.

15. What are the top ten selling herbs in the U.S. health food stores?[20]

Ginkgo biloba	Saw palmetto
St. John's wort	Kava kava
Ginseng	Horse chestnut seed extract
Garlic	Cranberry
Echinacea	Valerian root

16. For which conditions are herbs most commonly used?

Colds, burns, headaches, allergies, rashes, insomnia/stress, premenstrual syndrome, depression, diarrhea, and menopause.[21]

17. Can children take herbal medicines?

Yes—but it is best to work with a knowledgeable herbalist or pediatrician or family practice physician who can assist you with the dosing requirements. Little children are not "small adults." Some botanical preparations, such as ginseng, probably should not be used in children because they can affect hormonal secretion. Unfortunately, one of the hardest areas of study is the use of herbal remedies in children. Most academic centers find this area difficult to fund because of the inherent risk to children. In addition, glycerites are often used in herbal preparations for children for fear of exposure to the small quantities of alcohol in other extracts, but glycerin may not be as effective in concentrating some active botanical components.

18. How long should botanical products be used to judge their effectiveness?

It depends on the half-life of the active ingredients. In general, because of the smaller doses and less concentrated nature of botanical preparations, it seems reasonable to allow several months before reassessing the therapeutic effects. As with all medications, some botanicals have a more rapid effect. For example, kava (*Piper methysicum*) produces relaxing effects within hours, and stinging nettles (*Urtica dioica*) may relieved allergic symptoms as quickly. However, a few months may be required to see the full effects of saw palmetto (*Serenoa repens*) for prostate hypertrophy or St. John's wort (*Hypericum perforatum*) for minor depression.

19. What is the story on red yeast rice? How is Cholestin related to lovastatin?

The story of Cholestin brings up the thorny side of botanicals as supplements under DSHEA. Cholestin, a proprietary product, is made from a pulverized strain of rice (*Monascus purpureus*) that is fermented with red yeast and ground into a dark brick-colored powder and placed in capsules. The rice is imported from China, where it has been used for thousands of years as an herbal remedy for digestion and "relief of liver stasis."[22] Approximately 7 years ago, Pharmanex, a small nutraceutical company, marketed this product as an agent for reducing cholesterol. When tested, it was found to contain compounds (monacolin K) similar to those found in the drug lovastatin patented by Merck and Company (from the yeast found on the rice). It was shown in many clinical studies to lower cholesterol.[23]

The classification of Cholestin as a dietary supplement came under scrutiny by the FDA, which filed a legal challenge against Pharmanex. Over a 5-year period, in a test case of the DSHEA, Pharmanex argued that Cholestin should be considered a supplement because it is a naturally occurring ingredient in red yeast rice and has been used for thousands of years in a traditional setting. Furthermore, it was argued that the content of monacolin K (the ingredient that is synonymous with lovastatin) was only 0.2% that of the Merck product Mevacor. In 1998, Pharmanex won the right to continue production of Cholestin. Merck challenged the ruling. Merck and the FDA argued that Cholestin should be considered a drug because it had similar compounds to lovastatin and reduced cholesterol by similar pharmacologic effects on hepatic enzymes (HMG -CoA reductase). Therefore, it should be removed from the supplement market and subjected to rigorous testing and registered like its pharmaceutical counterpart as a new drug. In 2001, the FDA and Merck won their case against Pharmanex. The product was ordered by the court to be withdrawn from the supplement market.[24]

20. How can one verify the potency of a botanical preparation?

Often one cannot tell from the packaging whether an herbal product contains the indicated percentages of active components. This problem makes purchasing botanicals off the shelf a potential nightmare for consumers and health care providers alike. Many people rely on word of mouth, trust the GMP of the botanical company, or scout out information about products from consumer advocacy groups. Good advice is to look for standardized products with guarantees from the manufacturer. Another option is to contact the company that manufactured the product and request a certificate of analysis. Sometimes the certificates are sent to the store with the products (one per shipment). In this case, talking with a store representative and requesting to see the certificate of analysis may be useful.

Information from independent laboratory testing is available on a limited basis. Products can be tested at several places. One of the oldest and best known labs is Consumer Labs.com. Another independent testing site, sponsored by U.S. Pharmacopoeia, is still under development. The best way to identify a reputable independent laboratory testing site is to contact the American Herbal Products Association or the American Botanical Council, which regularly assess quality control information about botanical products.

21. What resources are available for more information about botanicals?

- American Botanical Council
  PO Box 201660
  Austin, TX 78720
  www.Herbalgram.org

- Herb Research Foundation
  1007 Pearl St, Suite 200
  Boulder, Co 80302
  http://herbs.org

Internet sources
- Herbmed: www.herbmed.org (has links to PubMed articles)
- National Institutes of Health Dietary Supplement Database: http://www.nal.usda.gof/fnic/IBIDS
- New York Botanical Garden: http://www.nybg.org
- PhytoNET (operated by the European Scientific Cooperative on Phytotherapy): www.escop.com
- U.S. Department of Agriculture Phytochemical and Ethnobotanical Databases: www.ars-grin.gov/duke

Periodicals
- Herb Quarterly
  Long Mountain Press
  Box 548
  Boiling Springs, PA 17007

- Journal of Ethnobotany
  Elsevier Science
  PO Box 945
  New York, NY 10159-0945

- HerbalGram (see American Botanical Council]

Reference guidelines for practitioners
- Blumenthal M, Busse W, Goldber A, et al (eds): The Complete German Commission E Monographs. Austin, TX, American Botanical Council, Boston Integrative Medicine Communications, 1998.

- Fetrow C, Avila J: The Complete Guide to Herbal Medicines New York, Simon & Shuster, 2000.
- Pizzorno J, Murray MT: Textbook of Natural Medicine, vols. 1 and 2, 2nd ed. Edinburgh, Churchill Livingstone, 1999.
- Shultz V, Hänsel R, Tyler V: Rational Phytotherapy: A Physician's Guide to Herbal Medicine, 3rd ed. New York, Springer-Verlag, 1998.
- Weis RF. Herbal Medicine. Beaconsfield England, Beaconsfield Publisher, 1988.

REFERENCES

1. Foster S, Duke J: A Field Guide to Medicinal Plants: Eastern and Central North America, Boston, Houghton Mifflin, 1990.
2. Eisenberg DM, Kessler RC, Foster C et al: Unconventional medicine in the United States: Prevalence, costs, and patterns of use. N Engl J Med 328:246–252, 1993.
3. Eisenberg DM, et al: Trends in alternative medicine use in the United States, 1990–1997. JAMA 280:1569–1575, 1997.
4. Johnson B: One-third of nation's adults use herbal remedies: Market estimated at $3.24 billion. HerbalGram 40:49, 1997.
5. Blumenthal M: Herbal sales up 1% for all channels of trade in 2000. HerbalGram 53:63, 2001.
6. Fetrow C, Avila J: The Complete Guide to Herbal Medicines. New York, Simon & Shuster, 2000.
7. United States Congress: Dietary Supplement Health and Education Act of 1994, Public Law 103-417. 108 Stat. 4325–4333. Oct. 25, 1994.
8. Davidoff F: The heartbreak of drug pricing. Ann Intern Med 134:1068–1071, 2001.
9. Ang-Lee MK, Moss J, Yuan CS: Herbal medicines and perioperative care. JAMA 286:208–216., 2001
10. McGuffin M: Issues of quality: Analyzing herbal materials and the current status of methods validation. HerbalGram 53:44, 2001.
11. Huang WF, et al: Adulteration by synthetic therapeutic substances of traditional Chinese medicines in Taiwan. J Clin Pharmacol 37:334–350, 1997.
12. Robergs RA, Griffin SE: Glycerol.Biochemistry, pharmacokinetics and clinical and practical applications. Sports Med 26(3):145–167, 1998.
13. Bennet DA, Phun L, Polk JF, et al: Neuropharmacology of St. John's wort (Hypericum). Ann Pharmacol Ther 32:1201–1208, 1988.
14. Hobbs C: Handbook for Herbal Healing. Loveland, CO, Botanica/Interweave Press, 1994.
15. McGuffin M, Hobbs C, Upton R, Goldberg A: American Herbal Product Association's Botanical Safety Handbook. Boca Raton, FL, CRC Press, 1997.
16. Blumenthal M, Goldberg A, Brinckmann J (eds): Herbal Medicine: Expanded Commision E Monographs. Newton, MA, Integrative Medicine Communications, 2000.
17. Hirono I, et al: Carcinogenic activity of *Symphytum officinale*. J Natl Cancer Inst 61: 865–869, 1978.
18. Sheik NM, et al: Chaparral-associated hepatoxicity. Arch Intern Med 157:913–919, 1997.
19. Haller CA, Benowitz NL: Adverse cardiovascular and central nervous system events associated with dietary supplements containing ephedra alkaloids. N Engl J Med 343:1833–1838, 2000.
20. Blumenthal M:Herb sales down 3% in mass market retail stores—sales in natural food stores still growing, but at lower rate. HerbalGram 49:68, 2000.
21. Http://www.powerpak.com/CE/Dietary/tables.cfm Guidelines for Recommending Natural Supplements to Patients. Accessed 12/23/01; last revised 1/04/02.
22. www.virtualhealthinfo.com/her/red_yeast_rice.htm accessed 12/17/01.
23. Heber D, Yip I, Ashley JM, et al: Cholesterol-lowering effects of a proprietary Chinese red-yeast-rice dietary supplement Am J Clin Nut 69:231–236, 1999.
24. Pharmanex, Inc: Administrative Proceedings, Docket no 97P-0441; Final Decision. Department of Health and Human Services, Food and Drug Administration, Rockville, MD 20087.

19. NUTRITION

Wendy Kohatsu, M.D., and Stefanie Shaver, M.D.

1. How important is nutrition in health and illness?

Eating habits and food choices have a tremendous impact on health. Nutrition plays a contributing role in approximately 70% of diseases leading to premature death. Specific nutritional interventions have been shown to affect many diseases significantly, including hypertension, heart disease, cancer, diabetes, depression, and attention deficit hyperactivity disorder (ADHD). Despite the progress made in nutritional science during the past century, dietary habits of most Americans have declined. Shelves of grocery stores are crammed full of more and more products with less and less nutrition, and rates of obesity in the U.S. continue to rise.

Food defines who we are from the molecular to the spiritual level. We rely on adequate intake of macro- and micronutrients to grow, build, repair, and fuel our bodies. Through food we express our culture, caring, togetherness, family life, religion/faith, philosophy, and personal style. Healthy eating is a blend of all of these elements.

2. What can other cultures and systems teach us about nutrition?

Many cultures embrace Hippocrates' advice to "consider food thy medicine." In traditional Chinese medicine and other forms of Asian medicine, proper eating is a vital component of therapy. For example, cooling foods such as watermelon and yogurt direct energy inward because of their yin nature and may be prescribed for a pathologic yang condition. Ayurveda recommends certain types of food according to the person's dosha. For example, a "kapha" person should avoid dairy and sweets and is encouraged to eat bitter and astringent foods to stay in energetic balance. Fasting is a routine custom in many of the world's religions.

Studies conducted in the U.S. since the 1930s show consistent longevity benefits from calorie-restricted diets. Some of the oldest people in the world live on the Japanese island of Okinawa. One of the Okinawan secrets to long life is "hara hachi bu,"[1] which loosely translates as "eat until you are eight parts full [out of ten]." A simplistic form of caloric restriction, this approach basically means to leave a little room at the end of the meal and not to eat until the stomach is bursting at the seams. Because it takes the stretch receptors in the stomach about 20 minutes to register fullness, it seems wise to allow time to let the brain register the body's sensations.

Drastic shifts from traditional ways of eating has proved harmful to the Pima Indians of Southwest Arizona. At the turn of the last century, when the native diet centered on corn, beans, cactus buds rich in soluble fiber, and vegetables, diabetes was virtually unheard of. With the introduction of "white man's food"—sugar, saturated fats, and other refined products—rates of diabetes skyrocketed. Nearly 50% of Pima adults have type 2 diabetes. Small studies show that restarting a more traditional diet may reverse some of the disease. In the same vein, population studies of immigrants moving from Japan to Hawaii to mainland America, each with progressive adoption of a typical American diet, show increasing rates of breast and prostate cancer as well as heart disease. Honoring traditional ways of eating may have physical as well as cultural benefits.

3. Is a vegetarian diet healthy?

A vegetarian diet includes no meat and no seafood. A lacto-ovovegetarian diet includes eggs and dairy products. A vegan diet is exclusively plant-based, with no animal products. Variations of the vegan diet include a macrobiotic diet, which originated in Japan and emphasizes certain foods and methods of preparation, and a raw diet, which emphasizes raw foods. Generally, vegetarianism is chosen for health benefits, ethical reasons (animal cruelty, environmental concerns), or religious reasons. Most studies of vegetarianism in the U.S. include Seventh Day Adventists, who are vegetarian as part of their faith. This research has shown that a vegetarian diet is healthy. In fact, a large body of research indicates that vegetarians have a decreased risk of chronic disease compared with meat eaters. For example, vegetarians have a 24% reduction in mortality due to heart disease and a 40% reduction in cancer mortality compared with meat eaters.[2] Nut consumption, prevalent in many plant-based, Mediterranean, and Asian diets, seems to be particularly protective against ischemic heart disease.[3]

4. What are the benefits and risks of a vegan diet?

In general, the health **benefits** of a vegan diet are even more pronounced than those of a lacto-ovovegetarian. For example, the average cholesterol level of a vegetarian is 156, whereas the average cholesterol level for a vegan is 133. Of note, studies show that every 1% drop in cholesterol is associated with a 3–4 % drop in heart disease.[4]

Potential **risks** of adhering to an exclusively vegan diet include deficiencies of vitamin B_{12} and essential fatty acids. However, if one consumes B_{12}-fortified foods and foods rich in omega-3 fatty acids (e.g., flax oil, walnuts), this is not an issue.

5. To dairy or not to dairy?

Despite the highly publicized campaigns for milk, it does not benefit all people. For many cultures, cow's milk is not a traditional food, and digestibility varies amongst different ethnic groups. Some of these cultures have rates of osteoporosis far below that of the U.S., Canada, and Sweden—countries with the highest dairy intake.[5] Lactose intolerance is a considerable concern. About 5–15% of Caucasians and 60–90% of non-Caucasians show some degree of lactose intolerance, which can be manifested by abdominal bloating and discomfort, flatulence, and diarrhea. Proteins found in cow's milk have a complex antigenic structure and can cause a wide variety of allergic reactions in many people. Milk allergies have also been implemented in the genesis of type 1 diabetes in children,[6] irritable bowel syndrome, ADHD, chronic allergies, and asthma.

Dairy products also can be a considerable source of fat, especially saturated fat. An 8-oz glass of whole milk adds 150 kcal and 8 gm of saturated fat. Even in 2% milk, one-third of the calories come from fat (60% of which is saturated). Cow's milk and its individual components are not all bad, however—many people rely on milk as good source of bioavailable calcium, vitamin D, riboflavin, and protein. As with most food principles, moderation of intake is the key.

Luckily, for consumers who choose to exclude dairy, a growing number of soy, grain, and other nondairy "milks" and products are available—often fortified with the same nutrients found in regular milk. Because of the high prevalence of bovine growth hormone (BGH) use to increase milk yield and the widespread use of antibiotics in dairy cattle, organic dairy products are recommended.

6. What is the glycemic index?

The glycemic index measures carbohydrates with respect to how fast they cause the blood glucose level to rise compared with white sugar, which has a reference value of 100. The more rapidly the carbohydrate is absorbed from the gastrointestinal (GI) tract into the bloodstream, the higher the glycemic index. In general, the more processed a carbohydrate is from its original state, the higher its glycemic index. Both soluble and insoluble fibers slow down carbohydrate absorption. People are often surprised to find that a baked potato has a glycemic index of 121, higher than that of table sugar. A steep rise in blood glucose causes the body to produce an excess of insulin that can result in rebound hypoglycemia or lead to the development of insulin resistance.

Some studies have associated a low glycemic index diet with decreased rates of chronic disease such as diabetes and hypertension. However, the reality is that typically carbohydrates are not consumed in isolation. For example, a baked potato is usually eaten with a pat of butter or sour cream; bread is used in a sandwich with a protein. Like fiber, fats and proteins slow the breakdown of carbohydrates and stimulate the release of glucagon, which slows the rise in blood sugar; thus, the glycemic index of the combined foods is reduced. The glycemic index is a useful tool for research and for comparing carbohydrates but should not be the sole factor used to determine a carbohydate's worth. Indeed, other potential health benefits may be overshadowed by the fact that they have a high glycemic index. For example, cooked carrots may have a high glycemic index of 92 but are a good source of vitamin A. Because most high-glycemic foods are highly processed, the potential health benefit from eating a low-glycemic index diet may actually come from emphasizing foods that are less processed.

7. How helpful is fiber?

A growing body of research supports the benefits of dietary fiber in fruit, vegetables, and whole grains. Fiber is a complex mixture of substances and is categorized as water-soluble (e.g., legumes, oat bran, psyllium, pectin in grapefruit and apples, guar gum) or insoluble (e.g., cellulose, foods such as wheat bran). Based on epidemiologic evidence, lack of fiber in the diet has been implicated as a potential risk factor for development of colon cancer, heart disease, and diabetes. In particular, studies suggest the protective effect in a high fiber diet (particularly a diet high in wheat bran fiber) with respect to colon cancer.[7] Emerging evidence also indicates that vegetable fiber, more than grain fiber, may be protective in other types of cancer, particularly ovarian and possibly breast cancer. Increased dietary fiber is also useful in the management of irritable bowel syndrome, constipation, and hemorrhoids.

With respect to heart disease, water-soluble fiber exerts a beneficial effect on plasma cholesterol and triglyceride levels.[8,9] Many studies show not only preventive but also therapeutic benefits of increased dietary fiber on hypercholesterolemia as well as a reduced mortality rate for coronary artery disease. In type 2 diabetes, adequate dietary fiber in a meal slows the postprandial rise in blood sugar and the subsequent insulin response. In addition, a large study involving type 1 diabetics showed that a high-fiber diet improves glycemic control and reduces the number of hypoglycemic events.[10] Overall, it appears that water-soluble fiber has a greater effect on reduction of postprandial blood glucose, insulin, and serum lipid levels than insoluble fiber.

How much fiber is needed for health protective effects? Despite the lack of consensus, studies show benefits at a dietary fiber intake of 25–35 gm/day for patients with type 2 diabetes. This is a good target intake for other health problems as well. In addition, one study demonstrated that whole grain fiber is associated with a reduced mortality risk in comparison with a similar amount of refined grain fiber.[11] Any increase in dietary fiber intake should be accompanied by an increase in water intake.

8. How healthy are low-fat diets?

In the 1980s, Pritikin championed a low-fat diet, i.e., less than 10% of total calories as fat. Many national guidelines recommend around 30%. A 10%-fat vegetarian diet is one component of Ornish's well-known program for reversing CAD, which has shown impressive results. Other lifestyle interventions include exercise, stress reduction, and group support; thus, it is impossible to interpret the Ornish data exclusively with respect to a low-fat, plant-based diet. Studies by McDougall and others do show that a low-fat, plant-based diet alone effectively reverses coronary artery disease.

A "fatphobia" craze seems to have taken over the nation since the 1980s with the introduction of every possible low-fat, reduced-fat, and nonfat versions of all types of food—even fat-free mayonnaise (fat-free fat?). Unfortunately, since the obsession with decreased fat ingestion, the U.S. has seen a statistical increase in obesity. This increase probably is due to increased consumption of refined carbohydrates and overprocessed "nonfat" foods rather than complex carbohydrates. In fact, one study showed that the body mass index (BMI) was significantly lower for men and women on a high carbohydrate diet compared with those on a low carbohydrate diet.[12] Fat serves as a satiety indicator, and one may consume a whole pound of fat-free cookies before feeling the satiety associated with a small handful of nuts. A diet minimizing saturated fat, as found in meat and dairy products, and emphasizing moderate amounts of unsaturated fats, as found in olive oil, cold water fish, and nuts, is ideal.

9. What's the skinny on fats?

The quality of fats we eat is as important as the quantity. Much research has examined the specific effects of saturated, monounsaturated, and polyunsaturated fatty acids (PUFAs) on health. Every cell in the body is surrounded by a lipid bilayer that determines what goes in and out of the membranes and thus the function and health of the cell. Research has shown that unlike membrane proteins, which are genetically determined, and carbohydrates, which are extensively metabolized, the fat composition of cellular membranes is determined to a great extent by dietary intake. The old adage, "You are what you eat," certainly applies to fats.

There is no such thing as a pure saturated or pure polyunsaturated fat in nature. Every fat is composed of certain percentages of different kinds of fats. For example, olive oil is considered a good source of monounsaturated fat (about 70–77% of its composition, one of the highest known).

Flax oil is the richest source of omega-3 fatty acids at about 60% composition rate; salmon has about 30%. Note though that salmon also contains equal amounts of saturated fat.

Basic Facts about Fats

SATURATED	MONOUNSATURATED	POLYUNSATURATED
No double bonds	One double bond	Two or more double bonds
High % in lard, butterfat, coconut oil, hydrogenated fats	High % in olive oil, canola, avocados, almonds, hazelnuts	High % in (see below)
	Omega 9 (oleic acid)	Omega 6 (linoleic acid) in safflower, sunflower, corn, sesame
		Omega 3 (alpha-linolenic acid) in flaxseed, canola, fish, walnuts, dark leafy greens, purslane, hempseeds
Contributes to high cholesterol	Lowers low-density lipoprotein cholesterol	Multiple health benefits but spoil rapidly

Omega 3, 6, and 9 refers to the location of the first double bond (on the third, sixth, or ninth carbon molecule).

10. Explain more about omega-3 and omega-6 fatty acids.

The omega-6 and omega-3 fatty acids are essential and must be obtained from dietary sources because the body does not manufacture them. The problem is that in the contemporary American diet omega-6 fatty acids tend to be vastly overabundant compared with omega-3 fatty acids (ratios of 20:1 to 40:1). Although both are necessary, the dominance of omega-6 fatty acids leads to relative deficiencies of omega-3 fatty acids because they compete for the same enzyme pathways. In paleolithic times, this ratio is estimated to be closer to 4:1 or 2:1, and recent research suggests significant health benefits when dietary intake approximates these ratios. The former American Heart Association guidelines suggest 30% total fat intake, with no more than 10% saturated fat and approximately 10% each of mono- and polyunsaturated fats. Newer data call these guidelines into question.

Diets high in omega-3 fatty acids, such as the Mediterranean diet, have shown astounding results, including an approximately 70% reduction in the incidence of coronary heart disease.[13] Omega 3-rich diets also have significant impact on a wide variety of other diseases, including cancer, depression, diabetes, fatigue syndromes, and autoimmune disorders.[14]

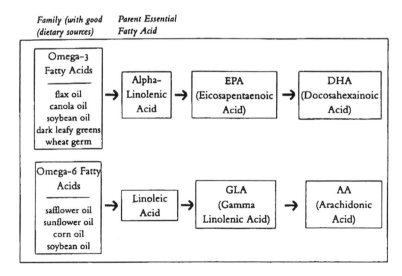

Essential fatty acid families. (From Melina V, Davis B, Harrison V: Becoming Vegetarian. Summertown, TN, Book Publishing Co., 1995, with permission.)

Food sources containing high amounts of omega-3 fatty acids include flax oil, soybeans, deep water fish, and wheat germ. Eicosapentaenoic acid (EPA) and dehydroacetic acid (DHA) are longer-chain omega-3 metabolites that have specific beneficial properties for nervous system health and contribute to anti-inflammatory series 3 prostaglandin production. Omega-6 fatty acids are abundant in easily obtainable sources such as corn and safflower oils as well as soybeans. Precursor omega-6 fatty acids can be converted into gamma-linolenic acid (GLA), which is the rare omega-6 fatty acid known to have particular anti-inflammatory benefits. Again, the challenge is to obtain the appropriate ratio of these oils in the diet.

11. What is an adequate intake of essential fatty acids (EFAs)?
The minimal intake of essential fatty acids, according to the World Health Organization, is 3% of total caloric intake as omega-6 PUFAs and 1% as omega-3 fatty acids. Note that this recommendation is an EFA minimum; a 4% total fat diet would be too extreme. For an adult on a 2000-kcal diet, this recommendation translates to 1.1 gm/day of pure alpha-linolenic acid. What is not known, however, is the amount of omega-3 fatty acids required for *maximal* benefit. Some clinical studies in children have required doses > 10 gm/day for therapeutic effects. This value should not be alarming; many junk foods easily contain 10 gm of "bad" fats in a single serving. Unfortunately, "bad" fats are nearly ubiquitous in processed snack foods and contribute to disease on a daily basis in the U.S.
Trans-fatty acids are the dark side of PUFAs. By definition, polyunsaturated fats contain more than one double bond, which makes them more vulnerable to oxidation from heat, light, and over time. Molecular chemistry reveals that these bonds can be in either cis- or trans- form. The fats in the human body membranes are all in cis- formation. Trans-fatty acids, often the byproduct of the chemical hydrogenation process used commercially to stabilize fats, are not recognized by the human body and have been independently implicated in higher rates of coronary artery disease and inflammatory states. Hydrogenated fats and partially hydrogenated fats (e.g., vegetable shortening) are hazardous to health, regardless of the original oil used, and should be avoided.

12. How healthy is the Mediterranean diet?
The term *Mediterranean diet* loosely refers to the range of diets in countries bordering the Mediterranean Sea. Extensive studies in the early 1960s indicate that the dietary pattern of Greece (more than other Mediterranean countries) includes high intake of fruits, vegetables (particularly wild plants), nuts and cereals, olive oil, and fish as well as lower intake of meat and dairy products (usually only as condiments) and moderate intake of wine. Analyses of the dietary pattern of the Greek isle of Crete show a number of protective substances, such as selenium, glutathione, a balanced ratio of omega-6 and omega-3 essential fatty acids, high amounts of fiber, antioxidants (especially resveratrol from wine and polyphenols from olive oil), and vitamins E and C, some of which have been shown to be associated with lower risk of cancer, including cancer of the breast.[15] As mentioned previously, dramatic improvements after adopting a Mediterranean diet have been documented in patients with heart disease and stroke; in addition, the diet reduces rates of cancer and many other diseases despite a total higher percentage of fat intake (about 40% compared with the recommended 30%).

13. How healthy is a high protein diet?
The 1990s have seen a slew of low-carbohydrate, high-protein/high-fat diets. Examples include the Atkins, Sugar Busters, Protein Power, and Stillman diets. These diets are appealing because of the short-term weight loss due to induction of metabolic ketosis. They claim health benefits from the stabilization of blood sugar, and therefore insulin levels, through consuming a majority of calories as protein and fat, and avoiding high-glycemic index carbohydrates. With respect to stable blood glucose, an exclusively plant-based diet emphasizing low-glycemic index food choices probably accomplishes the same goal, and certainly available data about the long-term vitality of cultures that emphasize this way of eating are more extensive. Furthermore, one study demonstrated that a complex carbohydrate diet fed to insulin-resistant people over 3 weeks led to a 30% reduction in insulin blood levels; cholesterol and triglyceride levels were reduced by 20%.[16]
At this point, no sound data support a high-protein, high-fat diet as cardioprotective or indicate a reduction in mortality or morbidity related to any chronic disease—nor has the safety of long-term

consumption of high-protein, high-fat diets been established. A diet high in saturated fat may increase the risk of cardiovascular disease, and the excessive excretion of calcium in urine secondary to high protein intake may contribute to osteoporosis. The indiscriminate consumption of a diet high in known disease-promoting substances (e.g., saturated fat, cholesterol, oxidants) and devoid of health-protective substances (e.g., phytonutrients, vitamins, fiber) is questionable in light of the substantial amount of research and epidemiologic studies supporting the health benefits of a predominantly plant-based diet.[17] Alternatively, one may choose leaner free-range meats, which tend to have less saturated fat and a favorable unsaturated fatty acid profile compared with conventionally raised counterparts. Soy protein foods are another option.

14. How healthy are the paleolithic-type diets?

The paleolithic diet was first introduced by S. Boyd Eaton, M.D., in *The Paleolithic Prescription* (1988). Eaton proposed that people are programmed genetically to consume a diet based on neopaleolithic patterns for optimal health. He argued that the human genome has changed little in the past 40,000 years since the Stone Age and that nutritional requirements before the advent of agriculture remain unchanged. Ethnographic studies reveal that humans evolved on a diet that was approximately 35% plant-based and 65% animal-based.[18] Fundamental to the paleolithic diet is an emphasis on lean meat, vegetables, fruits, nuts, and seeds, with no grain or dairy products. Because the meat was wild game, it was relatively lean and had a greater percentage of unsaturated fat. Therefore, the diet contained low-to-moderate amounts of fat and had a favorable omega-6-to-omega-3 fat ratio of 1:1 to 1:3. According to proponents, the typical Western diet, which is high in cereal grains and saturated fat, contributes to many modern diseases. The "Zone" diet, which was popularized by Sears and promotes a precise dietary macronutrient ratio of 30% fat, 30% protein, and 40% carbohydrate for optimal health, is loosely based on the paleolithic diet.

Any diet that advocates an increase in fresh fruits and vegetables, foods rich in phytonutrients, a favorable omega fatty acid ratio, and a reduction in refined carbohydrates is healthful. Data from twentieth century hunter-gatherers cultures that consume traditional diets show that they are largely free of the diseases of modern civilization regardless of the plant:animal ratio. Some cultures emphasize wild animal foods (e.g., Canadian Eskimos), whereas others emphasize wild plant foods (e.g., the !Kung),or domesticated plant foods (e.g., the Yanomamo).[19] A higher ratio of low-fat dietary protein in place of carbohydrates may prove to be a healthful option for some people. However, no sound data support a diet high in protein as more healthful that a diet high in complex carbohydrates. In fact, studies support the opposite. Long-term clinical trials targeting a model paleolithic diet are needed to determine whether it truly produces positive health outcomes.

15. How valid is the popular diet "Eat Right for Your Blood Type?"

Like the paleolithic theory, this diet, created by D'Adamo, is based on evolution, specifically blood type evolution, and subsequent tolerance or intolerance to particular foods. According to D'Adamo, foods contain substances called lectins—diverse proteins similar to certain blood type antigens that can cause certain blood type cells to agglutinate in vitro. D'Adamo proposes that a similar process occurs in vivo: that is, if a person with blood type A drinks milk (which has blood type B lectins), the milk will have a mild agglutination effect on the blood cells. D'Adamo states that lectins are resistant to acid hydrolysis in the stomach and, once they enter the blood stream, target certain organs, agglutinate blood cells, invoke an immune response, and subsequently cause damage to the organ. Therefore, each blood-type diet emphasizes foods compatible with an individual's blood type.

Actual controlled clinical trials are needed to validate D'Adamo's yet unproven theory. People who follow any of his blood-type diets are likely to see health benefits because of the overall emphasis on lean protein, unsaturated fats, vegetables, fruits, fiber, and varying amounts of complex carbohydrates. Of note, according to D'Adamo, people with blood type O are most suited for animal protein. However,a large number of people with blood type O are healthy and thriving on a vegetarian diet.[20] Because the blood-type diet has reduced calories compared with the average diet, people who follow it also lose weight. At this point, it is difficult to attribute the potential health benefits exclusively to the choice of foods based on blood type.

16. How much dietary protein is truly necessary?

A fair amount of controversy surrounds the optimal amount of dietary protein. Optimal amounts vary with age, health status, and activity level. In general, a healthy adult needs approximately 25 gm/day of protein to avoid disease. The recommended amount is 50 gm to ensure intake of an adequate essential amino acid profile. The AHA guidelines recommend 50–100 gm/day of protein (15–20% of total caloric intake). The safe upper limit is defined as 1.5 gm/kg of body weight. Very young people, pregnant women, and particularly elderly people have additional protein needs. Athletes may also need more protein. Optimal results from weight training may require additional dietary protein. The health risks of high protein consumption include potential renal impairment due to increased workload over time, but this effect has not been documented in healthy people without renal disease.

The superiority of animal vs. plant-derived protein is also controversial. Meat contains different types of saturated fat—stearic fat is less well absorbed and therefore does not significantly affect lipid profiles. However meat also contains palmitic fat, which does significantly raise cholesterol levels. A diet high in animal protein leads to elevated blood homocysteine levels, which are associated with an increased risk of cardiovascular disease. Alternatively, studies show that soy protein consistently lowers cholesterol, and the micronutrients and phytochemicals decrease homocysteine levels.[21]

17. Are organic foods healthier?

Organic food is produced by farmers who emphasize the use of renewable resources to enhance environmental quality for future generations. Organic food is produced without using most conventional pesticides, petroleum- based or sewage sludge-based fertilizers, bio-engineering, or ionizing radiation. Organic meat, poultry, eggs, and dairy products come from animals that are given no antibiotics or growth hormones. Before a product can be labeled "organic" a government-approved certifier inspects the farm where the food is grown to ensure that the farmer is following all of the rules necessary to meet the organic standards of the U.S. Department of Agriculture.

Ninety percent of U.S. crops are produced with chemical fertilizers and pesticides. Of great concern is the decreased vitamin and mineral content in fruits and vegetables over the past 60 years. Reasons include soil depletion, residue effects of chemical fertilizers and pesticides, mass agricultural production methods, and global pollution. One study showed a 27% higher vitamin C content in organic fruits and vegetables compared with conventionally grown crops. Protein content is noted to be less in organic crops, but of greater quality and improved amino acid composition.[22] The Environmental Protection Agency states that approximately 90% of fungicides, 60% of herbicides, and 30% of insecticides in current use are potentially carcinogenic. They may be present in minute quantities, but their cumulative effects are unknown.

The concerns for meat products are similar. Recent attention has focused on the high use of antibiotics in livestock[23] and growing documentation of antibiotic resistance. As many as 90% of all antibiotics produced in the U.S. are given to animals. Drugs such as penicillins, tetracyclines, cephalosporins, and fluoroquinolones are routinely given to herd animals to prevent the multiple illnesses for which they are at risk in densely populated quarters and to promote feeding efficiency. Hormones and pesticides are also found at significant levels in animal products, including dairy products. Diethylstilbestrol (DES), a known carcinogenic hormone, was routinely used in 90% of American cattle to fatten them up.[24] Anabolic hormones fed to animals have been linked to at least two different types of cancer[25] and possibly premature onset of puberty.

18. What are "designer" foods?

"Designer" foods fall into a growing category of functional foods, also known as nutraceuticals, that are vaguely defined as whole, fortified, or enhanced foods ranging from natural fruits and vegetables to isoflavone-concentrated soy products to beverages laced with St John's wort. Needless to say, this is murky territory because labels on supplements can claim that gingko added to soft drinks "boosts thinking" but provide no documentation to identify exactly what is added.

"Designer" margarines use plant sterols (sitostanol from pine tree pulp and sitosterol from soy) that block cholesterol absorption and have been shown in clinical trials to reduce LDL cholesterol by 10–15% with or without additional statin therapy. From $\frac{1}{2}$ to 1 tablespoon of designer margarines (about 5–10 gm of fat) was ingested 3 times/day. Dose ranges required for benefits are 3–5 gm/day of plant sterol esters.[26] The margarines used in these studies also contain 5–9% omega-3 fatty acids.

19. What is the most underconsumed macronutrient?

Water. Although not a nutrient per se, water composes 60–70% of the human body. Most people do not drink the recommended 8 glasses of water per day. Proper hydration is needed for waste elimination, organ health, and optimal cell and metabolic functions. People may often eat when their bodies are really sending signals for pure water. Drinking adequate amounts of water can correct this problem and aid in proper weight management.

Controversy exists over the benefits of bottled water versus tap water. Chlorine, used to sanitize public water supplies, and fluoride, often added to prevent dental caries, can cause toxic side effects in large amounts. Sales of bottled water have tripled in the 1990s, but a sobering report has tempered some of that enthusiasm. A study conducted in 1999 revealed that one-third of bottled waters samples had significant levels of organic chemicals, lead, and arsenic. The study also found that 25% of bottled water samples were indeed just tap water with fancy labels.[27] The best bet is an adequate filtration system that removes chloride, lead, arsenic, organic chemicals, nitrates, and bacteria—the most common contaminants found in drinking water. Combination filter systems (reverse osmosis + activated charcoal or electrochemical filtration) are usually recommended to remove all of the above.

20. How important is the timing of meals?

People who consider themselves "grazers" nibble frequently through the day, taking in perhaps several (6–9) smaller meals. Others are "bingers" who consume their entire daily caloric content in 1–2 meals/day. Studies show that, although overall differences are not great, the same amount of food divided into only a few large meals per day increases the chance of gaining weight and increasing one's fat stores. The body's ability to absorb nutrients may be exhausted at a certain level; any food taken in excess will be converted into fat. Greater elapsed time between meals shifts the body metabolism toward the "starvation" mode, in which the body tries to conserve calories as fat, increasing fat synthesis and accumulation.[28]

It is important to honor individual body rhythms. Some people are naturally hungry on awakening, whereas others do not seem to get hunger pangs until late afternoon. Some alternative health systems, such as ayurveda and traditional Chinese medicine, believe that the body cycles follow an internal clock that has specific optimal periods for eating and digestion. The most important factor in the timing of meals is to listen to your own internal body clues for hunger signals. Many people eat when it is convenient (e.g., during the noon lunch break, grabbing a bowl of cereal before taking the children to school) rather than when their bodies tell them to eat.

21. How much should I eat? What constitutes a "serving"?

The basic concept of appropriate serving size is not familiar to most Americans. According to the USDA Food Pyramid Guide, examples of average servings of food are as follows:

Meat = 2–3 ounces, about equivalent in size to an average deck of playing cards

Leafy greens = 1 cup	Cheese = 1½ ounce
Vegetables = ½ cup, cooked	Apple = 1 medium

Given that most restaurants still cater to the big American meal, what many consumers consider as a single serving of meat (12 ounces of prime rib) actually equals more than four servings of meat, according to standard guidelines. A generous mound of Italian pasta may be the equivalent of three servings of carbohydrates (not including the sauce). Equally deceptive is the frequent misreading of Nutrition Facts on every food product label. While ingesting 9 grams of fat in a serving of corn chips may not seem too bad, most people fail to realize that the handy grab-bag of chips actually contains 2.75 servings, which totals about 25 gm of fat per bag.

The best advice is to read labels carefully and to use common sense. For patients who desire to lose weight, an understanding of portion size is critical. Practical advice includes separating out what a "portion" is—i.e., literally dividing the pile of pasta into three equal parts to get a visual sense of what it means to eat a portion of carbohydrates before devouring the whole plate.

22. How valid is the concept of food combining?

Food combining was first popularized by Francis Lappé Moore in her groundbreaking vegetarian book, *Diet for a Small Planet*. The popular book *Fit for Life* has further championed this style of eating. The fundamental concept is that it is not enough to eat nourishing food; of equal importance is the capacity to digest and assimilate food properly. A guiding principle of food combining is to avoid protein and carbohydrates in the same meal because protein requires acid for digestion, whereas carbohydrates require an alkaline environment. Consuming the two together leads to delayed emptying time and indigestion. Vegetables can be eaten freely with either carbohydrates or protein, because they are digested equally well in an acid or alkaline medium. Fruit, which is thought to ferment if it remains in the stomach for prolonged periods, is to be eaten in isolation or at least 20 minutes before any meal. No sound studies support or negate this style of eating.

23. What is an elimination diet? How does it work?

Food allergy or intolerance can play a significant role in many chronic conditions such as migraines, asthma, otitis media, ADHD, arthritis, and autoimmune diseases. Clinical trials have reported improvement rates as high as 75% (ADHD, irritable bowel syndrome). Commonplace symptoms, such as dyspepsia, flatulence, chronic fatigue, skin rashes, and joint aches and pains, have been linked to food sensitivities. Many holistic practitioners consider addressing dietary sensitivities as a critical first step to symptom amelioration for many diseases. **Major trigger foods** include dairy products, wheat and other glutinous grains, eggs, corn, soy and soy products, peanuts, citrus fruits, yeast, refined sugars, and artificial additives, preservatives, and colorings.

Although immediate IgE hypersensitivity allergies and anaphylaxis to certain foods are obvious, delayed hypersensitivity reactions (typically IgG) can be so subtle that they tend to be dismissed by mainstream physicians. Conventional laboratory tests, such as the radioallergosorbent test, enzyme-linked immunosorbent assay, and provocation tests, are not highly sensitive for food-induced allergies. An empirical elimination challenge is not only straightforward and cost-effective, but specific to the persons tested. An elimination diet removes potential trigger foods from the diet for a period of usually a few weeks to months, and clinical symptoms are followed for resolution. Suspected trigger foods are then reintroduced into the diet one at time to see if symptoms recur. The theory behind food allergy testing is simple, but because most of our diet consists of composite foods (pizza = bread/carbohydrates + tomato sauce + cheese/dairy + various meat and vegetable toppings), the elimination diet is often hard to practice, requiring diligence and patience. When it is properly done, however, results are extremely beneficial. A rotation diet is a variation of the gold standard elimination diet in which all suspect foods are avoided for at least 5 days, or long enough to clear all traces from the digestive tract, and then rotated back into the diet.[29] (For more specific studies, see Chapters 24, 30, 36, and 60.)

24. Explain body hunger vs. emotional hunger.

Mindless eating, cleaning your plate because of "starving people in Africa," binging on "comfort" foods from childhood, and late-night snacking while watching TV represent emotional and social reasons for eating. Attempts to control what we eat are commonplace; approximately 25–30% of Americans at any given time are on a diet. A big part of the problem for most overweight Americans is not that they lack awareness of good nutrition but that they eat without being attuned to true body hunger or on the basis of emotional needs. Distorted body image and eating disorders have been noted in girls as young as 9 years, many of whom feel that they are already overweight.

In *Feeding the Hungry Heart*, Roth explores many of these pertinent issues and suggests that simply being in touch with ourselves is a way out of using food for emotional needs:

> At a given moment, our hunger might indicate a yearning as simple as asking to be held—or as complex as the necessity to examine a set of attitudes and responses we have developed in the past that are no longer effective in our present situation . . . . Hunger is deeply personal—it is the unanswered side of our dreams; it is born of the need for completion, fulfillment and serenity.[30]

Compulsive eaters may turn to the refrigerator as a source for solace for unfulfilled psychological needs. The solution lies not in greater knowledge of nutrition, but in a deeper understanding of ourselves and how to nurture human needs.

25. Does chocolate actually have health benefits?

Current research suggests that chocolate, despite its high fat content, may have health benefits. Initial studies suggest that the compounds found in cocoa have strong antioxidant effects. Chocolate, or more specifically the cocoa found in chocolate, contains antioxidant compounds called procyanidins. Chocolate also contains the flavonoid catechins and epicatechins found in grapes and tea. The amazing point is how chocolate compares with other flavonoid rich foods in respect to antioxidant activity as measured by an oxygen radical absorbance capacity (ORAC) score. Vegetables and fruits typically have high scores: blueberries, 2400; spinach, 1260; and broccoli, 890. Dark chocolate, with a score of 13,120 per 100 mg, has one of the highest ORAC score of any known food, perhaps secondary to its concentrated form.[31] In addition, studies suggest that the fat in chocolate, mainly stearic triglycerides (C18:0), does not adversely affect lipid blood profiles.[32] In fact, the polyphenol compounds in chocolate may even decrease LDL cholesterol oxidation. Chocolate also contains phenylethylamine (PEA) and anandamide, both linked to mood enhancement.

At present there are not enough data to make definitive recommendations for chocolate intake. The high caloric content of chocolate should be considered in people who are overweight, and people prone to herpes should avoid chocolate because of its high arginine content. In addition, the high phenylalanine content may exacerbate migraine headaches. However, as with red wine, moderate consumption of cocoa may be added to the growing list of health-protective foods in a balanced diet.

26. What is the healthiest diet?

Ultimately a person's own body dictates the optimal diet. Eating a wide variety of foods in small quantities and paying attention to the body's reactions are superior to recommendations from any book. However, common themes arise despite widely different dietary theories, and a growing body of evidence supports certain basic nutritional concepts for good health. First, eat a variety of foods, particularly vegetables, fruits, whole grains, and legumes. This provides a wide spectrum of health-protective substances such as phytochemicals, fiber, and micronutrients. Second, emphasize whole vs. processed foods, particularly with respect to grains. Whole grains contain much more protein, fiber, and micronutrients than refined grains. Third, emphasize monounsaturated and omega-3 fats (as found in olive oil, nuts, seeds, and fish such as salmon) and minimize saturated fat (as found in meat and dairy products). Last, eat in a manner that keeps the blood sugar level stable. This means a high fiber diet with a balanced intake of protein, fat, and unrefined carbohydrates. The optimal ratio of macronutrients for any one person probably varies, based on individual biochemistry and activity level. Experiment with different foods to maximize enjoyment.

27. What resources are available for more information?

- Werbach MR: Nutritional Influences on Illness, 2nd ed. Tarzana, CA, Third Line Press, 1996.,
- Pitchford P: Healing with Whole Foods: Oriental Traditions and Modern Nutrition, rev. ed. Berkeley CA, North Atlantic Books, 1993.
- Erasmus U: Fats that Heal, Fats that Kill. Alive Books, Burnaby, BC, 1993.
- Davis B, Melina V: Becoming Vegan. Summertown, TN, Book Publishing Co, 2000.
- Kesten D: Feeding the Body, Nourishing the Soul: Essentials of Eating for Physical, Emotional, and Spiritual Well-being. Berkeley, CA, Conari Press, 1997.

REFERENCES

1. Willcox BJ, Willcox DC, Suzuki M: The Okinawa Program. Clarkson Potter, New York, 2001.
2. Key TJ, et al: Mortality in vegetarians and nonvegetarians: Detailed findings from a collaborative analysis of 5 prospective studies. Am J Clin Nutr 70:516S–524S, 1999.
3. Sabate J: Nut consumption, vegetarian diets, ischemic heart disease, and all-cause mortality: Evidence from epidemiologic studies. Am J Clin Nutr 70:500S–503S, 1999.
4. Law MR, et al: Systemic underestimation of association between serum cholesterol concentration and ischaemic heart disease. Br Med J 308:363–366, 1994.
5. Melina V, Davis B, Harrison V: Becoming Vegetarian. Summertown, TN, Book Publishing Co, 1995.

6. Harrison LC, Honeyman MC: Cow's milk and type I diabetes. Diabetes 48:1501–1507, 1999.
7. Scheppach W, at al: WHO consensus statement on the role of nutrition in colorectal cancer. Eur J Cancer Prev 8:57–62, 1999.
8. Bazzano LA, et al: Legume consumption and risk of coronary heart disease in US men and women: NHANES I Epidemiologic Follow-up Study. Arch Intern Med 161:2573–2578, 2001.
9. Anderson JW: Dietary fiber prevents carbohydrate-induced hypertriglyceridemia. Curr Atheroscler Rep 2:536–541, 2000.
10. Giacco R, et al: Long-term dietary treatment with increased amounts of fiber-rich low-glycemic index natural foods improves blood glucose control and reduces the number of hypoglycemic events in type 1 diabetic patients. Diabetes Care 23:1461–1466, 2000.
11. Jacobs DR, et al: Fiber from whole grains, but not refined grains, is inversely associated with all-cause mortality in older women: The Iowa women's health study. J Am Coll Nutr 19(3 Suppl):326S–330S, 2000.
12. Kennedy ET, et al: Popular diets: Correlation to health, nutrition, and obesity. J Am Diet Assoc 101:411–420, 2001.
13. De Lorgeril M, et al: Mediterranean diet, traditional risk factors, and the rate of cardiovascular complications after myocardial infarction: Final report of the Lyon Diet Heart Study. Circulation 99:779–785,1999.
14. Simopoulos A, 2nd AUTHOR: The Omega Plan, CITY, PUBLISHER, 1998.
15. Simopoulos AP: The Mediterranean diets: What is so special about the diet of Greece? The scientific evidence. J Nutr 131(11 Suppl):3065S–3073S, 2001.
16. St Jeor ST, et al: Dietary protein and weight reduction: A statement for healthcare professionals from the Nutrition Committee of the Council on Nutrition, Physical Activity, and Metabolism of the American Heart Association. Circulation 104:1869–1874, 2001.
17. Anderson JW, et al: Health advantages and disadvantages of weight-reducing diets: A computer analysis and critical review. J Am Coll Nutr 19:578–590, 2000.
18. Cordain L, et al: Plant-animal subsistence ratios and macronutrient energy estimations in worldwide hunter-gatherer diets. Am J Clin Nutr 71:682–692, 2000.
19. Milton K: Hunter-gatherer diets: A different perspective. Am J Clin Nutr 71:665–667, 2000.
20. Cousens G: Conscious Eating, 2nd ed. Berkeley, CA, North Atlantic Books, 2000.
21. Chait A, et al: Increased dietary micronutrients decrease serum homocysteine concentrations in patients at high risk of cardiovascular disease. Am J Clin Nutr 70:881–887, 1999.
22. Worthington V: Nutritional quality of organic versus conventional fruits, vegetables, and grains. J Altern Compl Med 7:161–173, 2001.
23. Gorbach SL: Antimicrobial use in animal feed: Time to stop. N Engl J Med 345:1202–1203, 2001.
24. Robbins J: Diet for a New America. Stillpoint Publishing, Walpole, NH, 1987.
25. Rose FJ. Carcinogenicity studies in animals relevant to the use of anabolic agents in animal production. Environ Qual Saf Suppl 5:227–237, 1976.
26. Cholesterol lowering margarines. Med Letter 41(1055), 1999.
27. www.nrdc.org/water/drinking/bw/bwinx.asp. Accessed April 12, 2002.
28. Wilhelmine PHG, et al: Influence of the feeding frequently on nutrient utilization in man: Consequences for energy metabolism. Eur J Clin Nutr 45:161–169, 1991.
29. Rockwell SJ: Rotation diet: A diagnostic and therapeutic tool. In Pizzorno JE, Murray MT (eds): Textbook of Natural Medicine. Edinburgh, Churchill Livingstone, 1999, pp 517–520.
30. Roth G: Feeding the Hungry Heart: The Experience of Compulsive Eating. New York, Signet/ Penguin, 1983.
31. Adamson GE, et al: HPLC method for the quantification of procyanidins in cocoa and chocolate samples and correlation to total antioxidant capacity. J Agric Food Chem 47:4184–4188, 1999.
32. Schramm DD, et al: Chocolate procyanidins decrease the leukotriene-prostacyclin ratio in humans and human aortic endothelial cells. Am J Clin Nutr 73:36–40, 2001.

20. SUPPLEMENTS

Wendy Kohatsu, M.D., and Matthew Flesch

1. Discuss the history of supplement use in the United States.

Botanical products were the mainstay of American apothecaries of the 19th century, accounting for 67% of entries in the first edition (1820) of the U.S. Pharmacopoeia (USP), whereas now they represent a mere 2%.[1] After World War II, pharmaceutical products synthesized in laboratories became widespread not only because of scientific advances but also because of the high economic profitability of patentable, isolated chemicals.[2] Over half of modern U.S. pharmaceuticals have been directly derived from, are the synthetic analogs of, or were developed based on chemistry originally found in natural sources. Examples include aspirin from white willow bark, colchicine from autumn crocus, and taxol from the Pacific yew tree.

Despite the shift toward isolated pharmaceuticals, consumers seek out natural remedies to augment health and to treat self-diagnosed ailments. Forty percent of the U.S. population reports taking at least one vitamin or mineral supplement during the past month.[3] In 1999 the supplement industry boasted sales of 9.5 billion dollars in the U.S.,[4] with approximately 4.2 billion from herbs alone. Although sales are growing at a slower rate than during the boom in the mid 1990s, such figures are still impressive.

2. What is a dietary supplement?

A dietary supplement is defined by the Dietary Supplement Health and Education Act of 1994 as "a product (other than tobacco) intended to supplement the diet that bears or contains one or more of the following dietary ingredients: a vitamin, a mineral, an herb or other botanical, an amino acid, or a dietary substance for use by man to supplement the diet by increasing the total dietary intake, or a concentrate, metabolite, constituent, extract, or combination of the above ingredients."[5] Dietary supplements are also called nutraceuticals, phytochemicals, and natural therapeutics; in addition to the above, they include megavitamins, enzymes, food concentrates (protein powders and super-foods), certain hormones, and probiotic bacteria.

3. Are supplements necessary for good health?

The answer is controversial. Some experts say that with healthy eating habits people should be able to meet daily requirements of necessary nutrients without supplementation. For example, an orange provides 75 mg of vitamin C, which exceeds the RDA for vitamin C. However, since the advent of mass production farming during the past century, soil quality has been vastly depleted and fruits and vegetables no longer have the same nutrient value as before.[6] An orange does not have the same nutritional value it had 100 years ago. Other foods also have been affected by modern production methods. For example, eggs from free-range chickens have 20 times more vitamin E than standard supermarket eggs.[7] Supplements, therefore, may be needed to replace lost nutrients.

Other experts argue that some nutrients are better left in their natural form. For example, capsules of broccoli in health food stores contain many nutrients, but lose the other healthful benefits of the whole food such as fiber, water content, "live" enzymes, and some vitamins that may be destroyed during dehydration and processing. Perhaps both good eating habits and supplementation are needed to ensure proper nutrition.

4. What are dietary reference intakes (DRIs)? How are they related to the recommended daily allowances (RDA)?[8]

DRI is a generic term used to refer to at least three types of reference values, including RDAs. In the past, the RDAs, published by the Food and Nutrition Board of the National Academy of Sciences, served as the benchmark of nutritional adequacy in the United States. The traditional role of the RDA is described by the definition adopted more than 20 years ago: the levels of intake of essential nutrients that are judged to be minimally adequate to meet the known nutrient needs of practically all healthy persons.

Scientific knowledge about the roles of nutrients has expanded dramatically since the inception of the RDAs. Contemporary studies address topics not just on the prevention of classical nutritional deficiency diseases, such as rickets, but now include the reduction of risk of chronic diseases such as osteoporosis, cancer, and cardiovascular disease. The Food and Nutrition Board responded to these developments by re-setting nutrient reference values. Dietary reference intakes (DRIs) are the result of this new approach. The website of the Institute of Medicine at www.nationalacademies.org/ includes answers to frequently asked questions about DRIs.

5. What is a vitamin?

A vitamin is an organic cofactor that is necessary for many enzymatic reactions throughout the body. Because most vitamins are not produced in the body, they must be taken in through the diet or supplementation. The following comprehensive list of vitamins includes daily value (DV), the amount of the nutrient needed to ward off serious disease states; optimal daily allowance (ODA), the minimal amount needed for optimal health; and a few characteristics of each vitamin.

Vitamins and Their Essential Characteristics

VITAMIN	DV	ODA	TOXIC DOSE	COMMENTS
Vitamin A (retinol)	5000 IU	5000 IU	Extended use of 50,000+ IU	Vitamin A is often supplemented in its less toxic form, beta carotene, which is converted to retinol in the body. Vitamin A supports proper ocular function and vision, stimulates immune system, provides antioxidant benefits, aids in treatment of Crohn's disease, ulcerative colitis, and menorrhagia. Pregnant women should not use > 4000 IU/day. Food sources: carrots, dark green vegetables, yellow fruits and vegetables.
Vitamin B$_1$ (thiamine)	1.5mg	5–10 mg	NA	Vitamin B$_1$ improves mood and supports normal nervous system, heart, and muscle function. It is useful in Alzheimer's disease, congestive heart failure, diabetes, alcoholism, and many neurologic disorders. Food sources: brewer's yeast, soybeans, fish, whole grains, egg yolks, vegetables.
Vitamin B$_2$ (riboflavin)	1.7 mg	5-10 mg	NA	Riboflavin is used for migraine headaches, cataracts, and depression. It supports healthy hair, skin, and nails. Food sources: dark green vegetables, liver, milk (fortified), eggs, fish, beans.
Vitamin B$_3$ (niacin, niacinamide)	20 mg	25–100 mg	300–600mg	Niacin is useful for diabetes (types 1 and 2), hyperlipidemia, rheumatoid arthritis, acne, Raynaud's syndrome, and other circulatory disorders. It can be beneficial in the prevention of heart attacks. Food sources: brewer's yeast, liver, fish, eggs, wheat germ, figs.
Vitamin B$_5$ (pantothenic acid)	10 mg	10–50 mg	NA	Vitamin B$_5$ helps to produce steroidal hormones. It can reduce serum lipid levels and promote wound healing. Food sources: brewer's yeast, wheat germ, dark green vegetables, nuts, whole grains.
Vitamin B$_6$ (pyridoxine)	2 mg	10–20 mg	250–1000 mg.	Vitamin B$_6$ is necessary for the metabolism of amino acids (especially homocysteine) and proteins. It helps synthesize neurotransmitters, and is helpful for many neurologic disorders. It synergizes with many other vitamins, herbs and nutriceuticals. Food sources: brewer's yeast, rice bran, wheat germ, seeds, nuts, and beans.

Continued on following page

Vitamins and Their Essential Charactderistics (Continued)

VITAMIN	DV	ODA	TOXIC DOSE	COMMENTS
Vitamin B$_{12}$ (cyanoco-balamin, methylco-balamin)	6 µg	10–500 µg	NA	Vitamin B$_{12}$ is essential for cell division, helps protect nerve cells, and supports their proper function. It is involved in proper metabolism of fats, proteins, and carbohydrates. Most pharmaceuticals deplete B$_{12}$, as does stress. Injections must be given to people with pernicious anemia, who lack the intrinsic factor necessary for GI uptake of B$_{12}$. Food sources: liver, red meat, fish.
Vitamin C (ascorbic acid, ascorbate, [mineral] Ester C)	60 mg	250–1000 mg	10 gm	Vitamin C, the most widely known and used vitamin, is used primarily to support immune function and as an antioxidant. It also promotes wound healing, reduces allergy symptoms, aids cholesterol management, and prevents scurvy. Food sources: citrus fruit, tomatoes, berries, melons, green vegetables.
Vitamin D (ergosterol [D$_2$], chole-calciferol [D$_3$])	400 IU	400 IU	25,000–60,000 IU	Vitamin D is produced in the body through direct exposure to sunlight; its deficiency causes rickets. It is a hormone precursor; aids absorption of calcium, magnesium, and zinc; helps prevent osteoporosis; promotes proper sleep cycle; and helps maintain proper thyroid function. Natural sources:sunlight, fish, milk (fortified), seafood.
Vitamin E (tocopherol)	8–10 IU	400 IU	NA	Tocopherol, the most important of the fat-soluble antioxidants, protects against oxidative stress from free radicals.It reduces platelet aggregation, prevents oxidation of low-density lipoprotein cholesterol, mitigates symptoms of Alzheimer's disease, reduces healing time of damaged skin, and can be used topically to minimize scarring as wounds heal. Food sources: wheat germ, nuts, eggs, soybeans, whole grains, vegetable oils.
Vitamin K (menadione) -	NA	65–80 µg	NA	Vitamin K is used primarily for blood clotting but is also beneficial in osteoporosis. Food sources: leafy green vegetables, broccoli, green tea.
Folic acid (folate)	400 IU	400 IU	NA	Folic acid, a water-soluble member of the B-vitamin family, must be replaced daily. It plays a role in many reactions, from neural cell function, to cell division and growth, to formation of red blood cells. It can lower homocysteine levels and protect the heart. It also protects the developing fetus against birth defects because of its essential role in DNA and RNA synthesis. Food sources: dark green vegetables, brewer's yeast, egg yolks, apricots.
Bioflavonoids (quercetin, rutin, hes-peridin)	NA	100 mg (per 500 mg vita-min C)	NA	Bioflavonoids (part of the vitamin C complex) synergize with vitamin C. They increase capillary strength, elasticity, and permeability; help resist infection; and retard oxidation of vitamin C. Quercetin synergizes with bromelain (a digestive enzyme) to slow production of excess mucous in sinus infections. Food sources: citrus fruit (inner rind), apricots, rose hips.

From LaValle JB, et al: Natural Therapeutics Pocket Guide 2000–2001. Hudson, OH, Lexi-Comp, 2001; Pizzorno J, Murray MT: Textbook of Natural Medicine, 2nd ed. Edinburgh, Churchill Livingstone, 1999; and Jellin JM, et al (eds): Natural Medicines Comprehensive Database, 3rd ed. Stockton, CA, Therapeutic Research Faculty, 2000.

6. Are supplements regulated by the Food and Drug Administration (FDA)?

A massive grassroots effort by concerned citizens across the country successfully lobbied Congress to vote in favor of the Dietary Supplement and Health Education Act (DSHEA) of 1994, which prevented the FDA from regulating supplements and vitamins sold over the counter. The amount of mail that Congress received about DSHEA was second only to the Vietnam War. The downside of DSHEA is that the lack of reliable standards for nutritional supplements confounds both patients and clinicians alike. The FDA can pull a supplement off the market only if harm has been proven. Unlimited access to supplements has proved hazardous in some situations. Ephedra (ma huang), an herb used safely for millennia in China, has been widely marketed as an "energy booster," weight loss herb, and sports supplement. One hundred forty cases of adverse effects have been reported to the FDA, including 10 deaths. Also concerning are the potential drug-herb-supplement side effects, the majority of which probably go undetected.

7. What health claims are supplement manufacturers allowed to make?

The supplement industry must adhere to strict labeling requirements but does not have to submit evidence of safety or efficacy. The burden of proof for safety falls on the FDA. Structure/function claims are allowed on supplements sold in the U.S., but manufacturers cannot make specific claims about efficacy. The frequent result is vague and watered-down labeling. A bottle of St. John's wort may claim that it "supports mood" but cannot specifically state that it is used to treat depression (despite the fact that it is a first-line treatment for depression in Europe). Other vague but acceptable structure/function claims include "alleviates fullness," "improves absentmindedness," and "maintains healthy lung function." Such labeling does little to help consumers make informed decisions.

8. What markers help consumers in assessing the quality of a supplement or company?

Unlike pharmaceutical products, uniformity is not guaranteed; supplement products may vary from manufacturer to manufacturer and even from batch to batch. Good manufacturing practice (GMP) standards exist for food, but the FDA has not established GMP for dietary supplements. Quality may depend on the part of the plant used, length of storage time, and how the product was processed and prepared. Some reputable supplement companies adopt GMP standards of their own. For example, in a plant that processes herbal supplements, a botanist may perform a gross inspection of the barrels of the crude herb, and laboratories may check for contaminants and perform gas chromatography and/or mass spectrometry to confirm quality and content during all phases of processing.

Many botanical products are standardized to contain a particular marker compound or "active" ingredient. For example, even though *Echinacea purpurea* has hundreds of natural components, it may be standardized only to the sesquiterpene esters. Of note, a different species (*E. angustifolia*), also hailed for its immunostimulating properties, is typically standardized to its echinanosides component. The multiple variables inherent in natural products pose obvious challenges in creating industry-wide standards. Consumers can ask for a certificate of analysis, which is a formal "report card" in which the components of a supplement are listed and the percent content verified, preferably by a third party.

9. Discuss current trends in the supplement industry.

Supplements are a profitable industry. In some countries, such as Germany, the government mandates and funds research on botanical products and regulates them just like pharmaceutical products. In the U.S., products are sold mainly in health food stores, large retail chains, catalogs, and, to a growing extent, via the Internet. The high prevalence of supplement use also reveals a salient message: Americans are willing to pay out of pocket, since supplements, for the most part, are not reimbursed by third-party payors. Large pharmaceutical manufacturers such as Rexall, Bristol Myers Squibb, and SmithKline Beecham have seen the silver lining in supplement sales and market their own brands.

10. Is there a difference between natural and synthetic vitamins?

In some ways the answer is yes; in others, no. Generally the molecule of the active component of the synthetic vitamin looks chemically identical to its natural counterpart. In such cases, synthetic and natural vitamins may work the same in the body. Large clinical trials using both natural and synthetic vitamins for various diseases have not answered the question of whether one form is superior to the other. For example, the B-vitamins are regularly synthesized because of the highly unstable nature of the food-derived species. Even when B-vitamins are derived from food sources, they must be synthetically complexed with HCl or some other acid for stability and proper utilization in the body. The same is true of natural vitamin E, which is generally complexed with succinate or acetate. These examples seem to blur the boundary between natural and synthetic.

There can be subtle differences between the structure of synthetic and natural vitamins. Synthetic beta carotene, for example, is produced only in its trans configuration, whereas natural forms are found primarily in the 9-cis conformation. The 9-cis form is far more bioavailable and effective as an antioxidant than the trans form. Another distinction is the issue of toxicity. Some vitamins have no toxicity in their natural forms, whereas the synthetic form may have a toxicity threshold at large doses. Vitamin K is an example. Phylloquinone (vitamin K_1), which is naturally derived from alfalfa, has no known toxicity, whereas menadione (synthetic vitamin K_3) may become toxic at doses ranging from 600 to 1000 mg.

The major difference is that natural vitamins often exist in a complex, whereas in synthteic vitamins only the active molecule is present. Examples include ascorbic acid (vitamin C), which in its natural form is complexed with many bioflavonoids as well as acid buffers , and tocopherol (vitamin E), which, when derived from wheat germ, is found in a complex of mixed tocopherols and tocotrienols that activate and synergize with the alpha tocopherol.[9–11] Indeed, the best formulation of vitamins may already be found in nature.

11. What are antioxidants? What do they do?

To understand the role of antioxidants, we must first take into account free radicals and their effect in oxidative stress. Under some conditions, a molecule loses one electron of its outer orbital and is said to be oxidized. The species of the molecule with one less electron than normal is known as a free radical; it is highly reactive, aggressively seeking to replace the lost electron. It does so by stealing an electron from the outer orbital of a neighboring molecule, thus creating a new free radical. Radical chain reactions can then ensue, in which millions of radicals can be formed in seconds, causing significant damage to the cells that the molecules compose. This process is known as oxidative stress. Reaction chains can be ended only when two radicals form a moderately stable molecule or when a new species is introduced that can donate an electron without becoming volatile. These species are known as antioxidants, because they stop the oxidation chain reaction without becoming radicals themselves.

Antioxidants are able to achieve this effect because of their profound structural stability. Even though, by necessity, they become radicals, they are not reactive because of intramolecular resonance stabilization and cooperative efforts between different antioxidants. For example a molecule of alpha tocopherol (vitamin E) can donate an electron to end a reaction and then stabilize itself to remain nonreactive. It can remain quiescent until a molecule of ascorbic acid (vitamin C) donates an electron so that it can end another chain. The oxidized vitamin C, now called dehydroascorbate, can stabilize itself as well, until it can be converted back into active ascorbic acid by glutathione and reduced nicotinamide adenine dinucleotide (NADH) through redox recycling.

Many free radicals attack the lipid membranes of cells and the proteins that allow active transport into the cell and, once inside the cell, its DNA. Free radicals can have a damaging, even mutagenic effect on the cells; hence the importance of antioxidants. Oxidative stress can be triggered by many environmental conditions (e.g., air pollution, ultraviolet light, nuclear radiation) as well as by internal factors (e.g., stress, pesticide-laden food, contaminated drinking water, cigarette smoke, and a host of other carcinogens). Without antioxidants to stem the tide of rapacious free radicals, vast amounts of damage could occur with even the smallest exposure.

Reducing the effects of oxidative stress and protecting the cells from mutation have earned antioxidants their reputation as rejuvenating and cancer-preventing agents. Numerous antioxidants are available on the market, such as the antioxidant vitamins, A, C, and E; bioflavonoids and carotenoids (including lutein and lycopene); selenium; pycnogenol and grape seed extract, both sources of oligomeric proanthrocyanidins; green tea, a source of polyphenols and catechins; superoxide dismutase (SOD); and coenzyme Q10.

12. What controversies surround the use of antioxidants?

Although antioxidants have far-reaching benefits and are generally safe in their whole-food form, overuse of supplemental forms hs raised concern. Excessive doses of vitamin C (> 5000 mg/day) can lead to stone formation in patients with preexisting renal failure. Two large trials[12,13] using synthetic beta carotene were surprisingly associated with an increased risk of lung cancer in smokers; the pathologic mechanism remains unknown. High doses of supplemental vitamin A (retinol) in excess of 50,000 IU/day are toxic to the body and teratogenic at much lower doses. These concerns, however, are not specific to antioxidants; any supplement or drug used above recommended levels or without expert guidance can have deleterious side effects. In their natural food form, these nutrients may yield greater benefits than in isolated concentrates.

A separate concern is the controversial use of antioxidants during chemotherapy, when oxidative damage is the goal. The intent is to destroy cancer cells, and concomitant use of supplemental antioxidants is designed to protect normal cells, but studies are divided as to whether cancer cells also receive this protection.[14]

13. What are probiotics?

Certain strains of bacteria are not harmful to the body and, in fact, are essential to its proper function. Adults carry about 4 -8 lb of friendly bacteria in the intestines. These strains of bacteria are called probiotics, which literally translates as "for life." Over 400 different strains of probiotic bacteria inhabit the gut environment. The first of these, *Bifidobacterium bifidum*, enters the newborn's sterile digestive tract with the first sip of breast milk.

14. How do probiotics promote health?

Probiotics help us function in a number of ways, not the least of which is by maintaining a healthy gut environment. Probiotics inhibit the growth of deleterious bacteria through many aggressive methods, including the production of hydrogen peroxide and a natural antibiotic called acidophilin. Probiotics help to maintain the functioning of the villae in the colon by cleansing them of fermenting matter. They also help reduce inflammation in the colon and small intestine. Oral probiotic supplements are largely used to replenish colonies lost to antibiotic usage. Used in this way, they can prevent the diarrhea and *Candida albicans* yeast overgrowth that may follow the use of antibiotics. They can also protect against urinary tract infections, Crohn's disease, and colon cancer.

Good colonization is the key to successful supplementation with probiotics. The supplement fructooligosaccharides (FOS) can aid a developing colony by providing a food source for the bacteria. Although FOS nourishes probiotics, it is an indigestible fiber in the human digestive system, thus providing a food source for which the probiotics do not need to compete. Many probiotic supplements contain FOS in their formulations. The patient should also be sure that the supplement contains pure, living probiotic bacteria, with a minimum of 4 billion live organisms per capsule at the time of expiration.[15] Most manufacturers produce probiotics that must be refrigerated even before opening. A few companies have created processes that ensure vitality without refrigeration. To allow the best chance for survival through the stomach to the small intestine, probiotic supplements should be taken 10–15 minutes before a meal.

15. What are amino acid supplements? How do they differ from protein supplements?

The difference between protein supplements and amino acid supplements is usually one of application. Protein supplements are generally used by people who feel that they need extra protein, either because their dietary restrictions (e.g., vegetarianism) do not provide proper protein intake through normal diet, or because they feel the need for more protein to help build or repair muscle tissue (usually body builders). Protein is, of course, broken down into amino acids, but the quantity of any one amino in a protein supplement is not high enough to achieve a specific effect.

Amino acid supplements, on the other hand, concentrate individual amino acids in sufficient quantity to achieve a particular effect. Essential amino acids are derived only through diet or supplementation (e.g., arginine, histidine, isoleucine, leucine, metionine, phenylalnine, threonine, tryptophan, valine). Amino acids are the building blocks of proteins used in the construction of enzymes, which are necessary for nearly every biologic reaction in the body. Each individual amino acid can have highly specific physiologic effects.

AMINO ACID	EFFECTS
L-Arginine	Used primarily by body builders and other athletes becaues of its stimulating effect on muscle generation and fat metabolism. Arginine also aids in the release of growth hormones and helps treat male sexual dysfunction.
L- Carnitine	Helps stimulate fatty acid and protein metabolism and may improve cardiac function. It is used by athletes and people interested in weight loss.
L-Glutamine	Useful in lower GI disorders (e.g., inflammatory bowel syndrome) because of its beneficial effect on cilia. It is also helpful in muscle regeneration and repair.
L-Glutathione	A major part of the detoxification enzyme pathways, especially for metals and carcinogens. It is a strong antioxidant, reducing free radical formation from radiation, and also has immunostimulatory properties.
L-Lysine	Used primarily to slow the development of lesions caused by herpes simplex; also has some effect on calcium absorption and utilization.
L-Methionine	When converted by the body into S-adenosyl methionine (SAMe), L-methionine can regulate serotonin reuptake and thereby stabilize moods. In this form, it can also have a positive effect on osteoarthritis.
N-Acetyl cysteine (NAC)	A strong antiviral agent; also to detoxify heavy metals. NAC provides antioxidant protection for cells. Its isomer also is used pharmacologically for treatment of acetaminophen overdoses and for its mucolytic effect in pulmonary disease.
L-Tyrosine	An important precursor to many neurotransmitters; used to combat depression and thyroid disorders.

From LaValle JB, et al: Natural Therapeutics Pocket Guide 2000–2001. Hudson, OH, Lexi-Comp, 2001; and Jellin JM, et al (eds): Natural Medicines Comprehensive Database, 3rd ed. Stockton, CA, Therapeutic Research Faculty, 2000.

16. What are "superfoods"?

Superfoods are a class of supplements that straddle the line between food and herb or nutriceuticals. Although they are considered foods because of their extremely high nutritional content (it is said that spirulina will yield 20 times the amount of protein as soybeans when grown on the same amount of land), they are called "superfoods" because they also induce specific effects in body functions.

A good example is bee pollen, a dense concentration of proteins and carbohydrates made up of flower pollen collected by bees. Bee pollen has significantly high levels of protein. It also can mitigate the symptoms and severity of seasonal allergies. Chlorella, a microalgae, is rich in amino acids and vitamins; it helps to raise serum albumin levels, detoxify the liver, and enhance the production of energy by stimulating the Krebs cycle. Spirulina, another microalgae, is one of the richest sources of amino acids and provides all of the essential amino acids. Spirulina is used to enhance the immune system, protect against ultraviolet radiation, and keep liver cells from mutating.

Other superfoods include royal jelly, wheatgrass, barley grass, brewer's (or nutritional) yeast, lecithin, propolis, kelp, garlic, and essential fatty acids (EFAs).

17. Are melatonin and DHEA the "fountains of youth" that the media imply?

The body's production of both melatonin and dehydroepiandrosterone (DHEA) declines as aging progresses. This finding has provoked the media to portray the two hormones as the "cure" for the aging process. Little evidence, either experimental or anecdotal, supports this claim. Melatonin and DHEA may have clinical value, but they do not alter or reverse the process of aging. Unlike other hormones that are also known to decline with age, melatonin and DHEA do not require a prescription; they are widely available over the counter.

Melatonin has been shown to regulate sleep patterns and to decrease the incidence and severity of periods of insomnia. It is also used as an antidepressant in seasonal affective disorder (SAD). Much of the recent interest in DHEA has been directed toward 7-keto DHEA, a more stable, and arguably safer, form of DHEA that, unike DHEA, is not synthesized into androgens and estrogens in the body. This form of DHEA has been shown to increase fat metabolism, furthering its use as a weight loss supplement. 7-Keto DHEA also increase thyroxine (T_3) levels and enhances immune system function by increasing interleukin 2 production and lymphocyte activity.[16]

18. What supplements can stimulate the immune system? How do they work?

Herbal and mushroom products with specific immune-enhancing properties have become popular recently. This trend is consistent with the more frequent adoption of a holistic perspective, which promotes healing not only by prescribing antibiotics to kill infections but also by boosting the body's natural defense mechanisms. In addition, because some cancers may have an immunologic component, studies have explored how some supplements may modulate specific activities of the immune system.

For many years we have known of the stimulatory effect of echinacea on phagocytosis and lymphocyte activity. Larch (*Larix occidentalis*) is receiving more attention through studies of its arabingalactans and their anticancer activity. Arabinogalactans increase the release of interferon gamma, tumor necrosis factor, and interleukins 1 and 6. They stimulate macrophage activity and natural killer (NK) cytotoxicity against tumor cells. Inositol hexaphophate (IP-6) is a B-vitamin with NK cell-stimulating potential. Mushroom extracts studied for use as supplemental cancer therapies include 1,3 beta d-glucans, which is derived from *Saccharomyces boulardii*; maitake (*Grifola frondosa*) D-fractions; reishi (*Ganoderma lucidum*); shiitake mushroom extracts; and MGN-3. Other supplements being reinvestigated for immunostimulatory effects are astragalus (*Astragalus membranaceus*), bovine colostrum, and selenium.[11]

19. What delivery systems are available in nutriceutical supplements?

The many commercially available delivery systems include capsules, tablets, sublingual tablets, powders, drink mixes, liquid suspensions, colloidal liquid suspensions, tinctures, teas, oral sprays, lipoceutical oral sprays, oral gel, sublingual liquids, nasal gel, topical creams, transdermal creams, and topical sprays. Each delivery method claims benefits in some way over the others.

One of the debates in delivery technology is whether tablets or capsules are more easily digestible. This issue becomes important when the digestive system has been compromised or is geneally weak; ease of digestion may make the difference between a full clinical dose or a subclinical dose. Currently, the trend tends to favor capsules because of the need for fewer inactive ingredients (tableting agents, glazes, and colors) and the fact that many commercial tableting procedures produce a pill that will not break down efficiently in the gut. Tablets, however, allow timed-release systems and enteric coatings.

Lipoceutical delivery systems are potentially more efficient than any other system. Lipoceutical supplements are liquid suspensions in which the supplement is enveloped in microscopic pouches of lipids. The lipid pouches can pass through membranes—specifically, the sublingual membranes. Thus supplement enters directly into the bloodstream without having to survive the harsh gut environment.

20. What do patients encounter upon entering a health food store?

Often patients go to a pharmacy, health food store, or a large retail chain that sells "health products" to purchase supplements. They may be faced with a staggering array of multiple brands and varying doses, delivery forms. and mixtures. Customers may be left to fend for themselves or get advice from the store clerks, some of whom may have never had formal training in botanicals or chemistry. One researcher, claiming to suffer from severe daily headaches of recent onset, spoke with personnel in 29 health food stores and recorded their responses. Less than 25% advised seeing a physician, and 42 different interventions were recommended.[17]

Of course, some health food stores specifically hire credible nutritional counselors to assist customers in making informed selections and to refer to medical practitioners when appropriate. Because it is difficult to keep up with medical literature as well as the rapidly changing supplement market, it may be wise to form an alliance with key staff members at venues where your patients shop. An incognito trip to familiarize yourself with available products and store personnel allows you to understand the patient's point of view.

21. How can physicians better educate themselves about supplementation? How can they facilitate patient education?

Patients often do not consider supplements as medications, and an estimated 15 million people take botanicals or high-dose vitamins in combination with prescription medications. Even when specifically asked on a comprehensive medical intake questionnaire, patients underreported their use of dietary supplements (30%) by half compared with a structured face-to face interview (60%).[18] This finding underscores the importance of directly asking patients about use of supplements—not only to prevent potential drug complications but also to align treatment with their personal philosophy. Many patients take vitamins and supplements to augment their health rather than treat disease. Supporting the proactive attitudes of your patients helps them achieve their goals.

22. List reliable sources for additional information.
- Office of Supplements at the National Institutes of Health [http://dietary-supplements.info.nih.gov/].
- LaValle JB, et al: Natural Therapeutics Pocket Guide 2000–2001. Hudson, OH, Lexi-Comp, , 2001. Easy-to-use information that is practical and fits in your pocket.
- Murray MT: Encyclopedia of Nutritional Supplements. Rocklin, CA, Prima Publishing, 1996.

REFERENCES

1. Williamson JM, Wyandt CM: An herbal update. Drug Topics 142:66–73, 1998.
2. LaValle JB, et al. Natural Therapeutics Pocket Guide 2000-2001, Hudson, OH, Lexi-Comp, 2001.
3. Balluz LS, et al: Vitamin and mineral supplement use in the United States: Results from the Third National Health and Nutrition Examination Survey. Arch Fam Med 9:258–262, 2000.
4. Vivian JC: Regulation of health claims for dietary supplements and foods. U.S. Pharmacist May:53–62, 2001.
5. Porter DV: Special report: dietary supplements—recent chronology and legislation. Nutr Rev 53:31–36, 1995.
6. Worthington V: Nutritional quality of organic versus conventional fruits, vegetables, and grains. J Altern Compl Med 7:161–173, 2001.
7. Simopoulos A, Robinson J: The Omega Plan. New York, HarperCollins, 1998.
8. www.nationalacademies.org/IOM. Accessed 4/8/02.
9. LaValle JB, et al: Natural Therapeutics Pocket Guide 2000-2001. Hudson, OH Lexi-Comp, 2001.
10. Pizzorno J, Murray MT. Textbook of Natural Medicine, 2nd ed. Edinburgh, Churchill Livingstone, 1999.
11. Jellin JM, et al (eds): Natural Medicines Comprehensive Database, 3rd ed. Stockton, CA, Therapeutic Research Faculty, 2000.
12. Goodman GE, et al: Risk factors for lung cancer and for intervention effects in CARET, the Beta-Carotene and Retinol Efficacy Trial. J Natl Cancer Inst 88:1550–1559, 1996.
13 Albanes D, Heinonen OP: Alpha-tocopherol and beta-carotene supplements and lung cancer incidence in the Alpha-Tocopherol, Beta-Carotene Cancer Prevention Study: Effects of base-line characteristics and study compliance. (ATBC study) J Natl Cancer Inst 88:1560–1570, 1996.
14. Prasad KN, et al: High doses of multiple antioxidant vitamins: Essential ingredients in improving the efficacy of standard cancer therapy. J Am Coll Nutr 18:13–25, 1999.]
15. Patient Information Sheet. Integrative Medicine Consult, Newton, MA, 2001.
16. http://www.humaneticscorp.com/7ketoabstracts.html. Accessed 4/7/02.
17. Vickers AJ, et al: Advice given by health food shops: Is it clinically safe? J R Coll Phys icians 32:426–428, 1998.
18. Hensrud DD, et al: Underreporting the use of dietary supplements and nonrprescription medications among patients undergoing a periodic health examination. Mayo Clin Proc 74:443–447, 1999.

21. EXERCISE AND FITNESS

Jeffry S. Life, M.D., Ph.D.

1. Define exercise.

Exercise is physical activity that is planned and structured for the sole purpose of improving, maintaining, or expressing a particular type(s) of physical fitness.[1] Exercise differs from physical activity, which is performed for purposes other than the specific development of physical fitness. Regular physical activity, however, can improve physical fitness.

Exercise includes two broad categories: aerobic and anaerobic. **Aerobic exercise** includes duration activities (e.g., running, bicycling, swimming) that extract energy more slowly from biochemical reactions that require oxygen. **Anaerobic exercise** includes activities such as sprinting and weight lifting, which utilize biochemical reactions that provide high levels of energy in the absence of oxygen.

2. Define fitness.

Fitness is a set of attributes related to a state of well-being that provides optimal performance for a given exercise or physical activity.[1] The many components to fitness include muscular strength, power, and endurance as well as cardiorespiratory endurance, flexibility, balance, and agility.

3. Does an improvement in level of fitness improve health outlook?

Numerous studies have demonstrated that behavioral changes, including improved level of physical fitness, delay all causes of mortality and extend life.[2] A study of Harvard alumni over an 11- to 15-year period demonstrated that men, regardless of their age, who were initially sedentary but adopted a more moderate-to-vigorous lifestyle of regular exercise activity had a 51% lower risk of death than men who remained sedentary. This study also revealed that becoming more physically active on a regular basis is of equal benefit in terms of reducing the risk of cardiac mortality as quitting cigarette smoking, reducing body weight, or controlling blood pressure.

The evidence continues to be overwhelming that even mild-to-moderate regular exercise, for both men and women, promotes good health, improves quality of life, and can significantly increase life expectancy. These results are achieved through a substantial reduction in the risk of death not only from heart disease but also from cancer and other degenerative diseases.

4. How does exercise affect lipid profiles?

Regular exercise improves lipid metabolism in men, and higher-volume aerobic exercise programs increase levels of high-density lipoprotein cholesterol (HDL-C) in both pre- and post-menopausal women.[3] Studies of resistance training found no increase in HDL-C levels. Levels of low-density lipoprotein cholesterol (LDL-C), total cholesterol, and body fat were reduced.

5. What should an adequate medical evaluation of a healthy person include before an exercise prescription is given?

Before any healthy person over the age of 35 years starts an endurance and strength-training program, the health care provider should undertake a complete evaluation, including physical exam, lab work, and possibly an exercise stress test. The lab work should include at least a fasting lipid profile (total cholesterol, LDL-C, HDL-C, and triglycerides), a metabolic panel to evaluate electrolyte status, liver and kidney tests, and a complete blood count.

6. How much aerobic exercise is necessary to achieve cardiovascular benefits?

The American College of Sports Medicine (ACSM) recommends that aerobic endurance exercise should be performed 3–5 days/week for 20–60 minutes continuously at 55–90% of maximal heart rat.[4] Sedentary people may have to exercise at the low end of the intensity range for a longer period than physically active people.

The Centers for Disease Control and Prevention (CDC) recommends that, at a minimum, adults engage in moderate-intensity physical activity in which they expend approximately 200 kcal/day (about 30 minutes/day). These activities can be outside a formal exercise program and also can be intermittent. Mild-to-moderate exercise is far better than none, but vigorous exercise is best of all.

7. How important are warm-ups and cool-downs?

Proper warm-ups and cool-downs are an essential part of a well-designed exercise program to ensure maximal performance and minimal injuries. A warm-up of 5–10 minutes of low-intensity calisthenic-type exercise, such as slow or brisk walking or light cycling, is ideal. A cool-down period of about the same duration provides gradual recovery from the endurance phase of both aerobic and anaerobic activities.

8. Are flexibility exercises important?

Flexibility diminishes with age, but no evidence indicates that this decrease is part of the aging process. Loss of flexibility is more likely due to diminished physical activity. Flexibility can be improved at any age through static stretching and range-of-motion exercises that promote elasticity of the soft tissues. Flexibility training should be performed at the end of an exercise program, when all of the tissues are warm, for 10–15 minutes on at least 2–3 days/week.[5]

9. How does exercise affect aging?

Exercise is undoubtedly the best "medication" that health care providers can prescribe. Increased fitness resulting from a regular exercise program can dramatically reduce the effects of aging that lead to functional decline and poor health.

A recent study of men in their 50s at the University of Texas Southwestern Medical Center in Dallas showed that just 6 months of aerobic exercise training, in which frequency, duration, and intensity were gradually increased, resulted in a return to the level of fitness that the men had at age 20 years.[6] This finding was confirmed by measuring aerobic power—the ability of the heart and lungs to supply oxygen to working muscles and cardiovascular performance. The researchers concluded that "no matter what your age, it's your current fitness level, not you're past fitness level, that really dictates how fit you are."

10. Why is it important to include resistance strength training in the exercise program?

Until recently, resistance training was believed to be appropriate only for young, healthy, male athletes. This mindset led many people to overlook the enormous benefits of resistance training for younger women, older men and women, and even children. Muscle strength begins to decline rapidly in sedentary people at about age 50.[7] This decline can be totally prevented and even reversed by simply incorporating resistance training into the person's lifestyle. Some studies have shown that just 2 months of strength training can reverse two decades of muscle loss.[8]

Improvement in the strength of elderly people also has important implications for health and quality of life. Balance and coordination are improved, and the risk of falls (a major cause of injury, fractures, and debilitation leading to death in elderly people) is greatly reduced. Strength training also helps to maintain and even increase bone density in both women and men of all ages, further reducing the risk for fractures.

11. What are "free weights"? Do they have any advantage over resistance machines?

Exercise with free weights involves dumbbells and barbells rather than the resistance machines seen in most commercial and home gyms. Athletes and strength coaches believe that free weights offer advantages that resistance machines do not provide. The athlete must completely control the lifted weight while maintaining balance. This process requires the recruitment of a greater number of motor units—not only in the muscles being trained, but also in stabilizing muscles. Many experts believe that free weights lead to greater muscle growth as well as increased strength compared with resistance machines. A good strength-training regimen incorporates both free weights and resistance machines.

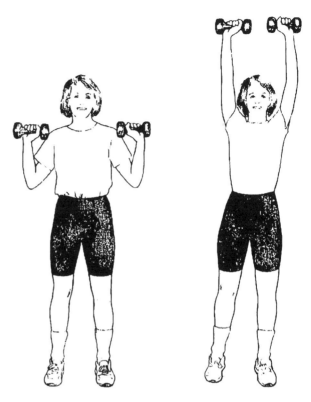

Use of free weights. (From Strong Women Stay Young by Miriam E. Nelson, Ph.D., and Sarah Wernick, Ph.D., copyright © 1997 by Miriam E. Nelson and Sarah Wernick. Used by permission of Bantom Books, a division of Random House, Inc.)

12. Does the ability to adapt to training decrease with age?

Recent studies in which older subjects were encouraged to train at higher intensities have shown that at any age people have considerable ability to increase endurance capacity and strength with proper training.[9] Exercise training can minimize or even reverse the syndrome of frailty, which is so prevalent among the most elderly people.

13. What is the best way to determine what a person should weigh?

Currently the body mass index (BMI), which is the ratio of weight to height squared, is used to determine whether a person is overweight or obese. A high BMI is associated with an increased prevalence of mortality from heart disease, diabetes, and cancer. This simplified approach works fairly well for most of the population, but since it looks only at weight and height, it does not assess body fat content—the factor that most increases the risk for diabetes, strokes, cancer, arthritis, and premature death. A much better assessment of health risks is the percentage of body fat. Height-weight tables should be avoided, and patients should be assessed as overfat rather than overweight.[10]

Fat and lean body mass can be measured by first determining body composition. The most common and widely used technique is measurement with calipers of skinfold thickness from selected sites. This method determines body fat percentage, which should be used to determine ideal body weight and degree of fatness.

14. What percentage of body fat is thought to be associated with good health and fitness?

Ideal body composition depends on age and gender. The following table lists the percentages of body fat for men[11] and women[12] that correlate with excellent to poor health and fitness ratings according to age. This table can be used as a guideline to determine ideal body weight. As a general rule, no man at any age should have > 18% body fat and no woman should exceed 25% for optimal fitness and health. Obesity and high health risk are defined as the accumulation of body fat > 25% for men and > 33% for women.

Percentages of Body Fat

HEALTH/FITNESS RATING	20–29 YR	30-39 YR	40–49 YR	50–59 YR	60+ YR
Men					
Excellent	< 11	< 12	< 14	< 15	< 16
Good	11–13	12–14	14–16	15–17	16–18
Average	14–20	15–21	17–23	18–24	19–25
Fair	21–23	22–24	24–26	25–27	26–28
Poor	> 23	> 24	> 26	> 27	> 28
Women					
Excellent	< 16	< 17	< 18	< 19	< 20
Good	16–19	17–20	18–21	19–22	20–23
Average	20–28	21–29	22–30	23–31	24–32
Fair	19–31	30–32	31–33	32–34	33–35
Poor	> 31	> 32	> 33	> 34	> 35

15. What is the best way to measure body fat?

There are numerous methods to assess percentages of body fat, but most require expensive and large pieces of laboratory equipment. Hydrostatic weighing has been considered the gold standard by which all other methods have been validated despite an error margin of ± 4%. Air-displacement plethysmography, a new, also costly method, is as accurate as hydrostatic weighing and appeals to people who are unable or reluctant to be submerged in water.

By far, the simplest and least expensive method for determining percentages of body fat is to measure subcutaneous fat at selected sites by measuring skinfold thickness with calipers. This technique provides a good estimate of body fat percentages (± 3–5% of hydrostatic weighing values) when done by trained, experienced people.[13]

16. What is $\dot{V}O_2$? Why is it important?

$\dot{V}O_2$ is an important number used by exercise physiologists to measure how much oxygen people use during exercise. The maximal ability to consume and utilize oxygen during exercise is called $\dot{V}O_2max$. $\dot{V}O_2max$ is determined by genetic make-up and exercise history. Most authorities regard it as the single best measurement of cardiorespiratory endurance and aerobic fitness. After the age of 25–30, $\dot{V}O_2max$ values decrease about 1% per year in people who remain sedentary.[14]

Fortunately, people can prevent this decline and actually increase $\dot{V}O_2max$ through endurance training (also called aerobic and cardio exercise)—at any age, regardless of physical condition.[16] In fact, the least fit people can achieve the greatest increase in $\dot{V}O_2max$ values.

17. What is the best endurance-training program to improve $\dot{V}O_2max$ (aerobic capacity)?

Two variables of endurance training play the key roles in increasing $\dot{V}O_2max$: volume (duration of training) and intensity (degree of difficulty of training). For a long time many authorities believed that gains in aerobic capacity and endurance were directly related to the volume of training. Consequently, people were advised to spend a great deal of time every day in slow, easy training. Recent research, however, has shown, that the intensity of the exercise directly improves aerobic capacity ($\dot{V}O_2max$) and enables people to reach maximal performance levels.[16]

Long-distance, low-intensity training does not produce the biochemical and physiologic changes needed to increase $\dot{V}O_2max$. High-intensity training (which can include intermittent high-intensity exercise or continuous exercise at near-competition pace) is required to maximize endurance performance and aerobic fitness.

Intermittent exercise (also called interval training) consisting of fast-paced, brief exercise bouts with short rest periods between bouts achieves the same aerobic benefits as long, continuous, high-intensity exercise without the boredom that many experience. Some people, however, prefer the near-meditative state associated with continuous training. The recommendation is to do one or the other or to combine the two, keeping in mind that intensity—not volume—is the critical factor in improving performance.

18. What is the best way to determine oxygen consumption levels?

The best and simplest way to determine the percentage of $\dot{V}O_2$max at which a person is training is to use heart rate as a guide.[17] First, determine the maximal heart rate by using the formula 220 – age = maximal heart rate (MHR). If the person is already in excellent physical condition, use 205 – $\frac{1}{2}$ age = MHR. MHR can be considered equivalent to $\dot{V}O_2$max, and the heart rate achieved during exercise can be converted into the percentage of MHR, which reflects the percentage of $\dot{V}O_2$max.

19. What heart rates should people attempt to achieve in order to burn the most body fat for a given amount of exercise?

The heart-rate zone of 50–65% of MHR is no longer believed to be the best range to burn fat. The target heart rate zone of 65–85% of MHR is now considered by most exercise physiologists to be the best level of intensity for improving endurance, achieving ultimate fitness, increasing $\dot{V}O_2$max, and getting rid of body fat.[18] If, however, a person is just beginning aerobic training, it is best to train in the 50–65% zone until he or she is ready to move into the target heart rate zone.

20. What is the best exercise program to increase cardiorespiratory endurance and physical fitness?

The best and most efficient method to increase aerobic fitness and cardiorespiratory endurance (the most important component of physical fitness) is to perform high-intensity training for 30 minutes 5 times/week after a 5-minute warm-up and before a 5-minute cool-down in the target heart rate zone.[16]

Resistance strength training must be included in the overall exercise program to achieve maximal health benefits. The most recently published guidelines for resistance strength training include using at least 8–10 different exercises, with a minimum of one exercise per major muscle group, 2–3 times/week on alternate days. Younger people should use 8–12 repetitions per set, and older people and cardiac patients should use 10–15 repetitions per set.[1] All sets should be performed at moderate-to-maximal effort.

Neither aerobic nor strength training programs should be started before the person has his or her doctor's approval.

21. How can people (especially men) get rid of their "spare tire"?

Abdominal obesity, a common problem for almost all men and many women, results mostly from deposits of fat inside the abdominal cavity—the so-called intra-abdominal fat. Abdominal obesity is the worst kind of fat because it not only adds inches to the waistline but also is one of the major causes of poor health.It does not simply hang out quietly inside the belly like subcutaneous fat under the skin; it is very much alive, actively producing harmful hormones and other chemicals that many scientists believe can cause cancer, elevate blood sugars, and produce insulin resistance that leads to hyperinsulinemia and diabetes.[19] This problem is of special importance to men because intra-abdominal fat increases the most with age.

Abdominal girth has been shown to be a better predictor of future coronary artery disease and type 2 diabetes than BMI—even though BMI is considered to be the gold standard and is used by doctors, nutritionists, and other health professionals to assess health risks. Unfortunately, many people with a normal, "healthy" BMI have significant amounts of disease-causing intra-abdominal fat.

Typically, a 1–4% reduction in overall percent of body fat occurs with endurance training in older adults, which is similar to that seen in younger adults. Of special note, however, in older men intra-abdominal fat is specifically targeted and can decrease by as much as 25% with exercise training.

22. Are there any contraindications to exercise testing and training for older men and women?

The contraindications to exercise testing and exercise training are the same regardless of gender or age. The major relative contraindications are recent ECG changes, recent myocardial infarction, unstable angina, uncontrolled arrhythmias, third-degree heart block, acute congestive heart failure, severe aortic stenosis, suspected dissecting aneurysm, myocarditis, thrombophlebitis, recent systemic or pulmonary embolus, acute infection, and significant emotional distress. The major relative contraindications for exercise testing include elevated blood pressures, cardiomyopathies, valvular heart disease, complex ventricular ectopy, and uncontrolled metabolic disease.

Adherence to the general ACSM guidelines for exercise testing, exercise recommendations, and medical supervision of both testing and recommendations is imperative.[20]

23. Are losses of muscle mass and strength and increases in body fat stores inevitable functions of aging?

Age-related loss of muscle mass (sarcopenia) accounts for the decreases in basal metabolic rate (BMR), muscle strength, and activity levels often observed in the elderly. Energy requirements decline as the BMR declines. When the decreased caloric need is not matched by an appropriate decrease in caloric intake, body fat content increases. Increased body fatness and the accompanying increase in abdominal obesity promote many disease states. The decrease in muscle mass is the direct cause of diminished strength. Decreased strength in the elderly is a major cause of disability.

Recent data suggest that such changes in body composition and aerobic capacity are not a function of aging. A study of endurance-trained people of different ages revealed that body fat stores and maximal aerobic capacity were not related to age but rather,to the total number of hours of exercise per week.[21]

Resistance strength training is also especially important in the elderly. It increases muscle size as a result of an increase in the number of muscle contractile proteins. As muscle mass increases, so does strength, which may enable an elderly person to ambulate without a cane, rise from a chair unassisted, or carry groceries. Although both aerobic and strength training are necessary, sarcopenia can be stopped and reversed only with strength training. Increased muscle mass and strength are the first steps toward reversing the syndrome of physical frailty and promoting a lifetime of increased physical activity, good functional capacity, and independence.

24. Does exercise help prevent osteoporosis?

Both aerobic exercise and weight-bearing physical activities are important in maintaining overall health as well as healthy bones, but it appears that strength training may be better at preserving bone density. High-intensity progressive strength training has been shown in several well-controlled studies to improve significantly the prevention and treatment of osteoporosis in both men and women.[22] Progressive resistance training helps premenopausal women achieve the highest peak bone mass possible and is also thought to help maintain or increase bone density in postmenopausal women. Studies continue to demonstrate that muscle mass, strength, balance, physical activity, and functional capacity are increased substantially with resistance training in men and women of all ages, including the very old.

25. What are the differences between aerobic endurance training and resistance strength training in terms of health and fitness?

Research has clearly shown that resistance training is essential for the development of muscle mass, strength, power. and endurance. Only recently, however, has the focus of importance of resistance training shifted from fitness to health and disease prevention. A recent symposium on resistance training for health and disease addressed the scientific evidence for the importance of strength training for the development and maintenance of muscle and bone and its importance in the prevention and rehabilitation of many chronic disease problems, such as physical dysfunction, obesity/metabolism, weight control, osteoporosis, low back pain, and disability.[23] Pollock and Vincent recently reviewed the effects of resistance training on health, as described in the following table.[24]

Comparison of the Effects of Aerobic Endurance Training and Resistance Strength Training on Health and Fitness Variables

VARIABLE	AEROBIC EXERCISE	RESISTANCE EXERCISE
Bone mineral density	↑↑	↑↑
Body composition		
% fat	↓↓	↓
lean body mass	↔	↑↑
Strength	↑↑	↑↑↑
Glucose metabolism		
Insulin response to glucose challenge	↓↓	↓↓
Basal insulin levels	↓	↓
Insulin sensitivity	↑↑	↑↑
Serum lipids		
HDL	↑↑	↔
Resting heart rate	↓↓	↔
Stroke volume	↑↑	↔
Blood pressure at rest		
Systolic	↓↓	↔
Diastolic	↓↓	↓↔
VO_2max	↑↑↑	↑
Endurance time	↑↑↑	↑↑
Physical function	↑↑	↑↑↑
Basal metabolism	↑	↑↑

From Pollock ML, Vincent KR: The President's Council on Physical Fitness and Sports Research Digest. Series 2, No. 8, December 1996.

26. What form of exercise has been shown to help with low back problems?

One of the best ways to treat chronic back injuries and chronic back pain is adherence to a program that includes both aerobic and strength-training exercises. This approach helps prevent future injuries by maintaining physical fitness and leanness throughout life. Back injuries occur 10 times less often in people who perform aerobic and resistance training.

Although all forms of exercise have been shown to benefit people with chronic low back pain, an intense, integrated approach that includes regular resistance training has been proven to be the most effective. This form of exercise not only improves endurance and activity tolerance but also increases the strength and flexibility of back muscles. In addition, it promotes weight loss (obesity is a major cause of acute and chronic back pain) and provides beneficial psychological effects.

A study by Nelson and colleagues was designed to determine whether patients with back pain for whom spinal surgery was recommended could avoid surgery through an aggressive strengthening program.[25] After following a 10-week intensive back-strengthening regimen, 57 of the 60 patients no longer required surgery and were virtually pain-free. Well over 100 other studies have shown that cardiovascular and strength-training exercises can alleviate chronic back pain by strengthening and increasing the flexibility of back muscles.

27. Is weight-lifting advisable for people with heart disease?

Recently an expert panel of scientists, organized by the American Heart Association, put to rest the age-old myth that weight-training and other forms of resistance exercise are bad for the heart. The committee advises physicians to recommend this form of exercise for healthy older patients as well as those with heart disease, including some people with recent heart attacks, as long as they are closely monitored and supervised by experienced health professionals.[26]

Patients with healthy hearts (regardless of age or gender) and patients with unhealthy hearts can now be encouraged to start using resistance training along with aerobic training as an important part of a heart disease prevention and/or treatment program. Indeed, some debilitated patients may need first to gain muscle mass in order to participate meaningfully in aerobic exercise.

28. What, if any, exercise restrictions should be instituted during pregnancy?

Despite the often publicized fears of exercise during pregnancy, ample evidence indicates that regular exercise is beneficial to both mother and fetus as long as certain guidelines are followed. The American College of Gynecology recommends aerobic exercise 3 times/week for up to 15 minutes. According to Lokey and others, no evidence indicates that exercise 3 times /week for up to 45 minutes at a heart rate of 144 beats/minute is harmful.[27] Exercise performed for longer durations, at higher intensities, at high altitudes, or during thermal stress (hot or humid conditions) may be harmful to the fetus. It is important to recognize that what may be beneficial to the mother may be detrimental to the fetus.

29. Do we need to worry about the present state of children's levels of fitness and health?

The Surgeon General's Report on Exercise revealed that nearly one-half of Americans aged 12–21 years are not vigorously active on a regular basis.[28] Participation in all types of physical activity has dramatically declined in recent years as age or grade in school increases. Daily enrollment in physical education classes dropped from 42% to 25% among high school students between 1991 and 1995 and is even lower now. Several large-scale studies of the upper-body strength of children have ranked them in the "very poor" category. American children, compared with children in Europe, Great Britain, Australia, and Canada, also have much poorer cardiovascular endurance.

Childhood physical inactivity has become a national crisis, contributing significantly to the current epidemic of childhood obesity.[1] The percentage of overweight and obese children and adolescents has more than doubled since the early 1970s, and much of this increase is blamed on physical inactivity, although poor nutritional habits play an equally important role. Every year that a child remains overweight, his or her chance of growing into an overweight adult increases. The single most important predictor of developing diabetes is overweight. Childhood and adolescent type2 diabetes, previously almost unheard of, has now become a major health problem in America, adding to the epidemic of type 2 diabetics in the adult population.

To make matters even worse, the origins of coronary artery disease, the number-one killer of Americans, start in childhood. As many as 40% of children aged 5–8 years have at least one heart disease risk factor (high cholesterol, physical inactivity, obesity, or high blood pressure).

Clearly, physical inactivity is an insidious disease affecting the quality of life of today's children and tomorrow's adults. Healthy lifestyle habits can reduce the risk of developing diabetes by > 90% and can also prevent the development of heart disease and other degenerative diseases. Healthy exercise and nutritional practices must be incorporated into the daily lives of children—and follow them into adulthood.

30. What principles of resistance training should be used in children?

Evidence continues to mount that children as young as 7 years of age can increase strength when they participate in a structured resistance training program. The safety and efficacy of resistance strength training for prepubescent children is well documented.[29] Recommendations to minimize the risks of injury include the following[1]:
- Medical clearance must be obtained.
- Proper supervision by trained experienced individuals is essential.
- The facility must be safe for children
- Maximal lifts, sudden explosive movements, and competition with others must be discouraged.
- Proper breathing and lifting techniques must be taught and used.
- Adequate rest includes at least 2 minutes between exercise sets.
- Adequate fluid intake is essential.
- Participation in a wide range of exercises should be encouraged to promote overall development.
- A brief warm-up should precede and a brief cool-down should follow the exercise session.
- Exercise sets should consist of high repetitions (12–15) and relatively low resistance to achieve the greatest improvement in muscle strength and growth with no adverse effect on bone, muscle, or connective tissue.

31. Is there any real benefit to hyped-up sports drinks?

Over the past few years an ever increasing number of sports drinks claim to provide not only fluid but also essential nutrients that improve muscle strength, endurance, and overall performance. In truth, there is nothing "magical" about any of these beverages. All contain carbohydrates, which have been clearly shown to be beneficial when muscle glycogen levels are near depletion and blood glucose levels are low. Research has shown, however, that carbohydrate ingestion is beneficial only during prolonged exercise. If pre-exercise nutrition is adequate, there is no metabolic or ergogenic (performance-enhancing) need to ingest carbohydrate during continuous exercise lasting less than 90 minutes. In fact, ingestion of carbohydrates during short-term exercise simply increases the calorie intake and interferes with efforts to get rid of body fat.

Only small amounts of electrolytes are lost during very heavy exercise and can easily be replaced by eating fruits or vegetables. Only endurance athletes who sweat heavily for extended periods need to replenish electrolytes during exercise .

It is important to consume plenty of water during exercise. People should drink more than they think that they need. People are notorious for underestimating the required amount of water.

32. Do any supplements enhance exercise performance?

Many supplements claim to enhance exercise performance, but only creatine has stood up to the rigors of scientific investigation.[30] Research confirms that creatine produces significant improvements in sports that demand high levels of strength, power, and speed in both men and women. Increases in lean body mass associated with creatine supplementation, once thought to be due to water retention, have now been shown to be due to actual gains in muscle tissue. Creatine truly is a major key to achieving greater strength, muscularity, and peak performance. Because creatine has been on the market for less than 10 years, however, long-term studies are unavailable.

How does creatine work? It is naturally produced by the kidneys and liver from three nonessential amino acids and then transported into muscle cells, where it is converted into creatine phosphate (CP). CP provides an instant source of additional adenosine triphosphate, the metabolic fuel needed to carry out most energy-consuming processes, including muscle contraction.

33. Can older people benefit from taking creatine?

A study by Pirola et al. in patients over 60 years of age with muscle atrophy after femoral fractures showed a 1.9-fold greater increase in thigh and leg muscle mass with daily ingestion of 500 mg of creatine for 20 days in conjunction with physical therapy compared with subjects not receiving creatine.[31] Other studies have shown that older people can demonstrate a significant reduction in muscle fatigue by taking creatine. In another study, Tarnopolsky gave creatine supplements to patients with neuromuscular diseases associated with muscle weakness and wasting and showed that creatine supplementation increased their strength.[32] He believes that creatine, when combined with an exercise program, also helps healthy elderly people to retain muscle strength and mobility. These studies demonstrate that highly trained athletes and young people are not the only people who can benefit from creatine. It appears that older people can get even more benefit from this supplement.

34. What are the psychological benefits of exercise?

Numerous studies have demonstrated that physical exercise of low-to-moderate intensity is associated with improvements in mood and well-being and reduces anxiety, depression, and stress.[34] Positive effects on self-concept, self-esteem, and self-assurance have also been reported.

Improvements in psychological functioning associated with exercise are poorly studied, but they are believed to result from the increased sense of mastery, control, and self-sufficiency that accompanies improved levels of fitness. Exercise is also a form of meditation that triggers an altered and more relaxed state of consciousness, which may provide additional help in dealing with stress. Exercise is a form of biofeedback that can teach self-regulation of the autonomic nervous system, thus improving control of emotional and psychological states. Health care providers have a significant responsibility to inform their patients about the physical and psychological benefits of physical activity and to motivate them to participate regularly.

REFERENCES

1. Robergs RA, Roberts SO: Fundamental Principles of Exercise Physiology for Fitness, Performance, and Health. New York, McGraw-Hill, 2000.
2. Paffenbarger RS, et al: Changes in physical activity and other lifeway patterns influencing longetivity. Med Sci Sports Exerc 26: 857, 1994.
3. Saltin B, Astrand PO: Free fatty acids and exercise. Am J Clin Nutr 57(Suppl):752S, 1993.
4. Brennan,FH: Exercise prescriptions for active seniors: A team approach for maximizing adherence. Physician Sportsmed 30(2):19–26, 2002.
5. Wilmore JH, Costill DL: Physiology of Sport and Exercise, 2nd ed. Champaign, IL, Human Kinetics, 1999.
6. Turning back the clock 30 years in 6 months. Tufts Univ Health Nutri Lett 19(11):1, 2002.
7. Lexell J: Ageing and human skeletal muscle: Observations from Sweden. Can J Appl Physiol 18:2, 1993.
8. Yarasheski KE, et al: Acute effects of resistance exercise on muscle protein synthesis in young and elderly adults. Am J Physiol. 65:210, 1993.
9. Klitgaard H, et al: Function, morphology and protein expression of aging skeletal muscle: A cross-sectional study of elderly men with different training backgrounds. Acta Physiol Scand 457(Suppl):1, 1990.
10. Life JS: Performance nutrition. Muscle Media Mag 80:32–33, 2000.
11. Jackson AS, Pollock ML: Generalized equations for predicting body density of men. Br J Nutr 40:497–504, 1978.
12. Jackson AS, et al: Generalized equations for predicting body density of women. Med Sci Sport Exerc 12:175–182, 1980.
13. Lohman TG: Advances in Body Composition Assessment. Champaign, IL, Human Kinetics, 1992.
14. Dehn MM, et al: Longitudinal variations in maximal oxygen intake with age and activity. J Appl Physiol 33:805, 1972.
15. Soina RJ, et al: Differences in cardiovascular adaptations to endurance exercise training between older men and women. J Appl Physiol 75:435, 1975.
16. McArdle WD, Katch FI, Katch VL: Exercise Physiology, 5th ed. Philadelphia, Lippincott Williams & Wilkins, 2001.
17. American College of Sports Medicine: Resource Manual for Guidelines for Exercise Testing and Prescription, 3rd ed. Philadelphia, Lippincott Williams & Wilkins, 1998.
18. Knight EL: Heart Rate Based Exercises for Preventive Medicine. ISC Division of Wellness, 2000.
19. Reaven GM: Pathophysiology of insulin resistance in human disease. Physiol Rev 75:473, 1995.
20. American College of Sports Medicine: Guidelines for Exercise Testing and Prescription, 5th ed. Baltimore, Williams & Wilkins, 1995.
21. Evans WJ: Exercise training guidelines for the elderly. Med Sci Sports Exerc 31:12–17. 1999.
22. Layne JE, Nelson ME: The effects of progressive resistance training on bone density: A review. Med Sci Sports Exerc 31(1):25–30, 1999.
23. Feigenbaum MS, Pollock ML: Prescription of resistance training for health and disease. Med Sci Sports Exerc 31(1):38–45, 1999.
24. Pollock ML, Vincent KR: The President's Council on Physical Fitness and Sports Research Digest. Series 2, No. 8, December 1996.
25. Carpenter DN, Nelson BW: Low back strengthening for the prevention and treatment of low back pain. Med Sci Sports Exerc 31(1):18–24, 1999.
26. Fletcher GF, et al: Exercise standards for testing and training: A statement for healthcare professionals from the American Heart Association. Circulation 104:1694–1740, 2001.
27. Lokey EA, et al: Effects of physical exercise on pregnancy outcomes: A meta-analytic review. Med Sci Sports Exerc 23:1234–1239, 1991.
28. Mahan KL, Escott-Stump S: Krause's Food, Nutrition & Diet Therapy, 10th ed. Philadelphia, W. B. Saunders, 2000.
29. Kraemer WJ, Fleck SJ: Strength Training for Young Athletes. Champaign, IL, Human Kinetics, 1993.
30. Williams MH, et al: Creatine: The Power Supplement. Champaign, IL, Human Kinetics, 1999.
31. Pirola V, Pisani L, Teruzzi P: Evaluation of the recovery of muscular trophicity in aged patients with femoral fractures treated with creatine phosphate and physiokinesitherapy. Clin Terapeut 139:115–119, 1991
32. Tarnopolsky M, Martin J: Creatine monohydrate increases strength in patients with neuromuscular disease. Neurology 52:854–857, 1999
33. Weyerer S, Kupfer B: Physical exercise and psychological health. Sports Med 17(2):108–116, 1994.

22. ENERGY MEDICINE

Joann D'Aprile, D.O.

1. Define bioelectromagnetics.

Bioelectromagnetics (BEM) is the science that studies how living organisms interact with electromagnetic fields.[1] All living organisms possess electrical phenomenon and, indeed, without them would die. Every cell of the body is made of atoms composed of subatomic energy particles in constant motion. When electric currents (no matter how small) flow, a magnetic field is generated.

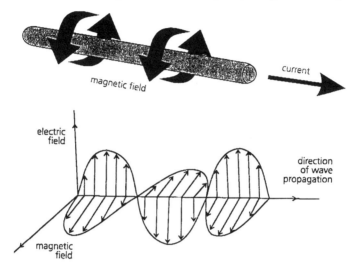

Top, An electric current in a wire produces a magnetic field in the space around the wire. *Bottom,* Electromagnetic theory showing a wave in which the electric field in perpendicular to the magnetic field and also to the direction of propagation. (From National Institutes of Health: Bioelectromagnetics applications in medicine. In Alternative Medicine: Expanding Medical Horizons. Washington, DC, Office of Alternative Medicine, National Institutes of Health, 1994 [NIH publication no. 94-066].)

The strength of the magnetic field depends on the amount of current flowing through the wire, nerve, or tissue. An electromagnetic (EM) field contains both an electric and a magnetic field. The EM spectrum spans from DC (zero frequency) waves, radio waves, microwaves, and visible light wavelengths to gamma and cosmic rays. Clearly exposure to ionizing, high-frequency radiation is harmful; even overexposure to ultraviolet light causes damage. Less appreciated is the fact that low- and extremely low-frequency waves can produce specific physiologic effects in the body. Evidence points to the cell membrane, often mildly electrochemically charged, as a primary area where applied EM fields act on cells. Medical applications of BEM is a growing field.

2. What is energy medicine?

Energy medicine is a broad concept based on the belief that "in addition to a system of physical and biochemical processes, the human being is made up of a complex system of energy."[2] Clinically, energy medicine is used every day in conventional medicine to diagnose and treat various conditions with methods such as radiation therapy, ultrasound, electrical muscle stimulation, and pacemakers. In addition to these more familiar techniques, there is a host of methods whose exact mechanisms have been more difficult to identify and qualify with available instruments. They are based on the belief that we are all surrounded by a field of energy that flows through and around us and is constantly interacting with the environment. In a state of wellness, energy flows freely. These methods may include diagnosis and healing that is less direct, or at a distance, from the intended subject.

3. How long and where has energy medicine been practiced?

Energy healing has been practiced by various cultures across the world for thousands of years. It is one of the oldest forms of healing. The idea of an energetic connection between every element of the physical world has been expressed in many ways, both in Eastern and Western cultures. In China, it is called *chi* or *qi*; in Japan, *ki*; in India and Tibet, *prana*; in the Jewish kabalistic tradition, *yesod*; and in Sufi tradition, *baraka*. In Eastern philosophy, the energy fields emanating from the body and mind are united. In the West, the body's innate energy flow also has special names. Pythagoras conceived of a life energy (*pneuma*) visible in the luminous body as early as the sixth century B.C. Other terms include *wakan* (Lakota tribes), *orenda* (Iroquois tribes), *megbe* (Ituri pygmies), and the Holy Spirit (Christians).[3]

4. Discuss the historical background for energetic healing.

Various healings are described in the Bible and other spiritual works all over the world. The "laying on of hands" (also known as therapeutic touch and healing touch) was practiced by Jesus. Evidence of fields of light surrounding Jesus and other spiritual figures is evident in religious paintings. The earliest writings describing the human energy field in Chinese culture date back 4000–5000 years to the *Yellow Emperor's Canon of Medicine*. This first textbook on internal medicine described the movement of qi in the body along meridians, or energy channels, and its relationship to health. Electricity from electric eels, used for healing the sick, was first documented about 2750 B.C.[4]

The first recorded mention of "vital" energy in Western literature was by the Pythagoreans around 500 B.C. *Vis medicatrix naturae*, or the healing power of nature, was described in Greece by Hippocrates (460–377 B.C.), who referred to using his hands to "pull and draw" aches and impurities away from his patients.[5] Paracelsus reported "a healing energy that radiates within and around man like a luminous sphere." He believed that this energy could cause and cure disease, work from a distance, and be influenced by magnets, planets, and stars. Some of the theories and practices of contemporary energy medicine reflect these earlier beliefs.

5. What types of healing systems and techniques are included in energy medicine?

Energy Medicine Techniques

THERAPY	THEORY
Acupuncture	Direct therapy involving stimulation of acupuncture points with thin needles to activate the body's own energies to restore health. Part of a whole system of traditional Chinese medicine.
Acupressure	Similar to above but uses finger pressure to stimulate points.
Qi-gong	The art of cultivating internal energy. A self-healing practice to help keep qi flowing through the body and to help connect body, mind, and spirit. Also applied by masters to help others heal.
Tai chi	A series of flowing exercise movements to build and circulate energy for health and healing.
Aikido	Japanese martial art that builds ki (chi). Practitioners learn to master the mind and body while learning the art of self-defense.
Yoga	Philosophy and practice of poses that teach balance of the body, mind, and spirit. Variations range from meditative to vigorous practice.
Polarity therapy	Touch therapy of balancing flow between positive and negative poles within the body.
Therapeutic touch	Indirect energy medicine technique derived from the laying on of hands and incorporated into nursing practice. The practitioner senses and treats by directing universal energies to the patient's auric fields.

Table continued on following page

Energy Medicine Techniques (Continued)

THERAPY	THEORY
Healing touch	Also founded by nurses, it contains elements of therapeutic touch but also involves direct physical contact with the patient.
Reiki	Another indirect energy medicine technique channeling universal life-force energy through the healer, using specific hand placements to promote physical healing.
Homeopathy	Homeopathic remedies are made by high dilution of substances that cause symptoms in their undiluted state. These substances retain the vibrational pattern of the remedy, which activates the body's vital force to stimulate healing.
Color, sound, and light therapy	Therapy based on using the various vibrations of color, light, or sounds to restore balance. Music is used to stimulate various brainwave frequencies to help induce healing. The Mozart effect is an example of music for relaxation and learning. Chanting or drumming may also induce therapeutic rhythms.
Prayer	A type of spiritual healing independent of any specific religion. A positive, pure thought form sent out to the universe, usually for the benefit of another.

From Baggott A: The Encyclopedia of Energy Healing. New York, Sterling Publishing, 1999, with permission.

6. Summarize the science behind energy theories.

Scientific models of mechanistic thinking, originating with Isaac Newton in the late 17th century, described atoms as the basic building blocks of the universe. Matter could be understood by reducing it to its smallest parts. In the early 19th century, electrical and magnetic phenomena were discovered. Newtonian physics, however, could not explain or be applied to these new discoveries.

Soon it was found that electric charges in motion, particularly electrons, gave rise to circular magnetic fields and electromagnetic forces. Eventually, instruments were created that could detect and measure these fields. Michael Faraday and James Clerk Maxwell were responsible for establishing the concept of a universe filled with force fields. Thus, field theory was born. Maxwell also discovered that light is actually a short electromagnetic wavelength. The first real break with classical physics occurred with the work of Max Planck, who discovered that matter absorbed heat and radiated light in chunks, which he termed quanta. He used this theory to explain the observed spectrum of a blackbody. Albert Einstein subsequently postulated that electromagnetic radiation could exist only in discrete units, called photons.

7. How did Einstein's theories change the concept of energy?

In the early 20th century, Einstein published the theory of relativity, which shattered all Newtonian concepts. His theory describes a four-dimensional space-time continuum and established the connection between space and time, which no longer were viewed as separate entities. His famous equation, $E = mc^2$, determined that all objects with mass have an amount of energy (E) that equals the objects mass (m) times the square of the speed of light (c^2). Even the smallest amount of matter, including the atoms and molecules that make up the human body, has an incredible amount of energy.

Because Einstein was able to bring together the concepts of mass and energy, his theory of special relativity established the union of time and space. His work was followed by the development of the de Broglie wavelength. Because both mass and light are forms of energy and light can be understood as a particle or a wave, Louis de Broglie theorized that matter could be seen as a particle or a wave. This theory established the concept of wave-particle duality. In quantum theory, waves and particles are not distinct entities; in fact, the wave is a packet of energy in its purest form. These wave functions have no definite frequencies and repeat themselves cyclically in space and time, carrying energy.[6]

Quantum theory forced physicists to accept the fact that the solid material world of classical physics dissolves at the subatomic level into wavelike probabilities of interconnectedness. In other words, subatomic particles are not things but interconnections among things. Nothing can be viewed as an isolated entity.[7] Modern medicine still relies heavily on Newtonian mechanistic concepts and reductionistic logic. Energy medicine continues to evolve from the profound insights of quantum physics. It seems that medicine has a lot of catching up to do.

8. What is the energy anatomy of the body?

There are at least three distinct forms of energy anatomy:

1. **Chakras.** The concept of chakras comes from Eastern philosophy and yogi doctrine; the name is derived from the Sanskrit word meaning "wheel." Traditionally, seven chakras have been described; they are centered over nerve plexuses and endocrine centers in the body, the area of the third eye in the forehead, and at the crown of the head. Eastern theory holds that the major chakras are associated with major body organs or systems. For example, the third chakra located at the solar plexus is associated with the adrenal glands and the energy of power; the fourth chakra, the heart, is associated with the energy of love.

2. **Meridians.** Energy (qi) also has been found to run along channels called meridians (see figure at left), which are used in traditional Chinese medicine (see Chapter 11).

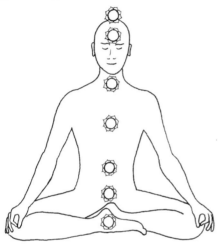

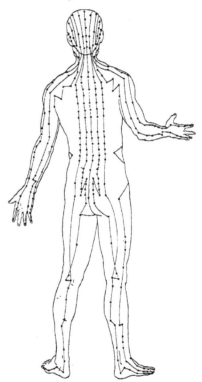

Above, The seven chakras are centered over nerve plexuses and endocrine centers in the body, the area of the third eye in the forehead, and at the crown of the head. (Drawing by Matthew Flesch.)

Right, Acupuncture points on meridians of qi. (From *Between Heaven and Earth* by Harriet Beinfield and Efrem Korngold, copyright © 1991 by Harriet Beinfield and Efrem Korngold. Used by permission of Ballantine Books, a division of Random House, Inc.)

3. **Auras.** The bioenergy field, or aura, does not end with the body's physical limits but moves within, extends outward, and surrounds us. It is the focus of many of the indirect energy medicine techniques. The aura is made up of layers of energies known as the subtle bodies, which include the etheric body, the astral/emotional body, the mental body, and the spiritual body. The closest layer to the physical body, the etheric body, is the most important in regard to energy healing because it is considered a perfect blueprint for the body (see figure on following page).

9. What does energy medicine tell us about the phantom limb phenomenon?

Some neurologists believe that the brain is encoded from birth with a map of the body and may be the reason why amputees still have the sensation of a missing, or phantom, limb. The sensation also may be due to the continuation of bioelectric and magnetic impulses along nerves that, by the laws of physics, continue to propagate outward even beyond the truncated anatomy. Other theories to explain phantom limb pain include the continuation of the body's energy fields through meridians and/or as an extension of the human aura within the etheric body.

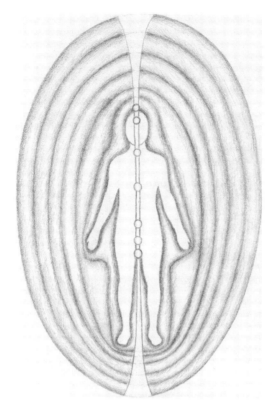

The seven levels of the auric field.

10. How do these energies relate to actual anatomic structures?

Robert O. Becker, an orthopedic surgeon, established the relationship between regeneration of body parts and electrical currents. While looking into the reason that some broken bones do not heal, he discovered that any injury to the body, such as a broken bone, registers abnormally as a positive magnetic field. (Remember that electric currents carry a negative charge). This positive electromagnetic signal goes to the brain, which responds by sending a negative electromagnetic signal to the injured area. The body then concentrates the necessary negative magnetic field at the injured site for healing. As healing begins, the affected area oscillates from electromagnetic positive to electromagnetic negative. If the body succeeds in sending enough electromagnetic current to the site of injury, it will heal itself.

Becker also found that acupuncture meridians conduct electrical current. Acupuncture needles, when placed in meridians, create electrical ion fluxes in those areas.[8] Many follow-up studies have replicated the acupuncture meridian electric measurements and their use in diagnoses. Of interest, stimulation of acupuncture points located on the small toe and associated with vision (corresponding to the traditional Chinese energy anatomy but not, of course, to the eye itself) caused the vision centers of the brain to light up on functional magnetic resonance scanning. Direct stimulation of the eyes with light produced similar results, but sham acupoints used as controls did not.[9] It seems that science is beginning to validate theories of energetic anatomy.

11. Do any instruments measure human energy?

Electrons, the main carriers of magnetism, move within the nervous system's direct current (DC) circuit, spinning either clockwise to form positive magnetic fields or counterclockwise to form negative magnetic fields. Modern instruments that have enabled scientists to detect some of the body's electromagnetic properties include nuclear magnetic resonance (NMR), magnetic resonance imaging (MRI), superconducting quantum interference (SQUID), magnetoencephalography (MEG), electroencephalography (EEG), electromyography (EMG), computed tomography (CT), and positron emission tomography (PET).

Most medical research thus far has tried to explain life in terms of gross electrical measurements, such as electrocardiograms (EKGs) of the heart, electroencephalograms (EEGs) of the brain, and electromyograms (EMGs) of muscles. In fact, surface electrodes anywhere on the body pick up all electrical activity in the body. Thus, recordings from the heart, which produce the strongest impulses, are present wherever electrodes are applied to the body. In addition, with an understanding of physics, we can recognize that this energy and information are continuously sent outward into the space around us. One researcher has measured heart frequencies at least 4 feet from the body.

Schwartz and Russek at the University of Arizona found a synchronization of cardiac energy between the subject's and experimenter's EKGs and EEGs from a distance of 3 feet as part of a follow-up to the Harvard Mastery of Stress study.[10] A similar, more recent study verified these results by providing evidence of an electromagnetic energy exchange by the heart, as demonstrated by the registering of the EKG signal of one subject in another subject's EEG when the two subjects were either touching or in close proximity.[11]

12. How has the human energy field been measured?

Dr. Valerie Hunt at the University of California, Los Angeles conducted studies of fields of energy distinct from other biologic activity. She has measured consistent waveforms and frequencies that correlate with the colors of the aura as reported by Rosalyn Bruyere, a well-known auric reader.[12] Physics teaches us that all matter is made of energy vibrating to a different frequency, creating the illusion of a material world perceivable through the five senses. The variety of intensity of these vibrations is expressed through the different colors of the electromagnetic spectrum and may be detected with electromagnetic measuring devices. This research may offer some explanation of the auric field.

How consciousness, and even nonlocality, may cause changes in these fields is under serious study. Elmer Green isolated subjects sitting in front of a copper wall from outside electromagnetic influence and explored possible electromagnetic correlates of the human energy field.[13] Green theorized that people in deep meditation may generate electrical voltages in their body. In a study of healers, he found that voltages increased with the intention to heal. Eventually he drew two conclusions from his experiments:

1. Whatever the type of energy is associated with healing, one of its connections is electrical. Green did not believe that electricity by itself was the cause of the healing.

2. Green came to accept distance healing as fact. He believed that enough research demonstrated the effects of prayer at a distance to support this conclusion.[13]

13. What is the energetic basis for illness?

Because all matter is energy, humans can be considered dynamic energetic systems that are affected by various forms of energy. As Gerber observes, "If we are beings of energy, then it follows that we can be affected by energy."[14] With this concept in mind, health can be viewed as a state of dynamic equilibrium when functioning is optimal. Disequilibrium, or dis-ease, can be viewed as an energy imbalance, excess, or deficiency. In other words, a deficient part of the system may need more energy, whereas an excessive part may have energy that needs to be released. We also can begin to understand how our own energy systems may be affected by subtle changes in the environment, diet, and even emotions. Much work that is under way to study the possible interactions between mind and matter (e.g., psychoneuroimmunology and direct neuropeptide links between the brain and the body) makes more "logical" sense.

Similarly, changes in biomagnetic energies on the quantum level may be responsible for physical and/or emotional changes. Early in the 20th century, Harold Saxton Burr at Yale did extensive research on the role of electricity in the development of disease. He studied energy fields of all living things, eventually writing a book called *Blueprint for Immortality: The Electric Patterns of Life*, later published as *The Fields of Life*. He believed that the energy fields of life reflected the physical and mental conditions of the person and so could be used to help diagnose illness. Burr measured surface potentials and changes in body potential and correlated them with disease states. He found that weakness in the life fields predated disease states.[15] His work was ahead of its time and contradicted established medical belief systems. Many of his theories are currently being studied again.

14. Discuss the conventional applications of energy medicine.

Various forms of energy have been used to diagnose and treat illness. Light energy is an accepted form of conventional healing with well-documented mechanisms. For example, bilirubin lights (phototherapy) are used to treat jaundice in the newborn, full-spectrum lights are used to treat seasonal affective disorder, and ultraviolet light is used to treat certain skin disorders (e.g., psoriasis) and for sterilization purposes. Laser beams are used to make incisions, stop bleeding, and correct diabetic retinopathy, to name a few.

Ultrasound, transcutaneous electrical nerve stimulation (TENS), diathermy, and other similar physical therapy modalities mostly use thermal effects, particle displacement, electrophoresis, or dielectric breakdown to help relax muscles in spasm and relieve pain. Similarly, transcranial electrostimulation (TCES) applies low currents to the brain externally for the treatment of depression, anxiety, and insomnia.[16] Electroshock therapy has been used to treat major depression. In addition, pacemakers, defibrillators, and electrical spinal stimulation are familiar in modern medicine.

Studies also have shown that vibrations from rhythmic sounds have a profound effect on brain activity. Music therapy had been used successfully for a variety of conditions, including stress, tension, mental distraction, and negative moods. One study found significant increases in hostility, sadness, tension, and fatigue after subjects listened to grunge rock music and significant increases in caring, relaxation, mental clarity, and vigor after they listened to music designed to have mood-lifting effects.[17] Music has been used in a wide variety of medical settings and has been shown to decrease anxiety before surgery, to improve cardiovascular function in intensive care patients, and to increase serum IgA in hospitalized children.[18]

15. Have any of the nonlocal EM techniques been found helpful in treating illness?

Many healing modalities involve contact or proximity between practitioner and patient, including therapeutic touch, healing touch, qi-gong, reiki, shiatsu, craniosacral osteopathic techniques, and polarity therapy. They are based on the assumption that an exchange of energy facilitates healing. Studies have demonstrated physiologic and psychological effects of many of these treatments, but we have not yet been able to pinpoint a mechanism to explain the effects. It is postulated that a tuned resonance pattern may develop between healer and patient. Many energy medicine techniques involve use of the healer's hands to work with energy fields several inches from the patient's body, while the patient either sits or lies comfortably. It is not the contact that produces the effects but the interaction of fields.

Therapeutic touch has one of the largest research bases of any of the energetic modalities. It has been the subject of numerous doctoral dissertations, master's theses, and postdoctoral studies, several of which have been funded by the National Institutes of Health. Early studies demonstrate evidence that therapeutic touch affects the patient's blood components and brain waves and generates an overall relaxation response.[19] Between 1971 and 1975 Krieger conducted a series of experiments in which she found that hemoglobin levels of patients who were ill rose significantly (up to 1.5 gm within 2 hours) after treatment by experienced healers.[20]

Studies also demonstrate increased weight gain among premature neonates treated with therapeutic touch. Because other studies have not been able to replicate consistent physiologic changes after therapeutic touch, it has been suggested that its effects may simply be psychological. However, when the electromagnetic fields of healers are measured, the increase in voltage seen is associated with the intent to heal. Intention, therefore, may be largely responsible for the benefits and changes found in earlier studies.

One study of hospitalized cardiac patients,demonstrated a significantly greater decrease in post-treatment anxiety compared with a control intervention in which nurses mimicked the movements of the therapeutic touch technique but did not focus their intention on helping the patients.[21] An extensive literature addresses nonlocal effects, prayer, and distance healing. Dossey has pointed out that the term "energy," as it is used here, may not be the appropriate term to describe nonlocal effects, which cannot be explained by conventional electromagnetic theory.[22]

16. How does one incorporate energy medicine into mainstream treatment on a day-to-day basis?

Although it is relatively simple to incorporate many of the familiar uses of bioelectromagnetics, such as EKGs and MRIs, most physicians have not yet learned how to use less conventional techniques such as therapeutic touch, prayer, or craniosacral therapy. The common factor that binds all of these techniques is that they are developed from natural human potentials and are available to anyone who chooses to learn and develop the skills.

Because of their natural tendency toward compassion, training in anatomy, and direct physical contact with patients, nurses were the first to incorporate touch therapies in mainstream medical settings. Because of its development in the nursing community, therapeutic touch has been primarily practiced in the nursing profession. However, even parents cuddling an upset baby are giving energy healing. Likewise, there are many instances in which physicians can learn to use various energy techniques on a daily basis. They do not take a lot of time and blend well with many clinical settings. Gently touching a shoulder while listening to heart sounds, using therapeutic touch or certain craniosacral techniques to help alleviate acute pain or anxiety in the hospital setting, or simply sitting and praying with patients are only a few such examples.

17. For what diagnoses is energy medicine most useful?

Energy medicine has been especially useful for pain control (both acute and chronic), anxiety, wound and incision healing, burn healing, fracture nonunion, immune system support, improved cardiovascular and respiratory function, anxiety and depression, and diabetic neuropathy. Success also has been reported with children's disorders such as attention deficit hyperactivity disorder, learning and speech difficulties, and ear complaints. Bioelectromagnetics (BEM) refers to the science of how living organisms interact with electromagnetic fields, including how those fields may affect physical systems both positively and negatively. Current studies of applications of EM fields include osteogenesis, wound healing, nerve stimulation, tissue regeneration, treatment of osteoarthritis, electrical stimulation of acupuncture points, and immune system stimulation.[23]

18. Are magnets part of energy healing?

Magnets have been used to promote healing for thousands of years. Lodestone, a naturally magnetic mineral, was claimed to have healing properties in early Chinese medical literature. Paracelsus reported treatments with magnetic fields at the University of Basil in 1530. In the late 17th century, Franz Anton Mesmer used magnets on patients but found that passing his hands above the patient's body could produce the same healing effects.

Permanent or static magnets have become increasingly popular in recent years, especially for pain relief. How they work is not exactly known. A popular theory is that magnets help relieve pain and increase healing time by improving blood flow and oxygen levels to the area to which they are applied. This process, in theory, helps flush out lactic acid and other inflammatory mediators, which, in turn, helps to decrease muscle spasm. Evidence also indicates that magnetic fields may block pain signals to the brain. Other proposed mechanisms include, induction of resonance of outer shell electrons, effects on cell membrane receptors, changes in the ion movement in cells, and release of endorphins and other hormones, antibodies, and neurotransmitters.

In one double-blind study of 50 people, a small magnet strapped to the most sensitive sore spots of postpolio patients reduced pain acutely. In the magnet therapy group, 76% of patients reported significant pain relief after 45 minutes of exposure to low gauss strength magnets, whereas only 19% of patients reported relief after they received inactive placebos.[24]

19. What other conditions may be helped with electromagnetic therapy?

Pulsed electromagnetic field (PEMF) therapy has been approved by the Food and Drug Administration for the treatment of delayed and nonunion fractures. The body part is exposed to magnets to which an electrical current is applied. This therapy evolved from the work of Becker (see question 10), who found that the body has a limited capacity to generate negative magnetic fields and thus cannot produce the necessary gauss strength to heal certain disorders.[25] In addition, magnetic stimulation of nerve and brain tissue has been studied as an alternative to electrical stimulation for the diagnosis and assessments of various neurologic conditions, including multiple sclerosis, amyotrophic lateral sclerosis, Guillain-Barré' syndrome, and other degenerative disorders. This approach may be a less painful, safer, and more accurate method of diagnosis. Evidence also supports increased peripheral nerve regeneration and function and promotion of angiogenesis.[26]

20. How does one learn to sense energy fields?

Some types of energy exist outside the usual range of sensory perception (e.g., microwaves, ultraviolet radiation). We trust that they exist. We must be open to the possibility that human energy fields and healing energy also exist. As mentioned earlier, all of us have the innate ability to sense the body's energy system. On walking into a room of people we may notice a tense atmosphere or, conversely, a warm mood. Or we meet someone and pick up good or bad "vibes." These are examples of the subjective experience of energy. We can perceive radio waves, not by sight, but by listening to the radio. In the same way, we can learn to recognize the subtle energies around the body through touch. Some people are even able to learn to perceive visually the subtle energy field around the body.

A helpful exercise is to hold the palms of the hands about two inches apart, facing each other. Relax the hands as much as possible. Closing both eyes may help to filter out visual distractions. Simply become aware of any sensations that you feel between your palms. This sensation may take the form of tingling or electricity, heat or cold. When you start to feel something, start to move the hands a bit further apart slowly, then closer together again. You may feel a pulling sensation. Try to see how far you can move your hands apart before you can no longer feel this sensation. You can also practice with a partner, taking turns holding your palms above your partner's palms. As with any concept or skill, the more you learn and practice, the better your ability to understand fully. Remember what C.G. Jung observed in 1919: "I shall not commit the fashionable stupidity of regarding everything I cannot explain as a fraud."

21. What resources are available for more information?
- Gerber,R: Vibrational Medicine. Santa Fe, NM, Bear & Co., 1996.
- Brennan B: Hands of Light: A Guide to Healing Through the Human Energy Field. Toronto, Bantam Books, 1987.
- International Society for the Study of Subtle Energies and Energy Medicine (ISSSEEM): an interdisciplinary organization for the study of the basic sciences and medical and therapeutic applications of subtle energies (http://www.issseem.org).

REFERENCES

1. National Institutes of Health: Bioelectric applications in medicine. In Alternative Medicine: Expanding Medical Horizons. Washington, DC, Office of Alternative Medicine, 1994, pp 45–48 [NIH publication no. 94-066].
2. Hurwitz W: Energy medicine. In Micozzi MS (ed): Fundamentals of Complementary and Alternative Medicine, 2nd ed. New York, Churchill Livingstone,2001, p 238.
3. Hurwitz W: Energy medicine. In Micozzi MS (ed): Fundamentals of Complementary and Alternative Medicine. New York, Churchill Livingstone, 2001, pp 238–256.
4. Oschman J: Energy Medicine: The Scientific Basis. London, Churchill Livingstone, 2000.
5. MacManaway B, Turcan J: Healing. Wellingborough, England, Thorsons, 1983.
6. Dardik I: The great law of the universe. Cycles Mar/Apr:265–277, 1994.
7. Capre F: The Web of Life. New York, Anchor Books, 1997.
8. Becker R: The Body Electric. New York, Quill, William Morrow, 1985
9. Cho ZH, Chung SC, Jones JP, et al: New findings of the correlation between acupoints and corresponding brain cortices using functional MRI. Proc Natl Acad Sci USA 95:2670–2673, 1998.
10. Russek L, Schwartz G: Interpersonal heart-brain registration and the perception of parental love: A 42 year follow-up of the Harvard Mastery of Stress Study. Subtle Energies 5(3):195–208, 1994.

11. McCraty R, Atkinson M, Tomasino D, Tiller WA: The electricity of touch: Detection and measurement of cardiac energy exchange between beople.In Pribram KH (ed): Brain and Values: Is a Biological Science of Values Possible. Mahwah, NJ, Lawrence Erlbaum Associates, 1998, pp 359–379.
12. Hunt V: Infinite Mind. Malibu, CA, Malibu Publishing, 1996.
13. Green E: Copper Wall Research: Psychology and Psychophysics, Subtle Energies and Medicine, vol. 10, sect. 3, 1999, pp. 238–243.
14. Gerber R: Vibrational Medicine. Santa Fe, NM, Bear & Co., 1996.
15. Becker R: The Body Electric. New York, Quill, 1985.
16. Shealy N, et al: Neurochemistry of depression. Am J Pain Manage 2:31–36, 1992
17. McCraty R, Barrios-Choplin B, Atkinson M, Tomasino D: The effects of different types of music on mood, tension, and mental clarity. Altern Ther Health Med 4:75–84, 1998.
18. Aldridge D: The music of the body: Music therapy in medical settings. Advances 9:17–35, 1993.
19. Krieger D: Therapeutic Touch. New York, Prentice Hall, 1986.
20. Krieger D: Healing by the laying-on of hands as a facilitator of bioenergetic change: The response of in-vivo hemoglobin. Int J Psychoenerg Syst 1:121, 1976.
21. Quinn J: Therapeutic touch as an energy exchange: Testing the theory. Adv Nurs Sci Jan:42–49, 1984.
22. Dossey L: But is it energy? Reflections on consciousness, healing and the new paradigm. Subtle Energies 3(3):69–82, 1992.
23. National Institutes of Health: Bioelectromagnetics applications in medicine. In Alternative Medicine: Expanding Medical Horizons. Washington, DC, Office of Alternative Medicine, 1994 [NIH publication no. 94-066].
24. Vallbonna C, Hazlewood CF, Jurida G: Response of pain to static magnetic fields in postpolio patients: A double-blind pilot study. Arch Phys Med Rehabil 78:1200–1204, 1997.
25. Becker R: The Body Electric. New York, William Morrow, 1985, pp 97–102.
26. Hallett M, Cohen L: Magnetism: A new method for stimulation of nerve and brain. JAMA 262:538–541,1998.

III. Diagnoses

23. ANXIETY

Roberta Lee, M.D.

1. Define anxiety.

Anxiety disorders include a number of conditions marked by irrational, involuntary thoughts and behavior. The different classifications are (1) generalized anxiety disorder (GAD), (2) panic disorder, (3) phobias, and (4) posttraumatic stress disorder (PTSD). A defining characteristic for all of these disorders is disruption of daily life by overt distress or difficulty in carrying out routine tasks—personal, social, or vocational. For a diagnosis of GAD, intense worrying must occur on a majority of days during at least 6 continuous months.[1] In addition, three of the following symptoms must be present: easy fatigability, difficulty in concentrating, irritability, muscle tension , restlessness, and/or sleep disturbance. Patients frequently present with physical symptoms, unaware that the problem stems from a mental disorder.

2. How are other types of anxiety specifically defined?

Panic disorder is defined by discrete, unprovoked episodes of intense fear. At least four of the following specific symptoms are required for the diagnosis: chest pain or discomfort, chills, hot flushes, derealization, diaphoresis, dizziness, unsteadiness, fear of losing control, fear of dying, nausea, palpitations, paresthesias, and sensation of choking or trembling. In addition, one or more of the following symptoms should be present: worry about the implications of panic, significant behavior change related to the attacks (avoidance of situations), and/or persistent concern about having another attack for at least 1 month.[2]

Phobias are irrational fears of a specific entity or situation. The most common phobias are agoraphobia, social phobia, and specific (simple) phobias (e.g., fear of snakes, heights, flying, crossing bridge). Social phobia is the fear of being humiliated in front of other people and leads to avoidance of ordinary events such as professional or social interactions.

PTSD is defined by a set of typical symptoms that develop after a person sees, is involved in, or hears an extreme stressor. The person later reacts with fear and helplessness and persistently relives the event. These persistent phenomenon must last for more than 1 month.

Symptoms from any one of these anxiety disorders can resemble a variety of medical conditions. A full work-up is necessary to make distinguish them from these medical conditions.

3. What is the prevalence of anxiety in the United States?

Anxiety disorders are the most common mental disorder in the United States and are typically underdiagnosed. The 1-year prevalence of these conditions is 13.3% of the population, or 19.1 million people. The causes seem to involve a network of genetic, environmental, biochemical, and experiential factors. Experts suggest people with anxiety are at increased risk for physical illness such as cardiovascular disease.[3]

4. Do patients with anxiety make more frequent visits to medical facilities?

In general, the average patient with an anxiety disorder consults ten health care professionals before a definitive diagnosis is made.[2] Specific anxiety disorders have different patterns. For example, patients with panic disorder use primary care services about 3 times as much as other patients.[4] The cost burden to the health care system is substantial; in 1994 anxiety disorders in the U.S cost nearly $65 billion, 31% of the total cost of all mental disorders.

5. Can kava be used for the treatment of anxiety?

Various herbal medicines can be helpful for mild anxiety. Kava (*Piper methysticum*), derived from the lateral roots of a tropical pepper plant species, has been used for centuries in many Pacific Island cultures. In Europe, it has been recognized by health authorities as an effective remedy for mild anxiety. Seven small clinical trials have evaluated the efficacy of kava in GAD.[5] The constituents considered to be most pharmacologically active for anxiety are a group of compounds called kavalactones. Of the 15 isolated kava lactone structures, six are concentrated maximally in the root and vary depending on the subspecies that is harvested. The mechanism of action of kava in GAD has not been completely elucidated, although it seems to be similar to that of benzodiazepines. Kava supplements are generally standardized to contain 33% or 55% kavalactones. It is generally recommended that kava *not* be combined with alcohol, benzodiazepines, and other sedating medications because the effects can be cumulative.[6]

6. Recently kava was reported in several European journals to cause liver damage. Is it safe?

There are 30 case reports of alleged hepatotoxicity associated with the use of kava. All of the products used thus far have been made in Germany or Switzerland. One report resulted in death, and four resulted in liver transplantation. Because of these reports, marketing of kava is under active re-evaluation in Germany. To date no reports of hepatotoxicity have been reported in the U.S., but the FDA is monitoring the situation closely.

In most reports of adverse effects, conventional drugs were used concomitantly with kava.[7] The exact nature of the problem is unclear. There is some conjecture that it may involve manufacturing issue (traditional vs. modern extraction techniques), whereas others believe that some genetic variation in liver functioning makes certain people vulnerable to the use of kava in its more concentrated botanical form.[8] Recommendations from Mark Blumenthal, executive director of the American Botanical Council, seem reasonable and prudent[9]: "Kava should not be used by anyone who has any liver problems or by anyone who is taking any drug product with known adverse effects to the liver or anyone who is a regular consumer of alcohol." Because the reports so far are associated with chronic use, Blumenthal suggests that kava should not be taken on daily basis for more than 4 weeks. In addition, Blumenthal noted that consumers should discontinue use if symptoms of jaundice (e.g., dark urine, yellowing of the eyes) occur.

7. Is valerian useful for anxiety?

Valerian (*Valeriana officinalis*) is another botanical alternative for the treatment of GAD. Its clinical efficacy has been established primarily for sleep disturbances. Valerian is a large perennial plant native to East India, China, Europe, and North America with a characteristic unpleasant "old sock" odor that provides an important method of empirical validation. Compounds called valepotriates, which are found in the roots, may be responsible for the anxiolytic activity. Valerian extracts seem to work in a similar manner as benzodiazepines by enhancing activity of gamma-aminobutyric acid (GABA), a sedative neurotransmitter. Products with Indian and Mexican valerian should be avoided because of the mutagenic risk associated with their higher concentrations of valpotriates and baldrinals (up to 8%), the active constituents of valerian root.[6]

8. Can meditation help anxiety?

Studies of the effects of meditation show immense benefit in people with or without anxiety. One study of 22 medical patients with anxiety defined by DSM-IV criteria showed significant improvement in symptoms after patients were taught mindfulness-based meditation for 8 weeks. Furthermore, the majority of patients continued the meditation on a 3-year follow-up survey.[10]

Meditation is among a variety of techniques that tap into what Benson, a noted Harvard researcher and cardiologist, calls the "relaxation response."[11] This physiological response engages the parasympathetic nervous system, which controls digestion, breathing, and heart rate during periods of rest and relaxation and gives a sense of peace and calm.

9. Which foods should people with anxiety avoid?

Caffeine, which is among the most commonly consumed stimulants in the U.S., is found in coffee, teas, colas and other soft drinks and is absorbed rapidly. Its effects can be seen within 30 minutes after consumption. Some studies indicate that the caffeine in two cups of coffee (approximately

300 mg) can produce stress in sensitive people.[12] Other foods associated with increased stress are tobacco, alcohol, and refined white sugar. Diets high in refined sugar have been linked to increased lactic acid production, which leads to nervousness and irritability, panic attacks, and tension headaches in susceptible people.[13] Both tobacco and alcohol have been shown to alter serotonin levels and to increase anxiety in susceptible people.[14,15]

10. Are mind-body techniques effective for treatment of anxiety?

Various studies of mind-body techniques show improvement in symptoms of anxiety. One review analyzing electroencephalogram (EEG) biofeedback as a treatment for anxiety noted that enhancement of specific brain-wave patterns—alpha, theta, and alpha-theta combinations—decreased anxiety more than placebo.[16] Alpha and theta brain waves have been associated with a more relaxed state of mind in many studies.[17] A study in 1996 involved teaching children biofeedback techniques over a 6-week period. The results revealed significant reduction in anxiety.[18] In another study, guided imagery, a form of focused awareness similar to hypnosis, was used 3 days before surgery, during anesthesia induction, and intraoperatively. It was found to reduce anxiety, and the intervention group used 50% less narcotic medications than the control arm.[19]

Mind-body modalities such as biofeedback, guided imagery, hypnosis, progressive relaxation, and meditation have been proved effective for many medical applications and should be considered as adjunctive treatments for anxiety.

11. When is counseling appropriate for people with anxiety?

On one hand there appears to be a reasonable biochemical explanation for the cause of anxiety—an overexaggerated chemical imbalance in the amygdala, the part of the brain thought to be the alarm center. This perspective highlights the need for medication—either a pharmaceutical or botanical agent. On the other hand, every change in the mind produces a corresponding change in brain chemistry and, ultimately, in the body. Thus, it makes sense that cognitive behavioral therapy (CBT) should be considered in the treatment of anxiety. A number of studies have shown improvement in anxiety with CBT alone and in combination with medications.[20,21] (See also the National Institutes of Mental Health website at http://www.nimh.nih.gov).

At times, however, anxiety is so overwhelming that immediate assistance from a professional is advised. Seek immediate care if the patient has any of the following symptoms:
- Sense of losing control or going "crazy"
- Feeling of panic with no one available for support
- Difficulty in breathing or pain in the chest
- Excessive need to use alcohol or drugs
- Suicidal feeling
- Great difficulty in performing normal daily tasks because of overwhelming anxiety

12. Does exercise help anxiety?

Exercise is a great reliever of stress and anxiety and has been shown in a number of clinical trials to be of benefit. In one report published in the *American Journal of Epidemiology*, mood was significantly improved with exercise.[22] This benefit may be due to the elevated production of endorphins, the body's natural opiates.[23] This is thought to be the biochemical mechanism for the mood elevation known as "runner's high."

13. Can depression and anxiety coexist?

Yes. Depression and anxiety frequently coexist. Depression can lead to anxiety, and anxiety can trigger depression as the patient's world becomes more confining. Approximately one of every three persons with GAD has panic disorder. In addition, half of people with panic disorder have an episode of clinical depression.

14. Are homeopathic remedies effective for anxiety?

According to Jonas and Jacobs in *Healing with Homeopathy*,[24] various homeopathic remedies have been classified for acute emotional problems such as stage fright, examination anxiety, or emotional trauma (acute). Choosing the appropriate remedies involves identification not only of the stressful state but also of particular symptoms or signs that may seem unrelated. To choose the proper remedy, it is advisable to work with a practitioner who is properly trained in homeopathy.

15. Does music calm anxiety?

Yes. Music can have measurable effects. In one study done in 1998, alert patients receiving mechanical ventilation in intensive care units received 30-minute intervals of music or a rest period. Heart rate and respiratory rate decreased over time for the therapy group compared with the control group.[25] In another study, a group of patients recovering from acute myocardial infarction received 20 minutes of music in a quiet and restful environment. More pronounced reductions in heart and respiratory rate were noted in the experimental group than in the control group. Furthermore, anxiety was measurably reduced, and the reduction was sustained 1 hour after the music had stopped, suggesting that music may be beneficial in recovery.[26]

16. What other modalities may be considered for patients with anxiety?

Therapeutic massage, yoga, and aromatherapy, to name a few. Many people seek massage for its relaxing effects, and clinical studies support its benefits. In a 1999 study, pregnant women were randomized to either massage or relaxation therapy. Only the massage group reported reduced anxiety, better sleep, and improved mood. In addition, urinary stress hormones decreased in the massage group compared with the control group, and the massage group had fewer labor complications.[27]

In 1996, a small study of five patients with obsessive-compulsive disorder (OCD), a subtype of anxiety, were taught a specific yogic breathing pattern followed by a 1-year course of therapy. Significant improvement was seen, and three patients were able to stop their medication (fluoxetine) after 7 months of treatment.[28]

REFERENCES

1. American Psychiatric Association: Diagnostic and Statistical Manual of Mental Disorders, 4th ed. Primary Care Version. Washington, DC,American Psychiatric Association, 1995.
2. Pozuclo L, et al: The anxiety spectrum: Which disorder is it? Patient Care 13:73–93, 1999.
3. Rozanski A, Blumenthal JA , Kaplan J: Impact of psychological factors on the pathogenesis of cardiovascular disease and implications for therapy. Circulation 99:2192–2217, 1999.
4. Ballenger JC: Panic disorder in the medical setting. J Clin Psychiatry 58(Suppl 2):13–17, 1997.
5. Pittler M, et al: Efficacy of kava extract for treating anxiety: A systematic review and meta-analysis. J Clin Psychopharmacol 20:84–89, 2000.
6. Shultz V, et al: Rational Therapy: A Physicians' Guide to Herbal Medicine. Berlin, Springer, 1998.
7. Stafford N: Germany may ban kava kava herbal supplement. Yahoo News, November 19, 2001 (http://dailynews.yahoo.com).
8. Bone K: Kava and liver damage. Press release by Reuters, November 2001.
9. Blumenthal M: American Botanical Council announces new safety information on kKava. News release, American Botanical Council, December 20, 2001.
10. Miller J, et al. Three-year followup and clinical implications of a mindfulness meditation-based stress reduction intervention in the treatment of anxiety disorders. Gen HospPsychiatry 17:192–200, 1995.
11. Benson H: The Relaxation Response. New York, William Morrow, 1975.
12. Chou T: Wake up and smell the coffee. Caffeine, coffee and the medical consequences. West J Med 157:544–553, 1992.
13. Murray M, Pizzorno J: Encyclopedia of Natural Medicine. Rocklin, CA, Prima Publications, 1998.
14. Alta C, Bennet B, Wallac R, et al: Glucocorticoid induction of tryptophan oxygenase. Biochem Pharmacol 32:979–986, 1983.
15 Goodwin FK: Alcoholism research: Delivery on the promise. Public Health Rep.103:569–574, 1988.
16. Moore NC: A review of EEG biofeedback treatment of anxiety disorders. Clin Electroencephalogr 31:1–6, 2000.
17. Freeman W: Making Sense of Brain Waves: The Most Baffling Frontier in Neuroscience. Available at http://sulcus.berkeley.edu/wjf/AG.EEG21stCentruy.pdf. Accessed 12/31/2001.
18. Wenck LS, Leu PW, D'Amato RC: Evaluating the efficacy of a biofeedback intervention to reduce children's anxiety. J Clin Psychol 42(4) :469–473, 1996.
19. Tusek D, Church JM , Fazio VW: Guided imagery as a coping strategy for perioperative patients. AORN J 66:644–649, 1997.

20. Barlow DH, Gorman JM, Shear MK, et al: Cognitive-behavioral therapy, imipramine or their combination for panic disorder: A randomized controlled trial. JAMA 283:2529–2536, 2000.
21. Barret PM: Evaluation of cognitive-behavioral group treatments for childhood anxiety disorders. J Clin Child Psychol 27:459–468, 1998.
22. Farmer ME, Locke BZ, Moscicki EK, et al: Physical activity and depressive symptomatology : The NHANES 1 Epidemiologic Follow-up Study. Am J Epidemiol 1328:1340-51, 1988.
23. Carr D, et al: Physical conditioning facilitates the exercised induced secretion of beta endorphin and betal-ipoprotein in women. N Engl J Med 305:560–565, 1981.
24. Jonas W, Jacobs J: Healing with Homeopathy: The Complete Guide. New York, Warner Books, 1996.
25. Chlan L: Effectiveness of a music therapy intervention on relaxation and anxiety for patients receiving ventilatory assistance. Heart Lung 27(3)169–176, 1998.
26. White JM: Effects of relaxing music on cardiac autonomic balance and anxiety after actue myocardial infarction. Am J Crit Care 8:220–230, 1999.
27. Field T, Hernandez -Reif M, Hart S, et al: Pregnant women benefit from massage. J Psychosom Obstet Gynecol 20:31–38, 1999.
28. Shanna Loft-Khalsa DS, Beckett LR: Clinical case report: Efficacy of yogic techniques in the treatment of obsessive compulsive disorders. Int J Neurosci 85(1–2):1–17, 1996.

24. ATTENTION-DEFICIT HYPERACTIVITY DISORDER

Mary Bove, N.D.

1. Define attention-deficit hyperactivity disorder (ADHD).

ADHD, currently the most common psychiatric disorder among children, is a syndrome of mental, physical, and emotional symptoms. The key traits are distractibility, confusion, faulty abstract thinking, inflexibility, poor verbal skills, aimlessness, perceptual difficulties, inattention to body states, constant movement, food cravings, sleep problems, coordination problems, self-centeredness, impatience, recklessness, and extreme emotionalism.[1]

Many studies estimate that roughly 3–8% of school-aged children worldwide are affected by ADHD. Diagnostic criteria set by the American Psychiatric Association include presence of symptoms for at least 6 months, onset of symptoms before age 7 years, and demonstration of at least six of the criteria symptoms.

2. What are the three subtypes of ADHD?

1. The **inattentive type** is characterized by symptoms such as forgetfulness, distractibility, losing things, poor organization, inability to follow through on tasks, poor listening, and inability to sustain attention to activities.

2. The **hyperactivity-impulsivity type** is characterized by symptoms such as fidgeting, restlessness, inability to sit still, difficulty with waiting for one's turn, excessive talking, interrupting, and inability to engage in leisure activities quietly.

3. The **combined type** is characterized by a combination of both types of symptoms.

3. How is ADHD diagnosed?

Experts recommend use of ADHD-specific questionnaires and critiera from *The Diagnostic and Statistical Manual of Mental Disorders*, 4th ed. (DSM IV) by both parents and teachers. ADHD is a clinical diagnosis, and no blood tests or imaging studies are needed. Developmental disorders, malnutrition, hypothyroidism, visual and hearing problems, and abuse should be ruled out. Symptoms need to be present in two or more settings (e.g., home and school). There is a high prevalence of comorbid psychiatric disorders, including oppositional defiant disorder (33%), conduct disorder (25–50%), and depression and anxiety (25% each).[2] The presence of comorbid diagnoses often makes ADHD more difficult to treat.

4. What predisposes a child to ADHD?

Recent research and modern neurological imaging techniques have shed new light on ADHD. It is not a disorder of attention per se, as previously assumed, but is linked to genetic predisposition, poor brain development, and faulty brain chemistry. Studies of relatives of children with ADHD show genetic links to ADHD. For example, children of a parent who has ADHD have up to a 50% chance of experiencing the same difficulties. Genes implicated in ADHD are involved with the neurotransmitter, dopamine. Dopamine is secreted by neurons in specific parts of the brain to inhibit or modulate the activity of other neurons, particularly those involved in emotion and movement.[3] Brain imaging studies have indicated that the brains of children with ADHD have attention-regulating regions that are smaller in size and exhibit slower brain activity level.[4]

Other factors linked to the development of ADHD are premature birth, poor maternal health, first pregnancy, mother under 20 years old, hypertension in pregnancy, maternal use of alcohol, tobacco, or marijuana, and extreme psychological stress during pregnancy. Finding ways to prevent these prenatal problems can help improve the odds for families at higher genetic risk of ADHD.

5. Is ADHD more common in boys or girls?

Studies show that more boys than girls are affected with ADHD. Boys with ADHD tend to be overactive, aggressive, and disruptive. One study found that boys with ADHD display more attention problems than girls with ADHD, regardless of the grade level.[6]

6. Do children outgrow ADHD?

It was once thought that ADHD eased with age, but in many children it continues into adulthood, leading to adjustment problems at work, in school, or in other social situations. Adults with ADHD suffer from low self-esteem; limited social skills; career difficulties; absentmindedness and daydreaming; difficulty with reading, learning, concentration, and memory; and forgetfulness. They seek out constant stimulation, change, and immediate gratification.[7]

7. Should stimulant medications (e.g., methylphenidate, dextroamphetamine) be used for ADHD?

Evidence from medical literature points to the efficacy of stimulant medications for children with ADHD, especially in measures of attention. Some clinicians believe that severe cases should be treated initially with medications, whereas others favor behavioral interventions or both. However, many parents may favor a nonpharmacologic approach, and more than 90% of pediatricians in one survey reported that parents asked about alternative therapies for ADHD.[7]

A large, randomized trial[8] sponsored by the National Institutes of Mental Health concluded that a combination of medication with behavioral intervention yielded no significantly greater benefits than medication alone for treatment of ADHD symptoms, but the combined treatment did result in similar positive outcomes with significantly lower medication doses. In areas such as aggression, internalizing symptoms, social skills, parent-child relations, and academic achievement, behavioral treatments fared as well as medication alone. Seventy percent of the children receiving behavioral treatment were successfully maintained without medication during the 14-month study period.

Side effects from stimulant medications used for ADHD include insomnia, decreased appetite, abdominal pain, headache, blood pressure elevation, and rebound of ADHD behaviors when medication wears off. Of interest, use of stimulant medication for ADHD is 10–30 times higher in the United States than in other countries[9], so this phenomenon may be in part cultural.

8. Does sugar cause or worsen ADHD?

Sugar is not a cause of ADHD, but whether it contributes to symptoms is a topic of debate. Studies of the effects of sugar on children with ADHD have shown conflicting results. Because 30–40% of parents of children with ADHD strongly believe that sugar causes their child's behavior to deteriorate,[1] the need for further research is great.

Sugar is one of the foods most craved foods by children with ADHD, perhaps because their brains do not receive sufficient amounts of blood glucose as fuel for brain function. Foods high in sugar do not necessarily give the brain more fuel. It is clear that simple sugars in any form are not helpful in maintaining a stable level of blood sugar metabolism. Langseth and Dowd performed 5-hour oral glucose tolerance tests in 261 hyperactive children and found that 74% displayed abnormal glucose tolerance curves. The predominant abnormality was a low, flat curve indicative of hypoglycemia.[10] Low blood sugar obviously promotes hyperactivity via increased adrenalin secretion. Refined carbohydrate consumption appears to be the major factor in promoting reactive hypoglycemia. (i.e., hypoglycemia due to a quick elevation in blood sugar for 1 or 2 hours, followed by a severe drop in blood sugar levels).[11] Because refined sugar also may promote dental caries and is a source of "empty" calories, it makes sense to limit sugar intake.

9. Do artificial food colorings or preservatives cause or worsen ADHD?

In 1973 Feingold presented the theory that food additives are a causative factor in hyperactivity; his theory has been hotly debated ever since. At first it appeared that the majority of double-blind studies designed to test the Feingold hypothesis found no link between food additives and hyperactivity. However, on closer examination of these studies and further investigation into the literature, it becomes evident that food additives, in fact, play a major role in hyperactivity.[12] Studies of the Feingold hypothesis in Canada and Australia confirm this finding. Many parents report improvement in their child's symptoms with use of the Feingold diet, which eliminates all food additives, colorings, and preservatives. Results from more recent studies designed to test the effects of the yellow dye tartrazine on the behavior of hyperactive children show a clear dose-response effect, causing reactions such as restlessness, irritability, and sleep disturbances. Parents of the children in one study reported behavioral improvement with the diet and subsequent deterioration of behavior on introduction of the foods containing artificial colors.[13]

Secondly, many food additives and preservatives deplete minerals and other important nutrients in the body, such as zinc, magnesium, and essential fatty acids. Because deficiency of these nutrients can contribute to behavioral symptoms of ADHD, this is another reason to avoid exposure to artificial additives.

10. Is ADHD the result of poor parenting skills?

No. But research clearly shows that orderly family processes and firmness help a child with ADHD adjust successfully.[1] Parenting skills such as encouragement, time-management techniques, and learning from mistakes can help the child overcome feelings of low self-worth and nurture self-esteem.

11. Can parents learn effective behavioral techniques to help their child with ADHD?

The American Academy of Pediatrics strongly recommends that the health care provider work with the parents, child, and school personnel as a collaborative team. Children with ADHD have low self-esteem as a result of feeling driven, confused, victimized, rejected, uncontrolled, angry with others, and angry at themselves.[14] Parents can learn effective techniques to help their child deal with some of the personality traits and to manage both the child's and their own life. Education about ADHD through reading, support groups, workshops, and counseling is the first step.

Suggested behavioral techniques for parents include praising positive behavior; taking one step at a time and keeping it simple; setting limits and being consistent; choosing nonstimulating activities; maintaining good communication; cultivating a sense of humor; fighting only the big battles; and not letting the ADHD destroy their happiness, sanity, and marriage.

Raising a child with ADHD can be a great challenge for the family. Family harmony, routine, and structure can deteriorate slowly over time. Family counseling, marriage counseling, and support groups offer constructive ways to recognize these problems and work toward rebuilding family harmony. Early identification of trouble spots early, maintenance of open and complete emotional communication, and lots of love can lessen the difficulties that may arise.

12. What dietary or nutritional measures can help a child with ADHD?

Some studies show that most children with ADHD have some mineral deficiency, which may contribute to their symptoms. Research reveals that a high percentage of children with ADHD are deficient in calcium, magnesium, zinc, and iron.[15] Current studies of magnesium deficiency and ADHD showed that 9% of children had lowered magnesium levels in serum, red blood cells, or hair.[16] In another study of 50 children with ADHD and documented magnesium deficiency, supplementation with 200 mg of magnesium daily led to a significant decrease in hyperactivity.[16] Yet another study found significantly lower serum levels of zinc in children with ADHD compared with controls.[17]

Deficiency of essential fatty acids (EFAs) has been found to be a factor in some children with ADHD. Several studies report that boys with ADHD have a lower blood level of EFAs, accompanied by dry skin, frequent urination, and excessive thirst, all of which are symptoms of EFA deficiency.[18] Many brain proteins undergo specific interactions with EFAs in the cell membrane to facilitate proper neuron communication. A diet high in EFA-rich foods, such as cold-water ocean fish, seaweed, algae, nuts, seeds, beans, and raw vegetable oils, is necessary for normal brain metabolism, improves immune function, and aids in healthy skin and hair growth.

13. Are food allergies or sensitivities a factor in ADHD?

This topic also has been highly debated, because early study results showed no connection. However, better designed studies published in the 1980s and 1990s[19] reported that food sensitivities are a major cause of ADHD symptoms in many children (more than 70%).[4] Many parents of ADHD children report that eliminating food allergens from the diet is helpful in reducing the symptoms of ADHD. The most common offenders were additive-containing foods, chocolate, cow's milk, oranges, and cheese.[20] Salicylate-containing foods also have been linked with ADHD disorder,[21] including fresh raspberries and strawberries, canned plums and prunes, tomatoes, peppers, almonds, peanuts, honey, peppermint, and many spices, such as cinnamon, curry, oregano, rosemary, paprika, and pepper.

An elimination diet removes potential trigger foods (e.g., refined sugar, dairy products) for a period of usually a few weeks, and clinical symptoms are followed for resolution. Several studies reported improvement of symptoms such as headaches, abdominal pains, and seizures.[22] Two double-blind, placebo-controlled studies using food challenges confirmed the negative effects of food additives and food allergies on behavior and mental performance. In the first study, 19 of 26 children responded favorably to the elimination diet; in the second study, 59 of 78 children responded favorably.[23]

14. Are there any herbal alternatives to medications such as methylphenidate (Ritalin) or dextroamphetamine (Dexedrine)?

No. If a child is doing well on prescription medications, there is no need to discontinue them. Some herbal medicines, however, may be useful. Parents and practitioners may choose to avoid prescription medications altogether, to decrease drug side effects, or to choose therapeutic regimens more consistent with their philosophy of healing. The herbal approach does not mimic prescription medications but looks at the whole person and uses herbs to treat the different aspects of the disorder.

15. What herbal medicines are used in the treatment of ADHD?

Nervine (neurologically tonifying) herbs have been used traditionally in the treatment of hyperactivity. However, use of botanicals in children is advisable only under the supervision of a trained practitioner. Of the many herbs that may be used for ADHD, a few deserve particular mention[24]:

- Wild oat (*Avena sativa*) is calming, restoring, and relaxing; it also strengthens the nervous system and nerve tissue.
- Lemon balm (*Melissa officinalis*) calms nervous irritability, sensitivity, and excitement. Its warm aromatic lemony scent enhances mood and sleep.
- Passionflower contains several compounds with mild calming effects and mood-enhancing action; it also helps to improve concentration.
- Skullcap deserves mention for its strong tonifying effect on the nervous system; it relaxes muscle, soothes nerve agitation, and calms the mind.
- Gotu kola can be a helpful stimulating herb for children with ADHD. It enhances mental functions such as concentration, memory, and alertness and also has mild antianxiety and relaxing effects.
- Adaptogen-acting herbs, such as *Eleutherococcus senticosus* and *Withania somnifera,* help to build up the nervous system and promote the body's ability to deal with the effects of stress. Withania has the reputation in traditional use of promoting learning and memory.

16. Discuss the relationship between ADHD and toxic heavy metal poisoning.

Several different biologic factors, which may be different in different children, are believed to trigger ADHD. The heavy metals, lead and aluminum, have been linked to ADHD.[1] Lead is a toxic metal that substitutes for essential minerals such as calcium, iron, and zinc in the body; its presence disturbs a number of important physiologic reactions that depend on these minerals.[4] Aluminum and lead can be measured in the blood, urine, or hair. Other heavy metals that have been questioned for a possible link to ADHD are mercury and fluoride.[25]

17. Can children taking prescribed medications also use alternative therapies?

Many of the complementary and alternative therapies can be used as part of a program for a child with ADHD who is taking prescription medications. Therapies such as dietary changes, massage, homeopathy, sensory-motor therapy, allergy/elimination diets, and ruling out aggravating biologic factors such as heavy metal toxicity or chemical sensitivities can be used. Use of therapies such as nutritional supplementation, amino acids and botanical medicines in conjunction with prescribed medications depends on the specific supplement and the specific medication as well as the individual child. Supervision by a physician, naturopathic physician, or practitioner knowledgeable in this area is recommended.

18. Can homeopathy be helpful?

Yes. Homeopathy is safe, natural, and without side effects. It attempts to treat the whole person, often using a single remedy to match the patient's symptom pattern and improve the patient's condition physically, emotionally, and mentally (see Chapter 13.) Use of homeopathic treatment for ADHD is essential for at least 1–2 years.[26]

The Lamont study (1997) of 43 children with ADHD showed statistically significant results that corroborated the superiority of homeopathic treatment to placebo.[25] Homeopathic physicians base their evidence for effectiveness on clinical results with many patients.

19. Do regular physical activity and exercise help in the management of children with ADHD?

Physical activity and exercise help develop coordination, balance, concentration, and self-esteem while uplifting the child's mood. In general, children with ADHD do better in less competitive, more individualized sports, such as skiing, swimming, dance, bicycling, and martial arts. The central focus of well-taught martial arts is self-control, the hallmark of goals for helping a child or adolescent with ADHD.

20. Discuss the role of massage in the treatment of ADHD.

Because many children with ADHD have trouble in differentiating between touch that is gentle and touch that is threatening, the type of massage therapy is important. Often light or gentle touch can be more painful, whereas paradoxically deep-pressure massage and heavy touch are more tolerated by the child. One study compared deep-pressure massage with relaxation training in a group of adolescents with ADHD on 10 consecutive school days. Compared with the relaxation-trained group, the massaged group showed a greater decrease in fidgetiness after sessions, spent more time on tasks, and experienced a greater decrease in overall level of hyperactivity at school.[27]

21. Give an example of an integrated wholistic treatment plan for ADHD.

After a complete history and intake to become familiar with the child's personality traits, family, and general health, the practitioner may suggest a few lab tests to rule out contributing factors. Examples include heavy metal testing via hair, blood, or urine; allergy testing for airborne or food sensitivities with enzyme-linked immunosorbent assays; serum amino acid testing; and complete digestive stool analysis.

Treatment should be tailored to the patient to incorporate test results, general ADHD guidelines, and individual aspects. A diet eliminating food allergens, colorings, preservatives, and aggravating foods such as chocolate, oranges, and cow's milk is initially recommended. Further dietary suggestions include more nondairy protein and sufficient omega-3 and omega-6 raw oils as well as limited amounts of simple carbohydrates and salicylate-containing fruits and vegetables.

Supplementation with vitamins, minerals, amino acids, and essential fatty acids or a homeopathic remedy may be prescribed. Biweekly massage or cranial-sacral therapy, along with physical activity such as tai chi, may be helpful. Herbal medicines may be used to support digestive function, to desensitize allergens, to calm overexcitement and aid in sleep, to strengthen the nervous system, and to support immune function. The goals of the plan are to limit contributing biologic factors and to improve brain chemistry, immune function, digestive function, and physiologic stress adaptation mechanisms. Optimizing theses functions eases emotional and mental stress.

REFERENCES

1. Taylor J: Helping Your ADD Child, 3rd ed. Rocklin, CA, Prima Publishing, 2001.
2. Smucker WD, Hedayat M: Evaluation and treatment of ADHD. Am Fam Physician 64:817–829, 2001.
3. Barkley R: Attention deficit hyperactivity disorder. Sci Am 279(3): 66-71, 1998.
4. Stevens L: 12 Effective Ways to Help Your ADD/ADHD Child. New York, Avery/Penguin Putnam, 2000..
5. DuPaul G, Barkley R: Situational variability of attention problems: Psychometric properties of the Revised Home and School Situation Questionaires. J Clin Child Psychol 21:178–188, 1992.
6. Wender, Paul: Attention Deficit Hyperactvity Disorder in Adults, New York, Oxford University Press, 1995.
7. Ambulatory Care Quality Improvement Program: Monitoring Children with Attention Deficit Hyperactivity Disorder. Elk Grove, IL, American Acadamy of Pediatrics, 1997.
8. MTA Cooperative Group: A 14-month randomized clinical trial of treatment strategies for attention-deficit/hyperactivity disorder. Arch Gen Psychiatry 56:1073–1086, 1999.
9. Taylor EB: Development of clinical services for attention-deficit/hyperactivity disorder. Arch Gen Psychiatry 56:1097–1099, 1999.
10. Lanseth, L, Dowd J: Glucose tolerance and hyperkinesis. Food Cosmet Toxicol 16:129–133,1978.
11. Murray M: In Defense of the Feingold Diet. Natural Medicne Journal Aug/Sept. 1(7): 1-5, 1998.
12. Mattes J: The Feingold diet: A current reappraisal. J Learn Disabil 16:319–323, 1983.
13. Rowe KS, Rowe KJ: Synthetic food coloring and behavior: A dose response effect in a double-blind, placebo-controlled, repeated measures study. J Pediatr 125:691–698,1994.
14. Reichenberg-Ullman J, Ullman R: Ritalin Free Kids, 2nd edition, Rocklin CA, Prima Health, 2000, pp19-21.
15. Kozielec T et al: Deficiency of certain trace elements in children with hyperactivity. Psychiatr Polska 28:345–353, 1994.
16. Kozielec T, Starobrat-Hermelin B: Assessment of magnesium levels in children with ADHD. Magnes Res 10 (2):143–156, 1997.
17. Toren P, et al: Zinc deficiency in attention deficit hyperactivity disorder. Biol Psychiatry 40:1308–1310, 1996.
18. Mitchell EA, et al: Cinical characteristics and serum essential fatty acid levels in hyperactive childen. Clin Pediatr 26:406–411, 1997.
19. Egger J, Stolla A, McEwen LM, et al: Controlled trial of hyposensitization in children with food-induced hyperkinetic syndrome. Lancet 339:1150–1153, 1992.
20. Carter CM: Effects of a few foods: Diet in attention deficit disorder. Arch Dis Child 69:564–568 1993.
21. Swain A, Soutter A, et al: Salicylates, oligoanthigenic diets and behavior. Lancet ii:41–42, 1985.
22. Egger J, Carter C, Gramham P, et al: Controlled trial of oligoantigenic treatment in the hyperkinetic syndrome. Lancet i:540–545, 1985.
23. Boris M, Mandel FS: Foods and additives are common causes of attention deficit hyperactive disorder in children. Annals Allergy 72: pp462-7, 1994.
24. Bove M (ed): Encyclopedia of Natural Healing for Children and Infants, 2nd ed. New York, Keats Publishing, 2000, pp 143–144.
25. Reichenberg-Ullman J, Ullman R: Ritalin Free Kids, 2nd ed. Rocklin, CA, Prima Health, 2000.
26. Lamont J: Homeopathic treatment of attention deficit hyperactivity disorder. Br Homeopath J 86(10):196–200, 1997.
27. Field T, et al: Adolescents with attention deficit hyperactivity disorder benefit from massage therapy. Adolescence 33:103–108, 1998.

25. DEPRESSION

Craig Schneider, M.D.

1. Is it always necessary (or realistic) to make a precise diagnosis of the specific depressive disorder?

No. Although a specific diagnosis often helps tailor treatment, studies suggest that the major subtypes of depression, including major depressive disorder, dysthymia, recurrent brief depression, and minor depression are actually quite fluid. Depression is more accurately viewed as a disease spectrum rather than discrete subtypes.[1] Many people seen in primary care settings do not meet the criteria for many of the well-known depression categories but fall under the DSM-IV category, "depressive disorder not otherwise specified (NOS)." Such patients still may benefit from treatment. For specific categories see the *Diagnostic and Statistical Manual of Mental Disorders*, 4th ed., Primary Care Version. Washington, DC, American Psychiatric Association, 1995.

2. Which came first—neurochemical imbalance or symptoms?

It is still unclear whether depression results from alteration in neurotransmitter levels or whether neurotransmitter levels are altered by psychological states. Current understanding of the pathophysiology of depression stresses the biochemical imbalance of biogenic amines (e.g., neurotransmitters such as serotonin, norepinephrine, dopamine) in the brain. It is clear that most people with depression do experience such biochemical change. Interestingly, an experiment conducted by psychologist Martin Seligman in the 1960s demonstrated that dogs taught "learned helplessness" also experienced these biochemical changes. When the helpless dogs were subsequently taught control, the biochemical changes corrected. This model has been applied to other animals and was used subsequently by researchers to study antidepressant medications.

3. With so many effective antidepressant pharmaceuticals available, why should complementary/alternative medicine (CAM) approaches be considered?

Patients and practitioners choose not to use conventional antidepressants for multiple reasons. A recent National Institute of Mental Health survey suggests that approximately 70% of depressed people go untreated, and mood disorders account for between 60–75% of deaths by suicide.[2] One important explanation of undertreatment is social stigma. The mentally ill still experience discrimination at an institutional level with regard to health care benefits.[3] Because mental illness conveys unacceptable images to a large segment of society, people may avoid care for fear of being labeled "socially undesirable." Thus, many patients do not seek assistance from the conventional health care system, which they fear will place this label on them. They may seek CAM approaches on their own or with alternative practitioners.

Additionally, many people fear the side effects of conventional treatment more than the symptoms of depression. Although newer antidepressants are no more effective than older agents, they offer the advantage of significantly improved side-effect profiles. Nonetheless, some studies suggest that up to 40–50% of patients taking selective serotonin reuptake inhibitors (SSRIs) complain of sexual side effects, and a recent study showed that over 50% of patients treated with an SSRI or tricyclic antidepressant (TCA) by their general practitioner had discontinued use by 6 weeks.[3] Concern is also emerging that effective short-term pharmacologic therapy for depression in fact may worsen long-term outcomes.[4,5]

4. What is the advantage of an integrative approach to treating depression?

In this patient-centered approach, psychological as well as spiritual, cultural, and physical aspects of life and current situation are routinely assessed. Dietary habits, physical activity, substance abuse, relationships, and support are examined, along with images of health, significant stresses, available coping mechanisms, and meaning derived from symptoms. This approach minimizes the social stigma often associated with mental illness, and is often successful in eliciting the patient's world view so that the most appropriate, effective treatment can be recommended, increasing the potential for adherence and positive outcomes. The appropriate recommendations may be conventional medications, alternative approaches, or a combination. The integrative approach is more closely aligned with a significant portion of the population that avoids conventional medicine, because it does not mesh well with their philosophical approach to life[6]; thus, a broader population of depressed people may be attracted to effective medical care.

5. How well does St. John's wort treat mild-to-moderate depression?

While the exact mechanism of action of St. John's wort remains unknown, several meta-analyses have demonstrated that it is more effective than placebo for treating mild-to-moderate depression.[7] St. John's wort appears to be as effective as conventional antidepressant medications. Side effects in most of the trials were significantly fewer than with conventional pharmaceuticals (TCAs and SSRIs) and included GI upset, allergic reactions, fatigue, dry mouth, restlessness, and constipation. St. John's wort is one of the best studied botanical medicines in use, but legitimate criticisms of these studies include variance in extract potency across studies, lack of long-term studies, and heterogeneity of the populations studied.

A recent study involving 200 patients concluded that St. John's wort was not effective for the treatment of major depression, but was found to be well tolerated.[8] Although this study has been reported in the lay press as proof that St. John's wort is not an effective treatment for depression, this conclusion is misleading. Critics of the study point out that St. John's wort is not indicated for major depression, as the study simply confirms. Prescribed by both Hippocrates and Galen, St. John's wort was used in Europe throughout the middle ages for a number of conditions, including those that today are recognized as depression. Licensed in Germany as a prescription medicine in 1984, it is widely prescribed for treating mild-to-moderate depression. Three million prescriptions for St. John's wort are filled yearly in Germany, nearly twice the number of prescriptions written for other antidepressant medications.

6. Can St. John's wort be recommended to patients taking pharmaceutical drugs for conditions other than depression?

Yes, but because emerging evidence indicates cytochrome P450 induction by St. John's wort, it is advisable to use caution when recommending its use in combination with other drugs metabolized along the P450 pathway. Cytochrome P450 3A4 appears to be induced significantly. Interactions between St. John's wort and other medications metabolized along this pathway, including indinavir, cyclosporine, and ethinyl estradiol, have been documented.[10] Many commonly prescribed drugs are P450 3A4 substrates, including midazolam, lidocaine, calcium channel blockers, and serotonin receptor antagonists.[10] St. John's wort has been reported to reduce the anticoagulant effect of warfarin (a P450 2C9 substrate)[11] and also affects the pharmacokinetics of digoxin, perhaps via the induction of P-glycoprotein transporter.[12]

7. What is the active antidepressant component in St. John's wort?

As with many botanicals this is not a simple question. Most studies demonstrating the efficacy of St. John's wort used extracts standardized to 0.3% hypericin, which was believed to be the active ingredient. Recently hyperforin has been identified as more active than hypericin.[13] St. John's wort standardized to 5% hyperforin reportedly demonstrates superior efficacy compared with formulations standardized to 0.3 % hypericin. Some experts postulate that the clinical efficacy of St. John's wort may be attributable to the combined contribution of several mechanisms, each one too weak by itself to account for the end effect.[14] Evidence indicates that St. John's wort has weak serotonin, dopamine, and norepinephrine reuptake-inhibiting action in addition to weak monamine oxidase inhibition in vitro.[13] Some evidence also suggests that St. John's wort may inhibit interleukin-6, increasing cortisol production and resulting in an additional indirect antidepressant effect.[15]

8. When recommending St. John's wort, do I need to advise my patients to avoid consuming certain food items?

No. This concern arises because St. John's wort has been found to possess monoamine oxidase (MAO)-inhibiting action in vitro. Concomitant use of MAO inhibitors with foods high in tryptophan or tyramine (e.g., beer, wine, cheese, preserved fruits, meats, vegetables) can precipitate hypertensive crisis. The MAO-inhibiting action of St. John's wort is now believed to be insignificant in vivo in common therapeutic dosage.[13]

9. What is the role of SAM-e in the treatment of depression?

A number of open and randomized controlled trials suggest that S-adenosylmethionine (SAM-e) is an effective and well-tolerated antidepressant, and its onset of action is more rapid than that of standard pharmaceutical antidepressants (most patients respond within 1 week).[16] SAM-e functions as the body's major methyl donor and is essential to the metabolism of multiple neurotransmitters, including norepinephrine, serotonin, and dopamine.[20] Both intravenous and oral supplementations result in increased levels of biogenic amines in the brain and appear to increase synaptic membrane fluidity and improve binding. Note that SAM-e may cause hypomania or mania in bipolar patients and should be avoided in this population.

10. Name a stable oral form of SAM-e.

The most stable oral form appears to be 1,4 butanedisulfonate, which should have a room temperature shelf-life of 2 years. Recommend an enteric-coated form. To avoid GI upset, start with 200 mg daily and gradually adjust upward over 1–2 weeks to a dosage of up to 800 mg twice daily.

11. Are there any concerns about combining dietary supplements such as St. John's wort and SAM-e with conventional pharmaceutical medications for treating depression?

Yes. Because both supplements and available pharmaceutical drugs for treating depression appear to alter the levels of biogenic amines in the brain, their combined use may result in additive effects, potentially leading to problems such as serotonin-syndrome. It may be appropriate to use particular combinations, but this must be done under the close supervision of a knowledgeable physician. Because SAM-e appears to have a more rapid onset than other dietary supplements or pharmaceutical approaches, it is sometimes started concurrently with another antidepressant and then weaned as the second agent begins to take effect.

12. Can exercise play a role in the treatment of depression?

Definitely. Multiple studies demonstrate that regularly performed exercise is as effective an antidepressant as psychotherapy (which is as effective as pharmaceutical therapy). Aerobic and anaerobic activity appear to work equally well.[18] It appears that participation in an exercise regimen rather than level of fitness achieved is a better predictor of antidepressive effect.[19] As with psychotherapy, the combination of exercise and antidepressant medication is superior to either alone.[18]

13. Describe the rationale for using exercise as therapy in depression.

Exercise probably works in a multifactorial manner, involving alteration of neurotransmitter levels, endorphins, and psychological factors.[20] Participating in an exercise program requires patients to take an active role in their recovery. As strength and body image improve, so do self-confidence, self-esteem, and a sense of mastery—at least in many patients. Another theory suggests that increasing body temperature leads to a more relaxed state as muscle spindle activity is decreased and electrical activity in the cerebral cortex is synchronized. Research will undoubtedly yield additional mechanisms.

14. Is exercise useful for preventing recurrence of major depressive disorder?

A recent study at a major U.S. university medical center suggests that exercise is at least as effective in preventing recurrence as sertraline (Zoloft) over 4 months, and was more effective 6 months after the study had concluded.[21]

15. What lifestyle factors should people with depression avoid?

Tobacco, alcohol, and excessive caffeine and sugar. Tobacco use is one of the major factors contributing to premature morbidity and mortality in the U.S. Regardless of condition, all patients should be advised against its use. It may affect mood disorders through nicotine stimulation of cortisol secretion, which in turn activates tryptophan oxygenase. As a result, less tryptophan reaches the brain and serotonin levels are diminished.[22] Alcohol transiently increases the turnover of serotonin, but over time decreased levels of serotonin and catecholamines result.[23] Although moderate alcohol use may offer a degree of cardiovascular protection, its use should be discouraged in patients with depression, because alcohol dependence is an independent risk factor for suicide. Some evidence also suggests that excessive caffeine and refined sugar intake are associated with depression.[24,25]

16. State the most common symptom of folic acid deficiency.

Depressed mood. Some estimates of borderline or low folate levels in depressed adults are as high as 35%.[26] Patients with low levels of folic acid respond more poorly to therapy with SSRIs, and folic acid supplementation significantly improves response to SSRI therapy.[27] Vitamin B_{12} supplementation should accompany folic acid replacement to avoid masking B_{12} deficiency. Other B vitamins are also essential to the normal manufacture of neurochemicals. Recently the government has mandated folic acid fortification of a number of staple foods, which probably will reduce significantly the rates of folic acid deficiency.

17. What other nutritional factors may be relevant to depressed patients?

A growing body of epidemiologic data suggests that a deficiency of omega-3 fatty acids or an imbalance in the ratio of omega-6 and omega-3 fatty acids correlates with increased rates of depression.[28] It is hypothesized that alterations in fatty acids may lead to abnormalities in synaptic membrane fluidity, thus interfering with the synthesis, binding, and uptake of neurotransmitters.[29] Clinical trials remain to be conducted, but increasing the ratio of omega-3 fatty acids to omega-6 fatty acids is safe and has other demonstrated benefits, including cardiovascular health.

18. Is there any reason to believe that omega-3 fatty acids may play a role in treating bipolar disorder?

Yes. It is believed that omega-3 fatty acids inhibit neuronal signal transduction pathways in a similar manner as lithium carbonate and valproic acid. Recently a small randomized, controlled trial demonstrated that the addition of omega-3 fatty acids to usual treatment was well tolerated and improved the short-term course of the illness.[30]

19. Is there a relationship between food intolerance and depression?

Little evidence in the literature supports such an association, but many practitioners and patients report improvement in symptoms after the identification and avoidance of certain foods via elimination or rotation diets. A trial of one of these diets is reasonable.

20. Does 5-hydroxytryptophan (5-HTP) play a role in the treatment of depression?

5-HTP is a precursor in the metabolism of serotonin, and a number of open and randomized controlled trials suggest that it may be as effective as standard antidepressants.[31] Tryptophan appeared promising as a treatment for insomnia and depression but was removed from the market when a contaminated batch was linked to an outbreak of eosinophilic myalgia syndrome (EMS) in people with abnormal activation of the kynurenine pathway. Although 5-HTP is not metabolized along this pathway, case reports have linked 5-HTP to an EMS-like syndrome. The problem appears to be related to a family of contaminants, known as peak X, that is commonly found in commercially available 5-HTP.[32] Because of the uncertainty surrounding 5-HTP, it appears prudent to avoid recommending its use until further information emerges.

21. Can acupuncture have an effect on neurotransmitter levels?

Acupuncture has been used for centuries in Asia for the treatment of virtually all known disease states. Although the exact mechanism of action by which acupuncture relieves depression remains unknown, both human and animal studies demonstrate that the stimulation of certain acupuncture points can alter neurotransmitter levels.[38] The World Health Organization recognizes acupuncture as effective in treating mild-to-moderate depression. Case series indicate that acupuncture is promising in treating depression, and this finding is supported by several uncontrolled and controlled studies. Electroacupuncture has proved equally effective as amitriptylene in two randomized, controlled trials of 5 and 6 weeks' duration. Follow up at 2–4 years revealed no difference in rates of recurrence.[34] Larger, well-designed trials are under way.

22. When does relaxation training have a role in the treatment of depression?

When a component of anxiety is involved. Various methods that induce the "relaxation response" (e.g., decreased sympathetic arousal resulting in muscle relaxation, reduced blood pressure, lower pulse rate) can be useful. Examples include meditation, biofeedback, autogenic training, hypnosis, progressive muscle relaxation, and breathing techniques. Although well-designed studies investigating the role of these techniques in depression without anxiety are limited, they are generally safe, pleasant, and potentially useful adjunctive treatments.

23. Describe the role of phototherapy in treating depression.

Phototherapy is an accepted treatment for seasonal affective disorder (SAD), and small randomized controlled trials also suggest that it may be an effective adjunct to pharmacotherapy in both unipolar and bipolar depression.[35]

24. Can hormones be used to treat depression?

Possibly. A number of small trials suggest that estrogen replacement can improve symptoms in peri- and postmenopausal women with depression. Larger, well-designed trials will answer this question more definitively.

25. What is transcranial magnetic stimulation (TMS)?

TMS uses topographically selective mild electrical stimulation to specific areas of the brain. It requires no general anesthesia and appears to have minimal side effects. It is currently being studied as a promising alternative to electroconvulsive therapy.

REFERENCES

1. Angst J, Sellaro R, Merikangas JR: Depressive spectrum diagnoses. Compr Psychiatry 41(2Suppl 1):39–47, 2000.
2. Frank E, Thase ME: Natural history and preventative treatment of recurrent mood disorders. Annu Rev Med 50:453–468, 1999.
3. Lawrenson RA, Tyrer F, Newson RB, Farmer RD: The treatment of depression in UK general practice: Selective serotonin reuptake inhibitors and tricyclic antidepressants compared. J Aff Dis 59:149–157, 2000.
4. Fava GA: Do antidepressants and antianxiety drugs increase chronicity in affective disorders? Psychother Psychosom 61:125–131, 1994
5. Thase ME, Kupfer DJ: Recent developments in the pharmacotherapy of mood disorders. J. Consult Clin Psychol 64(4):1–14, 1996.
6. Astin J: Why patients use alternative medicine: Results of a national study. JAMA 279:1548–1553, 1998.
7. Linde K, Ramirez G, Marlow CD, et al: St. John's wort for depression: An overview and meta-analysis of randomized clinical trials. Br Med J 313(7052):253–258, 1996.
8. Shelton RC, Keller MB, Gelenberg A, et al:. Effectiveness of St John's wort in major depression: A randomized controlled trial. JAMA 285:1978–1986, 2001.
9. Piscatelli SC, Burstein AH, ChaittD, et al: Indinavir concentrations and St. John's wort. Lancet 355:547–548, 2000.
10. Ang-Lee MK, Moss J, Yuan CS: Herbal medicines and perioperative care. JAMA 286:208–216, 2001.
11. Yue QY, Bergquist C, Gerden B: Safety of St. John's wort. Lancet 355:576–577, 2000.
12. Johne A, Brockmoller J, Bauer S, et al: Pharmacokinetic interaction of digoxin with an herbal extract from St. John's wort (*Hypericum perforatum*). Clin Pharmacol Ther 66:338–345, 1999.
13. Delle et al: Presented at Sixth World Congress of Biological Psychiatry, Nice, France, June 22–27, 1997.
14. Bennet DA, Phun L, Polk JF, et al: Neuropharmacology of St. John's wort (Hypericum). Ann Pharmacother 32:1201–1208, 1998.

15. Lake J: Psychotropic medications from natural products: A review of promising research and recommendations. Altern Ther 6(3):36–60, 2000.

16. Bressa GM: SAMe as antidepressant: Meta-analysis of clinical studies. Acta Neurol Scand Suppl 154: 7–14,1994.

17. Chavez M: SAMe: S-adenosylmethionine. Am J Health Syst Pharm 57:119–123, 2000.

18. Martinsen EW, Hoffart A, Solberg O: Comparing aerobic with nonaerobic forms of exercise in the treatment of clinical depression: A randomized trial. Compr Psychiatry 30:324–331, 1989

19. Moore K: Exercise training as an alternative treatment for depression among older adults. Altern Ther 4(1):48–56, 1998.

20. Carr DB, Bullen BA, Skrinar GS, et al: Physical conditioning facilitates the exercised-induced secretion of beta-endorphin and beta-lipoprotein in women. N Engl J Med 305:560–565, 1981.

21. Babyak M, Blumenthal JA, Herman S, et al: Exercise treatment for major depression: Maintenance of therapeutic benefit at 10 months. Psychosom Med 62:633–638, 2000.

22. Alta C, Bennett B, Wallace R, et al: Glucocorticoid induction of tryptophan oxygenase. Biochem Pharmacol 32:979–984, 1983.

23. Goodwin FK: Alcoholism research: Delivering on the promise. Public Health Rep 103:569–574, 1988.

24. Christensen L, Somers S: Comparison of nutrient intake among depressed and nondepressed individuals. Int J Eat Disord 20:105–109, 1996.

25. Kreitsch K, et al: Prevalence, presenting symptoms, and psychological characteristics of individuals experiencing a diet-related mood disturbance. Behav Ther 19:593–604, 1988.

26. Murray M, Pizzorno J: Affective disorders. In Textbook of Natural Medicine, 2nd ed. New York, Churchill Livingstone, 1999, pp 1039–1057.

27. Coppen A, Baily B: Enhancement of the antidepressant action of fluoxetine by folic acid: A randomised, placebo controlled trial. J Aff Dis 60(2):121–130, 2000.

28. Bruinsma KA, Taren DL: Dieting, essential fatty acid intake, and depression. Nutr Rev 58(4):98–108, 2000.

29. Maes M, et al: Fatty acid composition in major depression: Decreased n-3 fractions in cholesteryl esters and increased c:20:4n6/c20:5n3 ratio in cholesteryl esters and phospholipids. J Aff Dis 38:35–46, 1996b

30. Stoll AL, Severus WE, Freeman MP, et al: Omega 3 fatty acids in bipolar disorder: A preliminary double-blind, placebo-controlled trial. Arch Gen Psychiatry 56:407–412, 1999.

31. Meyers S: Use of neurotransmitter precursors for treatment of depression. Altern Med Rev 5:64–71, 2000.

32. Klarskov K, Johnson KL, Benson LM, et al: Eosinophilia-myalgia syndrome case-associated contaminants in commercially available 5-hydroxytryptophan. Adv Exp Med Biol 467:461–468, 1999.

33. Han J: Electroacupuncture: An alternative to antidepressants for treating affective diseases? Int J Neurosci 29:79–92, 1986

34. Ernst E, et al: Complementary therapies for depression: An overview. Arch Gen Psychol 55:1026–1032, 1998.

35. Beauchemin KM, Hays P: Phototherapy is a useful adjunct in the treatment of depressed in-patients. Acta Psychiatr Scand 95:424–427, 1997.

26. ATHEROSCLEROSIS

Robert Bugarelli, D.O.

1. Define atherosclerosis.

Atherosclerosis is a systemic inflammatory disease of the vascular system, primarily the arterial tree. It leads to coronary artery disease (CAD), cerebrovascular disease (CVD), and peripheral vascular disease (PVD). Atherosclerotic plaques occur principally in medium and large elastic, muscular arteries— most commonly in arteries supplying the heart, kidneys, brain, and extremities. These lesions begin to develop in childhood and slowly (in most instances) grow in size and number over time. The initial event leading to atherosclerotic plaque formation is endothelial dysfunction.

2. What causes endothelial dysfunction?

Many causes of endothelial dysfunction have been demonstrated, including hyperlipidemia, hypertension, diabetes, free radicals from tobacco ingestion, elevated levels of plasma homocysteine, and infectious agents such as *Chlamydia pneumoniae*. These agents cause injury to the endothelium, and the inflammation that results from the body's attempt to heal leads to plaque formation. Leukocytes, smooth muscle cells, cytokines, vasoactive peptides, and growth hormones become activated. The endothelium becomes more permeable, and low-density lipoprotein (LDL) cholesterol is deposited.

Oxidation of LDL causes more inflammation, and the ultimate result is a plaque, which has a lipid-rich core. Under stress—physical, emotional, chemical, neurohormonal, or psychosocial—more damage at the site of these plaques causes microtears in the endothelial cap covering the lipid-rich cores. When the lipid core is exposed to the bloodstream, platelet aggregation occurs and clot can form over the plaque rupture, resulting in an unstable coronary syndrome or myocardial infarction.

3. Explain is the scope of the problems associated with atherosclerosis.

Atherosclerosis and its complications are the major causes of mortality in the U.S. and the Western world. Over 500,000 Americans die of heart disease annually. Over 6 million Americans have CAD, and over 1.5 million heart attacks occur yearly. Eighty percent of patients with CAD die from the disease. Data collected in 1994 demonstrate that the cost of CAD in the U.S. is in excess of 53 billion dollars. Approximately 20 billion of those dollars were spent on interventional procedures such as angioplasty and bypass surgery.

4. What are the classic risk factors for the development of arteriosclerosis?

- Elevated blood cholesterol
- Hypertension
- Smoking
- Diabetes
- Physical inactivity
- Family history

These risk factors are additive with respect to overall risk for CAD . The more risk factors, the greater the incidence of CAD. Patients with three or more risk factors have over a 700% incidence of CAD compared with age-matched counterparts who are free of risk factors. Of interest, family history was not determined to meet Framingham criteria for independent risk, and the effects of exercise and stress were not added to the Framingham risk assessment because of potential difficulty in quantifying their effects.

5. List the novel risk factors for CAD.

- Low high-density lipoprotein (HDL)
- Elevated triglycerides
- Elevated homocysteine
- C-reactive protein (CRP)[1]
- Fibrinogen
- Lipoprotein a (LPa)[2]
- Total cholesterol–HDL ratio
- Apoprotein A-1 and B-100
- LDL particle size
- Interleukin 6 (IL-6)[3]

6. Why is it important to consider heart disease in women?[4]

Heart attacks are the number-one killer of women, greater than breast, ovarian, lung, and colon cancers combined. Unfortunately, women often do not seek attention early enough for some of the more interventional treatments for acute coronary disease, and there is a disturbing history of preferential vigilance in men (women presenting with vague chest symptoms are more likely to be diagnosed with anxiety than men). In addition, many of the medications and diagnostic studies used to detect and treat CAD were previously studied only in men. Women have smaller hearts, finer arteries, and, of course, a different hormonal milieu that may not allow simple generalization of data derived from men. It was not until 1993 that Congress passed legislation requiring that women be included in all clinical trials. Up to 20% of women with myocardial infarction (MI) do not have the classic symptoms of crushing substernal chest pain and radiation down the left arm; instead, they may have more vague symptoms of high abdominal pain, fatigue, and shortness of breath. Treadmill tests are less accurate for women, with a 25% false-positive rate. For adequate cardiac protection, HDL may be a more important factor in women for protection from MI (levels > 45 vs. > 35 for men). With all of these factors in mind, it is important to be vigilant and to seek early and appropriate diagnosis and treatment for women presenting with cardiac symptoms. WomenHeart is a national patient advocacy organization for women with heart disease, founded by women heart attack survivors, that works to improve the health and well-being of women heart patients. For more information, see www.WomenHeart.org.

7. What is considered the standard of care for CAD in traditional Western medicine?

Aspirin, beta blockers, angiotensin-converting enzyme (ACE) inhibitors, and statin therapy have been demonstrated in large multicenter, randomized, controlled trials to decrease morbidity and mortality from CAD. The 2001 guidelines from the American Heart Association/American College of Cardiology (AHA/ACC) address these issues and more. See www.aha.org for the full guidelines.

8. What are the most important components of a lifestyle intervention program for CAD?

1. Diet and weight management
2. Exercise
3. Smoking cessation
4. Stress management
5. Group support

9. Do lifestyle changes really work?

Yes. Ornish and his group at the Preventative Medicine Research Institute in Sausalito, CA, have demonstrated that a truly comprehensive program incorporating all of the above elements not only decreases the symptoms of coronary artery disease but also decreases the need for revascularization procedures. In the Lifestyle Heart Trial,[5] patients maintaining adherence to this year-long intervention had 91% reduction in angina. The program has been proved to lead to microscopic regression of atherosclerotic plaques by angiographic follow-up. A 4.4% reduction in absolute percent diameter stenosis was seen at 1 year and a 7.8% reduction at 4 years. These angiographic changes were associated with improvements in myocardial perfusion, as demonstrated by positron emission scan.. Patients also had a 37% reduction in LDL cholesterol without statin therapy.[5,6] Currently, a large Medicare-funded trial is under way to see if the Ornish lifestyle reversal program works for an older patient population.

10. Of the many diets out on the market, which is the best for patients with CAD?

The Mediterranean diet is the only diet that has been clinically proven (with striking results) to reduce cardiovascular mortality significantly. The Lyon Diet Heart, a 4-year secondary prevention study, compared a Mediterranean diet with the AHA step 1 diet in post-MI patients. Subjects eating a Mediterranean diet demonstrated a 76% reduction in fatal and non-fatal MIs compared with controls at 4 years. The diet is plant-based with large quantities of fruits and vegetables and limited quantities of dairy and red meat. The relatively high percentage of fat intake (approximately 40%) a is derived mostly from olive oil, along with the consumption of oily fish such as salmon.[7] For more information about the Mediterranean diet, visit the following website: http://www.old wayspt.org.

11. **Describe the differences between "good fats" and "bad fats" with respect to atherosclerosis.**
    Good fats include both monounsaturated fats and omega 3 fatty acids.
    • Monounsaturated fats help to lower total cholesterol and LDL (especially when it replaces saturated fats) without affecting the level of HDL. Sources include olives and olive oil, avocado, and certain nuts (almonds and cashews).
    • Omega-3 fats are found in cold-water fish, including salmon, mackerel, herring, sardines, and kippers as well as flax seed, flax oil and walnuts. The mechanism of action of omega-3 fatty acids is the production of anti-inflammatory prostaglandins that help to inhibit blood clot formation. They have been shown to help reduce the risk of sudden cardiac death, arrhythmia, and hypertension.[8]
    Bad fats include saturated fats, trans-fatty acids, and some polyunsaturated fats.
    • Trans fatty acids are probably the worst form of fat that humans ingest. The sources include margarine, shortening, hydrogenated vegetable oils, and deep fried foods as well as just about every brand of snack food on the market. Trans-fatty acids increase LDL and decrease HDL; they are form of fat associated with the highest risk of heart disease.[9]
    • Saturated fats tend to be very high in cholesterol content and are derived primarily from animal and dairy sources as well as fried foods. They are linked closely not only to heart disease but also to other chronic degenerative diseases such as cancer and diabetes. It is clear from many studies that reduction in total fat, in particular saturated fat, is extremely important in the treatment and prevention of coronary heart disease.[10]
    • Polyunsaturated fatty acids (PUFAs). Sources include corn, safflower oil, and cottonseed oil—oils frequently used in commercial food products. PUFAs typically contain omega-6 fatty acids, which overall tend to promote the production of inflammatory mediators and inflammatory prostaglandins. These fats are also prone to oxidation, which produces toxins and directly damages cell membranes. They also have been demonstrated to lower HDL.[11]

12. **Name natural dietary measures that have been proved to help control cholesterol.**
    1. **Change in dietary fat consumption** (see previous question).
    2. **Increase in fiber consumption.** Fiber consumption and lowering of cholesterol have been extensively studied. Most common fiber products include oat, psyllium, pectin, and flax. Soluble fiber found in legumes, fruits, and vegetables is highly effective in lowering cholesterol levels naturally. They also augment low-fat diets by helping to reduce cholesterol levels even further. In a large review of the benefit of fiber on serum lipids, 88% of studies demonstrated significant reductions in cholesterol. These effects were dose-dependent, and intake of about 35 gm/day was associated with up to 23% reduction in total cholesterol. Oat bran and oatmeal are the best-studied soluble fibers.[12] Psyllium and flax are insoluble fibers and lower cholesterol to a lesser degree than soluble forms.[13]
    3. **Increase in garlic consumption.** Garlic is best eaten in its raw form or very lightly cooked; recommended intake is 1–2 cloves/day. Garlic consumption has been shown to help reduce blood pressure as well as total cholesterol by 9–12 % in small randomized, controlled trials. Some controversy surrounds prepared garlic supplements such as powders and capsules; the evidence-based literature for both of those preparations is mixed.[14]
    4. **Increase in flax consumption.** In addition to its fiber content, flax (*Linum usitatissimum linaceae*) is high in omega-3 fatty acids. Cardiovascular benefits from flax come from its cholesterol-lowering, platelet inhibition, and mild estrogenic effects. The whole seed offers all of these benefits but needs to be ground up to break through the tough, indigestible outer hull. The dose used to lower cholesterol is 2.5 teaspoons 3 times/day,[15] but some nutritionists recommend up to 4 tablespoons/day.

13. **Does Chinese red yeast rice lower cholesterol?**
    Chinese red yeast rice (*Monascus purpureas*) is a traditional food product dating back to the Tang Dynasty (800 A.D.) in China. It naturally contains the molecule lovastatin, which is estimated to provide about 50% of its inherent HMG-CoA reductase activity. Red yeast rice is sold under the brand name Cholestin, and in a large trial at Tufts University, Cholestin reduced total cholesterol by 16% and LDL by 21%; HDL increased by 15% rise. The usual dose of red yeast rice is 1.2 gm 2 times/day.[16]

This product has aroused significant controversy, because the manufacturers of synthetic lovastatin (Mevacor) claim a patent on the molecule, and Cholestin, which can be bought at about $20–30 per month, is much less costly than the average $187 for lipid-lowering medications. Sale of red yeast rice was prohibited by the Food and Drug Administration (FDA) in 1998 as an unapproved "drug," but it subsequently won approval as a "dietary supplement." After much continued legal battle, the FDA and the manufacturer won their case, and red yeast rice was ordered to be withdrawn as an over-the-counter supplement.

14. What is known about guggul?

Gugulipid (*Commiphora mukul*), also known as simply guggul, is derived from the myrrh tree native to India and is used extensively there. Guggul increases hepatic uptake of LDL cholesterol from the blood yet does not appear to have any significant side effects. More large studies are needed to confirm its safety. At least two randomized, controlled trials demonstrate a 10–12% reduction in total cholesterol and 25% reductions in LDL. Gugulipid also lowers triglycerides by up to 27% and raises HDL by 16–20%.[17] The recommended dose of gugulipid is 500 mg 3 times/day, standardized to at least 5% guggulsterone extract per tablet.

15. What is the evidence for the use of antioxidants? How do they help reduce the risk of atherosclerosis?

This issue is controversial, and data are mixed. Antioxidants help prevent arteriosclerosis by inhibiting the oxidation of LDL cholesterol by free radicals. LDL is oxidized in the arterial walls; therefore, antioxidants help to stabilize vascular endothelial function. Combination use of antioxidants appears even more effective than use of any single agent. Multiple long-term observational and epidemiologic studies of dietary intake of antioxidants have demonstrated consistently a lower incidence of CAD.[18] Results of randomized, controlled trials, however, have been mixed, particularly with vitamin E. Supplement-drug interactions are beginning to surface, and one study recently concluded that supplementing a synthetic antioxidant combination unexpectedly blunted the therapeutic effects (usually an increase in HDL) of simvastatin and niacin.[19]

In general, antioxidant supplementation does not appear to be as beneficial or as cost-effective as ensuring adequate dietary intake from flavonoid-rich foods, such as colored fruits and vegetables, dark leafy greens, and tea.

16. Discuss the vitamin antioxidants.[20]

Vitamin C (ascorbic acid) is a water-soluble vitamin that works within the extracellular spaces, plasma, and lymphatics. It is the first line of antioxidant defense. It enhances the effects of vitamin E and is particularly beneficial in smokers. Doses of 200–500 mg/day have been demonstrated to stabilize endothelial function and assist with cholesterol metabolism.21

Vitamin A (retinol) and **vitamin E** (α-tocopherol) are fat-soluble vitamins that work in some membranes within the plasma cell membranes and mitochondria and within plasma lipoproteins. They prevent lipid hydroperoxides, which form during cardiac stress within both LDL and cell membranes. The standard dose range for vitamin A is 15,000–50,000 IU of mixed carotenoids; for vitamin E, 400 –800 IU. Observational studies have suggested for more than 20 years that antioxidants may be beneficial for the prevention and treatment of CAD. Randomized, controlled trials using various doses and forms of supplemental vitamin E have shown inconsistent results. Despite favorable results in CHAOS,[22] the GISSI[23]and HOPE trials[24] showed no benefit. The CHAOS trial used 400–800 IU of natural α-tocopherol, whereas the other trials used lower doses and/or synthetic vitamin E as well as a second active drug in the comparison group. (See also Chapter 20.)

17. What about other antioxidants for CAD?

Coenzyme Q10 (CoQ10, ubiquinone) is an essential compound in mitochondrial oxidative phosphorylation, in which it assists electron transfer in the production of adenosine triphosphate (ATP). CoQ10 is depleted in elderly patients, patients who are malnourished and patients who are taking statin drugs and beta blockers. It is also a very strong lipid antioxidant. CoQ10 has been demonstrated to be much a stronger antioxidant than even vitamin E, and data suggest that the ratio

of CoQ10 to total cholesterol may have more significance than the ratio of HDL to total cholesterol.[25] CoQ10 has been proved in multiple studies to help reduce symptoms of angina and improve
exercise tolerance particularly in patients with congestive heart failure (CHF). (See Chapter 27.)

Grape seed extract is an excellent source of procyanidolic oligomers (PCOs), which are potent
plant flavonoid antioxidants. PCOs have greater antioxidant activity than either vitamin C or vitamin
E and have been shown to lower cholesterol and inhibit platelets and vascular constriction. Dietary
flavonoid intake has been strongly associated with decreased death from CAD.[26]

18. What other minerals are of benefit in preventing arteriosclerosis?

Essential minerals such as magnesium, potassium, selenium, zinc, and calcium are important
cardioprotectors. They are of particular importance in malnourished and institutionalized patients.

Magnesium and **potassium** are critical in preventing heart disease and stroke. They are also important in rhythm stabilization, blood pressure regulation, and management of congestive heart failure. The intravenous form of magnesium has been shown to help in the treatment of acute MI. Both
minerals are available in whole foods (tofu, legumes, seeds, nuts, green leafy vegetables).[27,28]

Selenium helps to maximize plasma glutathione peroxidase activity, which neutralizes hydrogen peroxide radicals and decreases lipid peroxidation. Selenium also potentiates the action of vitamin E[29] and is often taken at the same time.

19. Discuss the relationship between homocysteine and B vitamins.

Homocysteine is an intermediate in the conversion of methionine to cysteine. When a patient is
deficient in folic acid, vitamin B_6, or vitamin B_{12}, this conversion is inefficient and results in an increase in plasma homocysteine, which has been directly linked to atherosclerosis through endothelial damage of vessel wall collagen. Homocysteine levels above 10 µg/dl are an independent risk
factor for heart disease stroke and peripheral artery disease. Supplementation with B complex vitamins has been shown to be effective in reducing homocysteine levels and subsequently risk.[30,31]

20. What are the beneficial effects of green tea in the natural treatment and prevention of ar-
teriosclerosis?

The health benefits of green tea stem from its high content of polyphenols, which are naturally
occurring antioxidants. Polyphenols and green tea have been shown to be approximately 100 times
more effective in neutralizing free radicals than vitamin C and approximately 25 times more successful in reducing free radicals than vitamin E. Cardiovascular benefits include antioxidant properties, ability to limit clotting, and favorable cholesterol profile with reductions in LDL and total
cholesterol as well as increases in HDL.

21. What about soy?

Soy-based food and products are rich in phytoestrogens called isoflavones. Sound evidence
links regular consumption (30–50 mg/day) with lower rates of heart disease and breast and prostate
cancer as well as beneficial effects on menopausal problems such as hot flashes and osteoporosis.
With respect to atherosclerotic arterial occlusive disease, the benefits arise from a more favorable
cholesterol profile, including reductions in total cholesterol and LDL and a significant increase in
HDL. A meta-analysis by Anderson[32] demonstrated a 9–13% reduction in total cholesterol, a 13%
reduction in LDL, and an 11% reduction in triglycerides in over 38 studies. The greatest percent
changes (20%) were seen in patients with total cholesterol levels > 200.

In 2000, the FDA recognized soy protein as a food source that may reduce the risk of heart disease. Soy phytoestrogens have been used as an alternative hormone replacement regimen in postmenopausal women (see Chapter 38).

22. What is the benefit of drinking alcohol, specifically red wine, for the prevention of arte-
riosclerosis?

Over 60 studies in a variety of settings and designs consistently demonstrated a cardiovascular
risk benefit from moderate alcohol consumption. Across the board these studies have shown that
moderate drinkers have one-half the risk of nondrinkers. Epidemiologic controversy exists over the

definition of "moderate." The U.S. government states that < 2 drinks/day constitutes moderate intake (one drink is defined 25g ETOH = 1 beer, 1 shot of spirits, one 4- to 6-oz glass of wine). The United Kingdom, on the other hand, defines < 5 drinks/day as moderate consumption. In general, mortality begins to rise somewhere between 3 and 6 drinks/day.[33]

Cardioprotective effects of alcohol include increased HDL (20%), antiplatelet activity, decreased fibrinogen, decreased C-reactive protein, increased tissue plasminogen activator, and decreased smooth muscle proliferation. Alcohol in small amounts also helps with vasodilatation, blood pressure-lowering, and reduction of perceived stressors.[34] National population surveys demonstrated no difference in mortality based on alcohol preference, but there was a trend toward decreased hospitalizations in red wine drinkers. This trend may be attributable to an overall better state of health consciousness.

23. What is the "French paradox?"

Like green tea, grapes, and grape juice, red wine is loaded with anthocyanins and proanthocyanidins, which are other forms of plant-based sterols, another class of polyphenols. They demonstrate the same strong antioxidant effect as the polyphenols found in green tea. In Europe, red wine is considered to be the most cardioprotective beverage because countries with the highest rates of consumption (France, Italy, Spain, and Switzerland) have very low incidences of cardiovascular disease despite consumption of relatively high-fat diets, particularly in France. Many explanations to have been proposed to account for the mortality difference. Proponents of red wine as the "cardiac guardian" have shown that red wine can negate the endothelial dysfunction that occurs with the consumption of high fat diets.[35] The protective value of the high-antioxidant polyphenols concentrated in red grape skins seems to confirm this theory.

Opponents of the red wine theory account for the paradox through a "time lag" in the overall consumption of high-fat meals in France compared with countries such as the United Kingdom. They postulate a future increase in the incidence in CAD in France.[36] Others postulate that the paradox stems from the French custom of undercoding cardiovascular disease on death certificates. The debate continues.

24. What herbs are used in the management of atherosclerotic disease ?

Hawthorne (*Crataegus oxyacantha*) contains oligomeric procyanins, flavonoids, and catechins. Clinical trials strongly support use of hawthorne for mild (New York Heart Association class 1 and 2) CHF. It has also been shown to help reduce blood pressure, lower cholesterol, and reduce ischemia as well as improve exercise capacity. These benefits may be due to ACE inhibitor-like effects, moderate diuresis, and an increase in vagal tone. Hawthorne is usually standardized to 2.2% flavonoids or 20% procyanidins. the German Commission E does not indicate any herb-drug interactions, even with cardiac glycosides such as digitalis.[37]

Panax notoginseng contains saponins, which act as calcium ion channel antagonists. It increases the systemic amount of tissue plasminogen activator and thus improves fibrinolytic function. It limits the proliferation of smooth muscle and promotes coronary vasodilatation. There are no demonstrable drug-herb interactions, but ginseng use should be attenuated in patients who are prone to anxiety disorders, insomnia, and hypertension and avoided in combination with stimulants such as caffeine. The usual dose is 200–500 mg/day standardized to 5% ginsenocides.

Salvia miltiorrhiza (dan-shen) is a Chinese sage plant. Its active substances are tanshinones, which are potent antioxidants that produce coronary vasodilatation and inhibit platelet aggregation. Patients who are taking warfarin sodium should avoid dan-shen because it can potentiate the anticoagulant effect of warfarin.

Garlic (see question 12).

Gugulipid (see question 14).

Ginger (*Zingiber officinale*) works as an antiplatelet agent and improves cholesterol profile by limiting cholesterol absorption. There are no known drug-herb interactions with ginger. Ginger is taken as a tea and a common culinary herb. As a supplement, ginger is standardized to 4% volatile oils and usually taken with food.

Shiitake (*Lentinus edodes polyporaceae*) has cholesterol-lowering action primarily due to a compound called eritadenine, which helps increase the rate at which the body eliminates blood cholesterol. The mushrooms are also full of dietary fiber, which further reduces cholesterol levels. Reports of blood-pressure lowering and platelet inhibition have also been documented.[38]

25. Does stress really play a role in the pathogenesis of arteriosclerosis?

Yes. It has been demonstrated that post-MI patients with high levels of perceived stress have three-fold cardiac mortality rates in the 5 years after infarct compared with controls.[39] Stress is not "only in the mind" but truly affects the hard-wired fight-or-flight mechanisms in a multitude of ways that have direct and indirect effects on the cardiovascular system. The direct effects stem from abrupt changes in adrenergic and sympathetic tone, including increases in heart rate and blood pressure, arterial vasospasm, increased platelet aggregation, and decreased cholesterol metabolism. Reductions in the normal beat-to beat variability of heart rate, a measure of parasympathetic innervation from the vagus nerve to the heart, is a strong predictor of sudden death. Anxious, depressed, or hostile patients have been shown to have lower heart rate variability.

The indirect effects of stress on the heart include overeating, underexercising, increased addictive behavior (e.g., smoking, drinking), sleep difficulties, poor nutrition practices, and engaging in high risk behaviors as seemingly benign as not wearing a seatbelt. Finding healthy ways to reduce stress can help not only to reduce the physiologic response to stressors but also to improve quality of life.

26. What other psychosocial factors increase a patient's risk of arteriosclerosis?

Type A behavior is characterized by time urgency ("hurry sickness"), free-floating anger or hostility, and intense competitiveness. Since the 1950s type A behavior has been established as a demonstrable risk not only for coronary artery disease but also for early mortality from all causes. Type A behavior is more prevalent in men.

Social isolation (in many forms, including lack of religious affiliation) is often associated with depression and anxiety, both of which have been shown to increase cardiovascular as well as all-cause mortality. Several large retrospective and prospective studies have reported a 3–5 times increased risk of premature death in patients who have a low level of social connection.

Depression also has been established as an independent, reliable predictor of heart disease incidence.The most significant factor is duration rather than severity of depressive symptoms. Patients who have rated themselves as having moderate-to-severe depression had a 72–84% increased risk of cardiovascular death for as long as 10 years after the episode.

Anxiety is often included with depression and is associated with a similar prospectively determined independent risk for the development of heart disease. This finding is particularly well studied in survivors of sudden cardiac death with automatic defibrillators.

Conversely, **optimism** has been shown to result in 50% reduction in surgery and CAD-related rehospitalization compared with pessimistic attitudes.[40] The take-home point is the need for careful assessment of psychosocial factors as part of the cardiac risk profile in patients, with institution of appropriate intervention.

27. Describe mind-body interventions that are helpful for patients with arteriosclerosis.

Meditation of various types has been widely studied and shown to lower blood pressure, aid smoking cessation, lower cholesterol, and lower the effects of chronic perceived and oxidative stress in patients with heart disease. In a recent study at Duke University, post-MI patients randomized to meditative stress management techniques had a 75% reduction in events compared with standard medical care and/or exercise. Follow-up demonstrated that meditation is highly cost-effective.[41]

Guided imagery has been shown to be particularly useful because of its low cost and ease of delivery. It uses the patient's imagination to help bring about a sensorial change, including relaxation and changes in perception. Imagery has been documented to reduce stress and postoperative pain associated with cardiovascular procedures.[42] Other effects achieved through imagery include reductions in hypertension, tachycardia, onset of dysrhythmia, and incidence of arrhythmia in defibrillator patients (some of the most angst-ridden patients in all of medicine).

Group support has been demonstrated to correlate with improved outcomes and lower risk of mortality in patients with various diseases, including ischemic heart disease and hypertension.[43] It is an integral component of the Ornish lifestyle intervention program (see question 9).

Yoga, tai chi, cognitive behavioral therapy, and **music therapy** have also shown measured physiologic benefits and decreased markers of stress in cardiovascular patients.

28. Discuss the role of spirituality in the prevention and treatment of atherosclerosis.

Many studies have documented the beneficial effects of spirituality and religiosity on health. Patients who attend prayer or religious services regularly have lower risks of death from ischemic heart disease and have better outcomes after MI, angioplasty, and coronary artery bypass grafting (CABG).[44] Patients who consider themselves to have high levels of faith report lower anxiety and depression scales and higher estimation of perceived well-being. Many religious groups encourage diets that are more heart healthy and are associated with lower rates of substances abuse from either tobacco or alcohol. Religious and/or spiritual patients tend to have improved and higher levels of social support, and several studies have found improvement in multiple clinical endpoints in patients who have been prayed for, whether they were aware of it or not. Although hard to rationalize, the arguments for tapping into prayer to connect spirit to mind and body are persuasive. A randomized trial recently demonstrated the benefit of intercessory prayer (from 8 different faiths) directed toward cardiac patients either in intensive care units or before, during, and after coronary interventions.[45]

29. What are the benefits of exercise on CAD?

The beneficial effects of exercise have been clearly demonstrated time and time again. The benefits are probably due to multiple factors, including improved oxygen supply to the myocardium, weight reduction, mood enhancement, improved lipid profile, and improved glycemic control in diabetes. Patients engaged in long-term exercise are also more likely to adhere to other healthy lifestyle programs. Death risk from CAD is doubled in physically inactive patients compared with active counterparts.[46]

Exercise is a consistent factor in following patients who have undergone long-term successful weight loss. Exercise is the most effective way to raise HDL cholesterol. One of the proposed mechanisms is improved lymphatic circulation and cholesterol transport. Because muscles utilize free fatty acids in the first 24 hours after exercise, triglycerides drop precipitously. Even light activity is better than none. Emerging data also suggest that cumulative daily activity is as cardioprotective as session or block-time exercise several times weekly.

30. How important is standard cardiac rehabilitation?

Unfortunately, doctors have done an inadequate job of enrolling patients with CAD in structured cardiac rehabilitation. Less than 20% of eligible patients are enrolled.[47] One of the problems is socioeconomic inequality, which favors the more affluent. Bias in the referral patterns of physicians also has been demonstrated against women and elderly patients. A final obstacle is the need for specific coding of MI/CABG patient classification index to ensure reimbursement and enrollment. Patients with diagnoses of chronic angina and CHF, who may be able to prevent further complications of their disease, are not covered for rehabilitation.

There are many benefits of standard cardiac rehabilitation, which focuses primarily on exercise. Exercise capacity and duration consistently have been shown to improve by 30–50% with just 3 months of exercise 3 times/week. Angina class decreases, mood improves, activities of daily living become easier, heart rate and blood pressure improve, glucose metabolism improves, insulin resistance decreases, weight decreases, and, most importantly, the all-cause mortality rate decreases by 25% at 3 years.[48] In the absence of intense nutritional counseling, lipid effects are modest with the exception of improved HDL. Therefore, an integrative approach is optimal for complete risk factor modification. Components of a comprehensive cardiac rehab program include lipid management, hypertension management, smoking cessation, weight reduction, diabetes management, psychosocial management, and exercise.

31. Are any integrative modalities effective specifically for cerebrovascular disease?

All of the modalities that lower the risk of coronary artery disease work throughout the body to decrease atherosclerosis systemically. Several modalities have been proved helpful in the treatment of stroke and its sequelae, including seizures, depression, memory and learning impairments, peripheral nerve injuries, and sexual dysfunction. Of these, two of the best studied are ginkgo biloba and acupuncture.

Ginkgo biloba has been the subject of over 300 scientific papers and 40 double-blind studies. Its active components, ginkgolides and lactones, improve cognitive function by altering arterial and vascular elasticity, have demonstrable active antiplatelet effects, and have been shown in several studies to reduce the effects of short-term memory loss and attention deficit after cerebrovascular injury, thereby enhancing stroke recovery.[49,50] The dose is 40 mg 3 times/day, standardized to 24% ginkgo flavone glycosides and 6% terpene lactones.

Acupuncture has been demonstrated to be effective in improving sensory stimulation and consolidation and coordination of motor function after stroke. It helps improve activities of daily living, ability to demonstrate functional capacity with respect to balance and mobility, and perceived quality of life, as measured by self-report scales.[51]

32. What about integrative approaches to peripheral vascular disease (PVD)?

Walking is one of the best therapies for claudication associated with PVD and has been demonstrated to be more effective than medication or surgery in many cases. Improvement is due to the development and maintenance of rich collateral circulation. A meta-analysis of 33 studies demonstrated a 179% increase in walking distance with a simple walking program alone.[52]

Gingko biloba has been demonstrated in multiple studies to help improve arterial blood flow through its antiplatelet and vasodilatory properties. Demonstrable improvements in walking distance and diminished symptoms of claudication have been shown despite documented changes in the arterial brachial indices.[53]

33. What nonconventional therapies are available for venous disorders of the peripheral vascular system?

The most well described alternative treatment for venous insufficiency and varicose veins is horse chestnut (*Aesculus hippocastanum*). Its active constituent is aescin, a mixture of various saponins. It is used primarily for the treatment of hemorrhoids, varicose veins, and chronic venous insufficiency. Horse chestnut prevents edema by limiting capillary fragility and adding structural support to the capillary walls. Its side effects include pruritus, nausea, headache, dizziness, and leg spasms. The usual dose is 300 mg twice daily, standardized to 50 mg aescin.[54] Horse chestnut extract is available in oral form as well as topical preparations.

34. Which herbs and/or vitamins used in the systemic treatment of atherosclerosis should be used cautiously with anticoagulants because of their antiplatelet/antithrombotic activity?

Bilberry, cayenne, dong-quai, flax oil, garlic, ginger, ginkgo biloba, gugulipid, shiitake mushroom, and turmeric. These substances have a theoretical additive effect on bleeding, especially if the patient is taking conventional anticoagulant or antiplatelet therapy. We should caution patients, carefully weigh the risks and benefits, and take careful histories.

35. Is chelation therapy helpful in the treatment of atherosclerotic vascular disease?

Chelation therapy is a widespread, popular, and costly CAM therapy used in the prevention and treatment of atherosclerosis. The word *chele* means "to claw" in Greek. Chelation reportedly uses ethylenediamine tetraacetic acid (EDTA) to remove heavy metals from atherosclerotic plaques. Patients undergo a series of intravenous infusions of EDTA 2 times/week (4 hours per session) for a total of 20 or more treatments. The average cost is approximately $100/infusion.

Chelation therapy was first used as front-line treatment for heavy metal intoxication. Patients with CAD treated for heavy metal toxicity anecdotally reported decreased angina; thus the practice began. Several historical postulates have been touted to explain the potential mechanism of action, including the "roto rooter" hypothesis proposed to remove calcium from arterial plaques. The parathyroid hormone (PTH) theory states that as calcium is removed from the blood, PTH is stimulated, resulting in bone remineralization. The calcium used to replenish the bone remineralization was supposed to have been derived (according to theory) from arterial plaques. Another theory states that free radical inhibition prevents some mutation.

Chelation also has been examined for treatment of ischemic cerebrovascular disease and PVD. Approximately 37 years of literature about EDTA chelation therapy are available, consisting generally of poor-quality, small case studies.[55] The risk of hypocalcemia is significant, because calcium is leeched not only from plaque but also systemically.

Randomized control data do not support chelation therapy as standard practice for the treatment of coronary disease, peripheral vascular disease, or stroke However, in case reports and anecdotal nonrandomized studies, the vast majority of patients have reported dramatic symptom relief with chelation therapy. The rush of warmth and good feeling may be due to intravenous vitamin therapy, which is often given with EDTA. Presently a pilot study examining chelation therapy for post-MI patients (PACT) is under way; it is the precursor to a large, hopefully NIH funded multicenter trial (TACT) to settle the question of chelation therapy once and for all.

REFERENCES

1. Ridker PM, Stamper MJ, Rifai N: CRP and other risk factors for CAD. JAMA 285:2481–2485, 2001.
2. Scanu et al: LP(a): A genetic risk factor for CAD. JAMA 267:3326–3329, 1992.
3. Lindmark V, Diderholm D, Wallentin L, Siegbahn A: Relationship between interleukin 6 and mortality in patients with unstable coronary artery disease. JAMA 286:2107–2113, 2001.
4. McAuliffe K: Women and heart attacks. Available at www.womenheart.org. Accessed 4/13/02.
5. Ornish D, et al: Can lifestyle changes reverse coronary atherosclerosis?:Lancet 336:129–133, 1990.
6. Ornish D, et al: Intensive lifestyle changes for reversal of heart disease. JAMA 28:2001–2007, 1998.
7. de Lorgeril M, et al: Mediteranean alpha linoleic acid rich diet in secondary prevention of heart disease: The Lyon Diet Heart Study. Lancet 343:1454–1459, 1994.
8. Harper CR, et al: The fats of life: The role of omega-3 fatty acids in the prevention of coronary heart disease. Arch Intern Med 161:2185–2192, 2001.
9. Ascherio A, et al: Trans fatty acids and coronary heart disease. N Engl J Med 340:1994–1998, 1999.
10. Hu F B, et al: Dietary fat intake and risk of CAD in women: The Nurses Health Study. N Engl J Med 337:1491–1499, 1997.
11. Mattson F, et al: Comparison of effects of dietary saturated, monounsaturated and polyunsaturated fatty acids on plasma lipids and lipoproteins in man. J Lipid Res 26:194–202, 1985.
12. Ripsin CM, et al: Oat products and lipid lowering: A meta-analysis. JAMA 267:3317–3325, 1992.
13. Gore SR, et al: Soluble fiber and serum lipids: A literature review. J Am Diet Assoc 94:425–436,, 1994.
14. Silagy CA, et al: A metaanalysis of the effect of garlic on blood pressure. J Hypertens 12:463-468, 1994.
15. Bierenbaum ML: Reducing atherogenic risk in hyperlipidemic humans with flax seed supplementation. J Am Coll Nutr 12:501–504, 1993.
16. Heber D, Yip I, Ashley JM, et al: Cholesterol-lowering effects of a proprietary Chinese red-yeast rice dietary supplement. Am J Clin Nutr 69:231–236, 1999.
17. Pizzorno J, Murray M: Atherosclerosis. In Textbook of Natural Medicine, 2nd ed. Edinburgh, Churchill Livingstone, 1999.
18. Lonn EM, et al: Is there a role for antioxidant vitamins in the prevention of cardiovascular diseases? An update on epidemiological and clinical trials data. Can J Cardiol 13:957–965, 1997.
19. Cheung MC, Zhao XQ, Chait A, et al: Antioxidant supplements block the response of HDL to simvastatin-niacin therapy in patients with coronary artery disease and low HDL. Arterioscler Thromb Vasc Biol 21:1320–1326, 2001.
20. Institute of Medicine, Panel on Dietary Antioxidants and Related Compounds of Food and Nutrition: Dietary Reference Intakes for Vitamin C, Vitamin E, Selenium and Carotenoids from Available at www.nap.edu/books/0309069351/html/.
21. Simon JA, et al: J Am Coll Nutr Vitamin C and cardiovascular disease: A review. J Am Coll Nutr 11:107–125, 1992.
22. Stephens N, et al: Randomized, controlled trial of vitamin E in patients with coronary disease: Cambridge Heart Antioxidant Study (CHAOS).Lancet 347:781–786, 1996.
23. GISSI Investigators: Dietary supplementation with n-3 polyunsaturated fatty acids and vitamin E after MI. Lancet 354:447–455, 1999.
24. Yusuf S, et al: Vitamin E supplementation and cardiovascular events in hgh risk patients: Heart Outcomes Prevention Evaluation Study (HOPE). N Engl J Med 342:154–159, 2000.

25. Hanaki Y, et al: Co-enzyme Q-10 and coronary artery disease. Clin Invest 71(8):S112–S115, 1993.
26. Hertog MG, et al: Dietary antioxidant flavonoids and the risk of coronary heart disease: The Zutphen Elderly Study. Lancet 342:1007–1011,1993.
27. Mclean RM, et al:Magnesium and its therapeutic uses: A review. Am J Med 96:63–76, 1994.
28. Shechter M, et al: The rationale of magnesium supplementation in acute myocardial infarction. Arch Intern Med 152:2189-2196, 1992.
29. La Valle JB, et al: Selenium. In Natural Therapeutics Pocket Guide.Hudson Ohio, Lexi-Comp, 2001, p 502.
30. Glueck CJ, et al: Evidence that homocystein is an independent risk factor for atherosclerosis in hyperlipidemic patients. Am J Cardiol 75:132–136, 1995.
31. Ubbink JB, et al: Hyperhomocystenemia and the response to vitamin supplementation. Clinic Invest 71:993–998, 1993.
32. Anderson JW, et al: Meta-analysis of the effects of soy protein intake on serum lipids. N Engl J M ed 333:276–281, 1991.
33. Pearson T: Alcohol and heart disease: AHA Medical/Scientific Statement. Circulation 94 3023–3025, 1996.
34. Rimm EB, et al: Moderate alcoholintake and lower risk of coronary heart disease: Meta-analysis of effects on lipids and haemostatic factors. Br Med J 319:1523–1528, 1999.
35. Cuevas AM, et al: High fat diet induces and red wine counteracts endothelial dysfunction in human volunteers. Lipids l35:143–148, 2000.
36. Law M, et al: Why heart disease mortality is low in France: The time lag explanation. Br Med J 318: 1441–1447, 1999.
37. Hobbs C, et al: HerbalGram Hawthorne: A literature review. HerbalGram 2:19–33, 1990.
38. Jong C: Medicinal and therapeutic value of shiitake mushrooms. Adv Appl Microbiol 39, 1993.
39. Roganski A, et al: Impact of psychological factors on the pathogenesis of cardiovascular disease and implications for therapy. Circulation 99:2192–2217, 1999.
40. Scheier MF, et al: Optimism and rehospitalization after coronary artery bypass graft surgery. Arch Intern Med 159:829–835, 1999.
41. Blumenthal J, et al: Usefulness of psychosocial treatment of mental stress induced myocardial ischemia in men. Am J Cardiol 89:164–168, 2002.
42. Miller K, et al: Relaxation technique and postoperative pain in patients undergoing cardiac surgery. Heart Lung 19:136, 1990.
43. Germ W, et al: Social support in social interaction: A moderator of cardiovascular reactivity. Psychosom Med 54:324–328, 1992.
44. Levin S, et al: Religious factors in physical health and prevention of illness. Prev Hum Sci 9:41–64, 1991.
45. Krucoff MW, Crater SW, et al: Integrative noetic therapies as adjuncts to percutaneous interventions during unstable coronary syndromes: The Monitoring and Actualization of Noetic TRAining (MANTRA) feasibility pilot. Am Heart J 142:760–769, 2001.
46. Berlin RA, et al: A meta analysis of physical activity in the prevention of coronary artery disease. Am J Epidemiol 132:612–628, 1990.
47. Pashkow FJ, et al:Issues in contemporary cardiac rehabilitation: A historical perspective. J Am Coll Cardiol 21:822–834, 1993.
48. O'Connor GT et al: An overview of randomized trials of rehabilitation with exercise after myocardial infarction. Circulation 80:234–244, 1989.
49. Kleijnen J: Gingko biloba. Lancet 340:1136–1139, 1992.
50. Kleijnen J: Gingko biloba for cerebral insufficiency. Br J Clinical Pharmacol 34:352–358, 1992.
51. Hu HH, et al: A randomized controlled trial on the treatment of acute partial ischemic stroke with acupuncture. Neuroepidemiology 12:106–109.
52. Gardner AW, et al: Exercise rehab programs for the treatment of claudication pain. JAMA 274; 975–980, 1995.
53. Peters H, et al: Demonstration of the efficacy of gingko biloba special extract 761 on intermittent claudication: Aplacebo-controlled, double-blind multicenter study. Vasa 27:106–110, 1998.
54. Pittler MH, et al: Horse-chestnut seed extract for chronic venous insufficiency: A criteria based systematic review. Arch Dermatol 134:1356-1360, 1998.
55. Grier MT, et al: So much writing, so little science: A review of 37 years of literature on edetate sodium chelation therapy. Ann Pharmacother 2:1504, 1993.

27. CONGESTIVE HEART FAILURE

Russell H. Greenfield, M.D.

1. With all the advances in cardiology over the past two decades, why even discuss the integrative approach to heart failure?

Recent medical advances have markedly improved the overall prognosis of people with heart disease, but morbidity and mortality associated with heart failure remain high, and even when medical therapy is maximized, quality of life suffers. Consider the following sobering statistics:

- One type of heart failure (congestive cardiomyopathy) represents the lone form of cardiovascular disease with an increasing prevalence.[1,2]
- An estimated 4.8 million people in the US have heart failure. 400,000–700,000 people will receive a new diagnosis of heart failure this year, and half will die within 5 years.[3]
- Heart failure is the leading cause of hospitalization for patients over the age of 65.[4]
- Direct medical expenditures associated with treatment of heart failure exceed $20 billion annually.[5,6]

Heart failure is associated with 3 million hospitalizations and 250,000 deaths each year.[1,5,7,8] The incidence of chronic heart failure probably will grow as the population ages and as more people survive heart attacks. Experts say that we should equate the war on heart failure with the war on cancer.

Clearly, there is a need for a shift in emphasis. Practitioners and health policy must focus on means of *preventing* heart failure. In patients with established heart failure, we must use effective means, both conventional and complementary, to stem progression of the disease.

2. What is the best integrative approach to chronic systolic heart failure (left ventricular ejection fraction < 45%)?

Prevention is the foundation of integrative cardiology, especially in the setting of heart failure. Heart failure most commonly develops as a consequence of longstanding cardiovascular disease, especially hypertension and coronary artery disease. Key components of an integrative approach include:

- Smoking and alcohol cessation
- Appropriate dietary recommendations, including limited intake of saturated fat, partially hydrogenated fats, polyunsaturated oils, and fast foods[9–11] and increased intake of fruits and vegetables,[12–14] monounsaturated fats,[15] fiber,[16] and foods high in essential fatty acid content.[17–21]
- Adequate B vitamin intake[22,23]
- Increased intake of soy in the presence of elevated total and LDL cholesterol[24]
- Adequate intake of antioxidants[25–27]
- Exercise and weight management
- Stress management[28–38]
- Regular spiritual practice[39–42]

Concurrent illness, such as coronary artery disease, diabetes mellitus, hypertension, and kidney or liver disease must be addressed, and the use of medication that may adversely affect heart function minimized (e.g., nonsteroidal anti-inflammatory drugs, calcium channel blockers, certain antidysrhythmic agents).

3. What causes heart failure?

The pathophysiology of heart failure is complex and multifactorial. Initially helpful compensatory mechanisms ultimately contribute to functional and clinical deterioration. Pathophysiologic features include[4,43–45]:

- Left ventricular dilation and structural remodeling
- Reduced wall motion
- Systemic vasoconstriction

• Sodium retention and circulatory congestion
• Neurohormonal activation

4. How is heart failure classified?

The New York Heart Association classification of heart failure defines severity of illness by functional capability:

Class I: Physical activity is not limited by symptoms like shortness of breath, fatigue, or palpitations.

Class II: Physical exertion is mildly limited, with symptoms of shortness of breath, fatigue, or palpitations developing with typical daily activities.

Class III: Physical activity is severely curtailed as symptoms of shortness of breath, fatigue, or palpitations develop with any kind of activity.

Class IV: Symptoms and physical discomfort are present even at rest.

Rates of morbidity and mortality increase as people with heart failure move from lower to higher NYHA classifications.

5. What other diagnoses should be considered?

Heart failure should be considered in any patient presenting with fatigue, shortness of breath, palpitations, or leg swelling. Prompt recognition and intervention can significantly improve both quality of life and long-term prognosis. Other serious disorders involving the lungs, liver, and kidneys share similar presenting signs and symptoms. The differential diagnosis includes:

• Venous insufficiency
• Respiratory disorders (chronic obstructive pulmonary disease, asthma, pulmonary embolus)
• Kidney failure
• Allergic reaction
• Liver failure
• Obesity

6. Describe the integrative evaluation.

All the components of a traditional history and physical examination, as well as laboratory, echocardiographic and radiologic studies, are included in an integrative evaluation. Additional inquiry and lines of investigation include:

Medications. Include questions about present and past use of botanical medicines, vitamins, and supplements.

Social history. Ask about family and community ties, and be sensitive to feelings of isolation or strained family relations. Ask about the use of alcohol, tobacco products, and illicit drugs. Inquire about stress, its primary source, and how patients cope.

Diet. Get a general sense of the person's daily intake of nutrients. Is the intake of fruits and vegetables optimal (5–9 servings daily)? Do foods high in saturated and trans fats comprise a significant proportion of daily caloric intake? What is the person's relationship with food? (Does the patient enjoy meals or rush through them? Does the patient know the person preparing his or her food, or does the patient eat out all of the time?)

Exercise. Inquire into a person's relationship with exercise. Is it a pleasure or drudgery? How does the person define exercise? Is walking exercise, or is only weight lifting considered exercise?

Spirituality. Most people appreciate being asked about spirituality. Appropriate inquiries include:
• As your doctor, is there anything you would like me to know about your spiritual beliefs or practices?
• Where do you turn when challenged by difficulty?
• What activities provide you with inspiration?

Moods. Ask about feelings of depression, anxiety, or anger.

7. What is the integrative approach to treating people with acute pulmonary edema?

The management of acute cardiogenic pulmonary edema falls squarely under conventional Western medical therapy. Certain techniques, such as guided imagery or hypnosis, may help minimize anxiety, but the focus must be conventional Western therapy. Once the patient has been stabilized, other options may be entertained. There is no acceptable rationale for forgoing rapid institution of intravenous access, pharmacologic support, and aggressive airway management for the treatment of people experiencing acute cardiac decompensation.

8. Describe the integrative approach to the treatment of chronic systolic heart failure.

For patients with stable heart failure, as with most forms of significant chronic disease, the approach is multidisciplinary. Conventional pharmaceutical intervention remains the cornerstone of management, but there are many potentially beneficial, easily initiated complementary interventions. One must tailor the approach to the individual, combining the best of conventional Western medical therapy with the specific complementary interventions that fit the person's goals and value system.

Before instituting therapy, it is important to identify and address contributing or complicating factors, such as hypertension, diabetes mellitus, anemia, and valvular cardiac disease.

9. Do angiotensin-converting enzyme (ACE) inhibitors have a place in the integrative approach to heart failure?

Absolutely. Early and maximal use of ACE inhibitors not only slows progression of heart failure but also improves quality of life and long-term prognosis.[46-48] Most patients, unfortunately, do not receive the maximal beneficial dosage. Anyone with heart failure who can tolerate ACE inhibitors should take them at maximal dosage. For those who develop side effects, such as chronic cough, angiotensin receptor blockade or vasodilator therapy is considered an appropriate option.

10. What about salt restriction?

Sodium restriction improves cardiac function and symptoms in patients with NYHA class II or higher heart failure.[49] The degree of restriction need not be severe in the early stages of heart failure (avoiding added salt should suffice). With progressive worsening of heart function, it may be necessary to limit sodium intake to 2–3 gm/day.

11. What about diuretics?

Diuretics lessen cardiac workload by decreasing the amount of fluid that the heart must pump. Loop diuretics are the most commonly prescribed, especially in the presence of congestion, but thiazide diuretics can be used with milder disease. Periodic blood tests are mandatory to evaluate electrolyte balance. Some botanicals, such as dandelion leaves, celery, oat straw, and uva ursi, traditionally have been used as natural diuretics, but good studies of their efficacy are lacking. Many over-the-counter "water-loss" preparations contain caffeine or ephedra as diuretic agents and may be harmful to patients with heart disease. Diuretic teas containing juniper berries or horsetail should be avoided because of renal toxicity and neurotoxicity, respectively.[50]

12. Is it still appropriate to use digitalis?

Yes. Digoxin has been a mainstay of medical care since the common foxglove plant (*Digitalis purpurea*) was first used to treat heart failure over 100 years ago. A positive inotrope, digoxin also possesses beneficial neurohormonal activity. Although digoxin administration does not affect overall mortality due to heart failure, it improves symptoms, enhances exercise capacity, improves quality of life and clinical status, and reduces hospitalization rates when added to the standard regimen of ACE inhibitors and diuretics.[51-54]

Some physicians institute digoxin therapy early in the course of heart failure, whereas others prescribe it only in the presence of moderate-to-severe left ventricular dysfunction. Almost all patients with heart failure should take an ACE inhibitor and use other interventions, as described above, along with digoxin.

13. What about supplements for congestive heart failure (CHF)?

Coenzyme Q10 (CoQ10), carnitine, and hawthorn may be useful adjuncts to the pharmaceutical treatment of heart failure. Patients should know that these supplements do not act quickly, that 4–6 weeks may pass before clinical benefit is evident, and that they are most effective in people with less severe disease (NYHA classes II–III). Reliance on them is not appropriate in the setting of acute cardiac decompensation.

14. What is CoQ10? Does its use have any support in the literature?

CoQ10, also known as ubiquinone, has been studied and used for decades as a nutritional supplement for cardiovascular disease. A naturally occurring substance that behaves like a vitamin, CoQ10 is synthesized within the body from tyrosine. Highest concentrations are found within the mitochondrial membranes of organs with significant energy requirements, especially the heart. CoQ10 is necessary for adequate energy production and also possesses antioxidant[55] and membrane-stabilizing effects.[56]

Plasma and myocardial CoQ10 levels have been shown to be lower in patients with heart failure than in controls.[57–59] The more severe the degree of heart failure, the greater the deficiency of CoQ10. Exogenous administration of CoQ10 can correct demonstrated deficiency.[57,60]

Available studies of CoQ10 vary in quality, and many were performed before the widespread use of ACE inhibitors, beta blockers, and aldosterone antagonists in heart failure. The majority of the published data, however, suggest a supportive role for CoQ10, with beneficial effects on ejection fraction,[61–63] end-diastolic volume index,[62,64] development of pulmonary edema and hospitalization rate,[65] and symptoms.[63,66,67] Withdrawal of CoQ10 supplementation in the setting of heart failure results in worsening cardiac function.[68] Although a small number of studies suggest a survival benefit when CoQ10 is added to a conventional therapeutic regimen,[69,70] two recent studies failed to show clinical efficacy.[71,72] Large, multicenter trials of CoQ10 in heart failure are needed to determine its true efficacy.

15. What are the side effects of CoQ10? How is it dosed?

CoQ10 is essentially free of significant side effects. Some interactions with pharmaceutical drugs have been seen. Procoagulant activity in patients taking warfarin has been reported.[73] Patients taking HMGCoA-reductase inhibitors (statin drugs) also may benefit from CoQ10 supplementation, because statin drugs disrupt the production of CoQ10 to a significant degree.[74,76]

Optimal dosages of CoQ10 for heart failure have yet to be determined. Studies have used 30–600 mg/day, but most practitioners initially prescribe 100–200 mg/day, taken with a small amount of fat to aid in absorption. Softgel capsules appear to provide superior bioavailability of CoQ10.[77]

16. What about carnitine?

Another vitamin-like substance, carnitine moves fatty acids required for energy production from the cytoplasm into the mitochondria. Myocardial carnitine is concentrated within the left ventricle.[78,79] Depletion of myocardial carnitine impairs myocyte membrane function and results in weakened myocardial contractility. Carnitine levels are generally low in patients with heart failure.[80, 81]

Only the L-form of carnitine should be used therapeutically. Propionyl L-carnitine (PLC), which is created through esterification of L-carnitine, appears most effective because it is highly lipophilic.[82] PLC improves muscle metabolism,[83] stimulates the Krebs cycle,[84] and improves contractility in animal models.[85] Human studies with L-carnitine have shown improved cardiac performance and exercise tolerance in patients with ischemic heart disease and peripheral vascular disease.[86,87] Chronic administration of PLC improves ventricular function and reduces systemic vascular resistance.[88, 89] One notable study showed a significantly reduced 3-year mortality rate in patients with heart failure who take PLC.[90] Another well-done study[91] documented no significant benefit with PLC but demonstrated a trend toward beneficial effects in patients with somewhat preserved heart function (ejection fraction = 30–40%), and confirmed the safety of PLC.

The literature strongly suggests that PLC is safe for patients with heart failure. The dosage used in most studies is 2 gm/day (range: 1–3 gm).

17. Should we recommend hawthorn (*Crataegus laevigata* or *monogyna*) for heart failure?

Hawthorn is a slow-acting cardiac tonic whose active constituents are thought to be flavonoids, such as vitexin and rutin, and oligomeric proanthocyanidins (OPCs). The leaf and flower of the hawthorn plant are the parts recommended for therapeutic use by the German Commission E. Beneficial effects, based on both animal and human studies, include[92–94]:

- Improved coronary artery blood flow
- Enhanced contractility
- Antioxidant activity
- Phosphodiesterase inhibition
- ACE inhibition
- Antidysrhythmic effects (lengthens the effective refractory period)
- Mild reduction in systemic vascular resistance

Placebo-controlled trials have reported both subjective and objective improvement in patients with mild heart failure (NYHA classes I–III).[93,95] Hawthorn use compared favorably with captopril in a study of comparable groups of people with heart failure. There was no difference between the two treatment arms in regard to improvements in exercise capacity compared with baseline.[96] The investigators, however, used a relatively low dosage of captopril. Other studies have shown improvement in clinical symptoms, pressure-rate product, left ventricular ejection fraction, and subjective sense of well-being.[97–99]

Few side effects are associated with hawthorn use, but one drug interaction is important to keep in mind. Hawthorn may enhance the activity of digitalis glycosides, even though the plant does not contain digitalis-like substances. Reflexive avoidance of hawthorn in people taking digitalis for heart failure is unnecessary. An integrative approach considers using hawthorn to lower the therapeutically effective dosage of digitalis, thereby minimizing side affects and potential toxicity.

Hawthorn is commonly standardized to its content of flavonoids (2.2%) or OPCs (18.75%). Most practitioners agree that therapeutic efficacy is greater with higher dosages (600–900 mg/day).

18. What about patients with progressively worsening heart failure?

Once contraindicated in the setting of heart failure, beta blockers have clearly been shown to benefit all patients but those in the most severe functional classes of heart failure.[100–102] Beta blockers not only improve ventricular function and provide autonomic balance but also counteract specific neurohormonal processes that contribute to impaired cardiac function. Use of beta blockade is associated with increased left ventricular ejection fraction, reduced hospitalization rate, and decreased incidence of sudden death.[102] Many cardiologists now recommend early (NYHA class II) institution of beta blockade in the setting of heart failure but remain wary of its use in class IV heart failure, although the results of the COPERNICUS (CarvedilOl ProspEctive RaNdomIzed CUmulative Survival) trial may allay these concerns.

Studies[104–106] show a reduced hospitalization rate and decreased risk of sudden death when the diuretic and aldosterone antagonist spironolactone is added to standard pharmaceutical therapy for heart failure. Spironolactone appears especially useful in the most severe stages of heart failure (NYHA classes III–IV).

People with advanced stages of heart failure are at increased risk of life-threatening dysrhythmias and thromboembolic phenomena. Antidysrhythmic agents and anticoagulation may be recommended.

People with end-stage heart failure may be considered for surgical intervention, including placement of implantable defibrillators, left ventricular assistance devices, or even heart transplantation. Even people in this extreme situation, however, can benefit from relaxation therapy, engaging in spiritually inspiring activities, and watching movies that make them laugh.

19. What are future therapeutic options for heart failure?

Angiotensin receptor blockers	Intravenous immunoglobulin therapy
Arginine (an amino acid)	Nesiritide (recombinant B-type natriuretic peptide)
Artificial hearts	Parvalbumin
Biventricular pacing	Taurine (an amino acid)
Dacron cardiac "wrap"	Tumor necrosis factor alpha blockade
Dofetilide (class III antidysrhythmic agent)	Vasopeptidase inhibitors
Endothelin receptor antagonists	Vascular endothelial growth factor
Growth hormone	

REFERENCES

1. Ghali JK, Cooper R, Ford E: Trends in hospitalization rates for heart failure in the United States 1973–1986. Arch Intern Med 50:769–773, 1990.
2. Schocken DD, Arrieta MI, Leaverton PE, et al:Prevalence and mortality rates of congestive heart failure in the United States. J Am Coll Cardiol 20:301–306, 1992.
3. American Heart Association: 1998 Heart and Stroke Statistical Update. Dallas, American Heart Association, 1997.
4. Young JB: Contemporary management of patients with heart failure. Med Clin North Am 79:1171–1190, 1995.
5. Massie BM, Shah NB: Evolving trends in the epidemiologic factors of heart failure: Rationale for preventive strategies and comprehensive disease management. Am Heart J 133:703–712,1997
6. O'Connell JB, Bristow MR: Economic impact of hear failure in the United States: Time for a different approach. J Heart Lung Transplant 13:S107–S112, 1994.
7. Graves EJ: National Hospital Discharge Survey: Annual Summary, 1993. Vital and Health Statistics. Series 13. Data from National Health Survey. Washington ,DC, U.S. Government Printing Office 121:1–63, 1995.
8. Centers for Disease Control and Prevention: Cerebrovascular disease mortality and Medicare hospitalization—United States, 1980–1990, MMWR 41:477–480, 1992
9. Zock PL, Katan MB: Trans fatty acids, lipoproteins, and coronary risk. Can J Physiol Pharmacol 75:211–216, 1997.
10. Ascherio A, Willett W: Health effects of trans fatty acids. Am J Clin Nutr 66(Suppl):1006S, 1997.
11. Williams MJA, Sutherland WH ,McCormick MP, et al: Impaired endothelial function following a meal rich in used cooking fat. J Am Coll Cardiol 33:1050, 1999.
12. McCarron DA, Oparil S, Chait A, et al: Nutritional management of cardiovascular risk factors. Arch Intern Med 157:169–177,1997.
13. Ness AR, Powles JW: Fruit and vegetables, and cardiovascular disease: A review. Int J Epidemiol 26:1–13, 1997.
14. McDougall J, Litzau K, Haver E, et al: Rapid reduction of serum cholesterol and blood pressure by a twelve-day, very low fat, strictly vegetarian diet. J Am Coll Nutr 14:491,1995.
15. de Lorgeril M, Salen P, Martin JL, et al: Mediterranean diet, traditional risk factors, and the rate of cardiovascular complications after myocardial infarction: Final report of the Lyon Diet Heart Study. Circulation 99:779, 1999.
16. Wolk A, Manson JE, Stampfer MJ, et al: Long-term intake of dietary fiber and decreased risk of coronary heart disease among women (The Nurses' Health Study). JAMA 281(21):1998–2004, 1999.
17. von Schacky C, Angerer P, Kothny W, et al: The effect of dietary omega-3 fatty acids on coronary atherosclerosis: A randomized, double-blind, placebo-controlled trial. Ann Intern Med 130:554, 1999.
18. Hu FB, Stampfer MJ, Manson JE, et al: Dietary intake of alpha-linolenic acid and risk of fatal ischemic heart disease among women. Am J Clin Nutr 69:890, 1999.
19. Daviglus ML, Stamler J, Orencia AJ, et al: Fish consumption and the 30-year risk of fatal myocardial infarction. N Engl J Med 336:1046–1053, 1997.
20. Connor WE: Do the n-3 fatty acids from fish prevent deaths from cardiovascular disease? Am J Clin Nutr 66:188–189, 1997.
21. Albert CM, Hennekens CH, O'Donnell CJ, et al: Fish consumption and risk of sudden cardiac death (The US Physicians' Health Study). JAMA 279:23–28, 1998.
22. Rimm EB, Willett WC, Hu FB, et al: Folate and vitamin B6 from diet and supplements in relation to risk of coronary heart disease among women (The Nurses' Health Study). JAMA 279:359–364, 1998.
23. Malinow MR, Bostom AG, Krauss RM: Homocyst(e)ine, diet, and cardiovascular diseases: A statement for healthcare professionals from the Nutrition Committee, American Heart Association. Circulation 99:178, 1999.
24. Krauss RM, Eckel RH, Howard B, et al: AHA Dietary Guidelines. Circulation 102:2284, 2000.
25. Tribble D: AHA Science Advisory. Antioxidant consumption and risk of coronary heart disease: emphasis on vitamin C, vitamin E, and beta-carotene: A statement for healthcare professionals from the American Heart Association. Circulation 99(4):591, 1999.
26. Spencer AP, Carson DS, Crouch MA: Vitamin E and coronary artery disease. Arch Intern Med 159:1313, 1999.
27. Diaz MN, Frei B, Vita JA, et al: Antioxidants and atherosclerotic heart disease. N Engl J Med 337:408–416, 1997.
28. Mann SJ: The mind/body link in essential hypertension: Time for a new paradigm. Altern Ther Health Med 6(2):39–45, 2000.
29. Alexander CN, Schneider RH, Staggers F, et al: Trial of stress reduction for hypertension in Older African Americans. II: Sex and Risk Subgroup Analysis. Hypertension 28:228–237, 1996.

30. Barnes VA, Treiber FA, Turner JR, et al: Acute effects of transcendental meditation on hemodynamic functioning in middle-aged adults. Psychosom Med 61:525, 1999.
31. Castillo-Richmond A, Schneider RH, Alexander CN, et al: Effects of stress reduction on carotid atherosclerosis in hypertensive African Americans. Stroke 31:568–573, 2000.
32. Luskin FM, Newell KA, Griffith M, et al: A review of mind-body therapies in the treatment of cardiovascular disease. Part 1: Implications for the elderly. Altern Ther Heath Med 4(3):46, 1998.
33. Spence JD, Barnett PA, Linden W, et al: Lifestyle modifications to prevent and control hypertension. 7: Recommendations on stress management. Can Med Assoc J 160(9 Suppl):S46, 1999.
34. Ortho-Gomer K, Horsten M, Wamala SP, et al: Social relations and extent and severity of coronary artery disease. Eur Heart J 19:1648–1656,1998.
35. Kulkarni S, O'Farrell I, Erasi M, et al: Stress and hypertension. West Med J 97:34, 1998.
36. Jain D, Shaker SM, Burg M, et al: Effects of mental stress on left ventricular and peripheral vascular performance in patients with coronary artery disease. J Am Coll Cardiol 31:1314–1322, 1998.
37. Dembroski TM, MacDougall JM, Costa PT Jr, et al: Components of hostility as predictors of sudden death and myocardial infarction in the Multiple Risk Factor Intervention Trial. Psychosom Med 51:514–522, 1989.
38. Gallacher JE, Yarnell JW, Sweetnam PM, et al: Anger and incident heart disease in the Caerphilly study. Psychosom Med 61(4):446, 1999.
39. Koenig HG, et al: Attendance at religious services, interleukin-6, and other biological parameters of immune function in older adults. Int J Psychiatr Med 27:233–250, 1997.
40. Levin J: How prayer heals: A theoretical model. Altern Ther Health Med 2:66–73, 1996.
41. Oman D, Reed D: Religion and mortality among the community-dwelling elderly. Am J Pub Health 88:1469–1475, 1998.
42. Waldfogel S: Spirituality in medicine. Prim Care 24:963, 1997.
43. Packer M: How should physicians view heart failure? The philosophical and physiological evolution of three conceptual models of the disease. Am J Cardiol 71(S):3C–11C, 1993.
44. Francis GS, et al: The neurohormonal axis in congestive heart failure. Ann Intern Med 101:370-377, 1984.
45. Packer M: The neurohormonal hypothesis: A theory to explain the mechanism of disease of disease progression in heart failure. J Am Coll Cardiol 20:248–254, 1992.
46. SOLVD Investigators: Effect of enalapril on survival in patients with reduced left ventricular ejection fractions and congestive heart failure. N Engl J Med 325:293–302, 1991.
47. CONSENSUS Trial Study Group: Effects of enalapril on mortality in severe congestive heart failure. N Engl J Med 316:1429–1435, 1987.
48. Collaborative Group on ACE Inhibitor Trials: Overview of randomized trials of angiotensin-converting enzyme inhibitors on mortality and morbidity in patients with heart failure. JAMA 273:1450–1456, 1995.
49. Kotchen TA, McCarron DA: Dietary electrolytes and blood pressure: A statement for healthcare professionals from the American Heart Association Nutrition Committee. Circulation 98:613–617, 1998.
50. Herbal Diuretics. In DerMarderosian A (ed): The Review of Natural Products, St Louis, Facts and Comparisons, 1998.
51. Haji SA, Movahed A: Update on digoxin therapy in congestive heart failure. Am Fam Physician 62:409–416, 2000.
52. Riaz K, Forker AD: Digoxin use in congestive heart failure: Current status. Drugs 55:747–758, 1998.
53. Hauptman PJ, Kelly RA: Digitalis. Circulation 99:1265–1270, 1999.
54. Digitalis Investigation Group: The effect of digoxin on mortality and morbidity in patients with heart failure. N Engl J Med 336:525–533, 1997.
55. Frei B, Kim MC, Ames BN: Ubiquinol-10 is an effective lipid-soluble antioxidant at physiological concentrations. Proc Natl Acad Sci USA 87:4879–4883, 1990.
56. Ondarroa M, Quinn P: Proton magnetic resonance spectroscopic studies of the interaction of ubiquinone-10 with phospholipid membranes. Int J Biochem 155:353, 1986.
57. Folkers K, Vadhanavikit S, Mortensen SA: Biochemical rationale and myocardial tissue data on the effective therapy of cardiomyopathy with coenzyme Q10. Proc Natl Acad Sci USA 82:901–904, 1985.
58. Littarru GP, Ho L, Folkers K: Deficiency of coenzyme Q10 in human heart disease. Part II. Int J Vit Nutr Res 42:413–434, 1972.
59. Mortensen SA, Kondrup J, Folkers K: Myocardial deficiency of coenzyme Q10 and carnitine in cardiomyopathy: Biochemical rationale for concomitant coenzyme Q10 and carnitine supplementation. In Folkers K, Littarru GP, Yamagami T (eds): Biomedical and Clinical Aspects of CoEnzyme Q10, vol. 6. Amsterdam, Elsevier, 1991, pp 269–281.
60. Langsjoen PH, Vadhanavikit S, Folkers K: Response of patients in classes III and IV of cardiomyopathy to therapy in a blind and crossover trial with coenzyme Q10. Proc Natl Acad Sci USA 82:4240–4244, 1985.
61. Langsjoen PH, Langsjoen PH, Folkers K: Long-term efficacy and safety of coenzyme Q10 therapy for idiopathic dilated cardiomyopathy. Am J Cardiol 65:521–523, 1990.

62. Judy WV et al: Double blind double crossover study of coenzyme Q10 in heart failure. In: Folkers K, Yamamura Y (eds): Biomedical and Clinical Aspects of Coenzyme Q, vol 5. Amsterdam, Elsevier, 1986, pp 315–322.
63. Langsjoen PH, Langsjoen AM: Overview of the use of CoQ10 in cardiovascular disease. Biofactors 9:273–284, 1999.
64. Soja Am, Mortensen SA: Treatment of congestive heart failure with coenzyme Q10 illuminated by meta-analyses of clinical trials. Mol Aspects Med 18(suppl):S159–S168, 1997.
65. Morisco C, Trimarco B, Condorelli M: Effect of coenzyme Q10 therapy in patients with congestive heart failure: A long-term multicenter randomized study. Clin Invest 71(Suppl):s134–s136, 1993.
66. Baggio E, Gandini R, Plancher AC, et al: Italian multicenter study on the safety and efficacy of coenzyme Q10 as adjunctive therapy in heart failure. Molec Aspects Med 15:287–294, 1994.
67. Langsjoen PH, Langsjoen AM: Coenzyme Q10 in cardiovascular disease with emphasis on heart failure and myocardial ischemia. Asia Pac Heart J 7:160–168, 1998.
68. Judy WV, Hall JH, Folkers K: Coenzyme Q10 withdrawal: Clinical relapse in congestive heart failure patients. In Folkers K, Littaru GP, Yamagami T (eds) Biomedical and Clinical Aspects of Coenzyme Q. Amsterdam, Elsevier, 1991, pp 283–298.
69. Langsjoen PH, Folkers K, Lyson K, et al: Pronounced increase of survival of patients with cardiomyopathy when treated with coenzyme Q10 and conventional therapy. Int J Tissue React 12(3):163–168, 1990.
70. Judy WV, Folkers K, Hall JH. Improved long-term survival in coenzyme Q10 treated chronic heart failure patients compared to conventionally treated patients. In Folkers K, Littarru GP, Yamagami T (eds): Biomedical and Clinical Aspects of Coenzyme Q, vol 4. Amsterdam, Elsevier, 1991, pp 291–298.
71. Watson PS, Scalia GM, Galbraith A, et al: Lack of effect of coenzyme Q10 on left ventricular function in patients with congestive heart failure. J Am Coll Cardiol 33:1549–1552, 1999.
72. Khatta M, Alexander BS, Krichten CM, et al: The effect of coenzyme Q10 in patients with congestive heart failure. Ann Intern Med 132:636–640, 2000.
73. Spigset O: Reduced effect of warfarin caused by ubidecarenone [letter]. Lancet 344:1372–1373, 1994.
74. Folkers K, Langsjoen P, Willis R, et al: Lovastatin decreases coenzyme Q10 levels in humans. Proc Natl Acad Sci USA 87:8931–8934, 1990.
75. Mortensen SA, Leth A, Agner E, et al: Dose-related decrease of serum coenzyme Q10 during treatment with HMG-CoA reductase inhibitors. Molec Aspects Med 18(Suppl):s137–s144.
76. Ghirlanda G, Oradei A, Manto A, et al: Evidence of plasma CoQ10-lowering effect by HMG-CoA reductase inhibitors: A double-blind, placebo-controlled study. J Clin Pharm 3:226–229, 1993.
77. Chopra RK, Goldman R, Sinatra ST, et al: Relative bioavailability of coenzyme Q10 formulations in human subjects. Int J Vit Nutr Res 68(2):109–113, 1998.
78. Nakagawa T, Sunamori M, Suzuki A: The myocardial distribution and plasma concentration of carnitine in patients with mitral valve disease. Surg Today 24:313–317, 1994.
79. Pierpoint ME, Judd D, Goldenberg I, et al: Myocardial carnitine in end-stage congestive heart failure. Am J Cardiol 64:56–60, 1989.
80. Suzuki Y, Masumura Y, Kobayashi A, et al: Myocardial carnitine deficiency in congestive heart failure. Lancet 1:116, 1982.
81. Regitz V Shug AL, Fleck E: Defective myocardial metabolism in congestive heart failure secondary to dilated cardiomyopathy and coronary, hypertensive and valvular heart disease. Am J Cardiol 65:755–760, 1990.
82. Paulson DJ, Traxler J, Schmidt M, et al: Protection of the ischaemic myocardium by L-propionyl-carnitine: effects on the recovery of cardiac output after ischaemia and reperfusion, carnitine transport and fatty acid oxidation. Cardiovasc Res 20:536–541, 1986.
83. Tassani V, et al: Anaplerotic effect of propionyl-L-carnitine in rat heart mitochondria. Biochem Biophys Res Comm 199:949–953, 1994.
84. Di Lisa F, Menabo R, Siliprandi N: L-propionyl-carnitine protection of mitochondria in ischemic rat hearts. Mol Cell Biochem 88:169–173, 1989.
85. Ferrari R, Di Lisa F, de Jong JW, et al: Prolonged propionyl-L-carnitine pretreatment of rabbit: Biochemical, hemodynamic and electrophysiological effects on myocardium. J Mol Cell Cardiol 24:219–232, 1992.
86. Cherchi A, Lai C, Angelino F, et al: Effects of L-carnitine on exercise tolerance in chronic stable angina: A multicenter, double-blind, randomized, placebo controlled crossover study. Int J Clin Pharmacol Ther Toxicol 23:569–572, 1985.
87. Brevetti G, Chiariello M, Ferulano G, et al: Increases in walking distance in patients with peripheral vascular disease treated with L-carnitine: A double-blind, cross-over study. Circulation 77:767–783, 1988.
88. Mancini M, Rengo F, Lingetti M, et al: Controlled study on the therapeutic efficacy of propionyl-L-carnitine in pts with congestive heart failure. Arzneimittelforschung 42(II):1101–1104, 1992.
89. Caponnetto S, Canale C, Masperone MA, et al: Efficacy of L-propionyl-carnitine treatment in patients with left ventricular dysfunction. Eur Heart J 15:1267–1273, 1994.

90. Rizos I: Three-year survival of patients with heart failure caused by dilated cardiomyopathy and L-carnitine administration. Am Heart J 139:S120–S123, 2000.

91. Anand I, Chandrashekhan Y, De Giuli F, et al: Study on propionyl-L-carnitine in chronic heart failure. The Investigators of the Study on Propionyl-L-Carnitine in Chronic Heart Failure. Eur Heart J 19:70–76, 1999.

92. Busse W: Standardized Crataegus extract clinical monograph. Q Rev Nat Med Fall:189–197, 1996.

93. Schussler M, Holzl J, Fricke U: Myocardial effects of flavonoids from *Crataegus* species. Arzneimittelforschung 45(8):842-845, 1995.

94. Weihmayr T, Ernst E: Therapeutic effectiveness of *Crataegus*. Fortschr Med 114:27–29, 1996.

95. Tauchert M, et al: Effectiveness of hawthorn extract LI 132 compared with the ACE inhibitor captopril: Multicenter double-blind study with 132 NYHA stage II patients. Munch Med 136(Suppl 1):S27–S33, 1994.

96. Schmidt U, et al: Efficacy of the hawthorn (*Crataegus*) preparation LI 132 in 78 patients with chronic congestive heart failure defined as NYHA functional class II. Phytomedicine1:17–24, 1994.

97. Weikl A, Assmus KD, Neukum-Schmidt A, et al: Crataegus Special Extract WS 1442: Assessment of objective effectiveness in patients with heart failure. Fortschr Med 114:291–296, 1996.

98. Leuchtgens H: Crataegus Special Extract WS 1442 in NYHA II heart failure: A placebo controlled randomized double-blind study. Fortschr med 111:352–354, 1993.

99. Tauchert M, Gildor A, Lipinski J: High-dose Crataegus extract WS 1442 in the treatment of NYHA stage II heart failure. Herz 24:465–474, 1999.

100. Constant J: A review of why and how we may use beta-blockers in congestive heart failure. Chest 113(3):800–808, 1998.

101. Packer M. Do beta-blockers prolong survival in chronic heart failure? A review of the experimental and clinical evidence. Eur Heart J 19(Suppl B):B40–B46, 1998.

102. Frantz RP: Beta blockade in patients with congestive heart failure. Why, who and how. Postgrad Med 108(3):103–118, 2000.

103. Dahlstrom U, Karlsson E: Captopril and spironolactone therapy in patients with refractory congestive heart failure. Curr Ther Res 51:235–248, 1992.

104. RALES Investigators: Effectiveness of spironolactone added to an angiotensin-converting enzyme inhibitor and a loop diuretic for severe chronic congestive heart failure (The Randomized Aldactone Evaluation Study [RALES]). Am J Cardiol 78:902–907, 1996.

105. Pitt B, Zannad F, Remme WJ, et al: The effect of spironolactone on morbidity and mortality in patients with severe heart failure. Randomized Aldactone Evaluation Study Investigators. N Engl J Med 341:709–717, 1999.

106. Soberman JE, Weber KT: Spironolactone in congestive heart failure. Curr Hypertens Rep 2:451–456, 2000.

28. HYPERTENSION

Victoria Maizes, M.D.

1. What is the prevalence of hypertension?

At least 50 million adult Americans have hypertension (24% of the general population) The prevalence increases with age and is higher among African Americans compared with other ethnic groups. Ninety-five percent of diagnosed cases are termed essential hypertension. Much of what we call essential is probably due to diet, obesity, inactivity, stress, and alcohol consumption.

2. How well do the conventional and integrative medicine approaches mesh in treating hypertension?

Conventional hypertension treatment fits well with the philosophies of integrative medicine. Conventional treatment stresses lifestyle modification and a step-wise approach to treatment. The Joint National Committee VI (JNC VI) guidelines for hypertension released in November 1997 placed increased emphasis on lifestyle modification.[1] In patients with blood pressure measurement above 140/90 mmHg (stage 1) and no other risk factors, lifestyle interventions are indicated as initial treatment. Examples include weight loss, sodium restriction, moderate exercise regimens, and moderation of alcohol intake. They can be continued for as long as 1 year before drug treatment is initiated. However, drug therapy should be started immediately if comorbid conditions such as dyslipidemia or diabetes are present. Strong evidence indicates that the greatest benefit of antihypertensive drug treatment is in patients with hypertension and additional risk factors for cardiovascular disease.

3. What questions can be asked to assess the patient's experience of hypertension?

Assessment begins with discovering the patient's experience of hypertension by asking a series of questions such as the following:
- What does it mean to you to have high blood pressure?
- How has it affected your life?
- What insight has it given you?
- How do you feel about taking medication?
- What are your fears or concerns about hypertension?

Understanding the impact of hypertension on the patient deepens understanding and helps guide therapeutic choices.

4. Can people with hypertension successfully stop their medication by changing their diet?

The Hypertension Control Program (HCP) tested a nutritional intervention program. HCP focused on three main factors: weight, excess dietary sodium, and excess alcohol intake. This 4-year trial looked at whether people with hypertension could successfully discontinue their medications. Thirty-nine percent of participants in the nutritional intervention group were able to maintain normal blood pressure off medications compared with 5% in the control group.[2] The lifesteyle changes made were not huge, but the cumulative effect was substantial.

5. What is the DASH diet?

The Dietary Approaches to Stop Hypertension (DASH) trial was an 11-week, multicenter randomized feeding trial that tested the effects of dietary patterns on blood pressure. Nearly 460 subjects were divided between three groups: control, increased fruit and vegetables, and a combination diet (rich in fruits and vegetables, low-fat dairy, and reduced saturated fat.) In hypertensive subjects the combination diet led to a mean reduction in blood pressure of −11.4 systolic and −5.5 diastolic. Blood pressure reductions occurred in the setting of stable weight and sodium intake of approximately 3 gm/day. Subjects ate whole foods, not supplements. Limitation: the study only lasted 8 weeks.[3,4]

6. Do vegetarians have less hypertension?

Vegetarians have lower blood pressure and a lower incidence of hypertension and other cardiovascular diseases than nonvegetarians. There is no significant difference in sodium consumption in the two groups. Vegetarian diet contains more potassium, complex carbohydrates, essential fatty acids, fiber, calcium, magnesium, and vitamin C and less saturated fat and refined carbohydrate.

7. What is the appropriate ratio of potassium (K) to sodium (Na) in a healthy diet?

The current K:Na ratio in a typical American diet is 1:2. The ideal ratio may be 5:1. Most fruits and vegetables have a K:Na ratio of at least 50:1. Sodium restriction may be especially important in elderly Caucasians, African Americans, and Latinos. Recommend < 2.4 gm/day (1 tsp of table salt).

8. Do monounsaturated fatty acids protect people from hypertension?

The Mediterranean diet, which is rich in olive oil, has been found to be associated with lower levels of serum lipids and blood pressure compared with the typical American diet. Ferrara et al, did a double-blind, randomized, controlled trial in which 23 people with hypertension were assigned to a MUFA (monounsaturated fatty acids) or PUFA (polyunsaturated fatty acids) diet for 6 months and then crossed over to the other diet.[5] Systolic and diastolic blood pressures were significantly lower after the MUFA than after the PUFA diet (127 vs. 135 mmHg systolic and 84 vs. 90 mmHg diastolic). Medication dosage was significantly reduced during the MUFA but not the PUFA diet. The mechanism for the blood pressure reduction induced by olive oil is not known.

9. Can omega 3 fatty acids lower blood pressure?

Yes. Sixty double-blind studies have shown that fish oil or flaxseed oil supplements are effective in lowering blood pressure. The fat found in fish is omega 3 fatty acid, mainly eicosopentaenoic acid (EPA) and docosahexanoic acid (DHA). EPA competitively inhibits synthesis of thromboxane A_2, a vasoconstrictor that promotes platelet aggregation. Both EPA and DHA interfere with prostaglandin synthesis in platelets and blood vessels.[6]

10. Can soy lower blood pressure?

The data are mixed. A significant reduction in diastolic blood pressure was observed in a study of 51 nonhypertensive perimenopausal women. The women took a soy protein supplement twice daily as part of a placebo-controlled trial.[7] However, a randomized controlled trial of people with high normal blood pressure found no reduction in blood pressure with soy.[8]

11. What is the relationship between fiber and blood pressure?

There is an inverse relationship between fiber intake and blood pressure in both men[9] and women.[10] Soluble fibers such as those found in oatmeal, oat bran, and psyllium are usually recommended.

12. What is the evidence for using coenzyme Q10 (CoQ10) to treat hypertension?

Nearly 40% of people with hypertension have been shown to be CoQ10-deficient. Some evidence indicates that over 4–12 weeks CoQ10 lowers blood pressure in people with hypertension. A small randomized, controlled trial revealed improvement in blood pressure in patients treated with 60 mg of CoQ10 twice daily for 8 weeks.[11] In a study of 109 patients with hypertension, overall New York Heart Association functional class improved from a mean of 2.40 to 1.36 (p < 0.001), and 51% of patients discontinued between one and three antihypertensive drugs at an average of 4.4 months after starting CoQ10.[12] The mechanism appears to be a decrease in total peripheral resistance and probably reflects a direct impact of CoQ10 on the vascular wall. The recommended dose of CoQ10 is 100–200 mg/day. To maximize absorption, CoQ10 should be taken with meals that contain some fat, and dosages over 100 mg/day should be divided.

13. Which people with hypertension seem to benefit most from calcium supplementation?

The effect of calcium on blood pressure is controversial. Calcium may reduce blood pressure in African Americans, pregnant women and salt-sensitive people. For women with a calcium intake of at least 800 mg/day, the relative risk of hypertension was 0.78 compared with an intake of less than

400 mg/day.[13] Leanness may be a predictor of response to calcium supplementation in men who have a low baseline calcium intake.[14] In trials of calcium supplementation, blood pressure was reduced in people with hypertension, although in some studies this effect was seen only in a subset of participants. A 1996 meta-analysis pooled the data and showed a small effect.[15] The recommended dose is at least 800 mg/day of calcium carbonate or calcium citrate.

14. Describe the relationship between magnesium and hypertension.

There is a highly significant inverse relationship between magnesium and both systolic and diastolic blood pressure. A low level of magnesium was found to be the dietary factor most strongly associated with high blood pressure in the Honolulu Heart Study and the Nurses' Health Study.[16] For women with magnesium intake of at least 300 mg/day, the relative risk of hypertension was 0.77 compared with women whose intake was less than 200 mg/day.[17] Supplementing magnesium has had mixed results in studies. There may be a subgroup of responders, or the impact of long-term dietary intake may be different from short-term supplementation. Dose is 200–400 mg/day.

15. Is potassium supplementation a good idea in hypertension?

A meta-analysis of 33 studies revealed that potassium decreases blood pressure about half as much as drug therapy.[18] Ideally, one increases dietary intake of potassium by consuming foods such as bananas, grapefruit, dried beans, peas, broccoli, spinach, pumpkins, and squash. If this is not possible, the dose of supplemental potassium is 1.5–3 gm/day, usually as potassium chloride. Side effects can include nausea, vomiting, diarrhea, and ulcers.

16. Can vitamin C or B$_6$ lower blood pressure?

Population studies reveal that the higher the vitamin C intake, the lower the blood pressure. Preliminary studies show a modest blood pressure-lowering effect from vitamin C supplementation, which may be due to promoting the excretion of lead.[19] One small study of 20 people revealed reductions in systolic and diastolic blood pressure when vitamin B$_6$ was supplemented at 5 mg/kg.[20]

17. What is the current recommendation for exercise in patients with hypertension?

Exercise is a longstanding recommendation to reduce blood pressure. Exercise also has a favorable effect on stress, lipids, diabetes, weight, and other cardiovascular disease risks. Mean changes in blood pressure with mild-intensity cycle ergometer (50% maximal oxygen uptake, 60 min 3 times/week for 10 weeks) in controlled studies was –11 systolic and –6 mmHg diastolic. The American College of Sports Medicine recommends endurance training, 20–60 minutes 3–5 days/week at 50–85% maximal oxygen uptake.

18. What degree of weight loss is suggested to normalize blood pressure?

Modest loss of approximately 10% of body weight can normalize blood pressure.

19. What evidence supports mind-body approaches to the treatment of hypertension?

Biofeedback, relaxation, meditation, deep breathing, yoga, progressive muscle relaxation, autogenic training, imagery, hypnosis, and stress management have a modest effect on lowering blood pressure. A wealth of published literature supports the use of biofeedback in the treatment of high blood pressure. Unfortunately, many of the studies were poorly designed or had small numbers of participants. Taken as a whole, evidence indicates that biofeedback may be useful in some people with high blood pressure, but exactly what biofeedback techniques are best and which people are most likely to respond are not as clear.[21] A meta-analysis by Eisenberg et al. reviews the methodologic limitations of the studies and concludes that these interventions are superior to no therapy but not to credible sham techniques.[22] In this meta-analysis, however, only 3% (26 of 857) of the studies were deemed fit for inclusion.

20. Is garlic a good antihypertensive agent?

Garlic (*Allium sativum*) has a long history of traditional use in heart disease. The active ingredient appears to be allicin. A meta-analysis of eight clinical trials including 415 subjects, most of whom received a dried powdered extract with standardized allicin, revealed moderate benefit in lowering blood pressure.[23] The evidence, however, is mixed because of methodologic shortcomings in study design.[24] The dose of fresh garlic is 1–2 cloves/day. Add garlic at the end of the cooking process to retain its active properties, or use 300 mg of the dried garlic extract 3 times/day.

21. Are any other herbs effective for treating hypertension?

Relatively few herbs lower blood pressure; garlic is the most effective. Hawthorn (*Crataegus monogyna*) is widely used by physicians in Europe for hypertension, angina, arrhythmias, and congestive heart failure. It is considered a cardiovascular tonic. However, the blood pressure-lowering effect of hawthorn is mild.

22. Which herbs should be avoided in patients with hypertension?

Contraindicated herbs include licorice, ephedra, caffeine, and Panax ginseng, all of which can raise blood pressure.

23. Which homeopathic remedies are used for treating hypertension?

A constitutional remedy chosen by an experienced homeopathic prescriber is the most appropriate way to treat hypertension. For example, *Argentum nitricum* is used if blood pressure rises with anxiety and nervousness. *Aurum metallicum* is sometimes indicated for serious people, focused on career and accomplishment. *Calcarea carbonica* is often helpful to people with high blood pressure who tire easily and have poor stamina.

24. What evidence supports homeopathic treatment of hypertension?

There are few studies of homeopathy in hypertension. A small German randomized, double-blind, crossover study of 10 patients compared the effects of antihypertensive medication with homeopathic treatment. The blood pressure-lowering effect of medication was clearly superior to that of homeopathy. Of interest, the subjective complaints of the patients resolved equally well with medication and homeopathic treatment.[25] Homeopaths consider younger patients with short duration of hypertension the most effective patients to treat.

25. Have any randomized, controlled trials compared traditional Chinese medicine and Western medication?

No randomized controlled trials are available. A 1991 study by Wong et al. compared the efficacy of Chinese traditional treatment with Western medical regimen in 50 matched patients with hypertension.[26] Treatment of the 26 patients in the Chinese medicine group depended on gyan yan kan or sing yin shu diagnoses. The authors followed the patients for 23 days and concluded that both treatments were effective, but the Western approach was more effective. Given that many herbal therapies can take up to 2 months to achieve full effect, the duration of treatment may not have been adequate to compare the therapies fully.

26. Which are the first-line medications used in treating hypertension?

Treatment with a diuretic or beta blocker is the usual initial medication recommended by the Joint National Committee VI (JNC VI), particularly as they are the only agents proven to reduce mortality. However, studies of the efficacy of other antihypertensives are being conducted. Angiotensin-converting enzyme (ACE) inhibitors also are often used as first-line treatments, because of their lower side-effect profile, longer duration of action, and increased adherence rates.[27] If first-line agents do not achieve adequate control, tailor therapy to the patient's individual needs, and realize that a layered, stepwise approach may be necessary.

27. In patients with concomitant diseases, advanced age, or African-American ancestry, which are the recommended medications?

- Diabetes: ACE inhibitors
- Heart failure: ACE inhibitors or diuretics
- Myocardial infarction: beta blockers or ACE inhibitors if left ventricular dysfunction is present
- Isolated systolic hypertension (elderly): diuretics
- African Americans: diuretics or calcium channel blockers

28. Can a patient discontinue medications by using complementary/alternative medicine therapies?

Many motivated patients are able to reduce or eliminate medications gradually. Switching to a vegetarian or very low fat diet can be a particularly effective strategy. The most successful patients are those who make marked lifestyle changes, especially in dietary and exercise habits.

REFERENCES

1. www.nhlbi.nih.gov
2. Stamler R, Stamler J, Grimm R, et al: Nutritional therapy for high blood pressure: Final report of a four-year randomized controlled trial-the hypertension control program. JAMA 257:1484–149,1987.
3. Appel LJ, Moore TJ, Obarzanek E, et al: A clinical trial of the effects of dietary patterns on blood pressure. DASH Collaborative Research Group. N Engl J Med 336:1117–1124, 1997.
4. www.heartinfo.org
5. Ferrara L, Raimondi AS, d'Episcopo L, et al: Olive oil and reduced need for antihypertensive medications. Arch Intern Med 160:837–842, 2000.
6. Fish oil for the heart. Med Lett Drugs Ther 29(731):7–9, 1987.
7. Washburn S, Burke GL, Morgan T, Anthony M: Effect of soy protein supplementation on serum lipoproteins, blood pressure and menopausal symptoms in perimenopausal women. Menopause 6:7–13, 1999.
8. Hodgson JM, Puddey IB, Beilin LJ, et al: Effects of isoflavonoids on blood pressure in subjects with high-normal ambulatory blood pressure levels: A randomized controlled trial. Am J Hypertens 12:47–53, 1999.
9. Ascherio A, Rimm EB, Giovannucci EL, et al: A prospective study of nutritional factors and hypertension among U.S. men. Circulation 86:1475–1484, 1992.
10. Witteman JCM, Willett WC, Stampfer MJ, et al: A prospective study of nutritional factors and hypertension among U.S. women. Circulation 80:1320–1327, 1989.
11. Singh RB, Niaz MA, Rastogi SS, et al: Effect of hydrosoluble coenzyme Q10 on blood pressures and insulin resistance in hypertensive patients with coronary artery disease. J Hum Hypertens 13:203–208, 1999.
12. Langsjoen P, Langsjoen P, Willis R, Folkers K: Treatment of essential hypertension with coenzyme Q10. Mol Aspects Med 15(Suppl):S265–S272, 1994.
13. Witteman JCM, Willett WC, Stampfer MJ, et al: A prospective study of nutritional factors and hypertension among U.S. women. Circulation 80:1320–1327, 1989.
14. Ascherio A, Rimm EB, Giovannucci EL, et al: A prospective study of nutritional factors and hypertension among U.S. men. Circulation 86:1475–1484, 1992.
15. Allendar PC, Cutler JA, Follmann D, et al: Dietary calcium and blood pressure: A meta-analysis of randomized clinical trials. Ann Intern Med 124:825–831, 1996.
16. Ascherio A, Rimm EB, Giovannucci EL, et al: A prospective study of nutritional factors and hypertension among U.S. men. Circulation 86:1475–1484, 1992.
17. Witteman JCM, Willett WC, Stampfer MJ, et al: A prospective study of nutritional factors and hypertension among U.S. women. Circulation 80:1320–1327, 1989.
18. MacGregor SA, et al: Moderate potassium supplementation in essential hypertension. Lancet 2:567–570, 1982.
19. Ayback M, et al: Effect of oral pyridoxine hydrochloride supplementation on arterial blood pressure in patients with essential hypertension. Arzneim Forsch 45:1271–1273, 1995.
20. Simon JA. Vitamin C and cardiovascular disease: A review. J Am Coll Nutr 11:107–125, 1992.
21. Patel C, Marmot MG, Terry DJ. Controlled trial of biofeedback-aided behavioural methods in reducing mild hypertension. Br Med J 282:2005–2008, 1981.
22. Eisenberg DM, Delbanco TL, Berkey CS, et al: Cognitive behavior techniques for hypertension: Are they effective? Ann Intern Med 118:964–972, 1993.
23. Silagy CA, Neil HA: A meta-analysis of the effect of garlic on blood pressure. J Hypertens 12:463–468, 1994.
24. Mashour NH, Lin GI, Frishman WH: Herbal medicine for the treatment of cardiovascular disease. Arch Intern Med 158:2225–2234, 1998.
25. Hitzenberger G, Korn A, Dorcsi M, et al: Controlled randomized double-blind study for the comparison of the treatment of patients with essential hypertension with homeopathic and with pharmacologically effective drugs [in German] Wien Klin Wochenschr 94(24):665–670, 1982.
26. Wong ND, Ming S, Zhou HY, Black HR: A comparison of Chinese traditional and Western medical approaches for the treatment of mild hypertension. Yale J Biol Med 64:79–87, 1991.
27. http://www.harrisonsonline.com

29. ACNE

Roya Kohani, M.D.

1. What is the most common cutaneous disorder in the United States?

Acne vulgaris, which affects more than 17 million Americans, accounts for over 10% of all patient encounters with primary care physicians and over 4.8 million patient visits per year.[1]

2. How common is acne in different age groups?

The prevalence of comedones during adolescence approaches 100%. In fact, 90% of girls and 100% of boys have some form of acne during puberty. Acne can affect all age groups, from neonates to senior citizens. The number of patients over the age of 25 with either late-onset or persistent acne vulgaris is increasing. Acne affects 8% of 25- to-34 year-olds and 3% of 35- to 44-year-olds.[2]

3. Why is it imperative for physicians to be familiar with acne and its treatment?

Patients with acne often experience severe psychological morbidity and, on rare occasions, mortality due to suicide. Embarrassment, shame, anxiety, and low self-esteem have immense psychological effects on both social lives and employment.

4. What is known about the pathogenesis of acne?

Acne is a disease of multifactorial origin. External, metabolic, hereditary, and hormonal factors play a role in the pathogenesis of acne. However, four main factors have been recognized: retention hyperkeratosis, increased sebum production, presence of *Propionibacterium acnes* within the follicles, and inflammation. It is also postulated that patients with acne have a lower concentration of linoleic acid in their lipids compared with controls. This factor may play an important role in retention hyperkeratosis.[3,4]

5. Do vitamins help premenstrual acne in women?

Women with premenstrual aggravation of acne are often responsive to pyridoxine (vitamin B_6). Pyridoxine plays an important role in the normal metabolism of steroid hormones. In animal studies, a vitamin B_6 deficiency appears to cause an increased uptake and sensitivity to testosterone.[5,6]

6. Discuss the role of DHEA in the development of acne.

Dehydroepiandrosterone (DHEA) is an endogenous steroid hormone produced in the adrenal glands, ovaries, and testes. It is a stem hormone from which other sex hormones are synthesized. DHEA has received attention for its role in a variety of conditions. A study conducted by Lucky et al. found that premenarcheal girls with the highest levels of DHEA develop the most severe cases of acne. Higher levels of DHEA also were found in prepubertal girls with acne than in those without acne.[7] However, most patients with acne do not overproduce androgens. Instead, they probably have sebaceous glands that are locally hyperresponsive to androgens. Nevertheless, androgen excess due to a variety of conditions can cause acne.

7. Do oral contraceptive pills (OCPs) aggravate acne?

It depends on the pill. Oral contraceptives that are estrogen-predominant usually improve acne. Progestins with androgenic activities tend to aggravate acne. If an OCP contains an androgenic progestin, it probably will worsen acne. Currently eight types of progestins are used in OCPs with varying degrees of androgenicity. The progestins with the highest androgenic activities are levonorgestrel, norgestrel, and norethindrone acetate. For example, the most common side effect of Norplant (subdermal implants) is acne because norgestrel is used as the active ingredient. Patients need to know that individual responses to OCP are often unpredictable and differ from one person to another.

8. Can shaving cause acne vulgaris?

No. People who are genetically predisposed may develop pseudofolliculitis barbae rather than acne vulgaris. Pseudofolliculitis barbae can occur in all races, but it is more common among black men. The problem starts with an ingrown hair that produces an inflammatory reaction. The treatment is to avoid shaving, allow the inflammation to subside, and use an alternative method of hair removal.

9. Do chocolate and fatty foods cause acne?

The answer is not clear. Diet can definitely play a role in the development of acne. Certain cultures with diets that are markedly different from the Western diet have a lower incidence of acne. The interplay of diet and genetics over hundreds of years may have made these populations less susceptible. As a general rule, eating a diet rich in fresh fruits and vegetables and drinking 6–8 glasses of water per day may improve overall health and complexion, but the current thinking is that chocolate and Coca-Cola are not to be directly blamed for breakouts in teenagers. However, junk foods are deficient in essential nutrients that are important for good skin health. Foods rich in saturated fat and iodine (found in shellfish) also may tend to trigger breakouts in some people.

10. Does poor hygiene cause acne?

No evidence indicates that poor hygiene leads to acne. Washing and scrubbing do not alter the underlying condition. Of course, good hygiene is important in maintaining healthy skin, but a variety of factors, including diet, hormones, stress, and external factors, need to be examined carefully.

11. What dietary recommendations should you give to patients who are prone to acne?

A nutritious, well-balanced diet is important for the health of the skin. The Chinese believe that acne is tied to inefficient and incomplete digestion, which results in toxic metabolites that show up on the skin. The cleaner and simpler the diet, the more quickly the skin will heal. A skin-healthy diet emphasizes raw and lightly cooked vegetables, especially green leafy vegetables that contain valuable trace minerals and are rich in fiber. The menu should contain lean protein sources and complex carbohydrates, such as rice, whole-grain bread, potatoes, and legumes. These fiber-rich foods help ensure a clean gastrointestinal tract, which is especially important in the management of acne. In general, the following guidelines are effective for most otherwise healthy people who suffer from acne:

- Consume fresh green vegetables daily.
- Drink plenty of water to help flush toxins from the body.
- Eliminate or limit all animal fats and hydrogenated oils for at least 1 or 2 months. This category includes dairy products, margarine, fatty red meats, unskinned poultry, and all fried food. This step alone sometimes results in dramatic improvement.
- Eat three healthy meals daily to provide important nutrients and to decrease the cravings for sugary or greasy fried food.[8]

12. What drugs and pharmaceutical products can cause or aggravate acne?

- Steroid hormones (topical and systemic corticosteroids, testosterone, some progestins, and anabolic steroids)
- Antituberculosis drugs (isoniazid)
- Antidepressants (lithium)
- Antiepileptic drugs (phenytoin)[3,4]
- Certain cosmetic products, especially moisturizers that contain oils (e.g., mineral oils, petroleum) can block the comedones, which in turn can cause acne.
- Other culprits: ammonia, artificial colors, ethanol, ethylenediamine tetraacetic acid (EDTA), formaldehydes, nitrates, and artificial fragrances

13. Describe acne rosacea.

Acne rosacea is a chronic skin disease that often affects people in the third to fifth decade of life, although sometimes it affects elderly people and even adolescents. It is characterized by vascular dilatation of the central face, including the nose, cheek, eyelids, and forehead. It commonly presents with flushing, follicular papules pustules, and telangiectasia. Certain severe cases even present with rhinophyma and lymphedema. The cause is still unknown. Acne rosacea is more common in people of Celtic origin and less common among blacks. The disease is chronic, and control rather than cure is the goal of therapy.[3]

14. Does *Helicobacter pylori* play a role in the pathogenesis of rosacea?

A higher prevalence of *H. pylori* has been reported in patients with rosacea. One study noted an improvement in rosacea symptoms among *H. pylori*-positive patients in whom the infection was eradicated. However, there was no difference in rates of *H. pylori* seropositivity between patients with rosacea and those without it. The improvement in rosacea after treatment of *H.pylori* may be related to the use of metronidazole. The association at this time is not well supported by data.[9]

15. What are the main therapies used by most allopathic practitioners for treatment of acne?

Benzoyl peroxide, antibiotics, and retinoids are the mainstay of treatment. Retinoids are the single most important pharmaceutical medication used to treat acne vulgaris. Maximal benefits usually require about 12–16 weeks. The different preparations of retinoids, from topical to systemic, include Differin, Retin-A, Avita, Tazorac, and Accutane (the oral form of isotretinoin). Other topical agents include alpha-hydroxy acid, salicylic acid, and azelaic acid. Although no bacterial resistance has been reported with topical benzoyl peroxide or retinoids, more than 50% of patients using topical antibiotics develop resistance.[10–12]

16. How much does it cost to treat acne with systemic antibiotics for 1 year?[10]

- Minocycline: $1445.00
- Doxycycline: $280.00
- Erythromycin: $174.00
- Tetracycline: $45.00

17. How does complementary/alternative medicine (CAM) approach treatment of acne?

Acne is a multifactorial disease requiring an integrated therapeutic approach. Patients should be checked for treatable causes and underlying hormonal abnormalities. CAM focuses on integrated treatment of the underlying problem with nutrition, stress reduction via mind-body medicine, homeopathy, traditional Chinese medicine, vitamins, and supplements. A combination treatment involving botanicals, homeopathy, and nutritional supplement often yields good results, particularly in teenagers.

Depending on the definition of natural, one also may consider derivatives of vitamin A (e.g., retinoids, isotretinoin) as highly effective modes of treatment for acne when combined with proper diet and supplements. *Lactobacillus acidophilus* also has been recommended by some experts in restoring the friendly bacteria that are essential in maintaining healthy intestinal activity.[8] These probiotic bacteria are even more important in patients taking oral antibiotics chronically to treat acne.

18. Discuss some of the herbal remedies used in the management of acne.

Calendula officinalis (family: Asteraceae) is a common example. Calendula is also known as pot marigold (although it is not a true marigold). It is used in the form of a tincture, fluid extract, oil, ointment, lotion, and cream. One can also make a tea from the flowers and wash the skin with the tea. Bach flower crabapple also has been used topically to clear acne. Another effective agent is *Melaleuca alternifolia* (tea tree oil), an Australian plant from which an essential oil is extracted.[13] Another popular and efficacious naturally occurring product is azelaic acid, which has shown great effectiveness in the treatment of acne.

19. What is known about calendula?

The Commission E Monograph (1986) states that calendula flower preparations are used externally for wounds with poor healing tendency. Calendula promotes granulation and facilitates healing of skin inflammations, wounds, burns, eczema, and acne when used topically. Experiments in various wound models have demonstrated significant wound-healing properties, especially for a hydroalcoholic extract of the herb. A calendula ointment using 2–5 gm of the dried herb in 100 gm of a suitable base is applied externally. Oral administration is not recommended because of possible hepatotoxicity. No contraindications, side effects, or drug-drug interactions are known with the use of topical preparations of *C. officinalis*.[13,14]

20. How does tea tree oil improve acne?

Tea tree oil has antibacterial, antifungal, and antiviral properties. At least one study has shown improved healing of acne, scars, and boils from its actions against *Staphylococcus aureus*. An Australian study found that a 5% tea tree oil gel proved as effective against acne as a 5% benzoyl peroxide lotion.[15,16] A few drops of the oil applied two times daily to the affected areas is recommended for the treatment of acne. Tea tree oil is available at health food stores. Make sure that the label says that the product is 100% pure tea tree oil.[13,14] Tea tree oil has a minimal tendency to irritate skin despite its penetrating qualities. Occasionally it can cause contact dermatitis and irritation and needs to be diluted or even discontinued for a while.

21. How does azelaic acid work in patients with acne?

Azelaic acid is a nine-carbon dicarboxylic acid with antibiotic activity against *P. acnes*. Clinical studies with 20% azelaic acid creams have shown results equal to those achieved with benzoyl peroxide, retinoin, and oral tetracycline.[17] Azelaic acid is effective in all of the different forms of acne. A recent review found that topical cream containing 20% azelaic acid was as effective as 5% benzoyl peroxide, 4% hydroquinone cream, 0.05% tretinoin, and 0.5–1 gm/day of oral tetracycline in ameliorating comedonal, papulopustular, and nodulocystic acne. The authors suggest that the few side effects of topical azelaic acid and lack of overt systemic toxicity make it a better choice for chronic use than other agents. It should be applied to affected areas twice daily continuously for at least 4 weeks. Treatment usually has to be continued for at least 6 months to maintain the benefits produced after the first month.[18]

22. What is the role of traditional Chinese medicine (TCM) in treatment of acne?

According to case reports, various Chinese herbal treatments, both topical and systemic, have worked against acne when pharmaceutical drugs have failed. Chinese medicine focuses on restoring deficiencies and imbalances in different meridians. Two examples of these particular acne patterns include lung heat, which frequently appears on the forehead and nose as whiteheads and blackheads, or damp toxin with blood-stasis acne patterns that appear as deep, inflamed, and painful cysts involving the whole face, neck, and back. In general, the most common causes of acne, according to TCM, are dietary and emotional.[19] Consider consulting a practitioner of Chinese medicine with experience in treating acne (see Chapter 11).

23. What vitamins are known to be helpful in the treatment of acne?

Vitamin C and bioflavonoids help to clear acne by strengthening connective tissue and acting as a natural anti-inflammatory, respectively. The recommended dose for each is 250 mg 3 times daily for 1 month, followed by 250 mg once daily for 1 month (between meals). Vitamin A and vitamin E work in conjunction to reduce sebum production. Vitamin E helps regulate retinol levels in humans. Retinol (vitamin A) is effective in treating acne when used at high and potentially toxic doses of 300,000–400,000 IU/day for 5–6 months. Water-soluble beta-carotene, the precursor of vitamin A, although less toxic, does not seem to have the same acne-clearing benefits. Vitamin A at less than 25,000 IU/ day is safe and effective for the treatment of acne, especially when taken with zinc and vitamin E.[20] Use of retinol is contraindicated during pregnancy because of teratogenicity.

Pantothenic acid (vitamin B_5), which is physiologically active in the synthesis of cholesterol and steroid hormones, may be of value in high doses for the treatment of acne.[21] Pyridoxine (vitamin B_6) helps women with premenstrual aggravation of acne because of its role in the normal metabolism of steroid hormones.

24. Which minerals are known to be effective in treating acne?

Zinc is essential for the normal growth and development of the reproductive system; therefore, it is an important supplement during adolescence. A teenager can take 25 mg of zinc chelate or zinc picolinate twice daily for 2 weeks and then once daily for 2 months. Be careful not to exceed the recommended dose. Zinc is also important for proper metabolism of vitamin A.[22,23] Chromium helps balance blood sugar and decreases sugar cravings. The recommended dose is 100 µg of chromium picolinate twice daily for 1 month, followed by 100 µg once daily for 1 month.[24] Selenium and vita-min E work in conjunction to inhibit lipid peroxide formation in both women and men. Selenium is used at doses of 200 µg/day in treating acne.

REFERENCES

1. Kaminer MS, Gilchrest BA: The many faces of acne. J Am Acad Dermatol 32:S6, 1995.
2. Goulden V, Stables GI, Cunliffe WJ: Prevalence of facial acne in adults. J Am Acad Dermatol 41:577–580, 1999.
3. Fitzpatrick TB, Eisen AZ, Wolff K, et al: Dermatology in General Medicine. New York, McGraw-Hill, 1993.
4. Hurwitz S: Acne vulgaris: Pathogenesis and management. Dermatol Rev 15:47, 1994.
5. Snider V, Dieteman D: Pyridoxine therapy for premenstrual acne flare. Arch Dermatol 110:130–131, 1974.
6. Pizzorno J, Murray M: Acne vulgaris and acne conglobata. In Pizzorno J, Murray MT (eds): Textbook of Natural Medicine, 2nd ed. Edinburgh, Churchill Livingstone, 1999, pp 1033–1036.
7. Lucky AW, Biro FM, Huster GA, et al: Acne vulgaris in premenarchal girls: An early sign of puberty associated with rising levels of DHEA. Arch Dermatol 130:308,1994.
8. Rountree B, Walton R, Walton Z, Walton J: Smart Medicine for a Healthier Child. Garden City, NJ, Avery Publishing, 1994, pp 83–88.
9. Utas S, Ozbakir O, Trasan A, Utas C: *Helicobacter pylori* eradication treatment reduces the severity of rosacea. J Am Acad Dermatol 40:433, 1999.
10. Leyden JJ: Therapy for acne vulgaris. N Eng J Med 336:1156, 1997.
11. Cooper AJ: Systematic review of propionibacterium acnes resistance to systemic antibiotics. Med J Aust 169:259, 1998.
12. Ward A, Brogden RN, Heel RC, et al: Isotretinoin: A review of its pharmacological properties and therapeutic efficacy in acne and other skin disorders. Drugs 28:6, 1894.
13. Schulz T, Hansel H, Tyler S: Rational Phytotherapy: A Physician's Guide to Herbal Medicine. Berlin, Springer, 1998, pp 259–260.
14. Blumenthal J, Busse M, Goldberg S, et al: The Complete German Commission E Monographs.. Austin, TX, American Botanical Council, 1998.
15. Bassett IB, Pannowitz Dl, Barnetson RSC: A comparative study of tea tree oil versus benzoyl peroxide in the treatment of acne. Med J Austr 153:455–458, 1990.
16. Carson CF, Riley TV: The antimicrobial activity of tea tree oil. Med J Austr 160: 236, 1994.
17. Nazzaro P, Porro M: Azelaic acid. J Am Acad Dermatol 17:1033–1041, 1987
18. Nguyen Q, Bui TP: Azelaic acid: Phamacokinetics and phamacodynamic properties and its therapeutic role in hypepigmentary disorders and acne. Int J Dermatol 34:75–84, 1995.
19. Molony D, Molony MMP: The American Association of Oriental Medicine's Complete Guide to Chinese Herbal Medicine. New York,, Berkley , 1998.
20. Murray M, Pizzorno J: Vitamin A. In Pizzorno J, Murray MT (eds): Textbook of Natural Medicine, 2nd ed. Edinburgh, Churchill Livingstone, 1999, pp 1012.
21. Leung LH: Pantothenic acid deficiency as the pathogenesis of acne vulgaris. Med Hypoth 44:490–492, 1995.
22. Michaelsson G, Vahlquist A, Juhlin L: Serum zinc and retinol-binding protein in acne. Br J Dermatol 96:283–286, 1977.
23. Michaelsson G, Juhlin L, VahlquistA: Effects of oral zinc and vitamin A on acne. Arch Dermatol 113:31–36, 1977.
24. McCarthy M: High chromium yeast for acne? Med Hypoth 14:307–310, 1984.

30. ECZEMA

Roya Kohani, M.D.

1. Define dermatitis. How is it different from eczema?

Dermatitis refers to a specific group of inflammatory skin diseases. Many diagnoses fall into the category of dermatitis, such as contact and dyshidrotic dermatitis. Dermatitis literally means inflammation of the skin. Eczema is a Greek word meaning "boiling out." The terms *eczema* and *dermatitis* are frequently used interchangeably. When eczema is used alone, it usually refers to atopic dermatitis.

2. What is meant by atopy?

Atopy means "different." Atopic disorders refer to asthma, allergic rhinitis, and atopic dermatitis. Atopic disorders affect 8–25% of people worldwide. Patients with atopic disorders often have eosinophilia and increased IgE responses. They are highly sensitive to pruritic stimuli and may have immune system dysfunction. In fact, atopy is characterized by reduced cell-mediated immunity and defective antibody-dependent cellular cytotoxicity. Atopic disorders may occur in any race or geographic location, although the incidence seems to be higher in urban areas and developed countries, particularly in western societies.

3. Describe atopic dermatitis and its pathogenesis.

Atopic dermatitis is a chronic inflammatory skin disease that is considered familial and has allergic features. Psychologic, immunologic, genetic, and climactic factors may play a role in the pathogenesis of atopic dermatitis. Clinical studies demonstrate a higher risk if a child's mother rather than father has the disorder. Atopic dermatitis often occurs in patients with other atopic disorders. Fifty percent of patients with atopic dermatitis report a family history of respiratory atopy, whereas 85% have elevated serum IgE levels and show a positive immediate skin test result to various food and inhalant antigens. The exact immunologic mechanism is not completely understood, but it is known that, unlike asthma and allergic rhinitis, atopic dermatitis is not associated with the release of histamine. In fact, atopic dermatitis presents with a type IV hypersensitivity reaction as opposed to the type I reaction in asthma and allergic rhinitis.[1,2]

4. What factors are known to provoke or exacerbate atopic dermatitis?

The most common irritant is excessive washing without appropriate skin lubrication. Other common irritants include excessive perspiration, synthetic fabrics, solvents, and mineral oils. Airborne particles such as tobacco smoke, house dust mites, molds and animal dander can exacerbate disease in some patients, particularly infants with severe dermatitis.

5. How often do patients with eczema or psoriasis use alternative modes of therapy?

A 1990 survey by Jensen[3] found that 42.5% of patients with psoriasis (n = 506) and 51% of patients with atopic dermatitis (n = 444) had used alternative treatments. Patients with atopic dermatitis had most commonly used homeopathy, whereas patients with psoriasis most commonly used health food. Although the prevalence of alternative modalities clearly differs among different populations, many recent studies have shown a growing trend toward use of alternative therapy for a variety of diseases, including eczema and psoriasis.

6. Describe the link between emotional stress and atopic dermatitis.

There is a high association (81%) between emotional stress and provocation/exacerbation of atopic dermatitis. It is postulated that emotional stress can exacerbate a number of diseases that are affected directly by immune cells. Psychoneurodermatitis is a well known entity among dermatologists.[4]

7. Define contact dermatitis.

Contact dermatitis refers to any dermatitis that arises from direct skin exposure to a substance. The dermatitis is either allergic or irritant-induced. In allergic contact dermatitis, the trigger induces an immune response (type IV hypersensitivity reaction). In chronic cases, the dermatitis may be present for months or years; identifying the offending trigger may be difficult. Patients often react to agents to which they have recently been exposed, but sometimes they react to agents that they have used for months or years. In irritant contact dermatitis the trigger itself causes physical, mechanical, or chemical irritation of the skin.

8. What substances most commonly cause irritant contact dermatitis?

Soapy water, cleansers, rubbing alcohol, bleach, strong acids, and alkali are among the many common triggers. Most substances are used repeatedly on a daily basis. But some irritants can produce severe dermatitis after minimal exposure. Anyone can develop irritant contact dermatitis, but people with compromised skin (atopic dermatitis, dry skin) and people with light-colored skin are at higher risk.

9. What sensitizers in North America most commonly cause allergic contact dermatitis?

The plant oleoresin found in poison ivy, poison oak, and poison sumac. These agents cause an acute eczematous reaction at the contact sites with the plant leaves. Lesions can appear on other body parts through transfer of the plant resins by hands. Once the resin has been washed off the skin, the lesions do not spread. Other common sensitizers include nickel in jewelry, fragrances in cosmetics and perfumes, preservatives in topical cosmetics and medications, nail polish, chemicals in shoes (both leather and synthetic), and latex.

10. Which medications can cause allergic contact dermatitis?

Topical steroids and topical antibiotics (bacitracin, neomycin) are notorious for inducing contact dermatitis. Other agents include benzocaine and Thimerosal. In such cases, one form of dermatitis may be converted to allergic contact dermatitis when the lesions of the first disorder are treated with a topical medication.[5] Certain therapies in alternative medicine also cause allergic dermatitis. Some folk therapies advocate raw garlic as a topical anti-infective agent, and contact dermatitis is particularly common among people who apply undiluted essential oils to the skin; in some cases, application of tea tree oil can cause the same disorder.

11. Discuss the association between chronic venous insufficiency and allergic contact dermatitis.

Allergic contact dermatitis is common in patients with chronic venous insufficiency and difficult to diagnose because it mimics stasis dermatitis or cellulitis. Patients often experience failure to improve with treatment. The most common irritants are wool alcohols (lanolin), neomycin sulfate, parabens (preservative), and fragrances. More than 30% of patients with chronic venous insufficiency develop contact dermatitis to neomycin and 13% to bacitracin. Silver sulfadiazine is also a skin sensitizer.[6]

12. Describe dyshidrotic eczema.

Dyshidrotic eczema or dermatitis, also known as pompholyx from the Greek word for "bubble," accounts for 20% of cases of hand dermatitis. Typically patients develop acute episodes of intense pruritus on the palms and/or soles that progress to multiple small vesicles. The vesicles gradually desquemate over 1–2 weeks, leaving erosions and fissures that slowly resolve. This intensely pruritic chronic recurrent dermatitis of unknown etiology typically involves the palms and soles and lateral aspects of the fingers. The term *dyshidrotic* implies a malfunction of eccrine sweating, but this mechanism has not consistently been observed. In fact, one study has shown 2.5 times the perspiration volume on the hands of 25% of patients with dyshidrotic eczema compared with age-matched controls.[7]

14. What are the main differences in allopathic and alternative medicine guidelines for the treatment of eczema?

Dermatologists treat most cases of eczema with topical steroids. Although successful in the short term, steroids are suppressive rather than curative. In some cases, the immune system may weaken if higher doses of corticosteroids are used for a prolonged period. In contrast, complementary/alternative medicine (CAM) targets the immune-mediated processes that underlie most cases of eczema. For example, because stress is known to cause and exacerbate dermatitis via alterations in the immune system, stress reduction can be a highly effective intervention that addresses the underlying cause. CAM also incorporates nutrition, mind-body medicine, homeopathy, traditional Chinese medicine, botanicals, and supplements to treat eczema.

15. Discuss the role of essential fatty acids and prostaglandins in atopic dermatitis.

Metabolism of essential fatty acids (EFAs) and prostaglandins appears to be altered in patients with atopic dermatitis. Several analyses of fatty acids in plasma and blood cells in patients with atopic dermatitis have demonstrated a tendency toward higher levels of linoleic acid (precursor EFA) and relatively lower amounts of the longer-chain, beneficial polyunsaturated fatty acids (gamma-linolenic acid [GLA], eicosapentaenoic acid [EPA], dehydroacetic acid [DHA]). There may be a defect in a key enzyme, delta 6-desaturase, which converts linoleic acid to GLA. If such a defect exists, direct supplementation with GLA bypasses this enzymatic step and may be helpful.[8]

16. Which herbal remedies have been successfully used in the treatment of eczema?

Evening primrose oil, black currant oil, borage oil, calendula (also known as pot marigold) lotion or cream, tang gui, and gardenia formula (Chinese medicine) are among the main successful herbal remedies for dermatitis. Evening primrose oil must be used in doses of 3000mg/day to be effective. The following botanicals also have been used successfully in the treatment of eczema:
- *Arctium lappa* or dandelion (*Taraxacum officinale*) has been used as a dried root (2–8 gm), fluid extract (4–8 ml of 1:1 solution), juice of fresh root (1–2 tsp), or powdered solid extract (250–500 mg of 4:1 mixture).
- *Coleus forskolii* extract, standardized to 18% forskolin is dosed at 50 mg (9 mg of forskolin) 2–3 times/day.
- Licorice (*Glycyrrhiza glabra*) may be used as a powdered root (1–2 gm), fluid extract (2–4 ml of 1:1 solution), and dry powdered extract (250–500 mg of 4:1 mixture).

Among topical treatments consider chamomile and witch hazel preparations, which have support in the scientific literature and are also popular with patients.[9,10]

17. What evidence supports the role of GLA in the treatment of atopic dermatitis?

Several double-blind studies of evening primrose oil (at a dose of at least 3000 mg/day, which provides 270 mg of GLA) have shown benefit. However, overall results appear to be more favorable with omega-3 oil supplementation than with evening primrose oil.[11,12] Omega-3 oil is also less expensive. In 1989 Morse et al. performed a meta-analysis of four controlled parallel studies and five cross-over studies at various centers in which doctors and patients rated the efficacy of evening primrose oil in atopic eczema by scoring the degree of inflammation, dryness, scaliness, pruritus, and overall skin involvement. In the parallel studies both patient and doctor ratings showed a highly significant improvement in symptom scores relative to placebo. A positive correlation also was noted between improvement in clinical symptoms and rise in plasma levels of dihomo-gamma linoleic acid and arachidonic acid.[13]

18. Which preparations of GLA are most reliable?

Three products that vary in cost and amount of GLA are available in the United States: black currant oil, borage oil, and evening primrose oil. The most economic and effective form is black currant oil in doses of 500 mg twice daily. It takes 6–8 weeks to reach the desired effect.

In Germany, capsules containing 0.5 gm of evening primrose oil (corresponding to 40 mg of GLA) have been approved for the treatment and symptomatic relief of atopic dermatitis. The adult dose is 2–3 gm/day. Although this dose may seem large, 3 grams of oil constitute a small percentage of the usual total dietary intake of fat. Occasional side effects are nausea, digestive upset, and headache.

19. Discuss the role of vitamins and supplements in the treatment of eczema.

Several vitamins and supplements have been used successfully in patients with eczema. The most effective are the following:

- Vitamin A (50,000 IU/day)
- Vitamin E (400 IU/day of mixed tocopherols)
- Zinc (50 mg/day): decrease dose as condition clears;, take with food. Delta 6-desaturase, a critical enzyme in essential fatty acid metabolism, is zinc-dependent.
- Omega-3 fatty acids in the form of EPA and DHA (540 mg/day and 360 mg/day, respectively) or flaxseed oil (10 gm/day).[14,15]
- Quercetin, a bioflavonoid, appears to have antihistaminic effects (200–400 mg 3 times/day taken 5–10 minutes before meals).[16]

20. Discuss the role of food allergies in the pathogenesis of eczema.

Many studies have documented the major role of food allergy in atopic dermatitis. Food allergies are thought to be responsible for atopic dermatitis in children with a "leaky gut" (see Chapter 36). The increased antigen load on the immune system due to increased gut permeability increases the likelihood of developing additional allergies. Breast milk, on the other hand, has been known to prevent atopy. Many studies, including a 17-year follow-up study,[17] have shown that breast-feeding offers significant prophylaxis against atopic dermatitis.

Usually food allergy is best diagnosed via the elimination diet and challenge method. This approach is particularly effective in treating childhood eczema. In one study of patients with atopic dermatitis, the rate of recovery after 1 year was 26% for the five major allergens (egg, milk, wheat, soy, and peanut) and 66% for other food allergies.

21. How is a suspected food allergy treated in patients with eczema?

As a general recommendation, patients should start by using a 4-day rotation diet and eliminating all major allergens, particularly milk products, eggs, and peanuts, which are the offending foods in 81% of cases. As the patient improves, slowly introduce allergens and reduce the stringency of the rotation diet. Simple elimination of milk products, eggs, peanuts, tomatoes, and artificial colors and preservatives results in significant improvement in at least 75% of cases. Limit animal products, and add fatty fish such as salmon, mackerel, herring, and halibut.

22. What other CAM modalities are available to treat eczema effectively?

Visualization and hypnotherapy to take advantage of the mind-body connection is highly effective in allergic skin conditions and should be used in most cases of dermatitis. In Japan, doctors have achieved spectacular success with severe cases of eczema by the use of hot spring water and participation in group and individual counseling. No medications are used.[18]

23. How does traditional Chinese medicine treat dermatitis?

Tang-gui and gardenia formula are commonly used for skin conditions with associated symptoms of dryness, severe itching, and bleeding at site and traditionally have been used for "heat" conditions (see Chapter 11). Gardenia formula, a combination of eight herbs, clears heat, cools and activates blood, and disperses stagnant blood. It can be made into a tea or used in granular form.[19,20]

24. What clinical evidence supports the effectiveness of traditional Chinese medicinal plants in treatment of atopic eczema?

A placebo-controlled, double-blind trial of tang gui for treatment of widespread nonexudative atopic eczema was published by Sheehan et al. in 1992.[21] Thirty-seven children tolerated the treatment and completed the study. Response to active treatment was superior to response to placebo and was statistically significant. There was no evidence of hematologic, renal or hepatic toxicity. These findings anticipate wider therapeutic potential for Chinese medicinal plants.[21]

REFERENCES

1. Jones SM, Sampson HA: The role of allergens in atopic dermatitis. Clin Rev Allergy 11:471, 1993.
2. Ruiz RG, Kemeny DM, Price JF: Higher risk of infantile atopic dermatitis from maternal atopy than from paternal atopy. Clin Exp Allergy 22:762, 1992.

3. Jensen P: Alternative medicine for atopic dermatitis and psoriasis. Acta Dermatol Venereol 70:421–422, 1990.
4. Jordan J, Whitlock F: Emotions and the skin-the conditioning of scratch responses in cases of atopic dermatitis. Br J Dermatol 86:574–584, 1972.
5. Wilkinson SM: Hypersensitivity to topical corticosteroids. Clin Exp Dermatol 19:1, 1994.
6. Kulozik M, Powell SM, Cherry G, et al: Contact sensitivity in community-based leg ulcer patients. Clin Exp Dermatol 13:82, 1988.
7. Yokozeki H, Katayama I, Nishioka K, et al: The role of metal allergy and local hyperhidrosis in the pathogenisis of pompholyx. J Dermatol 19:964, 1992.
8. Manku M, Horrobin D, Morse N, et al: Reduced levels of prostaglandin precursors int the blood of atopic patients. Defective delta6-desaturase function as a biochemical basis for atopy. Prostaglandins Leukotrienes Med 9:615–628, 1982.
9. Pizzorno JE, Murray MT: Ectopic dermatitis. In Textbook of Natural Medicine, 2nd ed. Edinburgh, Churchill Livingstone, 1999, pp 1128–1131.
10. Sheehan MP, Atherton DJ: A controlled trial of traditional Chinese medicinal plants in widespread nonexudative atopic eczema. Br J Dermatol 126:179–184, 1992.
11. Bertj-Jones J, Graham-Brown RAC: Placebo-controlled trial of essential fatty acid supplementation in atopic dermatitis. Lancet 341:1557–1560, 1993.
12. Stewart JCM, et al: treatment of sever and moderately severe atopic dermatitis with evening primrose oil: A multicenter study. J Nutr Med 2:9–15, 1991.
13. Morse PF, Horrobin DF, Manku MS, et al: Relationship between plasma essential fatty acid changes and clinical response: Meta-analysis of placebo-controlled studies of the efficacy of Epogam in the treatment of atopic eczema. Fr J Dermatol 121:75–90, 1982
14. Bjorneboe A, Soyland E, et al: Effect of dietary supplementation of eicosapentaenoic acid in the treatment of atopic dermatitis. Br J Dermatol 117:463–469, 1987.
15. Soyland E, Funk J, Rajka G, et al: Dietary supplementation with very long chain n-3 fatty acids in patients with atopic dermatitis: A double-blind, multicentre study. Br J Dermatol 130:757–764, 1994.
16. Natural Therapeutics Pocket Guide 2000-2001. Hudson, OH, Lexi-Ccmp Hudson, OH, 2000.
17. Saarinen UM, Kajosaari M: Breastfeeding as prophylaxis against atopic disease: Protective follow-up study until 17 years old. Lancet 346:1065–1069, 1995
18. Weil A: Natural Health, Natural Medicine, Rev. Ed. New York, Houghton Mifflin. 1998.
19. Molony D, Molony M: American Association of Oriental Medicine Guide to Chinese Herbal Medicine. New York, Berkley Books, 1998.
20. Atherton D, Sheehan M, Rustin M, et al: Treatment of atopic eczema with traditional Chinese medicinal plants. Pediatr Dermatol 9:373–275, 1992.
21. Sheehan M, Rustin M, Atherton D, et al: Efficacy of traditional Chinese herbal therapy in adult atopic dermatitis. Lancet 340:13–17, 1992.

31. DIABETES MELLITUS

Scott M. Morcott, M.D., and Meg Landgraf, PA-C

1. Define diabetes mellitus.

Diabetes mellitus (DM) is a group of illnesses characterized by the presence of elevated blood sugar due to the body's inability to transport glucose efficiently from the bloodstream into cells. This inability is due to the destruction of pancreatic beta cells, decreased production of insulin, resistance to insulin, or a combination of the above factors.

There are three main types of DM: type 1, type 2, and gestational diabetes. Of increasing importance is the metabolic state known as impaired glucose tolerance (IGT), which predates type 2 DM by a few to several years.

2. Discuss the incidence and impact of diabetes in the United States.

There are approximately 16 million diabetics in the U.S. and 180 million in the world; 90–95% have type 2 diabetes, and 33% are undiagnosed. It is believed that an additional 10 million Americans are at risk for diabetes and that by the year 2025 approximately 9% of all Americans will have DM. Type 2 diabetes is related to lifestyle factors and is typically diagnosed after the age of 45 years, although its incidence in younger populations is on the rise due to the prevalence of obesity and sedentary lifestyles in U.S. culture. Complications of diabetes are thought to be due to poor long-term blood sugar control with resultant small vessel disease. Concerning statistics include:

- Over 18% of adults above the age of 65 have type 2 DM.
- Diabetes is the leading cause of blindness in adults.
- Diabetics are almost 4 times more likely to develop heart disease than nondiabetics.
- Diabetes is the most common cause of end-stage renal disease.
- Diabetics are more likely to develop impotence and neuropathy and to lose a limb because of vascular disease.
- Diabetes and its complications are one of the leading causes of death and disability in the United States.
- In 1996, Diabetes contributed to the deaths of over 193,000 Americans, and in 1997 diabetic costs were estimated at $98 billion dollars.[1]

3. How is diabetes diagnosed?

Measurement of a fasting blood glucose > 126 mg/dl on two separate occasions is the preferred way of diagnosing diabetes. Diagnosis also can be based on two random blood glucose measurements ≥ 200 mg/dl or an oral glucose tolerance test (OGT) with a blood glucose measurement ≥ 200 mg/dl 2 hours after a oral challenge with 75 gm of glucose in water.

4. What are the goals for managing diabetes?

One of the primary goals in diabetic management is to avoid secondary complications by maintaining the blood glucose in a normal range (70–110 mg/dl). The Diabetes Control Complications Trial (DCCT) and the United Kingdom Prospective Diabetes Study (UKPDS) demonstrated the long-term benefits of tight glycemic control in reducing several major complications, such as heart disease, stroke, kidney disease, and blindness.

5. What treatments are typically used to manage diabetes in western medicine?

Type 1 DM requires the use of insulin. Currently, insulin is either injected subcutaneously or administered through a pump via a catheter placed under the skin. Trials are currently under way to develop insulin that can be delivered through patches, inhalers, or pills.

Type 2 DM is most commonly treated with oral medication, although some patients require insulin therapy as well. Several classes of medications are designed to increase pancreatic production of insulin (sulfonylureas, repaglinide) or sensitivity of tissues to insulin (thiazolodinediones), to decrease the amount on glucose created by the liver (metformin), or to slow carbohydrate digestion (α-glucosidase inhibitors).

6. Can any alternative or complementary treatments replace insulin in type 1 DM?

No. Type 1 DM must be treated with insulin. Complementary treatments can be used in addition to insulin to help improve glycemic control and assist patients in coping with the disease.

7. What alternative therapies are recommended for type 2 DM?

A recent study revealed that over 60% of diabetic educators recommend or use alternative therapies. Common examples include physical activity, self-help, dieting, vitamins and supplements, herbal medicine, humor, relaxation therapies, prayer, imagery, meditation, massage, and music therapy.[2]

8. How does nutritional therapy benefit the treatment of diabetes?

Nutritional therapy is extremely important and, in combination with physical exercise, is first-line therapy for the prevention and treatment of diabetes. A diet that promotes consistent glycemic control is optimal for diabetics. Some diabetics can successfully control the disease through diet alone (so-called diet-controlled DM). Dietary management of cholesterol, low-density lipoprotein, and high-density lipoprotein can help decrease the likelihood of diabetic complications such as heart disease, peripheral vascular disease, and stroke. Maintenance of an appropriate body weight (body mass index [BMI] of 17–24) is also of prime importance, particularly for type 2 DM and people at risk of developing type 2 DM.

9. Discuss specific dietary recommendations for type 2 DM.

Because type 2 DM is often accompanied by obesity, caloric restriction and weight loss are common nutritional goals. In addition, caloric restriction (500 kcal less than calculated dietary need) has been shown to have beneficial effects on maintenance of normal blood sugar levels above and beyond the benefits associated with any weight loss. Moderate weight loss, regardless if whether ideal body weight is achieved, is beneficial for glucose control and should be encouraged. Dietary focus, however, should remain on good glycemic control and nutritionally sound intake.

10. Should diabetics avoid eating sugar or carbohydrates?

Sugar (sucrose) is not inherently worse than any other form of carbohydrate for diabetics. In fact, sucrose is broken down to glucose (glycemic index [GI] = 138) and fructose (GI = 32) during digestion, whereas starches are broken down only to glucose (see Chapter 19). As a result, sucrose is absorbed more slowly than other simple starches, such as a baked potato. Furthermore, diabetics who restrict intake of carbohydrates tend to eat a diet that is higher in fat, which may be related to elevated blood lipids. This is not to say that liberal amounts of sucrose are permissible because foods with high amounts of refined sugar tend also to be high in calories and fat and low in nutritional value (e.g., cookies, candy, desserts). The bottom line is moderation.[3,4]

11. What is the benefit of a high-fiber diet? Are any carbohydrates good for diabetics?

On the other side of the carbohydrate spectrum are complex carbohydrates with low GIs (lower GI = slower absorption). A high intake of fruits, vegetables, and whole grains rich in dietary fiber, particularly soluble fiber, not only lowers blood lipids (6.7%) but also improves glycemic control and decreases the degree of hyperinsulinemia in type 2 DM. Many diabetics fail to get the 24 gm of daily fiber recommended by the American Diabetes Association (ADA). An experimental diet that contained 50 gm of fiber, with half as soluble fiber, showed a reduction in hyperglycemia (8.9%) comparable to that typically seen with the addition of a hypoglycemic medication.[3] Whole foods were used rather than dietary fiber supplements.

12. Is there an optimal combination of fat, protein, and carbohydrate in a diabetic diet?

There are currently several conflicting theories about the benefits or concerns of dietary intake of carbohydrates, fats, and proteins. The ADA recommends that a diabetic diet consist of 10–20% of daily calories from protein, 30% or less from fat, less than 10% from saturated fat, and the other 50–60% from carbohydrates. The current controversy focuses on the appropriate amount of carbohydrate intake. Popular current strategies center on an increase proportion of caloric intake from protein and a decreased intake from carbohydrate, especially in diabetics with a high GI (e.g., Atkins, Bernstein, and Eades diets). Alternative approaches include focusing on a low total fat intake (10%) with increased intake of carbohydrate.

There is no one "diabetic diet," although recent evidence supports the encouragement of a diet high in fiber (50 gm), especially soluble fiber (25 gm). Dietary management should be based on individual needs, with the focus on glycemic control and weight management, and should involve the help of a registered dietician.

13. What foods contain a high content of soluble fiber?

Foods that are naturally rich in soluble fiber include cantaloupe, granola, grapefruit, lima beans, oat bran, oatmeal, okra, orange, papaya, raisins, sweet potato, winter squash, and zucchini.

14. Has the modern diet affected the increase in type 2 DM?

The Pima Indians of Arizona have the highest known prevalence of diabetes in the world. Fifty percent of adults have type 2 DM, which was virtually unknown a century ago. A small study of both Caucasians and Pima Indians found that changing from a traditional Pima diet high in complex carbohydrate and fiber (e.g., tepary beans, squash, cactus buds) to a modern high-fat diet caused decreases in beta cell function, glucose tolerance, and glucose effectiveness (increase in fractional disappearance of glucose/unit increase in glucose at a basal insulin rate) and an increase in plasma cholesterol concentration. This study suggests that dietary change can be partly responsible for an observed increase in prevalence of type 2 DM in Pima Indians over the past century. The study also observed that these changes were not racially defined and were equally noted in Caucasian counterparts.[5]

15. How important is regular physical activity in diabetes?

Very important. Obesity and sedentary lifestyles increase the risk of both type 2 diabetes and insulin resistance. Engaging in regular physical activity is an important component of any diabetic management program. Weight loss, in the form of fat, and development of lean muscle mass from exercise can improve the ability of muscle cells to utilize insulin and manage glucose more efficiently. Exercise training can improve HgbA1c, increase cardiovascular fitness, maintain appropriate weight for height and build, improve management of high blood pressure, lower cholesterol, LDL, and triglycerides, increase HDL, and improve stress management. No long-term trials have been conducted to evaluate the effect of improved diet and exercise habits on cardiovascular disease or other diabetic complications. The Look AHEAD (Action for Health in Diabetes) study is currently under way to examine how diet and exercise affect several major complications of type 2 DM.[6]

16. Can diet and exercise reduce the risk of developing type 2 DM?

The Diabetes Prevention Program (DPP), a major clinical trial undertaken at 27 centers nationwide, compared diet and exercise with metformin in 3,234 people with impaired glucose tolerance. The study revealed a 58% reduction in the risk of diabetes with lifestyle interventions vs. a 31% reduction with metformin alone. These results are encouraging for the over 10 million Americans with impaired glucose tolerance. This trial was the first U.S. study to demonstrate a reduced risk for diabetes with diet and exercise in a diverse, overweight population with impaired glucose tolerance.[6]

17. What complementary or alternative forms of movement have been shown to be effective in diabetes?

Qigong, a traditional Chinese form of exercise, has been studied in a small group of hospitalized diabetics and was shown to reduce postprandial plasma glucose without a significant rise in pulse. These effects were similar to those noted with conventional walking. In the U.S., tai chi is the best-known form of Qigong and is based on martial arts movements with roots in ancient military training. It is performed by completing a series of flowing movements that can improve balance, strength, and flexibility. The purpose of these movements is to balance the chi (life force), which in traditional Chinese medicine is considered a fundamental preventive health activity. Qigong is practiced by over 200 million people worldwide and does not require a significant level of fitness prior to participation.[7]

18. Is it possible that sleep deprivation plays a role in the development of diabetes?

Yes. Recent sleep research performed at the University of Chicago on 27 healthy, nonobese subjects demonstrated a 40% decrease in insulin sensitivity for "short sleepers" (5 hours/night) vs. "normal sleepers" (8 hours/night). This study suggests that insulin resistance, implicated as a risk factor for the development of type 2 DM, may be promoted by poor sleep hygiene.[1]

19. What vitamins, minerals, or supplements are helpful in the management of DM?

Studies have shown that chromium, magnesium, vanadium, biotin, and vitamins A, C, and E (among others) have a beneficial effect on blood glucose management.

20. What is chromium?

Chromium is an essential trace mineral for which no recommended daily allowance is currently available. The average dietary intake is about 30 µg/day or less. Research suggests that 500 µg of chromium picolinate twice daily has a beneficial effect on HgbA1c and control of fasting and 2-hour glucose and insulin levels.[8]

21. What role, if any, does chromium play in the management of type 2 DM?

Chromium's role in diabetes was not discovered until 1959 when it was recognized that diabetics receiving parenteral nutrition supplemented with chromium had lower blood sugars. Research suggests that type 2 diabetics have impaired chromium metabolism and tend to lose more chromium in their urine; furthermore, people with impaired fasting glucose were found to have diets low in chromium. These studies and observations suggest that lack of chromium may contribute to glucose intolerance. The mechanism of how chromium affects glucose metabolism is not fully understood, but it has been suggested that chromium may increase cell sensitivity to insulin, decrease insulin resistance, or help bind insulin to receptor sites. More studies are needed to confirm the therapeutic effect of chromium in diabetes, but some studies have supported its use. Chromium supplementation should be considered.[8,9]

22. What is the recommended dose and form for chromium supplementation?

Different studies have shown varied results. It appears that 500 µg twice daily is the most beneficial dose for controlling blood sugar. Chromium picolinate is thought to be utilized more efficiently than chromium chloride. Chromium is biologically active in the trivalent state, forming compounds with niacin and certain amino acids, collectively known as glucose tolerance factor or chromium polynicotinate.[10] The polynicotinate or picolinate forms of chromium are most frequently recommended for diabetes.

23. Discuss the safety of chromium supplementation.

The estimated safe and adequate daily dietary intake for trivalent chromium has been set at 200 µg/day, but no toxicity has been found in rats at dosages over 5000 times this amount. The Environmental Protection Agency suggests that long-term chromium exposure at doses 350 times the recommended amount of 200 µg/day is without appreciable risk of side effects over a lifetime. Isolated cases of possible chromium side effects include kidney/liver toxicity, thrombocytopenia, anemia, and weight loss. Few side effects were reported with the recommended dose of 500 µg twice daily.[11]

24. What is the association between hypomagnesemia and diabetes?

Magnesium deficiency is thought to be common in diabetics, and low magnesium levels may contribute to insulin resistance as well as a number of diabetic complications, such as retinopathy, heart disease, and hypertension. Diabetics should consider supplementation with 300–500 mg of magnesium aspartate or citrate per day. Good sources of dietary magnesium include green leafy vegetables, whole grains, tofu, seeds, and nuts.[12]

25. What role does vanadium play in the management of type 2 DM?

Unlike chromium, the trace mineral vanadium is not considered essential. It has no RDA, but the daily intake in humans is estimated to range from 10 μg to 2 mg. Vanadium can be found in a variety of food sources, such as lobster, skim milk, vegetables, and grains and cereals. In the late 19th century it was used to treat diabetes and remains a potential consideration. It appears to function as a cofactor in enzymatic activities that lower glucose levels (increased glycolysis, decreased gluconeogenesis). Vanadium can be toxic at high doses, and finding a readily absorbable and effective form has limited its current usefulness.[13]

26. What role does biotin play in the management of type 2 DM?

Biotin is in the B-complex family of vitamins, and deficiencies are rare because of its production by intestinal bacteria. It is important for the metabolism of fats, proteins, and carbohydrates. Biotin occurs naturally in many foods, including dairy products, egg yolks, meat, poultry, and soybeans. Toxicity is unlikely because of its water solubility. Although the mechanism is unclear, biotin appears to improve insulin sensitivity and may stimulate glucokinase, an enzyme involved in the utilization of glucose by the liver. Biotin levels actually tend to be higher in diabetics than in nondiabetics—a finding that suggests a possible dysfunction in the metabolism of biotin in diabetics. Studies have used supplements of 9–16 mg/day of biotin, but currently not enough information is available to support supplementation.[11]

27. What other vitamins may affect the development of diabetic complications?

Vitamin C. Supplementation with vitamin C (at least 100 mg/ day) may reduce the accumulation of sorbitol in red blood cells of diabetics as well as glycosylation of protein. Accumulation of sorbitol and glycosylation of proteins have been linked with diabetic complications such as nephropathy, neuropathy, and retinopathy. Whether supplementation with vitamin C reduces these complications is not yet known.[14]

Vitamin B_6 (pyridoxine). B_6 is a water-soluble vitamin that may improve glucose control and symptoms of diabetic neuropathy in insulin-dependent diabetics. B_6 is essential for the metabolism of tryptophan, which forms a complex with insulin, reducing its effectiveness. Insulin-requiring diabetics tend to have low levels of B_6, and supplementation has been suggested to improve glucose control. Diabetic neuropathy is a progressive, distal polyneuropathy with symptoms similar to those of B_6 deficiency. Several studies suggest a link between the two and have demonstrated improvement in diabetic neuropathy symptoms with B_6 supplementation (150 mg /day).[15]

Vitamin E. Vitamin E is a fat-soluble vitamin that has been found to be lower in some people with diabetes and diabetic complications such as retinopathy and nephropathy. Like vitamin C, vitamin E is an antioxidant and may help to reduce glycosylation of proteins. Oxidative stress has been implicated in the development of diabetic complications, but no clear evidence supports this hypothesis. High-dose vitamin E (1800 IU/day) supplementation has been shown to improve retinal blood flow and renal hyperfiltration in type 1 DM. The potential benefits should be studied further.[16,17]

28. What is alpha lipoic acid (ALA)? What role does it have in the treatment of diabetes?

ALA is a potent antioxidant with dual fat- and water-soluble properties. ALA has been studied and used in Germany for treating diabetic neuropathy for over 20 years. It has been shown to reduce the symptoms of numbness and pain in diabetic subjects with neuropathy when administered intravenously at a dose of 600 or 1,200 mg. Oral ALA has demonstrated modest improvement when used to treat cardiac autonomic neuropathy. Its likely mechanism of action is that of an antioxidant and aldose reductase inhibitor.[9]

29. What is gamma linolenic acid (GLA)? What is its role in treating diabetic neuropathy?

GLA is an omega-6 essential fatty acid used to treat the symptoms of diabetic neuropathy. In people with diabetes, impaired conversion of precursor fatty acids into GLA is thought to contribute to complications such as neuropathy. Studies of GLA supplementation (480 mg/day) have shown improvement in symptoms of diabetic neuropathy, presumably via increased blood flow to nerves and improved neurologic function. GLA is found in evening primrose oil, borage oil, and black currant oil.[12]

30. What nutrients may actually impair glucose control?

Zinc and iron.[11,12] Zinc is controversial in diabetics. It is a necessary mineral for insulin metabolism and also aids in diabetic wound healing. However, at doses above the RDA, zinc has been shown to interfere with glucose control. Two studies in particular indicated that the HgbA1c and fasting glucose levels in patients taking zinc supplements rose significantly. It is prudent to recommend that diabetic patients adhere to the RDA for zinc (15 mg/day). Elevated serum iron may also affect optimal glycemic control in diabetics, and blood sugar control may improve with a reduction in serum iron. Studies have shown that when a diabetic patient is given chelation medication that removes iron, there is a significant drop in fasting blood sugar and glycosylated hemoglobin. It is suggested that iron supplementation in diabetics be avoided if at all possible.

31. What herbal remedies may help control blood sugar?

Gymnema sylvestre has been studied in India, where it is known as "sugar buster," since the 1930s. Various studies have shown that it lowers blood sugar and glycosylated hemoglobin. Gymnema may stimulate regeneration of insulin-secreting cells in the pancreas as well as aid in the entry of glucose into cells, and decrease the absorption of intestinal glucose. The typical dose is 400–600 µg/day, standardized to contain 25% gymnemic acids per dose. Side effects are rare, but medical supervision is recommended because of the potential risk of hypoglycemia.[10]

Momordica charantia, or bitter melon, is a fruit that is widely used in Asia to lower blood sugar. It contains a substance called charantin and a plant insulin that closely resembles bovine insulin. A few studies have indicated that the juice, dried powder, and fruit may be helpful in lowering both fasting blood sugar and glycosylated hemoglobin. Limited animal studies have revealed that momordica may work by increasing glucose uptake by cells. The average dose of extract standardized to 5.1% triterpenes per dose is 100–200 mg 3 times /day. Momordica, although considered safe by Asian cultures, has not undergone any formal safety studies.[10]

Trigonella foenum graecum, commonly known as fenugreek, has been used for hundreds of years in India as both a culinary herb and medicine. The active component appears to be the fiber portion of the seed of the fruit. Studies have indicated that fenugreek is helpful in decreasing urinary glucose and fasting blood glucose and in controlling postprandial blood sugar elevations. It has been proposed that fenugreek works by inhibiting the absorption of glucose in the intestines (much like the alpha-glucosidase inhibitors), and oral glucose medications should be taken 2 hours before or after fenugreek because of possible interference with absorption. The average recommended dose is 25–50 gm/ day. The most common way to consume the herb is in the powered form of the defatted seed, mixed in a beverage.[11]

32. Does the plant sweetener stevia help to lower blood sugar? Should it be used in diabetics?

Stevia is a perennial shrub from South America that is commercially used as a natural sweetening agent and dietary supplement in the United States. Stevoside is the glycoside responsible for the sweet taste and is 300 times as sweet as table sugar or sucrose. A tiny amount (less than ¼ tsp) can sweeten an 8-oz. beverage, adding less than one calorie. Components of stevia have been shown to have hypoglycemic activity, thought to be due to inhibition of hepatic gluconeogenesis. Despite its widespread use, few human trials have evaluated the role of stevia in the management of diabetes. Several small trials have suggested a lowering of blood sugar in participants taking stevia. Because few long-term data are available, this supplement should be used with caution in diabetics.[18]

33. Does acupuncture have a role in the management of pain from diabetic neuropathy?

Yes. A small study was performed in diabetic patients with painful peripheral neuropathy unresponsive to standard medical therapy. After 8 weeks of treatment, patients reported an improvement in painful symptoms and ability to sleep at night. Acupuncture can be a useful adjunctive therapy for painful diabetic neuropathy.[19]

REFERENCES

1. American Diabetes Association at http://ada.yellowbrix.com/. Accessed in June 2001 and March 2002.
2. Sabo CE, et al: Use of alternative therapies by diabetic educators. Diabetes Educ 25:945–956, 1999.
3. Chandalia M, et al: Beneficial effects of high dietary fiber intake in patients with type 2 diabetes mellitus. N Engl J Med 342:1392–1397, 2000.
4. Jenkins DJ, et al: Diabetic diets: High carbohydrate combined with high fiber. Am J Clin Nutr 33:1729–1733, 1980.
5. Swinburn VL, et al: Deterioration in carbohydrate metabolism and lipoprotein changes induced by modern, high fat diet in Pima Indians and Caucasians. J Clin Endocrinol Metab 73:156–165, 1991.
6. Diabetes Prevention Program: Diet and exercise dramatically delay type 2 diabetes: Diabetes medication metformin also effective. http://www.niddk.nih.gov/welcome/releases/8_8_01.htm. Accessed on March 15, 2002.
7. Iwao M, Kajiyama S, Oogaki K: Effects of qigong walking on diabetic patients: A pilot study. J Altern Complement Med 5:353–358, 1999.
8. Anderson RA, et al: Elevated intakes of supplemental chromium improve glucose and insulin variables in individuals with type 2 diabetes. Diabetes 46:1786–1791, 1997.
9. Morelli V, Zoorob R: Alternative therapies. Part I: Depression, Diabetes, Obesity. Am Fam Physician 62(5):1051–1060, 2000.
10. La Valle JB, et al: Natural Therapeutics Pocket Guide. Hudson OH, Lexi-Comp, 2001.
11. Head K: Natural Treatments for Diabetes. Roseville, CA,. Prima Publishing, 2000.
12. Pizzorno JE, Murray MT: Diabetes mellitus. In Pizzorno JE, Murray MT (eds): Textbook of Natural Medicine. Edinburgh, Churchill Livingstone, 1999, pp 1201–1218.
13. Badmaev V, Prakash S, Majeed M: Vanadium: A review of its potential in the fight against diabetes. J Altern Complement Med 5:273–191, 1999.
14. Cunningham JJ, et al: Vitamin C: An aldose reductase inhibitor that normalizes erythrocyte sorbitol in insulin-dependent diabetes mellitus. J Am Coll Nutr 13:344–350, 1994.
15. Jones CL, Gonzalez V: Pyridoxine deficiency: A new factor in diabetic neuropathy. J Am Podiatry Assoc 68:646–653, 1978.
16. Bursell SE, et al: High-dose vitamin E supplementation normalizes retinal blood flow and creatinine clearance in patients with type 1 diabetes. Diabetes Care 22:1245–1251, 1999.
17. Jain SK: Should high-dose vitamin E supplementation be recommended to diabetic patients? Diabetes Care 22:1242–1244, 1999.
18. Cirigliano MD, Szapary PO: Stevia as a natural sweetener, hypoglycemic, and antihypertensive. Altern Med Alert 3(2):13–24, 2000.
19. Erwins DL, et al; Acupuncture: A novel treatment for painful diabetic neuropathy. In Hotta N, et al (eds): Diabetic Neuropathy: New Concepts and Insights: Proceedings of the 3rd International Symposium on Diabetic Neuropathy. Knagawa, 1994

32. OBESITY

Aubrey D. McElroy, M.D.

1. What causes obesity?

Simply put, obesity is caused by chronic ingestion of more calories than you burn. However, the type of foods that people eat can significantly affect the way in which they burn calories. Insulin is a storage hormone that stimulates storage of protein, fat, and sugars. Because sugar is toxic in high concentrations, the body changes sugar into glycogen and then into lipids. In addition, insulin allows sugar into muscle cells, where it is used for energy instead of lipids. Glucose stimulates insulin release. People who eat meals with high concentrations of simple carbohydrates change to the storage mode. In developed countries, most foods are highly processed. Most of the vitamins, fiber, and minerals are removed from white flour, leaving only simple starches that are quickly reduced to sugar by amylase. Table sugar has been processed into its purest form. Because people eat a large amount of these and other low nutritional sources of carbohydrates, their bodies tend to stay in the storage mode without receiving needed nutrients. When this problem is combined with low activity levels, endogenous steroids (from chronic stress), high density foods (high in fat), and constant availability of food, obesity results. As much as 70% of obesity may be due to this process. Many obese people also develop insulin resistance.[1]

2. Discuss the prevalence and impact of obesity.[2,3]

The frequency of obesity in adults (defined as 20% above ideal body weight) is currently 33%. This prevalence represents an increase over the past 40 years in both men and women to the point that many experts refer to "obesity epidemic." Just within the decade between 1980 and 1990, the prevalence of obesity rose by 40%. Even more concerning is the rising rates of obesity in children. Increased television watching, decreased physical activity, and diets high in sugar and poor quality fats contribute to the problem.

Obesity is more accurately defined as excessive body fat, not simply a matter of overweight. Muscular athletes may weigh more but are relatively lean. Obesity is defined as body fat percentages > 30% in women and > 25% in men. Obesity is not only highly prevalent but also associated with as much morbidity as poverty, smoking, and problem drinking.[4] Obesity is associated with increased risk for coronary heart disease, arthritis, diabetes, hypertension, dyslipidemia, and certain types of cancer. The good news is that even modest weight reductions can result in significant lifetime health and economic benefits.

3. What is insulin resistance?

Insulin resistance develops when people chronically ingest low nutritional carbohydrates and decrease activity levels. If stores of chromium, vanadium, and possibly other nutrients are depleted, the ability of striated muscles to respond to insulin is decreased. Chronic high glucose exposure can downregulate the muscle insulin receptors. Exposure to saturated fats can inflame the endothelium and cause endothelial dysfunction. People then require higher levels of insulin, which stimulate the production and storage of more lipids. This process is called insulin resistance. To add insult to injury, the increased amount of body fat makes people more resistant to insulin, and a vicious cycle results.[5,6]

4. Why is it so hard to lose weight?

In reality it is not hard to lose weight. Many patients have lost 100 or more pounds before asking for help. Unfortunately, many people lose the same 10 pounds over and over. The real problem is not to regain the weight. The body has several homeostatic mechanisms to return it to its previous high weight (set point). For example, leptin is released from fat cells when the cell membranes are stretched (when the fat cells are full). As people lose weight, the cell membranes are less tense and less leptin is released. When the serum leptin level decreases, appetite increases and metabolism slows. This process results in an overwhelming desire to eat carbohydrates and calorie-dense foods (high in fat). People lose about 10 pounds, their appetite increases, and they simply cannot pass a fast food restaurant without ordering a cheeseburger, cola, and French fries (supersized, of course). They then regain the lost 10 pounds plus a few more.

5. How can people lose weight naturally?
The most natural way to lose weight is by eating a healthy diet and increasing activity and basal metabolic rate. Because of the homeostatic mechanisms that try to return the body to its previous high weight, a great deal of will power and dedication is required to keep the weight off. Almost any diet program that decreases intake of calories, wastes calories in stool or urine, or increases burning of calories will work for a while. The real question is how to lose weight and keep it off in a healthy, effective, natural way. The most natural way to lose weight depends on healthy lifestyle changes, such as eating healthy foods, building muscle, and exercising regularly. Many people may require natural and/or allopathic therapies to lose weight and keep it off in a healthy manner.

6. What is the best diet to use?
Several healthy diets work very well. All have a few common denominators: high fiber intake, low intake of simple carbohydrates, high-quality protein, 20–30% of calories from healthy fats, and high nutrient content. These diets can be used during the weight loss phase and during the maintenance phase by simply increasing the number of calories. Each patient has different dietary requirements. The ratios of carbohydrates and proteins may change from diet to diet, but the percent of fat should always be around 20–30% for a lifelong healthy eating program. Whitaker has an excellent healthy eating plan.[7] Other good diets include Weight Watchers, Garden of Eden diet, the 40-30-30 plan, the Mediterranean diet, and the newer version of the American Diabetes Association's (ADA) high-fiber diet. The practitioner needs to evaluate the patient's likes and desires and select the best diet for each patient. The major downfall of many diets is too little natural soluble fiber. Such diets can be adjusted by exchanging high-fiber foods for low-fiber foods that are high in simple carbohydrates.

7. Why do patients initially do well on their diets and then become tired and fatigued?
A 300-pound woman begins a 1600-calorie, high-fiber ADA diet and walking program. For the first month she loses 22 pounds and feels great. She has more energy and wants to increase her exercise. During the next month she loses 10 pounds and feels tired. She has followed the diet strictly, as her husband confirms with his calorie count of her intake. On the tenth visit she has gained 2 pounds and feels more fatigued than before she started the program. Her husband watches her day and night and states that she is not cheating on her diet. The diet diary kept by her husband confirms that she has remained on the diet. Several factors may explain this phenomenon:

1. Her body kicked in with the homeostatic mechanisms in an effort to stem the weight loss and return her body to its previous high weight or set point.

2. She may feel under more pressure from her husband, who is keeping his own calorie count of her eating. This stress may cause an increase in endogenous steroids, which in turn causes insulin resistance, decreases metabolism, and inhibits lipolysis.

3. She has been on the same number of calories for the past 10 months. The lower leptin level attempted to lower her metabolism. If her level of exercise is not enough to raise her metabolism, her weight loss will slow and stop. This process is called a plateau. Her metabolism will decrease to the calorie intake to inhibit or slow further weight loss. Now she only burns 1600 calories per day. Before she started the program, she was burning more than 2500 calories per day.

8. How long should patients be treated for obesity?
In the past we treated obesity like an acute illness. The patient was given a medication and told to exercise and eat health foods. If the patient lost the desired amount of weight, the medication was stopped. Not surprisingly, such patients regained their weight. Obesity should be treated like diabetes or hypertension. Weight loss, healthy eating, regular exercise, natural therapies, and medications are used at the appropriate times. Once the desired or healthy weight has been obtained, the patient

needs to maintain it. This goal can be achieved only if lifestyle changes are continued. Some people may succeed with lifestyle changes; others require life-long medicinal therapy.[7]

9. What type of exercise program should I use for weight loss?

Any exercise is better than none. Each patient should be evaluated and prescribed an increased activity program. For some patients, the program may consist simply of turning off the television and walking around the house. Others may start a vigorous weight-lifting program. Whatever the exercise or increased activity level, it should be consistent and progressive. Thirty minutes of moderately vigorous exercise before breakfast each morning helps promote weight loss and good health. Exercising on an empty stomach turns on the body's mechanisms to burn stored energy (i.e., glycogen and lipids) and stimulates the basal metabolic rate for the rest of the day. Increased levels of activities of daily living, such as taking the stairs, walking the dog, or parking further from the door, can burn additional calories and stimulate the metabolism.[8]

10. What lifestyle changes are needed for weight loss?

Drink 10–14 oz of ice water per day; the body uses energy to warm the water. Eat high-fiber foods such as whole wheat, whole grains, nuts, seeds, vegetables, and fresh fruit with the skin. Eat high-quality proteins. Avoid simple carbohydrates such as sugars, white flour products, potato products, and refined white rice products. Avoid high-fat foods and saturated fats. Eat at least three healthy meals per day. Reduce stress, exercise daily, play more, and watch less television (e.g., computer, video games).[7,8]

11. Does ephedra help with weight loss?

Ephedrine *(Ephedra sinica)* has been used in China for centuries as a key ingredient in herbal formulations for lung problems. It is one of the most popular and successful natural weight loss therapies. However, people tend to think that "more is better." Many companies put too much ephedrine in their products, and many consumers take more than recommended. Since 1994, over 1000 adverse events and over 20 deaths have resulted from ephedrine. Almost all of these events were due to accidental overdose. Ephedrine helps in weight loss when used properly and accompanied by lifestyle changes. Eight milligrams of ephedrine works synergistically with about 100 mg of caffeine 2–3 times/day. It raises metabolism and suppresses appetite.

Ephedra should be used only in conjunction with healthy lifestyle changes. Caution should be used in patients with hypertension, heart disease, aneurysms, and other cardiovascular disease. Theoretical interactions may occur with monoamine oxidase (MAO) inhibitors, over-the-counter decongestants, thyroid medications, calcium channel blockers, beta blockers, and antiarrhythmics. Ephedra raises the blood pressure slightly, even at these low doses. Ephedrine comes from many different sources. Only products standardized to no more than 8 mg total ephedra alkaloids per dose should be used.[9] Successful weight loss and maintenance require lifestyle changes. Do not try to treat obesity with a "magic pill."

12. Can chromium picolinate help with weight loss?[11,12]

Yes, in select people. Chromium intake has decreased over the past 40 years because of low-fiber, highly refined foods. Serum levels of chromium are low in many type 2 diabetics. Chromium was shown in several sound studies to improve control of blood sugar. The dosage ranged between 200 and 1000 μg/day. In studies using chromium specifically for weight loss, however, results have not been as vigorous. Some people lose a modest amount of weight; only people with insulin resistance and low chromium levels have significant weight loss. Small increases in lean muscle have been seen and may enhance insulin sensitivity. Chromium picolinate works better than the salt forms; 400–800 μg/day is a safe dosage. Chromium must be used with caution in patients taking insulin or sulfonylureas because of potential hypoglycemia. The weight loss results from improvement in insulin resistance. Chromium must be used in conjunction with lifestyle changes.

13. Garcinia seems to help some people loss weight. How does it work?

Garcinia *(Garcinia cambogi)* contains hydroxy citric acid (HCA) and other compounds that appear to inhibit storage of fat through the inhibition of adenosine triphosphate citrate lyase. The sugar is then stored as glycogen. There may be a direct or indirect increase in metabolism. Animal studies have shown HCA to be a highly effective weight loss and muscle-building therapy. However, a recent well-designed, placebo-controlled study in humans found no significant weight loss with garcinia compared with placebo.[12] More human studies are needed before garcinia is dismissed as a weight loss therapy. It may be more effective when combined with other therapies. The most common regimen is 1500–3000 mg/day in divided dose with a product standardized to 50% HCA. Garcinia should be used with healthy lifestyle changes for best results. The long-term effects are not known. Caution is advised for diabetics, in whom doses of insulin and sulfonylureas doses may need to be decreased.

14. Does chitosan help with weight loss?

Chitosan (deacetylated chitin from crustacean shells such as lobster and shrimp) can ionically bind 5–10 times its own weight of lipids. A 1-gm capsule taken with a meal containing 20 gm of lipid can bind with up to 10 gm of lipids. However, not all of this fat will make it out of the body. The lipase can still act on the exposed lipid molecule, and bacterial lipases in the lower GI track can break down the fats. By itself, chitosan has not been highly effective in controlled studies. However, combination with a lipase inhibitor (e.g., Xenical) greatly reduces the side effects of the lipid inhibitors. Large amounts of chitosan may bind enough fat to make a difference. The only cautions are allergic reactions (to shellfish) and decreased absorption of some fat-soluble vitamins and healthy lipids.

15. Why do some people use 5-HTP for weight loss?

5-HTP (5-hydroxytryptophan), a modified amino acid, is a precursor for serotonin and can affect the levels of other neurotransmitters in the brain. It is most commonly used as an antidepressant but also has a slight effect on appetite. However, it works best as a weight loss therapy in people who are mildly depressed. Depression and anxiety can cause weight gain and prevent weight loss. Treating these disorders improves the efficacy of other therapies. The typical 5-HTP responder is a man or woman who is under constant stress, has evidence of mild-to-moderate depression, and has not responded to other modalities. The dose of 5-HTP is 50–100 mg 1–3 times/day. 5-HTP should not be used with MAO inhibitors, selective serotonin reuptake inhibitors, and possibly tricyclics. Some studies indicate that early satiety may play a roll in nondepressed patient.[10,13]

16. Does acupuncture help reduce weight?

Acupuncture is used for a number of health problems, including obesity, smoking, and addiction. Results vary with the patient as well as the acupuncturist. Motivated patients respond best. Acupuncture (with or without electrical stimulation) of the ear appears to help some patients. Best results may be obtained when it is used with other therapies and lifestyle changes.[14]

17. Do good fats help reduce weight?

Yes. Good fats such as conjugated linoleic acids (CLA) have profound effects in the body. The average American is deficient in CLA, which is essential for transporting dietary fat into muscle cells for use as an energy substrate and for building muscles. CLA is nontoxic with no known side effects and has strong antioxidant properties. A number of studies confirm its benefits in obesity, some immune dysfunctions, insulin resistance, high triglycerides, and (in animal studies) breast and prostate cancers. CLA may have many other suspected but not yet proven benefits. It is one of the few therapies that reduces obesity (improves the fat-to-lean ratio) without requiring significant lifestyle changes or using multiple modalities. However, the amount of fat loss can be significantly increased with lifestyle changes.

Some studies have not shown significant weight loss with CLAs, but they have shown improved body composition. CLA promotes muscle building and fat reduction. Because fat is less dense than muscle, patients lose inches and improve lean-to-fat ratios, although the body mass index (BMI) may stay the same. The typical regimen includes 1–6 gm/day in divided doses. CLA is found in small amounts in beef, milk, and cheese. CLA should be obtained as a supplement rather than in the diet. Beef and milk available in the U.S. are deficient in CLA. People would need to consume a large amount of unhealthy fats to obtain enough CLA.[7]

18. Do omega-3 fatty acids have a place in weight loss?

Omega-3 fatty acids are another form of good fat that helps with fat reduction. It is found in cold-water fish (e.g., salmon, sardines), some nuts (walnuts), and flaxseed. The U.S. diet is also deficient in omega-3 fatty acids. Americans consume far too many omega-6 and very few omega-3 fatty acids. The average ratio of omega-3 to omega-6 fatty acids is about 1:20. The ideal ratio is thought to be much closer to 1:3. Omega-3 fatty acids are used in building healthy membranes, incorporated into myelin, and function as an antioxidant. They are a precursor for anti-inflammatory prostaglandins[15] and also help with insulin resistance in prediabetics and diabetics. This benefit may be due to its anti-inflammatory effects. People who are deficient in omega-3 fatty acids may have problems with fatigue, hypertension, insulin resistance, asthma, tendinitis, and arthritis, all of which decrease activity levels. Therefore, omega-3 fatty acids can help.

Most sources of omega-3 fatty acids have other beneficial nutrients. Cold-water fish contain high-quality proteins; flaxseed contains ligans, fiber, and vitamins; and walnuts have protein, some fiber, and a great taste. The recommended dose depends on the source. The most common dosage is 1–2 tablespoons/day or 8–12 capsule/day. Omega-3 fatty acids break down with heat, time, and light. Flaxseed oil should be kept in a refrigerator[18] or freezer with a date on the label. If it is kept in the freezer, it will be as thick as molasses and will remain good for about 1 year. There are no known toxicities.

19. Do supplemental vitamins and minerals help with weight loss?

Supplemental vitamins and minerals do not directly promote weight loss. If the patient is already deficient in some vitamins and minerals, poor nutritional status may increase the difficulty of losing weight. The best diets have a variety of foods with high concentrations of a variety of vitamins and minerals. However, there may not be enough to provide for optimal health or to replaced low levels of vitamins. The recommended daily allowance (RDA) is the amount needed to prevent disease and deficiencies. Some studies indicate that certain vitamins and minerals can assist in losing weight. Physical exam and lab testing can reveal some vitamin deficiencies, which should be addressed like any other medical problem. Otherwise, a good multivitamin with minerals should be considered.

20. Does natural growth hormone help in weight loss?

Growth hormone (GH) is a large, fragile protein that works by directly stimulating lipolysis and indirectly stimulating muscle growth. It is used by many has an "anti-aging" therapy. GH can cause transient insulin resistance. Bovine and other animal sources have little biologic function in humans. GH is not absorbed through skin or mucous membranes and is broken down in the stomach. Homeopathic GH has not been proven effective in any well-designed, placebo-controlled studies. At present the only viable way of getting intact, active GH into the body is injection of a prescription-only, expensive human GH. Release of endogenous GH can be stimulated by exercise, high-protein meals, L-arginine, L-glutamine, and other amino acids in high doses. The best approach is to take the pharmaceutical grade of high-dose amino acids on an empty stomach. The doses of amino acids range from 1–10 gm. Combinations of amino acids can act synergistically.[17]

21. Should high doses of thyroid products be given for weight loss?

Thyroid products should not be used for weight loss, but they may be used to return hypothyroid patients to the euthyroid state. Induced hyperthyroidism can cause osteoporosis, tachycardia, psychosis, and other health problems. Therefore, therapeutic doses should be used only in patients with evidence of a poorly functioning thyroid gland.

22. How do I evaluate patients before placing them on a weight loss program?

A complete history and physical exam are required. Look for diseases that may cause obesity, prevent weight loss, or endanger the patient during exercise. Also evaluate the patient for vitamin deficiencies. Causes of obesity may include: hypothyroidism, Cushing-like syndromes, depression, insulin resistance, leptin resistance, arthritis, fibromyalgia, chronic fatigue syndrome, and other activity-reducing diseases. Problems that can prevent weight loss include vitamin or mineral deficiencies, anemias, depression, chronic stress, cardiovascular disease, psychiatric problems, posttraumatic stress syndrome (from childhood abuse), and neuromuscular diseases. Other diseases should be controlled, including hypertension, cardiovascular diseases, diabetes, osteoporosis, cancers, and anemias.

The BMI should be calculated. Other measurements may be used, such as percent body fat. Lab tests should include complete blood count, electrolytes, blood urea nitrogen, creatinine, liver function tests, EKG, thyroid-stimulating hormone, and urinalysis. Other tests may be ordered as indicated. A 3- to 5-hr glucose tolerance test may be helpful in some patients. After reviewing the data, decide whether the patient needs a weight loss program and what type. Options include lifestyle changes alone, lifestyle changes with natural therapies, or lifestyle changes with natural therapies and prescription medications. Remember that obesity is a chronic disease and should be treated as such.[18]

REFERENCES

1. Bray GA: Etiology and pathogenesis of obesity. Clin Cornerstone 2(3):1–15, 1999.
2. Kuczmarski R, et al: Increasing prevalence of overweight among US adults. JAMA 272:205–211, 1994.
3. Rippe JM, Crossley S, Ringer R: Obesity as a chronic disease:Modern medical and lifestyle management. J Am Diet Assoc 10(Suppl 2):S9–S15, 1998.
4. Strum R, Wells KB: Does obesity contribute as much to morbidity as poverty or smoking? Public Health 115:229–235, 2001.
5. Diamond FB: Newer aspects of the pathophysiology, evaluation, and management of obesity in childhood. Curr Opin Pediatr 10:422–427,1998.
6. Arner P: Insulin resistance in types 2 diabetes: Role of fatty acids. Diabetes Metab Res Rev 18(Suppl 2):S5–S9, 2002.
7. Whitaker J: Whitaker's Guide to Natural Healing: America's Leading "Wellness Doctor" Shares His Secrets for Lifelong Health. Rocklin CA, Prima Publishing, 1996.
8. Leermakers EA, Dunn AL, Blair SN: Exercise management of obesity. Med Clin North Am 84:419–440, 2000.
9. La Valle JB, et al: Natural Therapeutics Pocket Guide. Hudson, OH, Lexi-Comp, 2001.
10. Murray MT, Pizzorno JE: Obesity. In Pizzorno JE, Murray MT (eds): Textbook of Natural Medicine, Edinburgh, Churchill Livingstone, 1999, pp 1429–1439.
11. Anderson RA: Chromium, glucose intolerance and diabetes. J Am Coll Nutr 17:548–555, 1998.
12. Heymsfield SB; Allison DB et al: *Garcinia cambogia* (hydroxycitric acid) as a potential antiobesity agent: A randomized controlled trial. JAMA 280:1596–1600, 1998.
13. La Valle JB, et al: Natural Therapeutics Pocket Guide. Hudson, OH, Lexi-Comp, 2001.
14. Zhao M, Liu Z, Su J: The time-effect relationship of central action in acupuncture treatment for weight reduction. J Tradit Chin Med 20:26–29, 2000.
15. Talom RT; Judd SA, et al: High flaxseed (linseed) diet restores endothelial function in the mesenteric arterial bed of spontaneously hypertensive rats. Life Sci 64:1415–1425, 1999.
16. Cunnane SC, Ganguli S, et al: High alpha-linolenic acid flaxseed (*Linum usitatissimum*): Some nutritional properties in humans. Br J Nutr 69:443–453, 1993.
17. Scacchi M, Pincelli AI, Cavagnini F: Growth hormone in obesity. Int J Obes Rel Metab Disord 23:260–271, 1999.
18. National Task Force on the Prevention and Treatment of Obesity: Medical care for obese patients: Advice for health care professionals. Am Fam Physician 65:81–88, 2002.

33. OSTEOPOROSIS

Tamara Sachs, M.D.

1. Define osteoporosis.

Osteoporosis is a multifactorial disturbance of bone metabolism that manifests as a decrease in bone strength with a subsequent increased risk for bone fracture.

Bone strength is determined by a combination of bone quality and bone density. Bone strength reflects the integrity of the protein collagen matrix that contains many inorganic minerals in a structured and organized pattern. **Bone quality** refers to the microarchitecture, the amount of accumulated damage, the mineralization of the matrix, and the rate of bone turnover. **Bone** density is determined by the peak bone mass minus the cumulative amount of bone loss.

Bone growth and **bone remodeling** are regulated in poorly understood ways by numerous hormones and growth factors, notably parathyroid hormone (PTH), gonadal hormones, activated vitamin D, growth hormone, insulin and insulin-like growth factor, and various eicosanoids, especially prostaglandin E_2. Both men and women reach maximal skeletal bone mass around age 35 years, and both begin to lose bone mass at variable rates between ages 40 and 50. Up to 50% of **bone deposition** occurs during the pubertal years..

2. Discuss the demographics of osteoporosis.

Eight million American women and two million men have osteoporosis. Ten million more have low bone density (osteopenia), which is a reversible risk factor. Osteoporosis is responsible for more than 1.5 million fractures annually, including approximately 300,000 hip fractures, 700,000 vertebral fractures, 250,000 wrist fractures, and 300,000 other broken bones. Elderly people with hip fractures have a 25% 1-year mortality rate. Of those remaining, one-half need assistance in walking, and one-fourth of those who were living independently require long-term care.[1] The direct medical costs for osteoporosis and the 1.5 million associated fractures is $14 billion ($38 million/day), and the cost is expected to increase to over $60 billion by 2020 if nothing is done to change current trends.

The rate of osteoporotic fractures has increased markedly even after controlling for the increasing age of the population. A recent study of 200,000 women, age 50 and up, with no previous history of osteoporosis, found that 40% had osteopenia, resulting in a 1-year risk of fracture that was 1.8 times higher than normal. Fifty percent of women over the age of 50 will suffer a fracture of the hip, wrist or vertebra within their lifetime.[2] The risk of fracture in 50-year-old men is about 13% (about a 1 in 8 lifetime risk of fracture).[3] Older people fear hip fractures. The thought of falling can cause considerable anxiety and result in self-imposed restrictions on activities and outdoor excursions. This fear, of course, can result in isolation and depression, less sun exposure and hence less vitamin D as well as less exercise and a worsening of bone health.

3. What is the advantage of an integrative approach to osteoporosis?

According to the National Institutes of Health (NIH) Consensus Development Conference Statement on Osteoporosis,[4] future research must include a multidisciplinary and integrative approach to understand more clearly the complex and varied factors necessary for prevention and treatment of osteoporosis. The report specifically addresses "an urgent need for randomized clinical trials of combination therapy, which includes pharmacologic, dietary supplement and lifestyle interventions including muscle strengthening, balance, and management of multiples drug use, smoking cessation, psychological counseling, and dietary interventions." They further suggest that trials of dietary supplements are needed. In an integrative approach, conventional medications can be taken side by side with complementary and alternative medicine (CAM) therapies.

To reduce the incidence of fracture, a multidisciplinary approach is necessary. Goals of such a team include reducing falls, minimizing the physical impact of trauma on bones, and strengthening and preserving optimal function of many body systems—not only the skeleton but also the musculature that supports it and the brain, vision, reflexes, and proprioceptive and cerebellar functions that help maintain an upright position when we start to fall.

4. **What risk factors contribute to osteoporosis?**
   - Female-to-male ratio = 4:1   • Current cigarette smoker
   - Caucasian or Asian race   • Family history of osteoporosis (especially in mother)
   - Small and/or thin body type   • Early menopause
   - Advanced age up to 85 years

   From a CAM perspective, other risk factors include:
   - Macronutrient or micronutrient deficiencies
   - Less than 5–9 servings/day of fruits and vegetables
   - Excessive consumption of salt, especially in setting of low calcium intake
   - Excessive intake of refined carbohydrates and sugars
   - Inadequate essential fatty acids in diet (eicosapentaenoic acid, dehydroacetic acid)
   - High phosphorus intake (e.g., from large amounts of soda) with low calcium intake
   - Excessive caffeine, especially in the presence of low calcium
   - Deficiency of minerals and/or vitamin K, activated vitamin D, vitamin C
   - Chronic stress or chronic pain
   - Toxic exposures (e.g., aluminum, possibly lead, tin, cadmium)
   - High ratio of animal protein to vegetable protein
   - Frequent loss of significant amounts of body fat

5. **What are the secondary causes of osteoporosis?**
   Secondary factors also should be considered in the differential diagnoses for low bone mineral density and fragility fractures. Possible causes of secondary osteoporosis should be considered in newly diagnosed patients, young patients, and patients with no identifiable common risk factors. Determination of the Z-score can be helpful in this regard. The Z-score is similar in concept to the T-score, except that the bone mineral density is compared with an age-matched control group instead of a young healthy control group. A low Z-score may reflect bone loss not attributable to age alone and may suggest the possibility of secondary osteoporosis. The following problems may accompany or mimic osteoporosis:
   - Medications: excessive glucocorticoids (including steroid inhalers), phenytoin, phenobarbital, chronic heparin use, methotrexate, cyclosporine, chronic antibiotic use
   - Neoplasm
   - Renal disorders
   - Immobilization
   - Hyperthyroidism
   - Hyperparathyroidism

6. **What are the reversible causes of falls in elderly people?**
   Because fractures in patients with osteoporosis are associated with tremendous morbidity and mortality, it is important to address prevention of falls in the elderly. Reversible causes of falling include muscle weakness, gait unsteadiness, decreased flexibility and general level of fitness, and polypharmacology. Some geriatric experts define polypharmacology as more than four drugs. In addition to slower metabolism with multiple medications, there is also an increased risk of drug-drug side effects. Drugs of which clinicians should be especially wary include antihypertensives, sedatives, anticholingerics, some pain medications, and muscle relaxants.[5]

   Environmental hazards are a well-known cause of falls in the elderly. A home evaluation is invaluable to eliminate environmental hazards and to educate the patient and family about fall prevention. Avoid throw rugs, clutter, slippery floors, chairs without arm rests, storage of frequently used objects in high places, poor lighting, flooring or stairs in poor repair, and absent railing or grab bars in bathroom. Use night lights; consider use of a bedside commode and/or cane.

   Protecting the hip with special pads has been shown decrease hip fractures in a nursing home population by 60% (p < 0.002) The only problem was that some residents did not remember to wear them. If all participants had worn the hip pads on every day, an 80% decrease in hip fracture may have been realized. No reduction was seen in nonhip fractures, but there were no risks or side effects and the pads are cost-effective.

7. Can estrogen prevent or reverse osteoporosis?

Estrogen slows down and may even prevent bone loss associated with aging in women. Estrogen replacement therapy (ERT) preserves bone density for as long as it is taken, regardless of how many years after menopause it is started. It seems to take approximately 5 years of daily ERT to realize fully the beneficial bone effects, and when ERT is discontinued, the protective effects gradually cease. Five years after discontinuance of ERT, all preventative effects are gone; bones return to their pretreatment state. Two problems are involved with ERT:

1. The data are contradictory and sparse as to whether ERT prevents fractures and, if so, in whom and after how many years of use. The vast majority of studies (in fact, all studies until recently) looked only at bone density, bone markers, or calcium balance—not at fracture rates. Recent studies have had mixed results, but two of the better-quality studies reported no protection from fracture with ERT use.

2. Timing of ERT is also problematic. Women usually start ERT at menopause (50–55 years old). It is common for women to discontinue ERT or limit its use after 5 or 8 years (10 years maximum) because the evidence for ERT-induced breast cancer is strong after 10 years of use. Osteoporotic fractures occur mostly in the elderly (average age = 75). When protection is most needed, the estrogen effect is gone.

Recent studies have suggested that estrogen does not increase bone mineral density (BMD) in the normal sense but causes a kind of cortical swelling that looks radiographically like an increase in BMD. The real effect is on the microarchitecture of bone. This finding may explain much of the above data as well as the widely divergent results reported in the literature.

8. What are the general dietary recommendations for healthy bones?[6]

Bone is highly dynamic living tissue and has the same basic requirement for nutrition as other cells and tissues in the body. In addition, certain nutrients are specific to bone health.

- Consumption of vegetables and fruit has been associated with increased BMD and QTC and decreased bone turnover in both axial and peripheral bones.[7,8] This finding may be due to intake of naturally occurring vitamin K, which activates osteocalcin, a protein that anchors calcium into the collagen matrix. The Nurses Health Study found that those who ate a serving of lettuce a day had a 45% decrease in incidence of hip fracture compared with those who ate one or less servings per week. Vegetables and fruit are important sources of magnesium and potassium in addition to many other nutrients and may contain nonnutritional factors that aid in absorbing and assimilating minerals from foods.
- Magnesium, zinc, manganese, silicon, boron, and several other minerals are also part of the bone matrix and must be maintained in balance to make and deposit new bone.
- Human and animal studies consistently suggest that excessive salt can cause bone loss over time. Habitual excessive sodium causes increased renal excretion of calcium by its direct effect on the distal tubule as well as its indirect effect via PTH.
- Soft drinks should be discontinued or limited. They are high in phosphates, and frequent intake has been associated with decreased calcium level in adolescents. Limiting intake during this phase of life is especially important because maximal bone deposition occurs during adolescence.
- Increased consumption of omega-3 essential fatty acids.

9. How important is calcium in osteoporosis?

Calcium metabolism plays a critical role in bone development throughout life, especially during childhood and adolescence. If calcium intake is adequate, the effects of weight-bearing exercise are enhanced. Calcium blunts the loss of trabecular bone and during the first years of menopause slows loss of cortical bone more than trabecular bone. Supplementation with calcium may reduce fracture rates by 50%.[9]

In the United States, the recommended daily requirements of calcium are higher than in most other countries. The recommended doses are age-dependent and vary from 1000 to 1500 mg/day. This is calculated with the typical American diet in mind; high amounts of salt, refined sugar, and carbohydrates promote calcium loss. Many countries with a Mediterranean type of diet as well as those with traditional Asian diets ingest less calcium and have significantly lower rates of osteoporosis. Our long-time focus on calcium to the exclusion of other nutrients is regrettable, because proper bone formation requires a whole host of nutrients. Low calcium intakes also have been associated with low intake of magnesium, riboflavin, vitamins B_6 and B_{12}, and thiamine. A multifactorial deficiency may lead to increased rates of osteoporosis as well as calcium deficiency alone.

10. What are good sources of calcium?

Cow's milk remains the principal source of calcium in the U.S. diet. Nonfat, 2%, and whole milks have roughly the same amount of calcium and are frequently fortified with vitamins A and D. Oxalates in brassicas such as broccoli (70 mg/cup) and dark leafy greens such as collards (148 mg) and kale (94 mg) bind the calcium in these vegetables, but the absorbability of calcium is roughly the same as from cow's milk. For people who are lactose-intolerant or vegan or have food allergies to cow's milk, calcium-fortified nondairy options are available.[10] Other calcium-rich foods include figs, almonds, and sardines.

As for supplements, oyster shell calcium and bone meal have fallen out of favor because of their considerable lead content. Although calcium citrate (and other Krebs cycle chelates) is definitely a more soluble form of calcium with high uptake, a smaller total amount of calcium carbonate is required to obtain adequate amounts of elemental calcium. In addition, calcium carbonate is cheap and easily obtained by most people. Calcium citrate may be the preferred form for people with hypochlorhydria (inadequate gastric acid) or impaired renal function. Dividing the daily amount into small doses increases absorption up to 80%.

11. Discuss the role of magnesium in osteoporosis.[11]

In a survey of over 27,000 of Americans, only 25% had adequate dietary intake of magnesium. Magnesium is integral part of normal bone, and 50% of the body's magnesium is stored in bone. It is ubiquitously involved in 300 key cellular reactions, including formation of cyclic adenosine monophosphate, secretion of parathyroid hormone, and proper function of smooth and skeletal muscle. Magnesium also activates vitamin D, and a deficiency of magnesium leads to decreased levels of 1,25-dihydrovitmain D_3, the most active form. The recommended dose of magnesium is 400–800 mg/day. Ideally, magnesium is given with calcium at a ratio of 1:2 or even 1:1.

12. How does protein affect osteoporosis?

High-protein diets, especially those high in animal protein, have often been cited as causing both elevated urinary calcium excretion and decreased intestinal absorption of calcium. Increasing protein intake—from approximately 50 to 140 gm—doubled the urinary excretion of calcium in one study.[12] At the other end of the spectrum, very low levels of protein are also linked to osteoporosis. It seems that both extremes are associated with bone loss.

Recently an answer to protein-vegetarian dilemma has been suggested by several sources. A key factor in calcium balance is the ratio of animal protein to vegetable protein.[13] This finding makes evolutionary sense and may account for the multiplicity of different but healthy diets. It also explains the alkaline-ash theory of acid–base imbalance due to dairy and meat. Animal proteins and dairy products do not seem to create a negative calcium balance with adequate intake of vegetable proteins, including legumes, nuts, seeds, and large amounts of fruits and vegetables. Frequent consumption of vegetables and most fruits, regardless of protein content, also seems to prevent the negative effects of animal proteins.

13. Does soy help prevent osteoporosis?[14,15]

Phytoestrogens are plant compounds—nonsteroidal structures that resemble estradiol and that can behave in both an estrogenic and antiestrogenic manner. They are found in small amounts in many fruits, vegetables, and grains, but legumes are especially rich in the many types of phytoestrogens. The phytoestrogens found in legumes are called isoflavones. Of all foods, soybeans are the richest source of isoflavones. Studies have had mixed results, but it seems that the isoflavones, not the soy protein, create the positive effect on BMD. Studies with soy protein supplements and diets rich in soy have shown positive changes in bone markers consistent with bone formation, such as increased osteocalcin levels and a decrease in markers for bone resorption.

Soy foods can attenuate the normal bone loss that occurs during menopause, especially in vertebral bone. BMD in perimenopausal and postmenopausal women is improved when 90 mg/day of isoflavones is consumed over the course of 6 months. Because of the hormone-like properties of soy and isoflavones, it is advisable to limit soy supplementation to soy-based foods such as tofu and tempeh and to avoid concentrated isoflavone supplements or concentrated soy extracts. In food and at normal amounts, there is consistent evidence of protection from breast cancer, prostate cancer, and possibly colon and other cancers. At high doses in vivo, concentrated isoflavones have been shown to promote tumor growth in estrogen-sensitive tumors. The consumption of normal amounts (i.e., 1–2 servings/day) of foods rich in isoflavones appearS safe. Soy protein isolates and powders may cause unnaturally high levels of isoflavones with unknown long-term effects.

Soy was long thought to provoke hyperthyroidism, the treatment of which has been implicated in further bone loss. Recent randomized control trials have shown no association between soy supplementation and thyroid disease. There appears to be a noncausal association between these two common conditions in postmenopausal women. Theoretical concerns that soy can block the synthesis of thyroid hormone seem valid only in the presence of an iodine deficiency In the setting of existing goiter or history of goiter, soy foods or supplements should be used with caution. In addition, soy has several pharmacologic properties that modulate lipid metabolism, increasing HDL and preventing the oxidation of LDL in addition to improving arterial compliance. It also has antioxidant properties.

14. What is the role of vitamin D in osteoporosis?

$$\text{Vitamin D} \xrightarrow{\text{Sunlight}} \text{vitamin D}_3 \text{ (cholecalciferol)} \rightarrow \rightarrow \underset{\text{Active form}}{1,25\text{-OH vitamin D}_3 \text{ (calcitriol)}}$$

Vitamin D plays a significant role in maintaining BMD and preventing fractures. Vitamin D is necessary for calcium absorption from the gastrointestinal tract and for the deposition of calcium into the bone matrix. Low levels of vitamin D are common in institutionalized patients, nursing home residents, and inhabitants of northern latitudes in the winter. In the healthy elderly population, vitamin D levels have been noted to be low even in farmers and people taking daily multivitamins containing vitamin D. Occasionally elderly patients in particular are unable to convert vitamin D to its active form. This inability may be secondary to a liver or kidney problem or a genetic enzyme deficiency. Calcitriol is the active form of vitamin D available for use in this setting. It seems to have a role independent of calcium as well as working in association with calcium. Vitamin D rapidly lowers PTH levels and thus quickly inhibits bone resorption. One option for treatment of patients in extended care facilities and other settings is an annual intramuscular injection of vitamin D_2 (ergocalciferol) at a dose of 150–300,000 IU.[16] Recently vitamin D was shown to contribute to muscular function and perhaps balance, with less body sway and a significant decrease in the number of falls compared with controls. The elderly seem to have several reasons for decreased vitamin D levels and activity. Vitamin D is usually supplemented as D_3 at a dose of 400–800 IU/day.

15. How does exercise prevent osteoporosis?

Physical activity is an absolute prerequisite to strong bones. During childhood and adolescence, if enough calcium is present in the diet, physical activity becomes the most important predictor for bone formation. The benefits of exercise for patients with osteoporosis are multiple.[17] Weight-bearing exercise applies mechanical tension to muscle and bone, thus providing the stimulation to increase bone density by 2–8% per year. Types of weight-bearing exercise include brisk walking, running, dancing, and low- and high-impact aerobics. Elderly patients should have a physical exam before attempting to engage in any vigorous forms of exercise. The most important key is to start any form of exercise slowly and work your way up.

New evidence indicates that resistance training (weight lifting) is effective at increasing bone density.[18] Other advantages of resistance training include increased muscle tone, maintenance of a more finely tuned proprioceptive and kinesthetic system, increased endurance, and better mobility.

Even the very elderly have shown benefits with light weight training 2–3 times per week, adapted to their needs. Specific muscle groups targeted are hip and knee flexors.

16. Which CAM modalities are useful for osteoporosis?

Low-impact exercises such as yoga and tai-chi can improve balance and strength. This benefit is particularly important in the elderly, who may not be able to perform vigorous exercises,but need to reduce their risk of falls and fractures. In one study, tai-chi was shown to reduce the risk of falling by almost 50%.[19]

17. What resources are available for additional information?

- Gaby AR: Preventing and Reversing Osteoporosis. Roseville, CA, Prima Publishing, 1994.
- Nelson ME: Strong Women, Strong Bones. New York, J.P. Putnam's Sons, 2000.
- Northrup C: Women's Bodies, Women's Wisdom. New York, Bantam Books, 1994.
- Werbach MR, Moss J: Textbook of Nutritional Medicine. Tarzana, CA, Third Line Press, Inc., 1999.
- National Osteoporosis Foundation
  1232 22nd Street N.W.
  Washington, D.C. 20037-1292
  (202) 223.2226 www.nof.org

REFERENCES

1. National Osteoporosis Association: www.nof.org. Accessed 04/11/2002.
2. Siris ES, Miller PD, et al: Identification and fracture outcomes of undiagnosed low bone mineral density in postmenopausal women. JAMA 286:2815–2822, 2001.
3. Bilezikan JP: Gender specificity and osteoporosis. J Gen Spec Med Oct:6-11, 2000.
4. NIH Consensus Development Conference Statement on Osteoporosis Prevention, Diagnosis, and Therapy. Bethesda, MD, National Institutes of Health, 2000. March 23–27, 2000, volume 17, no. 1.
5. Leipzig RM, et al: Drugs and falls in older people: A systematic review and meta analysis. I: Psychotropic drugs. J Am Geriatric Soc 47:30–39, 1999.
6. Pizzorno JE, Murray MT: Osteoporosis. In Pizzorno JE, Murray MT (eds): Textbook of Natural Medicine. Edinburgh, Churchill Livingstone, 1999, p 1456.
7. Tucker KL, Hannan MT, et al: Potassuim, magnesium, and fruit and vegetable intakes are associated with greater bone mineral density in elderly men and women. Am J Clin Nutr 69:727–736, 1999.
8. New SA, Robins SP, et al: Dietary influences on bone mass and bone metabolism: Further evidence of a positive link between fruit and vegetable consumption and bone health? Am J Clin Nutr 71:142–151, 2000.
9. Reid IR: The role of calcium and vitamin D in the prevention of osteoporosis. Endocrinol Metab Clin North Am 27:389–398, 1998.
10. Weaver C, Proulx W, Heaney R: Choices for achieving adequate dietary calcium with a vegetarian diet. Am J Clin Nutr 70:543S–548S, 1999.
11. Abraham GE: The importance of magnesium in the management of primarily postmenopausal osteoporosis. J Nutr Med 2:165-178, 1998.
12. Licata A, et al: Acute effects of dietary protein on calcium metabolism in patients with osteoporosis. J Geront 36:14–19, 1981.
13. Sellmeyer DE, Stone KL, et al: A high ratio of dietary animal to vegetable protein increases the rate of bone loss and the risk of fracture in postmenopausal women. Am J Clin Nutr 73:118-122, 2001.
14. Alekel DL, et al: Soy protein and isoflavones: Their effects on blood lipids and bone density in postmenopausal women. Am J Clin Nutr 68(Suppl):1375S–379S, 1998.
15. Messina MJ: Legumes and soybeans: overview of their nutritional profiles and health effects Am J Clin Nutr 70:439-450, 1999.
16. Quesada Gomez JM, et al: Vitamin D insufficiency as a determinant of hip fractures. Osteopor Int Suppl 3:S42–S47, 1996.
17. Henderson NK, White CP, Eisman JA: The roles of exercise and fall risk reduction in the prevention of osteoporosis. Endocrinal Metab Clin North Am 27:369–387, 1998.
18. Nelson ME, et al: Effects of high-intensity strength training on multiple risk factors for osteoporotic fractures. JAMA 272:1909–1914, 1994.
19. Wolf SL, Sattin RW, et al: A study design to investigate the effect of intense Tai Chi in reducing falls among older adults transitioning to frailty. Control Clin Trials 22:689–704, 2001.

34. GASTROESOPHAGEAL REFLUX

Marcey Shapiro, M.D.

1. What is GERD?

GERD is an acronym for gastroesophageal reflux disease, a broad term that includes many symptoms, such as heartburn, bloating, belching, indigestion, and regurgitation. GERD is also known as dyspepsia. In GERD stomach contents, including acid, may back up through the esophagus, causing a burning or painful sensation. This sensation may be accompanied by an acid or bitter taste in the mouth and may mimic cardiac chest pain. When GERD reflux is frequent, the lining of the esophagus may become eroded and scarred because of contact with hydrochloric acid, or the cell lining of the esophagus may transform. This scarring can exacerbate the tendency to reflux.

2. Describe the pathophysiologic process underlying GERD.

Digestion of food begins in the mouth. When food is properly chewed, the enzyme ptyalin in saliva mixes with it and begins to break it down. This enzyme is particularly important for digestion of starches. Food then travels through the esophagus to the stomach. When food reaches the stomach, hydrochloric acid (HCl) and pepsin mix with the digesting food. As the chyme (liquefied, partially digested food) passes into the small intestine, pancreatic enzymes that further assist in digestion are secreted. Mucin-containing cells, which line the entire digestive tract to protect the mucosal lining, are especially prominent in the stomach, where normal pH is around 2.0 during digestion. HCl is particularly important for the digestion of proteins. A breakdown at any of these junctures can contribute to GERD, which can be seen as a back up of the contents in the plumbing.

3. What causes GERD?

Common causes of GERD include hiatal hernia, incompetence at the gastroesophageal sphincter, faulty esophageal peristalsis, and delayed gastric emptying,[1] which may be due to deficient stomach acid (see below). Nonsteroidal anti-inflammatory drugs can contribute to the suppression of mucin production in the stomach, causing the sensation of burning and leading to inflammation and possibly ulceration. The presence of parasites, overgrowth of candidal organisms, or bacterial infections (e.g., *Helicobacter pylori*) can result in symptoms. Both excessive and deficient stomach acid production, insufficient production of digestive enzymes, and environmental, food, or drug toxins can induce symptoms of GERD.

4. What is the prevalence of GERD?

In the United States, GERD affects 20% of adults at least once per week. Ten percent of adults report symptoms that occur daily, and about half of these have damage to the esophageal mucosa at endoscopy. Patients presenting with Barrett's esophagitis (in which the esophageal mucosal lining develops metaplastic cell structure resembling that of the stomach) have a 40-fold increased risk of esophageal cancer compared with controls.[1]

5. Discuss the role of excessive and deficient stomach acid in the pathogenesis of GERD from a CAM perspective.

The underlying question of why the factors that lead to GERD develop is a subject of much investigation in CAM. With ingestion of a typical high-protein, high-fat, high-calorie meal, the body's natural response is to secrete excessive hydrochloric acid to assist in digestion of this overload. If mucin production in the stomach is sufficient, the body should be able to handle occasional overindulgence in the normal manner. However when overindulgence is frequent, as in the standard American diet, excessive acid may irritate the sphincter between the stomach and esophagus. Stomach mucin production also may be compromised by ingestion of alcohol.

In contrast to popular belief, many people with GERD symptoms have either normal or deficient rather than excessive stomach acid. This finding may be due to drug-induced suppression of a normal gastric acid response, disease, or the aging process. The ability to produce stomach acid declines with age, in fact greater than 50% of persons over age 60 have low stomach acid production.[2] Many practitioners feel that burning symptoms are secondary to low mucin production in the stomach, rather than excess acid.[3]

GERD symptoms can occur when food is not digested properly because of low acid secretion is or food overload. The food remains churning in the stomach for an excessive amount of time. The remaining stomach acid then loosens the sphincter protecting the esophagus from the stomach, and stomach contents, including food, acid, and even bile, can ascend into the esophagus, causing the pathognomonic reflux symptoms. In the absence of ulceration, antacids are of no benefit in treatment of dyspepsia[4] and in fact are implicated in the pathogenesis of some diseases.

6. What tests can determine whether stomach acid is excessive, normal, or deficient?

The only irrefutable test is direct measurement of stomach acid collected after a standard meal.[5] This invasive test is not often done. A naturopathic shortcut is to give betaine HCl and pepsin capsules with the meal. Betaine is an amino acid that is used as a carrier for the HCl. One capsule, usually 300–600 mg of betaine HCl and 5–10 mg of pepsin, is given with each meal. If symptoms remain the same or improve, then after 1–2 days two capsules are given during or immediately after each meal. This pattern of increasing the number of capsules continues until the patient experiences heartburn or a warm feeling with ingestion of the capsules, at which point the patient should return to the number of capsules that alleviated symptoms without heartburn.

CAM practitioners have observed that if this test is not prolonged and the patient is careful in noting symptoms, there is little chance that the small amount of additional HCl/pepsin will cause significant damage, even if acid is truly excessive. If acid is deficient and the patient continues to work with betaine HCL/pepsin, eventually he or she may notice the symptoms of heartburn even with the previously therapeutic dose. Although the mechanism has not been studied, this therapy seems to prime the pump, restoring the body's own autoregulation of stomach acid. When heartburn occurs, patients should again decrease the number of capsules to a comfortable level.[6]

7. If stomach acid is low with meals, which herbs can help correct the situation?

Consumption of bitters, such as gentian, hops, angelica, goldenseal, and horehound, 20 minutes before a meal mildly stimulates endogenous hydrochloric acid production.[7,8] Usually these herbs are given as tinctures in small amounts (3–10 drops) for stimulation of stomach acid. In some cultures, a bitter drink is served as an aperitif to whet the appetite and stimulate the flow of gastric acid. Bitter tonics taken 20–30 minutes before a meal also stimulate the flow of saliva and bile. They work tonically only when used for a protracted period, usually several months.

8. Should *H. pylori* be ruled out as a contributor to GERD?

In many persons, *H. pylori* is a culprit in the pathogenesis of GERD. If infection is symptomatic, either as GERD or ulceration, it should be treated appropriately. Many holistic interventions for GERD, such as adding digestive enzymes, betaine HCl, or pepsin, are inappropriate if *H. pylori* is present and has not yet been eradicated because such therapies may precipitate ulceration.

9. Are any herbal or natural treatments effective against *H. pylori*?

Mastic gum, a crude drug obtained from the stem and leaves of *Pistacia lentiscus*, has been used for centuries for treatment of heartburn and GERD-type symptoms. A significant body of research shows that it is an effective therapy for *H. pylori*.[9] Usually it is given as a capsule, twice daily for 2–4 weeks. It can be administered with bismuth subsalycilate.

10. What is a demulcent?

A demulcent is a soothing, mucilaginous substance used for quieting inflammation in mucous membranes. Often demulcents are high in immune-supportive polysaccharides, which contribute to the demulcent properties of the herb. Examples of demulcents frequently used in treatment of GERD include slippery elm,[10] marshmallow root,[11] deglycerizinated licorice, plantain (lanceolate) herb, and plantain banana. Of these, slippery elm is an endangered species, only now recovering from the blight of Dutch elm disease. It is ecologically more sound to use any of the other three.

11. Discuss the appropriate use of aloe vera gel in GERD.

Aloe vera is a succulent plant native to Mediterranean climates. The central leaf consists largely of a gel that is rich in immune-tonifying polysaccharides. Just below the surface of the leaf is a yellow latex, which is high in aloin. Aloin is a potent anthraquinone glycoside that exerts its laxative effects by irritating the bowel wall and initiating free water secretion from the colon into the feces. Thus aloe, which is not aloin-free, is a cathartic laxative. Full-spectrum aloe is not appropriate in GERD. In contrast, aloe gel free of aloin is a soothing demulcent. It is usually given as 1–2 table-spoonfuls 2–3 times daily to quiet gastric or bowel inflammation and restore the immune system.

12. Is overgrowth of candidal organisms ever implicated in GERD?

There is much disagreement in the medical community about the significance of overgrowth of yeasts, including *Candida* species, in the pathogenesis of many GI disorders. In fact, stool testing often reveals an overgrowth of candidal organisms in persons suffering from GERD, gastritis, and inflammatory bowel disease. Treatment of the overgrowth often improves symptoms, although it is not known whether the excessive yeast is a cause or a result of the gastrointestinal inflammation.

13. Discuss the role of food allergies in GERD.

Many persons who present with symptoms or diagnosis of GERD have undetected food allergies. Although many methods can be used to determine food sensitivities, the best of these is probably an allergy rotation diet. The person writes down all of the foods that are consumed each day as well as all of the symptoms experienced on the same day. No food may be consumed more frequently than every 4 days, and every 7 days is an even better spacing, if possible. On the day of its consumption, a food may be eaten more than once. For example, if rice is the grain eaten on Thursday, rice cereal may be selected for breakfast, rice crackers for lunch, and basmati rice for dinner.

Patients and practitioners should know that symptoms of allergy or sensitivity are not always immediate; in fact, the initial symptoms of food sensitivity may not appear until 24 hours after a food is consumed. If a person has many allergies, a simplified diet at the onset of the allergy rotation diet is advised, with foods slowly added as they are shown to be tolerable. Allergy rotation diet can be used in conjunction with other methods of allergy testing, such as skin scratch testing or serum antibody testing. By eliminating offending foods from the diet as well as correcting intestinal permeability deficits, many people have recovered from chronic GERD.

14. Are herbs and nutrients safe to consume along with conventional drugs for GERD?

Conventional drugs for GERD include H_2 blockers (e.g., cimetidine [Tagamet], ranitidine [Zantac]) and proton pump inhibitors (e.g., omeprazole [Prilosec]). Currently no evidence suggests adverse cross-reactions or diminished efficacy of drugs with most herbs.[12] However, demulcents such as marshmallow root and slippery elm bark should be consumed at least 1 hour after medications (medications should be administered first), because they have been shown to "coat the stomach," potentially decreasing absorption of pharmaceuticals.[13]

15. Discuss the role of licorice in the treatment of GERD.

Licorice is one of the most widely studied herbs worldwide. A main constituent, glycyrrhizin, is 50 times sweeter than sugar. This fraction of licorice root has been proved effective in healing and preventing aspirin-induced gastric ulcers in animal models. Another constituent, glycyrrhizinic acid, is similar in molecular structure to adrenal cortical hormones. Because it may lead to water retention and increased blood pressure, this fraction is often removed. The resulting product is called deglycrrhizinated licorice (DGL). DGL can be given in capsules several times per day. It has been found to be comparable to cimetidine in the treatment of erosive esophagitis.[14] Its use is suggested if long term gastrointestinal (GI) ulcerogenic or irritant drugs are administered.[15] Other GI demulcents, such as marshmallow root, slippery elm bark, plantain bananas, and okra, are soothing to inflamed mucous and are quite safe for frequent use.

16. Which other herbs are useful in treating GERD?

Chamomile is probably the most commonly used herb in the treatment of GERD after licorice. Chamomile tea is frequently taken after meals as a digestive aid in European and North African cultures. It is soothing to infant colic, digestive upsets, gas, bloat, distention, and poor digestion. The ester bisbalol in chamomile has been found to help heal inflammatory processes in the GI tract, such as ulcers and gastritis, and its essential oil azulene is antiseptic, anti-inflammatory, and anodyne.[16] Chamomile helps with symptoms associated with overeating and soothes heartburn, particularly when mixed with ginger.

Ginger is a common culinary herb of the family Zingiberaceae. It has been traditionally used for treatment of nausea, flatulence, peptic ulcer, and other digestive disorders. It has anti-inflammatory, antifungal, and antiparasitic properties.[17] Smaller doses of ginger, as in fresh ginger tea or capsules containing 250–500 mg, can be used in treatment of GERD. Because some people find that the spiciness aggravates symptoms, a test dose should be tried before using ginger as an ongoing therapy.

Turmeric is another herb in the ginger (Zingiberaceae) family with marked anti-inflammatory activity. It is as potent as cortisone in short-term studies and is also renowned as an antimicrobial. In both ayurveda and Chinese medicine, this herb has long been used for numerous digestive disorders. In one placebo-controlled trial, 73% of patients with dyspepsia reported improvement with turmeric, although studies evaluating its use for ulcer healing have failed to show benefit.[17]

17. How are fatty acids used in the holistic treatment of GERD?

Essential fatty acids, especially the omega-3 group, are important modulators of inflammation. A diet rich in omega-3 fatty acids or supplementation of these nutrients helps decrease inflammation systematically, including the GI tract. For more information see Chapter 19.

18. Discuss the common dietary contributions to GERD.

Often people with GERD have difficulty in digesting grains, although proteins (especially meats), fats, and chocolate also may trigger symptoms. If GERD occurs particularly in the night or evenings, patients should try eliminating all grains from the evening meal. Gluten, in particular, seem to contribute frequently to GERD, whether in the refined or whole form. A diet eliminating gluten-containing grains (wheat, rye, barley, spelt, kamut, oats) for 6 weeks should determine whether they are a problem for a particular patient. In addition, acidic foods, especially tomatoes, and spicy foods are often implicated in GERD. Alcohol, of course, is another well known trigger of GERD symptoms. Patients should keep a diet and symptom diary to evaluate whether specific foods or food categories are triggers. Persons who suffer with GERD symptoms should drink plenty of water.

19. Is peppermint a good choice for easing digestion in persons with GERD?

No. Although peppermint is an excellent herb for correcting flatulence associated with poor digestion, it lowers tone in the pyloric sphincter and can actually exacerbate GERD.[18] Regular use of peppermint in persons with GERD can hasten erosion of the esophagus.

20. Can digestive enzymes be used in the presence of GERD?

Digestive enzymes containing high amounts of proteases, including pancreatic glandulars, are not advised in the presence of GERD. They have been known to cause ulceration of tissue that is already inflamed secondary to reflux. However, lipases and amylase are usually considered safe, and low protease mixed enzymes can be used with caution. Amylases may be quite helpful if starches trigger GERD, and lipases are similarly beneficial for people in whom fatty foods trigger reflux.[19]

21. Which homeopathic remedies[20] are commonly used in GERD?

Antimonium crudum: especially after overeating, generally with much eructation aggravated by acid substances such as wine or tomatoes.

Carbo vegetalis: used for bloating, gas, gas pains, and indigestion. Gas is the most prominent feature of disorders treated with carbo vegetalis.

Chamomilla: used for bitter taste in mouth, colic, crankiness, diarrhea, restlessness, irritability, and symptoms that worsen with heat or anger.

Ignatia: used for belching of sour material, problems that begin after upsetting news or trauma, and borborygmus.

Lycopodium: used for gas and belching and when stomach feels distended, even after a few bites; also helps heartburn that rises into the esophagus but not into the mouth.

Nux vomica: used for burping, sour or bitter taste, constipation, distention pain (up to several hours after eating), vomiting, and headache; especially helpful for symptoms due to rich food; stomach aches due to overindulgence in food and drink; symptoms that worsen after meals; symptoms due to, spicy food; and symptoms associated with cold that improve with warmth and rest.

Pulsatilla: used for dry mouth, flatulence, and lack of appetite; also helpful for abdominal distention, bitter taste in mouth, and heartburn that worsens with warmth and fatty foods but improves with coolness, fresh air, cold food, and drinks.

22. Does stress contribute to GERD?

Stress can contribute to GERD by many mechanisms. Stress can trigger impulses of the vagus nerve to the stomach, causing inappropriate secretion of hydrochloric acid. Stress also affects the immune system, endocrine system, and hepatobiliary system. It may weaken resistance to infections such as *H. pylori* or affect levels of digestive enzymes.

23. What other holistic modalities may be helpful in treatment of GERD?

- Many people report that adding vitamin E, which is a mild anti-inflammatory,[21] is soothing to symptoms. The general dosage range is 200–400 IU/day.
- Some practitioners find that oral use of probiotics (beneficial bacteria that populate the healthy colon) alleviates GERD symptoms.
- Mind-body techniques have shown benefit in management of many chronic conditions and may be excellent for alleviating symptoms of GERD.
- Manual lymph drainage can help to decongest lymphatics around the upper GI tract and stomach, improving elimination of wastes and immune function.
- Osteopathic manipulation can be helpful for hiatal hernia and structural problems in the GI tract.[22,23] Cranial osteopathy can quiet excessive vagus stimulation of stomach acid production.

REFERENCES

1. Tierney LM, McPhee S, Papadakis M (eds): 2002 Current Medical Diagnosis and Treatment. New York, Lange Medical Books/McGraw-Hill, 2002.
2. Vellas B, Balas D, Albarede JL: Effects of the aging process in digestive functions. Compr Ther 17(80): 46–52, 1991.
3. Lee L, Turner L, Goldberg B: The Enzyme Cure. Tiberon, CA, Future Medicine Publishing, 1998.
4. Nyrenn O, Adami HO, et al: Absence of therapeutic benefit from antacids or cimetidine in non-ulcer dyspepsia. N Engl J Med 314:339–343, 1986.
5. Stavney LS, Hamilton T, Sircus W: Evaluation of the pH sensitive telemetry capsule in the estimation of gastric secretory capacity. Am J Dig Disord ii:10, 1966.
6. Murray M: Encyclopedia of Nutritional Supplements. Rocklin, CA, Prima Publishing, 1996.
7. Glatzel H: Treatment of dyspeptic disorders with spice extracts. Hippokrates 40:916–919, 1969.
8. Deinenger R.: Amarum bitter principle remedies and their actio. Krankenpflege 29:99-100, 1975.
9. Huwez FU, Thirlwell D, Cockayne A: Mastic gum kills *Helicobacter pylori* [letter to the editor]. N Engl J Med 24:339:1946, 1998.
10. Boon H, Smith M: The Botanical Pharmacy. Quebec, Quarry Health Books, 1999.
11. Mills S, Bone K: Principles and Practice of Phytotherapy. Edinburgh, Churchill Livingstone, 2000.
12. Meletis CD, Jacobs T: Interactions between Drugs and Natural Medicines. Eclectic Medical Publications, 1999.
13. Brinker F: Herbal Contraindications and Drug Interactions. Eclectic Medical Publications, 1998.
14. Maxton DG, et al: Controlled trial of pyrogastrone and cimetidine in the treatment of reflux esophagitis. Gut 31: 351–354, 1990.

15. Rees WDW, Rhodes J. et al: Effect of deglycyrrhizinated liqourice on gastric mucosa damage by aspirin. Scand J Gastroenterol 14:569–607, 1979.

16. Bisset NG, Wichtl M: Herbal Drugs and Phytopharmaceuticals. Boca Raton, FL, CRC Press, 1994.

17. Schulick P: Ginger: Common Spice and Wonder Drug. Brattleboro, VT, Herbal Free Press, 1994.

18. Sigmund CJ, McNally EF. The action of a carminative on the lower esophageal sphincter. Gastroenterology 56:13–18, 1969

19. Lee L, Turner L, Goldberg B: The Enzyme Cure. Tiberon, CA, Future Medicine Publishing, Tiberon, 1998.

20. Panos M, Heimlich J: Homeopathic Medicine at Home. New York, Houghton Mifflin, 1980.

21. Zand J, Spreen A, LaValle JB: Smart Medicine for Healthier Living. Garden Park City, Avery, 1999.

22. Barral JP: Visceral Manipulation. Seattle, Eastland Press, 1988.

23. Barral JP: Visceral Manipulation II. Seattle, Eastland Press, 1989.

35. HEPATITIS

Marcey Shapiro, M.D.

1. What are the known types and known causes of hepatitis?

The known types of hepatitis are viral, drug-induced, and toxin-induced.

The **hepatitis A virus (HAV)** is highly contagious. Hepatitis A generally is caused by consuming food or water tainted with infected fecal matter; shellfish are a common vector.

The **hepatitis B virus (HBV)** is usually bloodborne; transmission is similar to that for hepatitis C (see below).

The **hepatitis C virus (HCV)**, an RNA virus, is the most common cause of cirrhosis, liver disease, and hepatocellular cancer in developed nations.[1] HCV is bloodborne and may be transmitted by blood transfusion, sexual contact (with exposure to blood through broken skin), intravenous drug use (with tainted needles), tattoos, perinatal exposure, and exposure to razor blades or toothbrushes of infected people (rare). The rate of perinatal transmission, which generally occurs at delivery, is 5%. The estimated rate of HCV transmission to noninfected partners in monogamous relationships is 1% per year.

Other viral causes include **hepatitis D, G,** and **E**; **Epstein Barr virus**; and **cytomegalovirus**. Many **drugs** can induce hepatitis; common examples are cyclosporine and fluconazole. **Chemicals** and **toxins** also can induce hepatitis (e.g., incorrect application of pesticides and herbicides). Of course, the most prevalent toxin causing hepatitis is abuse of alcohol.

2. Describe the natural history of hepatitis.

HAV and HBV usually have an acute onset. Symptoms include nausea, vomiting, jaundice, and diarrhea; fatigue can range from mild to severe. HAV is usually self limited, although it can be fatal in infants, immunocompromised patients, elderly patients, and peoples with concurrent HCV infection. Illness can take up to 1 month to present after infection.

About 7–10% of people infected with HBV become chronic carriers; in the remainder, the infection resolves, although the course may be slower than for HAV. Symptoms can take 2–4 months to develop after infection.

Serum RNA tests turn positive within 3 weeks of exposure. By 3 months, the vast majority of persons who have contracted the disease develop liver injury, but symptoms present acutely in only around 35% of patients. Eighty-five percent of people who contract HCV develop chronic infection,[2] but two-thirds remain asymptomatic for long periods. More than 30% eventually present with cirrhosis,[1] and 15–20% develop end-stage liver disease. In the U.S., 30% of patients diagnosed with hepatocellular carcinoma test positive for HCV.

The course of chemical- and drug-induced hepatitis depends on the severity and duration of exposure as well as the patient's underlying health.

3. What forms of primary prevention are available for prevention of hepatitis?

Vaccines are available for prevention of both HBV and HAV. Safer sex, including use of condoms and dental dams throughout sexual contact, is critical for prevention of HBV and HCV. Blood contact should be avoided through clean needle exchange and not sharing toothbrushes or razors with infected persons. People with hepatitis C should avoid shellfish because of the possibility of concomitant HAV infection.

4. How prevalent is HCV?

Hepatitis C accounts for 20% of cases of acute hepatitis in the U.S. Approximately 1.8% of Americans, or 4 million persons, are estimated to be infected. Worldwide cases are estimated at around 100 million.

5. **Discuss the conventional treatments for hepatitis and their success rates.**

For most forms of hepatitis, supportive and palliative care, including dietary modifications, is often all that is offered. Before disease develops, exposed contacts are treated with gamma globulin. Alpha interferon is sometimes used in the treatment of HBV with moderate success.

HCV is often treated with interferon, which is generally poorly tolerated and has a high prevalence of serious side effects, including psychosis, autoimmune thyroiditis, systemic lupus erythematosus, dilated cardiomyopathy, and sudden death.[1] Interferon results in long-term improvement in only a small percentage of patients. Ribavirin can be used in conjunction with alpha interferon or alone. Side effects include deep exhaustion, psychosis, hepatic fibrosis, cough, nausea, and vomiting. Combination therapy has resulted in decreased viral load and sustained improvement in a greater percentage of patients. Monotherapy with ribavirin improves levels of alanine aminotransferase (ALT) during treatment, but the improvement is not sustained after treatment is discontinued.

6. **Why should an integrative approach be considered in the overall management of hepatitis?**

For most types of hepatitis, complementary/alternative medicine (CAM) treatments are the only ones that have been shown to speed recovery and reduce inflammation in the liver. Even in patients with HBV and HCV to whom allopathic treatments, although less than perfect (see above), are offered, an integrative approach helps to minimize drug toxicity, support liver function and regeneration, and maintain total well-being.

7. **What is a cholagogue?**

Cholagogues are herbs that increase the flow of bile. Because bile is a natural laxative, cholagogue herbs loosen the stool. They are not habit-forming. Taken over time, cholagogues are believed to assist digestion and liver function and can prevent or dissolve gallstones. They are frequently advised for hepatic and gastrointestinal problems and include many fairly common tonic herbs, such as dandelion root, burdock root, licorice, and yellow dock. These herbs often are used during and after hepatitis.

8. **What is a choleretic?**

Choleretics are herbs that increase the amount of bile. These are used to strengthen the liver when it is not functioning properly because of insufficient bile production. Many choleretics are also cholagogues. Examples of choleretics include milk thistle (silymarin), dandelion (taraxacum), and artichoke. Some are used during hepatitis, and most are used during convalescence from hepatitis.

9. **Is acupuncture helpful in treating hepatitis?**

Yes. Both acupuncture and Chinese herbal medicine are helpful in chronic hepatitis, including hepatitis C. Acupuncture is most frequently used specifically to decrease inflammation in the liver.[3]

10. **Explain what is meant by phase 1 and phase 2 detoxification pathways.**

Through the detoxificateion pathways, the body converts lipid-soluble toxins into water-soluble compounds for excretion. **Phase 1** refers to the chemical reactions in the first phase of detoxification for most drugs and chemicals. The p450 cytochrome system uses oxygen to activate the compound for phase 2. This process results in intermediate detoxification products, which are not fully metabolized. Often the intermediates are more toxic to the liver than the original compound, and detoxification by phase 2 must be promptly completed or damage to the liver can ensue. **Phase 2** generally involves the addition of a water-soluble compound to the molecule via glucuronidation or sulfation.[4] Then the detoxified molecule can be more easily eliminated from the body through the stool. Phase 2 tends to be the rate-limiting step in most people, although both stages of detoxification can be impaired in liver disease.

11. **Why do people with chronic hepatitis often awake around 3 AM, unable to fall back asleep?**

According to the circadian cycle of the liver, bile production peaks in the morning, whereas activity for detoxification is highest in the evening. At approximately 3 AM, the liver switches its function to increased production of bile. If the liver is stressed, the person may be so sensitive that he or she awakes when the transition begins and is unable to fall back asleep. In the Chinese medicine model, 3 AM is the hour when the energy in the liver meridian starts to peak. The problem of early awakening, especially between 3 and 5 AM, is often successfully treated with acupuncture, often with a focus on entry/exit points of the liver and other meridians.

12. Why are persons with chronic hepatitis advised to consume organically grown foods rather than conventional foods, whenever possible?

Pesticides and herbicides used in growing conventional farm products often leave residues on the food. When the residues are ingested, typically they must be detoxified by the liver. Often they are complex molecules, requiring several stages of detoxification. If the residues are not detoxified, they can accumulate in tissues, potentially causing direct damage to cellular function. To break them down may exhaust hepatic detoxification pathways, including stores of glutathione, exposing vulnerable people to the possibility of further liver damage.

13. What is alpha lipoic acid? Why does it support the liver in hepatitis?

Alpha lipoic acid (ALA) is a hepatoprotective, antioxidant, detoxifying, and antiviral compound produced by a healthy liver. In patients with hepatitis it is hepatoregenerative, anti-inflammatory, and immunostimulating; it also stimulates production of glutathione and helps prevent the development of cancers by protecting intracellularly against DNA damage.[5] ALA production is impaired by hepatic dysfunction and the normal aging process. ALA is generally used in dosages of 100–300 mg 2 times/day for supportive treatment of hepatitis. It is considered safe in dosages up to 1800 mg/day. Because it may improve glucose control, blood sugar levels in diabetics should be monitored and medications adjusted appropriately.

14. What is NAC?

NAC is an acronym for the nutrient compound n-acetyl-cysteine. It has hepatoprotective,[6] antioxidant, and antiviral properties, including in vitro evidence of activity against HIV.[7] Along with selenium, it is a key constituent in the body's production of glutathione, a pivotal compound in phase 2 detoxification pathways. Some evidence indicates that endogenously produced glutathione is more effective for hepatoprotection than the orally administered form. Because it supports the rapid production of glutathione, the U.S. poison control center recommends NAC as the treatment of choice for overdose of acetaminophen.[8]

Over time, NAC may deplete both copper and zinc as well as other minerals, thus, for long-term use mineral supplementation is advised. NAC should be used with caution in patients with diabetes or gastritis and avoided in patients with peptic ulcer disease. Typical doses for long-term use in patients with hepatitis are 100–300 mg 2–3 times/day; higher doses are used acutely. Supplemental vitamin C supports the benefits of NAC.

15. How is the mineral selenium important to liver function?

Selenium is an important antioxidant and a key constituent of glutathione function, along with vitamin E and NAC. Selenium becomes depleted in HCV infection as well as in a number of other viral infections, including HIV and human herpes virus 6. The decline in selenium levels has been correlated with increased morbidity in these illnesses as well as in cirrhosis of the liver and hepatocellular carcinoma related to HCV.[9] The generally accepted therapeutic dose for supplementation is 200 µg/day. Excessive selenium can be toxic to the heart and liver, and overdose may present with nausea and vomiting.[10] Food sources include brazil nuts, butter, and whole wheat.

16. Which common over-the-counter (OTC) medication should people with hepatitis avoid or use with caution?

Large numbers of drugs can be dangerous or must be used in reduced dosages or with caution in people with liver compromise due to hepatitis. Patients should be aware that even common OTC drugs such as acetaminophen can be dangerous if the liver is not functioning properly, especially if used regularly or in the presence of other drugs or substances that affect hepatic function. This principle is especially true in patients with any problem or delay in phase 2 detoxification. Acetaminophen is metabolized by phase 1 detoxification into a biologically active intermediate that can damage the liver, causing inflammation and necrosis.

17. What foods and herbs should be used with caution in hepatitis?

Grapefruit contains the flavonoid narigenin, which slows metabolism in the p450 system. Although it is not contraindicated in hepatitis, patients should be made aware of potential interactions between grapefruit (including grapefruit juice) and prescribed medications. In patients with immune compromise (e.g., chronic active hepatitis B, chronic HCV, or acute hepatitis) raw fish (sushi), raw or partially cooked shellfish (e.g., oysters, clams), and raw meats should be completely avoided because of the risk of bacterial and viral contamination.

The herbs comfrey and coltsfoot also should be avoided because they contain minute amounts of known hepatotoxins. Chaparral has been documented to cause liver damage in high doses.

18. Can use of hormone-free meats benefit the liver?

Yes. The liver, of course, must metabolize any ingested hormones, just as it metabolizes prescription drugs. The U.S. Department of Agriculture places no restrictions on the timing of hormone administration in livestock relative to their slaughter. Theoretically, an animal may be injected with a high dose of steroid or a long-acting hormone on the day before it is slaughtered; thus, very high levels of hormone remain in its tissues. There is no way for consumers to know what levels or types of hormones are present in meats. Ingestion of meats that contain hormones may tax the liver's detoxification mechanisms in people with compromised liver function. If possible, it is prudent to avoid hormone-containing meat until more is known.

19. How can osteopathic manipulation help in the management of hepatitis?

Osteopathic medicine, especially visceral work, can help relieve inflammation, decongest the liver and surrounding tissues, and support overall function of the body during acute and chronic hepatitis.[11]

20. Compare the effects of coffee and green tea on the liver.

Both contain caffeine, which, despite its bad reputation because of overuse as a stimulant, actually is a phytochemical with potent antitumor activity. Green tea is a potent antioxidant and antiviral with activity against influenza, HIV, and several other pathogens. In both human and animal studies, inhibition of tumors of liver, lung, pancreas, breast, prostate, colon and others has been shown. The chemical constituents of green tea thought responsible for these actions are the catechins. In moderation, either coffee or green tea is safe in persons with hepatitis, but because of the added antioxidant and antiviral activity, green tea is of greater potential benefit as a caffeinated beverage.

21. What are bitters? Why are they relevant in hepatitis?

Bitters consist of a diverse number of herbs from various genera, all of which contain prominent compounds with a bitter taste. They are of benefit in convalescence from acute hepatitis. Initially milder bitters, such as artichoke or horehound, are used in small doses. Bitter tonics taken 20–30 minutes before a meal stimulate the flow of saliva and bile. They are used when the "digestive fire" (agni in ayurveda) is weak, as after an acute episode of hepatitis. Doses are quite small, and weaker people should begin with less potent bitters. Bitters should be used cautiously in chronic hepatitis and during acute hepatitis. Bitters are generally not isolated from plants; instead, they are taken as aqueous or alcohol extractions of whole plants.

Bitterness is gauged by several tasters, who then rate the minimal concentration of the plant that is required in aqueous solution to provide a bitter taste. This concentration is reported as the bitterness value of the plant. Gentian root, for example, is very bitter with a ratio of 1:20,000. The bitterness value is usually listed as the denominator; thus, gentian root is given a bitterness value of 20,000. Wormwood is half as bitter at 10,000, and artichoke or holy thistle has a bitterness value of only 1500. Bitters are found frequently in Compositae and Gentianiaceae families.

22. Summarize general dietary guidelines for people with hepatitis.

Avoid fats that require production of bile. Examples include cheese, whole eggs, and fatty dairy products,as well as fried foods such as French fries and potato chips. Egg whites, nonfat dairy products, and lean meats can be used. For the reasons discussed above, organic, nonprocessed, and hormone-free foods are probably a good choice. Consume plenty of whole grains, beans, vegetables, and fresh fruits. Root vegetables, greens, and artichokes are especially beneficial. If the person is ill, all fruits and vegetables should be cooked for ease of assimilation. Because people with or recuperating from hepatitis usually have decreased appetites, frequent small or tiny meals are recommended.

It is important to drink plenty of water. Fruit and vegetable juices are fine if consumed in moderation, although caution should be used with grapefruit juice. Pasteurized juices are generally safer for people with active hepatitis.

Avoid all alcohol during acute or chronic hepatitis. Also avoid iron supplements and foods high in iron during acute illness. When the liver is ill, it is difficult for it to process iron.

23. What herbs and herbal extracts can be safely used in acute hepatitis?

Dandelion has a long tradition of use in various cultures. In Chinese and ayurvedic medicine it is used to clear pathologic heat,[12] as in hepatitis, from the liver and gallbladder. It is a cholagogue with choleretic properties and an antioxidant. Dandelion is useful in all forms of hepatitis, including drug-induced.

Licorice is used traditionally in China for treating liver diseases; it has been demonstrated clinically to be effective against hepatotoxins such as strychnine and carbon tetrachloride.[13] It has antiviral and anti-inflammatory properties and is frequently used in China and Europe for treatment of chronic hepatitis.[14]

Milk thistle (see silymarin below).

Phyllanthus (*Phyllanthus amarus, emblica,* or *niruri*) is a hepatoprotective ayurvedic herb with antiviral activity against hepatitis, especially HBV[15] and HAV.[16] Several double-blind, placebo-controlled human studies, including one in children, have demonstrated efficacy,[17] but results are not consistent and more study is needed. It may be that only one variety is efficacious.[18]

Picrorrhiza (*Picrorrhiza kurroa*) is a Himalayan herb widely used in ayurvedic medicine. The standardized extract picroliv, which has been most widely studied form, was found to be more strongly hepatoprotective than silymarin.[19] The herb shows antioxidant, choleretic, immune-supportive, antihelminthic, and anti-inflammatory activity in oral extracts. Clinical studies in hepatitis showed improvement in liver function and more rapid recovery during acute illness.[18]

Schizandra is a Chinese herb used for centuries in patients with liver complaints. It has been shown to decrease inflammation and promote healing. It is often used in the recuperation stage of hepatitis, although extracts have been used successfully in China to treat fulminant hepatitis.[18]

24. What is silymarin?

Silymarin complex is the medicinally active constituent of the herb milk thistle, found in concentrations of 1–4 % in the fruiting body (often erroneously called the seed). Silymarin does not extract well into alcohol, and is best taken as a concentrated capsule of 70–90% silymarin. It is a complex of flavonolignans, including siliban, which is the most active ingredient.[20] Silymarin complex is hepatoprotective in viral, toxin (e.g., mushroom-induced),[21] and chemical hepatitis through several mechanisms: it increases glutathione stores in liver,[22] stabilizes hepatocyte membranes, and serves as an antioxidant. Silymarin is also hepatoregenerative; it increases de novo hepatocyte synthesis of RNA, stimulating ribosomal protein synthesis in the liver. Silymarin also inhibits hepatic fibrosis. Some studies indicate benefits of silymarin even in cirrhosis.[23] Generally, for daily protection 100 mg is sufficient; in acute or chronic illness, 250–500 mg/day may be helpful for an extended period.

25. What other nutrients may be helpful for people with hepatitis?

B complex vitamins are important to the functioning of the p450 cytochrome system. People with hepatitis or other forms of liver disease are often deficient in B complex. In addition to supporting detoxification, B vitamins have hepatoprotective and anti-inflammatory functions.[4] They are also important in lipid metabolism. B complex is a safe vitamin, best taken as a balanced formulation. Because B complex is water-soluble, excess is excreted in the urine and not stored by the body.

Vitamin E is another important antioxidant, protecting the liver against peroxidation and free radical damage. Vitamin E is also pivotal in lipid metabolism, and adequate amounts are necessary to maintain healthy cholesterol levels. Vitamin E supports the regeneration of glutathione and, of special importance for patients with hepatitis, protects cells from cirrhosis. Vitamin E is best taken as a natural supplement from food sources. Mixed tocopherols are advised. The generally accepted dosage is 400–800 IU. Vitamin E is best absorbed with a meal.

Zinc is often depleted in people with hepatitis, and low zinc levels are associated with suboptimal immune function.[24] Zinc is important for the proper functioning of glutathione. Zinc becomes depleted by supplementing NAC and must be added back into the diet. Copper should be taken with zinc; a typical dose is 1 mg of copper and 15–25 mg of zinc.

26. Which herb is a good choice for liver pain due to hepatitis?

The South American herb boldo (*Peumus boldus*) is highly regarded for alleviation of liver pain in hepatitis.[25] It also has anti-inflammatory and choleretic properties and helps decrease jaundice. Like milk thistle, it is a tonic for the kidneys as well as the liver. It is taken as a tea, tincture, or capsule. Boldo should not be used in patients with biliary obstruction.

REFERENCES

1. Hoofnagle JH: Hepatitis C: The clinical spectrum of disease. Hepatology 26(Suppl. 1):15S–20S, 1997.
2. Tong MJ, et al: Clinical outcomes after transfusion-associated hepatitis C. N Engl J Med 332:1463–1466, 1995.
3. Maciocia G: The Practice of Chinese Medicine. Edinburgh, Churchill Livingstone, 1994.
4. Bland J, et al: Clinical Nutrition: A Functional Approach. Gig Harbor, WA, Institute for Functional Medicine, 1999.
5. Berkson B: The Alpha Lipoic Acid Breakthrough. Rocklin, CA, Prima Publishing, 1998.
6. Harrison P, et al: Improvement by N-acetylcysteine of hemodynamics and oxygen transport in fulminant hepatic failure N Engl J Med 324:1852–1856, 1991.
7. Flanagan RJ, Meredith,TJ: Use of n-acetyl cysteine in clinical toxicology Am J Med 91(3c):131S–139S, 1991.
8. Prescott LF: Treatment of paracetamol (acetaminophen) poisoning with n-acetyl cysteine. Lancet ii:432–434, 1977.
9. Yu MW, Horng IS, Hsu KH, et al: Plasma selenium levels and risk of hepatocellular carcinoma among men with chronic hepatitis virus. Am J Epidemiol 150:367–374, 1999.
10. Garrison RH, Somer, E: The Nutrition Desk Reference, 3rd ed. Keats Publishing, 1995.
11. Barral JP: Visceral Manipulation. Seattle, Eastland Press, 1988.
12. Bensky D, Gamble A: Chinese Herbal Medicine: Materia Medica. Seattle, Eastland Press, 1986..
13. Fujita H, et al: Studies on the regulation by drugs against experimental hepatitis: The therapeutic effects of glycyrrhizinic acid, DL methionine and their complex against chronic liver injury in rats. Oyo Yakuri 16:637–669, 1978.
14. Eisenberg J: Treatment of chronic hepatitis B. Part 2: Effects of glycyrrhizinic acid on the course of illness. Fortsch Med 110(21):395–398, 1992.
15. Brook MG, et al: Effect of *Phyllanthus amarus* on chronic carriers of hepatitis B virus. Lancet 8616:1017–1018, 1988
16. Ott M, et al: *Phyllanthus amarus* suppresses hepatitis B virus by interrupting interactions between HBV enhancer 1 and cellular transcription factors. Eur J Clin Invest 27:908–915, 1997.
17. Antarkar DS, et al: A double blind clinical trial of aroga-wardhani, an Ayurvedic drug, in acute viral hepatitis. Ind J Med Res 72:589–593,1990.
18. Bone K: Clinical Application of Ayurvedic and Chinese Herbs. Queensland, Australia, Phytotherapy Press, 1996.
19. Ansari RA et al: Antihepatotoxic properties of picroliv: An active fraction from the rhizomes of *Picrorrhiza kurroa*. J Ethnopharmacol 34:61–68, 1991.
20. Flora K, Hahn M , Rosen H , Benner K: Milk thistle (*Silybum marianum*) for the therapy of liver disease. Am J Gastroenterol 93:139–143, 1998.
21. Desplaces A, et al: The effects of silymarin on experimental phalloidin poisoning. Arzneimittel-Forsch 25:89–96, 1975.
22. Valenzuela A, et al: Selectivity of silymarin on the increase of glutathione content in different tissues of the rat. Planta Med 55:420–422, 1990.
23. Ferenci P, Dragosics B, et al: Randomized controlled trial of silymarin treatment in patients with cirrhosis of the liver. J Hepatol 9:105–113, 1989.
24. Garrison RH, Somer E: The Nutrition Desk Reference, 3rd ed. New Canaan, Keats Publishing, 1995.
25. Buhner SH: Herbs for Hepatitis C and the Liver. Pownal, VT, Storey Books, 2000.

36. IRRITABLE BOWEL SYNDROME

Robert A. Weissberg, M.D.

1. How does allopathic medicine define irritable bowel syndrome (IBS)?

IBS is a functional bowel disorder, characterized by abdominal pain (often relieved by defecation), bloating, mucus in the stools, and irregular bowel habits, including diarrhea, constipation, or alternation of both. It is a common problem, found in 10–20% of the adult population, and has a female predominance of 60:40 or greater. IBS is distinct from inflammatory bowel and infectious bowel disorders. One of the most recent theories about the cause of IBS involves the hyperresponsiveness of serotonin-containing cells throughout the gut wall.[1]

2. How is IBS diagnosed?

There are a number of different systems for diagnosing IBS. First of all, it is important to rule out other diseases with similar symptoms, including cancer, diverticulitis, enteritis, inflammatory bowel disease, carcinoid syndrome, and lactose intolerance. Once other diagnoses have been ruled out, the Rome criteria[2] appear to be the most widely used and accepted: a functional disorder with at least 3 months of continuous or recurring symptoms of abdominal pain or discomfort that is relieved by defecation, change in frequency and/or consistency of the stool, and two or more of the following symptoms present on at least 25% of occasions or days:
- Altered stool frequency with onset of pain
- Altered stool form with onset of pain (lumpy/hard or loose/watery)
- Altered stool passage (strain, urgency, feeling of incomplete evacuation)
- Passage of mucus
- Pain relief with bowel action

3. Describe the allopathic approach to treating IBS.

Standard treatments include fiber supplements, antidiarrheals (e.g., loperamide), anticholinergic drugs, tricyclic antidepressants, and serotonin antagonists. In the past, phenobarbital and chlordiazepoxide were used. Unfortunately, recommendations for stress reduction, diet regulation, and lifestyle modification are generally viewed as secondary measures. To quote an IBS therapist: "With conventional medical treatment being of little proven benefit [for IBS], ... there is a need to look beyond treating the symptoms to addressing the cause. In the holistic view of illness, physical disease is only one of several manifestations of basic imbalance of the organism."[3] Allopathic treatments for IBS remain woefully inadequate, but fortunately IBS can be optimally treated with an integrative approach.

4. How do complementary and alternative practitioners view IBS?

The answer depends on which ones you ask. Complementary and alternative medicine (CAM) is made up of a multitude of disciplines and philosophies, each with its unique view of IBS. It is helpful to select a few of the most commonly encountered CAM disciplines for further discussion: mind-body or behavioral medicine, functional medicine, naturopathy and herbal medicine, traditional Chinese medicine, ayurvedic medicine, and homeopathy.

Each of these disciplines views IBS as more than just a problem with the gut. It is seen as indicating some form of imbalance in the patient's overall system, with primary symptoms expressed by the gut. The nature of the problem and its root causes depend on the theoretical system employed.

5. What is the mind-body view of IBS?

The whole-person approach is basic to the mind-body view of IBS, given the personal importance placed on gastrointestinal (GI) functions from alimentation to elimination. A full history is critical to a mind-body evaluation, taking into account key life events at the onset of symptoms or exacerbations, emotional responses to the symptoms, the role of IBS in the patient's total life experience, and personal gut metaphors. For example, if a person says "I can't swallow that," "it takes guts," or "I can't stomach my job," the metaphor may reveal a mind-body clue worthy of more exploration. A history of abuse and trauma and a dysfunctional family structure have been found to be associated with a incidence of IBS.[4] Effective treatment may depend on recognizing this and other associations for individual patients.

Stress is definitely known to trigger and worsen the symptoms of IBS. Patients with IBS are more likely than normal subjects to experience frequent and severe GI symptoms during times of stress. Stress produces measurable changes in colon motility and electrical activity.[5] Parasympathetic activity—via the vagus nerve, sacral parasympathics, and the intrinsic set of nerves within the GI tract known as the intramural plexus—enhances peristalsis as well as secretion of digestive enzymes. Overwhelming sympathetic "flight-or-fight" responses suppress this parasympathic flow and upset the normal digestive activity of the GI tract. In addition to the vagal (cholinergic) response, stress, also involves a serotonergic mechanism.

6. What is the brain-gut connection? How does it relate to IBS?

According to Dr. William B. Salt II, "The Mind-Body/Brain-Gut Connection is the key to understanding [IBS] and to the healing process.... There is a powerful 'connection' between the mind and the body/gut. Transmission is bi-directional: it is a two-way street. The gut affects the brain, and the brain affects the gut."[1] Many people with IBS, in fact, have enhanced sensitivity to sensations from the gut and other viscera. People with IBS also have a greater sensitivity and response to triggers, such as hormones, stress, seasonal changes, and psychological patterns. This heightened sensitivity can be turned around to serve a positive role as patients learn to recognize their GI symptoms as an immediate feedback tool and to apply mind-body techniques effectively after appropriate training.

7. Describe the mind-body treatments for IBS.

IBS was at one time considered a strictly psychosomatic disorder. Thus, it has a fairly long history of mind-body and psychological treatments, including some high-quality research. Potentially useful mind-body techniques include the following:

- Relaxation training
- Biofeedback
- Meditation (relaxation response, mindfulness)
- Stress management
- Hypnosis
- Guided imagery
- Psychotherapy

The following discussion focuses on the three mind-body treatments that have the most evidence for efficacy: relaxation training, stress management, and hypnosis

8. What is relaxation training? How well does it work for IBS?

Relaxation training includes a variety of methods with the common goal of inducing nonpharmacologically a state of reduced skeletal muscle tone, often with deeper respirations, and a deeply-relaxed state of consciousness. In pure relaxation training, the subject is asked to pay direct attention to his or her body tension and/or breathing. Progressive muscle relaxation, a technique originally developed by German physicians in the 1930s, involves first intentionally tensing, then relaxing all areas of the body in sequence. A number of controlled trials in a modest number of subjects with IBS indicate significant improvement in one-third to two-thirds of patients compared with conventional therapy.[6,7] In one or two small published studies, biofeedback combined with other relaxation techniques has been shown to improve IBS symptoms in up to two-thirds of subjects.[8]

9. Discuss the role of stress management.

Stress management is a multicomponent process by which a participant is taught a number of skills and tools and counseled how to handle effectively a number of life stresses. Components may include meditation, breathing exercises, assertiveness training, journaling, time management, and even exercise. In 1991, a small clinical trial comparing a six-session stress management program with conventional therapy for IBS showed a highly significant response rate of two-thirds for the stress management group compared with minimal responses in the conventional treatment group.[9] A more recent internal study done by an HMO in the Northeast with a comprehensive stress management program also showed improvement in IBS, among other illnesses, with a stress component compared with wait-listed subjects.[10] These methods have promise, but more studies should be done.

10. How is hypnosis used for treating IBS?

Hypnosis is described as a state of extremely focused awareness and attention. It may be self-induced or induced through an interpersonal interaction or taped instructions. During hypnosis, the subject is more open than usual to considering suggestions or affirmations. A few strategies that may be useful for IBS include reframing the unpleasant gut perceptions as more neutral or even positive and helpful; working with gut-based metaphors; suggesting reduced perception of gut stimuli; modifying the subject's experience of stress; and building a mini-vacation into which the patient may retreat when confronted with usual stresses.

Quite a number of studies, both uncontrolled and controlled, have shown definite improvements in a variety of IBS symptoms with hypnosis. In several controlled studies in England, Holland, Sweden, and the U.S. over the past 20 years, hypnotherapy led to significant improvements in overall quality of life and in the most troublesome symptoms of severe IBS.[11-13] One study indicated that a therapeutic audiotape, although useful, was not as effective as real-time hypnosis. Changes in colonic sensitivity and activity have been demonstrated with hypnosis. Despite these encouraging results, the lack of controls and small numbers in many of the studies must temper some of the enthusiasm. It is probably the case that hypnotherapy, if adapted to individual patient characteristics, can be a useful complementary therapy in many people with IBS.

11. Define functional medicine and explain its basic concepts.

According to the Institute for Functional Medicine, "Functional Medicine is a science-based healthcare approach that assesses and treats underlying causes of illness through individually tailored therapies to restore health and improve function." Functional medicine grew out of theoretical and applied nutritional biochemistry, holistic medicine, naturopathy, and the disciplines of immunology and cell biology. It uses standard and advanced assessment techniques and early intervention to improve and support the total functional state of the person rather than treating the diagnosis or pathology.

Key concepts and areas of focus in functional medicine include biochemical and phenotypic individuality, metabolic balance, ecologic approaches to the internal and external environment, homeodynamics (vs. homeostasis), and wellness orientation. Each person is considered to have a unique biochemical make-up, with more variation and needs for dietary environmental factors than current biomedicine assumes The definition of health includes a significant level of positive vitality, not simply the absence of disease. Homeodynamics extends the concept of homeostasis and assumes that the only steady state is constant change and adaptation, aiming at maximal survival and success. The individual patient, not the disease, is the focus of treatment,[14] which generally involves alteration of diet and activity as well as use of pharmaceutical doses of vitamins, minerals, metabolic factors, herbal pharmaceuticals, and functional foods. In some cases drugs also are used.

12. How are patients with IBS symptoms evaluated in functional medicine?

In functional medicine, the unique patterns of dysfunction for each patient are characterized by an understanding of IBS symptoms in terms of antecedents, triggers, and mediators and an understanding of the six areas of functional deficit described by the Institute for Functional Medicine (nutritional imbalance, immune and inflammatory imbalance, impaired detoxification, intestinal dysfunction, oxidative stress, and endocrine imbalance).

A thorough diet review is important, with particular attention to intake of fiber, common "problem" foods, habitual eating of certain foods, and levels of saturated fat, omega-6, and trans fatty acids. Clues are sought for non-IgE food sensitivity. Sometimes a "food-mood diary" is used for the diet review to help associate symptoms with particular foods. An elimination-challenge diet, in which several prevalent foods are eliminated for 1–3 weeks and then reintroduced one at a time, can be quite helpful.[17]

If you want to read more about this approach, Galland has written extensively about functional medicine, specifically in relation to GI disorders. He describes what are called the four vicious cycles of leaky gut: allergy, malnutrition, bacterial dysbiosis, and hepatic stress.[15] This field can be quite complex.

13. What special studies or tests are used for IBS in functional medicine?

Serum IgG food antibody panels are available to obtain further clues to possibly antigenic foods, although how closely these results correlate with symptoms is highly controversial.[16] Another important study is the comprehensive digestive stool analysis, including an assessment of flora in the stool. This test assesses fat digestion and absorption; level of pancreatic enzymes (chymotrypsin); short chain fatty acids and stool pH; measurements of the health of GI flora and levels of beneficial and potentially pathogenic flora, including protozoa; and the usual tests for occult blood, white blood cells, and standard pathogens. A gut permeability study, using lactulose and mannitol, and an assessment of hepatic detoxification and free radical levels, using acetaminophen, caffeine, and aspirin as challenge substances, may further characterize GI function and shed light on the etiology in individual patients.[15] Each of these studies leads to specific therapies to improve function and promote healing.

14. How valid are these tests?

All of the tests are based on known aspects of gut physiology and pathology. A variety of studies have shown associations between abnormalities in digestion, abnormal mucosal permeability, gut flora, food-related antibodies, detoxification, and measures of gut inflammation and the typical symptoms and problems of IBS.[17] There is a good deal of empirically based clinical experience over the past 20 years among practitioners of functional medicine in the use of these studies to guide successful therapy. There are, unfortunately, no large controlled studies comparing these approaches with conventional ones.

15. How does functional medicine treat IBS?

As with most systems, the treatment depends on the results of the evaluation. In general, a functional diagnosis of IBS assumes that four major dysfunctional mechanisms are active: impaired detoxification, oxidative stress, immune/inflammatory imbalances, and intestinal dysfunction. Each patient is prescribed a unique selection from the treatment choices in the following questions. Functional medicine offers a comprehensive view and often successful treatment plan for IBS.

16. How are detoxification problems treated with functional medicine?

Detoxification occurs as a normal physiologic function both in the liver and bowel wall. If detoxification is impaired, the main intervention is to decrease intake of potential food antigens (see below) and toxins and to increase intake of certain foods (e.g., cruciferous vegetables, legumes) that promote hepatic detoxification. Supplements or specialized medical food products to promote the major conjugation pathways and antioxidants to support cytochrome P-450 function are also available. Oxidative stress due to abnormally high levels of circulating free radicals may result from impaired detoxification in the liver and the bowel wall. Typical support in this area often includes large doses of vitamins C and E and carotenoids as well as supplementation of zinc, copper, selenium, N-acetyl cysteine, alpha lipoic acid. and proanthocyanidins. Many of these substances are known cofactors in detoxification and prostaglandin and cytokine synthesis or known free-radical scavengers. Anti-inflammatory herbs are sometimes given to reduce the further production of free radicals.[17]

17. How is food sensitivity in IBS treated?

In the case of suspected food allergy/sensitivity, the suspect food (for example, dairy or citrus foods) would be eliminated from the individual's diet for several weeks to months, then possibly rotated back in at no more than every 3-4 days, if tolerated. The patient notes whether or not IBS symptoms improve during the elimination phase, and/or flare up again with reintroducing the suspect food into the diet. Using elimination diets is a straightforward, individualized empiric approach which unfortunately is not well utilized by mainstream medicine. In addition to the elimination and rotation diets, use of sublingual and injected antigen dilutions to "neutralize" reactions have been promoted by pioneers in the field.

18. How does treatment of inflammation help patients with IBS?

Supplementation with omega-3 fatty acids, which are metabolized to anti-inflammatory leukotrienes and prostaglandin-3 series, can be helpful. Sources of these fatty acids are flax oil, 4–6 gm/day, and fish oils, 6–10 gm/day, depending on the eicosopentaenoic acid content. The omega-6 fatty acid gamma linolenic acid (GLA), found in oils of evening primrose, borage, and currant seeds, can help by providing precursors to the anti-inflammatory prostaglandin-1 series, and blocking arachidonic acid pathways. Typical doses supply 600 mg/day of GLA. Bromelain, a proteolytic enzyme complex from pineapple, also has an anti-inflammatory effect, especially when taken on an empty stomach. Extracts of turmeric (curcumin), ginger, and boswellia also have been used as anti-inflammatory agents because of their specific blocking actions in the prostaglandin synthesis pathways, including blockade of COX-2 activity.[17]

19. What other herbal products can be useful for IBS?

If gut spasm is a large factor, use of enteric-coated peppermint oil is a well-established therapy, supported by research.[18] The menthol in peppermint oil has a local calcium channel-blocking effect, which relaxes smooth muscle spasm in the colon. The usual dose shown to be effective in studies is 0.2 ml of the enteric-coated oil 3 times/day between meals. Note that the formulation with the enteric-coating is especially important because it allows the oil to travel to the site of action in the distal colon undigested and because peppermint in the stomach worsens reflux symptoms. Chamomile, caraway, cramp bark (*Viburnum opulus*), anise, and fennel are also useful.

Valerian, skullcap, lavender, lemon balm, and hops are sedative and relaxing herbs that can help stress-related irritable bowel symptoms. The bitter herbs, such as dandelion root, gentian, and milk thistle, are believed to stimulate digestion and empirically often improve IBS symptoms triggered by eating in general. Licorice root helps to stimulate and thicken the mucous layer in the gut and is useful for upper GI symptoms; it also enhances "digestive qi" in traditional Chinese medicine (see below). Astringent herbs, such as tormentil and agrimony, are useful in patients with diarrhea.

20. What is the 4-R program for IBS?

1. **Removal** or suppression of pathogenic or overgrown gut flora, including *Candida albicans*, certain bacteria, and protozoa. Agents such as nystatin, fluconazole, caprylic acid, enteric-coated garlic, uva-ursi, pau d'arco, oregano and thyme oils, goldenseal, and echinacea may be useful in suppression of pathogenic flora.

2. **Replacement** of deficient pancreatic and gastric digestive factors. If the stool analysis suggests inadequate digestion, digestive enzyme supplements, consisting of amylases, proteases, and lipases derived from pancreatic extract or vegetable sources, can help.

3. **Reinoculate** means adding to the gut potentially beneficial flora, such as various *Lactobacillus* species, bifidobacteria, and, in some cases, the yeasts *Saccharomyces cervesiae* and *boulardii* spp. These organisms compete with pathogenic flora, produce substances that support and nourish the gut epithelium, have anti-inflammatory effects, and also produce a favorable, slightly acidic pH in the colon. Prebiotic supplements such as soluble fiber, fructo-oligosaccharides, and N-acetyl D-glucosamine support their multiplication in the gut. Some evidence in the literature[20–22] and a good deal from clinical observation suggest that use of pro- and prebiotics can help IBS symptoms in many patients.

4. **Repair** refers to the addition of foods, herbs, or food derivatives, such as glutamine, butyrate, and fiber, that allow stressed or damaged gut epithelium to heal more quickly. Functional medicine practitioners believe that the gut epithelia are damaged by toxins found in food, inflammation (from allergic reactions), free radical cellular damage, radiation, and deficient colonocyte cellular nutrition. Zinc and pantothenic acid are particularly important for promotion of mucosal healing. Small bowel and colonic epithelia derive a large portion of their energy from glutamate and butyrate, respectively.[19]

21. How does traditional Chinese medicine (TCM) treat IBS?

In TCM, IBS is not viewed as an isolated diagnosis but as part of a pattern of dysfunction. Full TCM treatment of IBS may include dietary changes, herbs, acupuncture, therapeutic exercise, and massage, all tailored to the patient's specific diagnostic findings.[23] Because the GI organs are represented in four of the five Chinese elements (e.g., liver as wood yin, large intestine as metal yang), various forms of IBS present radically different diagnoses in TCM. Three of the more common ones are discussed below as examples.

TCM PATTERN	IBS SYMPTOMS	EXACERBATING FACTORS	TCM TREATMENT
Spleen qi deficiency	Fatigue Diarrhea Abdominal pain Gas and bloating	Overexertion	Acupuncture to nourish spleen qi
Spleen dampness	The above, plus: Feeling of heaviness Nausea Mucus in stool Sensation of incomplete stooling	Eating too much greasy food Overthinking Overworrying	Acupuncture to eliminate damp, nourish spleen Avoid dairy and sugar
Liver qi stagnation	Pellet-shaped stool Distending pain Nausea Belching or reflus	Stress	Acupuncture to restore liver qi Tai chi or qi gong exercises

22. Do any controlled clinical trials demonstrate that TCM works for IBS?

There are a number of Chinese studies, but most are not well controlled. A well-done, double- blind, controlled study[24] compared treatment with a preformulated herbal mixture, herbal treatment based on TCM diagnosis, and placebo. Major components in the fixed formula included ginger, licorice, arteme-sia, schizandra, poria, and angelica. An interesting result was that the group on the fixed formula initially had somewhat better results than the group on the customized formula, but 14 weeks after completion of the study, the customized group continued to improve, whereas the fixed-formula group tended to re-lapse. This study provides evidence supporting TCM treatment to reestablish balance and optimize GI function. Although small (35–42/group), this study provides a model for further research.

23. How does ayurveda view IBS?

In ayurveda, "ama," a pathologic substance produced by improper food and activity, is consid-ered the chief cause of disease. It is thought to block energy channels and to accumulate in weak organs and tissues. The ayurvedic analysis describes a pattern of blockage and imbalance in the con-text of IBS, with the dysfunction not limited to the gut, but involving the whole body. The dosha (body-mind type) of vata is connected with "wind" and is particularly associated in excess or imbal-ance with gut problems. The following quotation offers the flavor of this approach:

> Vata resides primarily in the colon, and when out of balance it creates erratic symptoms (especially gas and constipation). Like the wind, vatic conditions tend to have the qualities of dryness, coldness, and irregularity. These can manifest as coldness of the body, dryness of skin, eyes, and/or mouth, or dryness in the intestinal tract, which causes constipation (lack of lubrication leads to dry hard stool that doesn't pass readily). A vata imbalance also manifests as irregularity of symptoms, for example, variable digestive complaints, unpredictable menses, or fluctuating blood sugar.[25]

Ayurveda recognizes other forms of IBS as variants of "grahani," or disturbed function of the in-testine. The pitta type is associated with burning reflux, thirst, irritability, anger, and liquid foul smelling stools, whereas the kapha type is associated with nausea, phlegm, sluggishness and lethargy, constipation with mucous in stools, and belching with bad breath.

24. How does ayurveda treat IBS?

The treatment involves several levels, based on constitutional body-mind type and the ayurvedic diagnosis. The aims of treatment are to clear what are believed to be toxins and products of incom-plete digestion (ama), to restore functioning of blocked channels, and to rebalance the system ac-cording to the patient's constitutional type. A full ayurvedic treatment course for IBS may include panchakarma, dosha-specific dietary and herbal treatments, selective fasting, oil massage, strict reg-ulation of activity (perhaps specific yoga postures), and stress reduction measures.

25. What ayurvedic herbs are specifically used in IBS treatment?

Although the most effective ayurvedic remedies combine more than one herb, most manufacturers and distributors in the U.S. offer lines of single herbs. Below is a list of a few of the most popular.[26]

Amalaki (*Emblica officinalis*): Indian gooseberry contains more natural vitamin C than any other fruit.

Ardhrakam (*Zingiber officinale*): The antioxidant properties of ginger improve digestion, prevent nausea, and reportedly treat colds.

Arishta (*Azadirachta indica*): Neem is said to boost interferon production and improves the ability of lymphocytes to deal with immune system threats.

Haritaki (*Terminalia chebula*): Haritaki, one of three fruits found in the ayurvedic formula known as triphala, is said to relieve constipation, battle infections, and cleanse the colon. Haritaki may also destroy bacteria such as *Salmonella* species.

Yashtimadha (*Glycyrrhiza glabra*): Licorice can prevent and treat stomach ulcers and intestinal irritation.

Triphala powder, composed of 1 part haritaki, 2 parts bibhitaka, and 4 parts amalaki in ancient texts,and of equal parts of these components in more recent texts, has recently become popular in the West as a remedy for IBS, especially the constipated variety. No controlled clinical trials have been done, but case reports and the clinical experience of numerous ayurvedic practitioners over the centuries attest to its effectiveness. Triphala has a much broader application than the treatment of IBS-like symptoms. A recent review article[27] reports that triphala and its components have the following uses: general and digestive tonic, adaptogen and restorative, purgative, promotion of wound healing, and treatment of fever with cough and mucous, severe weakness or fainting due to illness, obesity (with guggul), chronic constipation, and gout (with guggul).

26. Describe the homeopathic approach to IBS.

In a homeopathic intake, a thorough history is taken, not only of IBS symptoms but also of constitutional factors that characterize the individual patient (e.g., quick temper, preference for warm weather, nervous constitution, craving for salt). These characteristics are used to select a remedy whose pattern most closely matches that of the patient.

Several homeopathic remedies may be used to treat the patient with IBS,[28] especially if matched with some of the following distinctive characteristics (partial list):

Argentum nitricum: Digestive upsets accompanied by nervousness and anxiety suggest the use of this remedy. Bloating, rumbling flatulence, nausea, and greenish diarrhea can be sudden and intense. The patient tends to be expressive, impulsive, and claustrophobic and may have blood sugar problems.

Asafoetida: A feeling of constriction all along the digestive tract (especially if muscular contractions in the intestines and esophagus seem to be moving in the wrong direction) strongly indicates this remedy.

Colocynthis: This remedy is indicated in the presence of cutting pains and cramping that make the person bend double or need to lie down and press on the abdomen.

Lycopodium: This remedy is often indicated for people with chronic digestive discomforts and bowel problems. Symptoms are typically worse between 4 and 8 PM. Despite so many digestive troubles, the person may have a ravenous appetite and may even awake in the middle of the night to eat. Problems with self-confidence, a worried facial expression, a craving for sweets, and a preference for warm drinks are other indications for lycopodium.

Nux vomica: Abdominal pains and bowel problems accompanied by tension, constricting sensations, chilliness, and irritability can indicate a need for nux vomica. Paients often crave strong spicy foods, alcohol, tobacco, coffee, and other stimulants—and usually feel worse after having them.

27. What overall recommendations for IBS can we draw from all of these approaches?

IBS is a highly prevalent and heterogeneous condition, for which there is no truly adequate treatment in conventional biomedicine. It is important, of course, to confirm the diagnosis of IBS, which must be and well differentiated from more serious conditions. CAM approaches often focus on what makes the patient unique and apply treatment accordingly. Each discipline has one or more significant contributions to offer in the treatment of IBS and often has something important to teach.

It makes sense to look at the patient's diet in detail, including history of food reactions, as well as lifestyle, stress pattern and history, and exposures to toxins, antibiotics, and other drugs. This information may suggest the elimination of specific suspect foods, testing for food sensitivity, abnormal gut flora, digestive deficiencies, and/or unbalanced detoxification. These results may suggest nutritional modifications and use of herbal and metabolic supplementation, especially agents such as *Lactobacillus* spp., glutamine, soluble fiber, peppermint, fennel, chamomile, and others, with proven efficacy.

Because stress is a common trigger for IBS, use of one or more mind-body therapies makes sense. Excellent, long-standing evidence supports the efficacy of relaxation training, biofeedback, meditation, stress management, and hypnosis. Psychotherapy may be extremely useful for selected patients, and approaches combining two or more therapies have support in the literature.

TCM, ayurveda, and homeopathy are three separate healing systems that have the advantage of taking a whole-person approach to the patient with IBS and may be the "best fit" for a particular patient. Even a practitioner rooted in the biomedical model and functional medicine can easily make use of a number of the concepts and treatments derived from these comprehensive systems.

REFERENCES

1. Salt WB II: Irritable Bowel Syndrome and The Mind-Body/Brain-Gut Connection. 1999.
2. Feldman M, et al: Sleisenger and Fordtran's Gastrointestinal and Liver Disease, 6th ed. 1998.
3. Mahoney M: Irritable Bowel Syndrome and Hypnotherapy. 2000. Available at http://www.healingwell. com/library/ibs/mahoney1.htm.
4. Drossman DA, et al: Sexual and physical abuse in women with functional or organic gastrointestinal disorders. Ann Intern Med 113:828–833, 1990.
5. Welgan P, et al: The effect of stress on colon motor and electrical activity in irritable bowel syndrome. Psychosom Med 47:139–149, 1985.
6. Creed F, Guthrie E: Psychological treatments of the irritable bowel syndrome: A review. Gut 11:1601–1609, 1989.
7. Blanchard EB: Relaxation training as a treatment for irritable bowel syndrome. Biofeedback Self Regul 18(3):125–132, 1993.
8. Schwarz SP, et al: Behaviorally treated irritable bowel syndrome patients: A 4 year follow-up. Behav Res Ther 28:331–335, 1990.
9. Shaw G, et al: Stress management for irritable bowel syndrome: A controlled trial. Digestion 50:36–42, 1991.
10. Ford P: Personal Communication, 1999.
11. Whorwell PJ: Use of hypnotherapy in gastrointestinal disease. Br J Hosp Med 45:27–29, 1991.
12. Francis CY, Houghton LA: Use of hypnotherapy in gastrointestinal disorders Eur J Gastroenterol Hepatol 8:525–529, 1996.
13. Vidakovic-Vukic M: Hypnotherapy in the treatment of irritable bowel syndrome: Methods and results in Amsterdam. Scand J Gastroenterol Suppl. 230:49–51, 1999.
14. http://www.healthcomm.com/fun_med/.
15. Galland L: Leaky Gut Syndromes: Breaking the Vicious Cycle. Available at http://www.healthy.net/asp/templates/Article.asp?PageType=Article&Id=425 Accessed 2000.
16. Rafel A, et al:Diagnostic value of IgG4 measurement in patients with food allergy. Ann Allergy 62:94–99, 1989.
17. Nichols T: Functional Medicine Adjunctive Nutritional Support for Irritable Bowel Syndrome. CITY, Institute for Functional Medicine, 1999.
18. Liu JH, Chen GH, Yeh HZ, et al: Enteric-coated peppermint-oil capsules in the treatment of irritable bowel syndrome: A prospective, randomized trial. J Gastroenterol 32:765–768, 1997.
19. Bland J: The 4R(tm) Gastrointestinal Support Program, (c) 2000. Available at http://www.healthcomm. com/functions/search/index.html.
20. King TS, Elia M, Hunter JO: Abnormal colonic fermentation in irritable bowel syndrome. Lancet 352:1187–1189, 1998.
21. Bernet MF, et al: *Lactobacillus acidophilu*s LA 1 binds to cultured human intestinal cell lines and inhibits cell attachment and cell invasion by enterovirulent bacteria. Gut 35:483–489, 1994.
22. Bouhnik Y, et al: Administration of transgalacto-oligosaccharides increases fecal bifidobacteria and modifies colonic fermentation metabolism in healthy humans. J Nutr 127:444–448, 1997.
23. Balfour T: Irritable Bowel Syndrome: A TCM Perspective. Available at http://www.balfourhealing.com/ treatment-ibs.html. Contact author at 881 Alma Real, Suite 316, Pacific Palisades, CA 90272, (310) 613-0387.
24. Bensoussan A, et al: Treatment of Rome Criteria diagnosed irritable bowel syndrome with Chinese herbal medicine. JAMA 280:1585–1589, 1998.
25. Demers C: Gut-Reaction: An Ayurvedic Look at Irritable Bowel Syndrome. (c)2000. Available at Himalayan Institute's YI Article Archive: http://www.himalayaninstitute.org/hiinstitute/archive.html.
26. Ayurvedic Medicine: Ancient Roots, Modern Branches. 1996.
27. Tillotson A, Khalsa KPS, Caldecott T: Triphala: Modern medicinal uses for a traditional ayurvedic formulation. Can J Herba 22(2):16–23, 42–44, 2001.
28. Homeopathic Remedies for Irritable Bowel Syndrome (IBS): http://www.healthwell.com/healthnotes/ Homeo/IBS_hm.cfm. Accessed 7/2100.

37. PEPTIC ULCER DISEASE

Susan Hadley, M.D.

1. List some of the factors that contribute to the development of peptic ulcer disease (PUD).

Cigarette smoking, alcohol, low-fiber diet, food allergy, stress, *Helicobacter pylori*, and medications such as aspirin and nonsteroidal anti-inflammatory drugs (NSAIDs).

2. What is the relationship between cigarette smoking and PUD? NSAIDs and PUD?

Cigarette smoking is thought to decrease bicarbonate secretion from the pancreas, increase bile salt reflux into the stomach, and hasten gastric emptying, all of which compromise the integrity of the gastric and duodenal mucosa. NSAIDs directly damage the lining of the stomach, compromising the integrity of the mucosa and allowing ulcer formation. In the United States as many as 7600 deaths and 76,000 hospitalizations each year are due to NSAID-induced gastric complications.[1]

3. Discuss the tests available for the diagnosis of *H. pylori*. What treatment is recommended once *H. pylori* is diagnosed?

H. pylori, a spiral gram-negative bacillus, is a known pathogen in PUD. *H. pylori* can be detected with a urease assay. A breath urease assay is noninvasive and also can be used in monitoring therapy. If biopsy via endoscopy is performed, a urease assay, histology, or culture is used for diagnosis; the urease biopsy assay is the most sensitive. Serologic studies can be indicated but unfortunately do not differentiate between acute and past infection. Stool antigen detection is used in some hospitals.

Treatment of *H. pylori* has been found to be most important in prevention of recurrent ulcers. No single agent is optimal in the treatment of *H. pylori*. Successful treatment includes one or more antibiotics (amoxicillin, clarithromycin, metronidazole, tetracycline) with a proton pump inhibitor (omeprazole); in some cases, bismuth or H_2 blockers are added.

4. How does food allergy play a role in the development of PUD?

Lesions of peptic ulcers and classic allergic reactions show similar microanatomic changes.[2] In addition to promoting allergic symptoms, histamine stimulates acid secretion from parietal cells. IgE-related allergic reactions induce damage in gastric and intestinal mucosa.[3] Food elimination diets have been successful in treating peptic ulcers.[4] The most common allergens are wheat and dairy. A single food or multiple foods can be eliminated for a 1-month period; then one food is reintroduced at a time, with close monitoring of symptoms. If the symptoms return, the food should be avoided because it may be a trigger for PUD.

5. Does fiber really make a difference in PUD?

The ability of fiber to promote mucin secretion and delay gastric emptying plays a role in the prevention and recurrence of peptic ulcers.[5,6] There are different classifications of dietary fiber. The noncellulose polysaccharides found in guar, legumes, and psyllium are responsible for the delay in gastric emptying. This delay promotes the initiation of digestion of proteins in the stomach, which decreases the possibility of allergy development as well as slows movement of food into the duodenum.

6. What about spicy foods?

Spicy foods, such as cayenne pepper, once were thought to worsen peptic ulcers but are now thought to help in their healing. In nonhemorrhagic ulcers, spicy foods draw blood supply to the gastric and duodenal mucosa, thus promoting the healing process. Cayenne pepper also has a local anesthetic effect. Patients can experiment with cayenne pepper tea. Add one-fourth teaspoon of cayenne pepper to 1 cup boiling water; steep for10 minutes. Alternatively, a capsule of the powder can be used.[7]

7. **Name two vitamins indicated in the treatment of PUD.**

Vitamins A and E are thought to maintain the integrity of the lining of the digestive tract. No literature to date supports a specific dosage of vitamin A and E supplementation in the treatment or prevention of PUD. Daily recommendations include vitamin E, 400 IU, and vitamin A. 50,000 IU. Of note, vitamin E is best absorbed in the d-alpha tocopherol form (check labels), and the remote chance of vitamin A toxicity can be avoided by taking the water-soluble precursor beta-carotene or mixed carotenes (50,000 IU). Zinc is thought to induce mucin secretion and also may be indicated in the treatment of PUD.

8. **Are over-the-counter antacids still recommended? What about the benefits of calcium in some of these preparations?**

Because of the rebound effect on gastric acid production, over-the-counter preparations are recommended only for short-term (no longer than 1 month) and intermittent use. Calcium-based antacids contain calcium carbonate, which is a poorly solubilized form. Calcium is better absorbed in the citrate form, which is preferred for patients with either renal impairment or hypochlorhydria (which is induced by antacid use). The sodium bicarbonate preparations may cause alkalosis in high doses, and the aluminum-containing antacids may cause constipation and aluminum toxicity as well as calcium and phosphorous depletion.

9. **What are the drawbacks to prescription medications such as H$_2$ blockers and proton pump inhibitors?**

These medications do not motivate patients to affect change in diet and lifestyle; thus they do not necessarily treat the root cause of the disease.

10. **List three botanicals used in the treatment of PUD.**

Licorice, chamomile, and slippery elm.

11. **Describe the mechanism of action of licorice.**

The active constituents in licorice have a variety of biologic activities. The most important in the treatment of PUD is glycyrrhizin. Glycyrrhizin has been shown to protect gastric mucosa (by regulating prostaglandin activity), increase plasma secretin and pancreatic bicarbonate output, decrease gastrin secretion, and inhibit in vitro replication of *H. pylori* and numerous viruses.[8] Because glycyrrhizin can negatively affect the aldosterone system, the deglycyrrhizinated (DGL) form is recommended. DGL has been shown to improve gastric mucosa longevity and increase mucosal blood flow. Several studies support the use of DGL in the treatment of PUD, and there are no known adverse side effects. As an example, one clinical study compared DGL with cimetidine.[9] DGL was found to be as effective as cimetidine and, because of its protective effects, to have a lower rate of relapse.

12. **What are the significant side effects and contraindications to the use of licorice?**

Because of its effect on corticosteroid metabolism, licorice is contraindicated in pregnancy, cholestatic liver disease, hypertension, renal disease, and concomitant use with potassium-lowering medications. However, because licorice is available in a deglycyrrhizinated form, side effects are minimal.

13. **How is licorice recommended to patients?**

In the DGL form, 2–4 380-mg chewable tablets can be taken 30 minutes before meals for 2–4 weeks. DGL is activated by enzymes in saliva and thus is recommended in a chewable (not capsule) form. Of note, ropes of candy licorice are often flavored with anise, not true licorice, and therefore do not have the same beneficial properties.

14. **What is the proposed mechanism of action of chamomile? What are the side effects? How is it recommended?**

Chamomile has antispamodic and smooth muscle-relaxing effects on the GI tract.[10] It also is known for its anxiolytic and anti-inflammatory effects. There are no known contraindications to chamomile, but allergy (although rare) has been reported as a side effect.[11] The recommended dose of chamomile is 3 gm of dried herb in 150 ml water 3 times/day as a tea.

15. What is known about slippery elm in the treatment of PUD?

Unfortunately, there are no good clinical trials for slippery elm. Traditional use of slippery elm is as a mucilage. When the herb comes into contact with intestinal membranes, it coats and soothes irritated mucosal surfaces, protects them from injury, and draws out toxins or irritants.

16. Is aloe vera recommended in the treatment of PUD?

Aloe vera is thought to inactivate pepsin, to inhibit the release of hydrochloric acid (by interfering with histamine binding to parietal cells), and to act as a healing demulcent.[12]

17. What is the role of bioflavonoids in PUD?

Ulcer-protective activity has been shown in animal and in-vitro studies for several flavonoids, which are naturally occurring compounds found in the human diet. This broad group includes anthocyanosides, genistin, quercetin, rutin, and silymarin - usually found concentrated in brightly pigmented fruits and vegetables. Proposed mechanisms of action include increase of mucosal prostaglandin content, decrease of histamine secretion from mast cells, inhibition of *H. pylori* growth, and free radical scavenging activity.[13]

18. Recommend integrative therapies for the treatment of stress.

Stress as a cause of certain illnesses remains controversial. However, studies do link stress to PUD.[14] Stress management techniques can include counseling, yoga, massage, reiki, and other modalities.

19. Name other forms of integrative therapies that may be used in the treatment of PUD.

Acupuncture, homeopathy, ayurveda, and other alternative systems have been used in the treatment of PUD. These modalities typically help the patient explore underlying factors and try to treat the root cause.

20. What is the bottom line of an integrative approach to PUD?

Integrative therapies can be first-line or adjunct treatments in PUD. First-line treatments include cessation of smoking, stress reduction, investigation of food allergens, and avoidance of other exacerbating factors. Use botanicals, and explore other modalities.

REFERENCES

1. Tamblyn R, Berkson L, Dauphinee D, et al: Unnecessary prescribing of NSAIDs and the management of NSAID-related gastropathy in medical practice. Ann Intern Med 127:429–438, 1997.
2. Siegel J: Gastrointestinal ulcer-arthus reaction! Ann Allergy 34:127–130, 1974.
3. DeLazzari F, et al: Specific IgE in the gastric and duodenal mucosa: An epiphenon pathogenetic mechanism of some forms of "peptic" ulcer. Minerva Gastroenterol Dietol 40:1–9, 1994.
4. Murray M, Pizzorno J: Encyclopedia of Natural Medicine. Rocklin CA, Prima Publishing, 1991, p 520.
5. Rydning A, Berstad A, Aadland E, Odegaard B: Prophylatic effects of dietary in duodenal ulcer disease. Lancet ii:736–739, 1982.
6. Misciagna G, Cisternino AM, Freudenheim J: Diet and duodenal ulcer. Dig Liver Dis 32:468–472, 2000.
7. Weil A: Natural Health Natural Medicine. New York, Houghton Mifflin, 1995.
8. Petry J, Hadley S: Medicinal herbs: Answers and advice. Part 2. Hosp Pract 36(8):57–58, 2001.
9. Morgan AG, et al: Comparison between cimetidine and Caved-S in the treatment of gastric ulceration, and subsequent maintenance therapy. Gut 23:545–551, 1982.
10. Petry J, Hadley S: Medicinal herbs: A primer for primary care. Hosp Pract 34(6):110, 1999.
11. Blumenthal M: The Complete German Commission E Monographs. Therapeutic Guide to Herbal Medicines. Austin, TX, American Botanical Council, 1998.
12. Murray M: The Healing Power of Herbs. Rocklin, CA, Prima Publishing, 1995.
13. Borrelli F, Izzo AA: The plant kingdom as a source of anti-ulcer remedies. Phytother Res 14: 589–591, 2000.
14. Anda R, Williamson D, et al: Self-perceived stress and the risk of peptic ulcer disease: A longitudinal study of U.S. adults. Arch Intern Med 152:829–831, 1992.

38. MENOPAUSE

Monica J. Stokes, M.D., FACOG

1. What should be a healthcare provider's first priorities when a patient presents with possible perimenopausal symptoms?

The perimenopause is a golden opportunity for health and well-being enhancement on all levels. It is also a time during which you will determine the quality and effectiveness of your relationship with your patient over the next many years. Risk profiles may be determined, screening test may be scheduled, and vaccinations and health promotion behaviors (e.g., nutrition, activity, supplements, stress reduction) may be recommended. Issues related to spirituality or sexuality may emerge. Your willingness to be open to the patient's questions and to consider alternative or integrative treatments or activities at different points during this stage of life will affect whether she will be open with you about what she is doing (or is considering) to treat herself. In addition, individual perimenopausal symptoms may mimic those of many illnesses; a differential diagnosis for the symptom must be kept in mind before assuming that the perimenopause is the only cause.

2. What is the difference between menopause and perimenopause?

Perimenopause refers to the transition between regular, ovulatory menses through the final months before menses terminate. It may last from 1 to 12 years and may be associated intermittently with a number of symptoms. Menopause is the complete cessation of menstrual bleeding for a period of 6–12 months in the absence of another cause for amenorrhea. The safer definition is 12 months, which more likely reflects complete cessation of reproductive capability. The age range at which natural menopause may occur is 40–58 years in our heterogeneous society. The age of actual menopause is made retrospectively. Smoking, hysterectomy, or persistent malnutrition may induce menopause 2–3 years earlier than it would have occurred otherwise. Menopause before age 40 should prompt considerable inquiry for the cause (e.g., autoimmune disease).

3. What symptoms may occur in perimenopause and menopause?

Different women experience the symptoms of perimenopause and menopause at varying levels of intensity, duration, and frequency and in various combinations. Symptoms may include vasomotor symptoms (hot flushes), sweating, vaginal dryness, atrophic vaginitis (associated with direct changes in sexual functioning), lower urinary tract mucosal atrophy with or without urge incontinence, reduced libido, reduced subdermal collagen integrity with sagging of skin, joint or muscle aches, memory deficits, sleep disturbances with associated mood fluctuations, emotional lability, or exacerbation of preexisting emotional or other psychiatric problems.

4. Why are women turning to complementary/alternative medicine (CAM) for help with symptoms of menopause?

Because of lack of confidence in the espoused benefits of conventional hormone replacement therapy (HRT) and the significant array of adverse side effects, fewer than 1 in 3 postmenopausal women choose to take HRT.[1] Fear of breast cancer is the most often cited reason for not starting estrogen. A frequent side effect of HRT is intermittent bleeding, and about half of women who start standard HRT discontinue it within 1 year. The North American Menopause Society estimates that more than 30% of women use acupuncture, natural estrogens, herbal supplements, or phytoestrogens.[2] Perhaps because of the known and feared side effects of conventional HRT, many women choose to explore CAM options for menopausal symptoms.

5. What long-term health risks may be associated with estrogen deficiency?

Osteopenia, osteoporosis (see Chapter 33), earlier onset of possible periodontal disease with tooth loss, earlier onset of age-related macular degeneration (the number-one cause of adult blindness in the U.S.), increased risk of primary coronary heart disease (controversial), and possibly stroke and earlier age-related cognitive decline.

6. What are the major potential risks and absolute contraindications of estrogen supplementation therapy?

Possible risks include increased risk of thromboembolic events, gallstone formation, a small increase in breast cancer risk (but a lower mortality risk), and increased risk of endometrial cancer (only in women with a uterus who do not receive appropriate adjunctive progesterone therapy).

Absolute contraindications include suspected estrogen-dependent cancers, current or recent breast cancer (withholding of estrogen is controversial in women who have been disease-free for longer than 10 years), undiagnosed genitourinary bleeding, active thrombophlebitis or thromboembolic disorder, active liver disease, or suspected pregnancy.

7. Can any one lab test reliably determine the presence of perimenopause?

No. Perimenopause is a time of wide fluctuations in estrogen levels during the day and over the month. Even follicle-stimulating hormone (FSH) levels fluctuate widely, depending on whether ovulation has occurred before the sample is drawn. If no ovulations have occurred for a few months, the FSH level may be temporarily in the lab's "menopausal range," although in fact the patient remains capable of reproduction and by definition, therefore, is not postmenopausal. One FSH measurement during one month is a poor test to determine whether a woman is possibly perimenopausal, as are estrogen levels. Saliva testing, although popular, is also a poor marker for similar reasons.

8. Can any lab test reliably confirm the postmenopausal state?

Clinical expertise recommends a combination of signs and symptoms, including age, 12 consecutive months of amenorrhea (in the absence of another cause), and a markedly elevated FSH level (60–100 mIU/L) on two tests repeated at least 1 month apart. This combination of signs and symptoms usually indicates the permanent loss of reproductive capacity. Use of less stringent criteria may be suggestive but not confirmatory. This error has resulted in many unplanned late-life pregnancies after a woman has been told that she no longer needs contraception. Continued periodic menstrual bleeding in a woman not on estrogen supplementation with a persistent, marked FSH elevation should provoke a postmenopausal bleeding investigation, which may include ultrasound evaluation of the endometrium, hysteroscopy, and/or endometrial tissue sampling.

Serial saliva testing for persistent hypoestrogenism is sometimes used as an alternative or adjunctive test. Saliva testing for estrogen levels has not yet been confirmed as a consistently reliable measure of estrogen levels for diagnostic purposes or for women on estrogen replacement therapy.

9. What are natural hormones? How do they differ from natural source or bio-identical hormones?

If *natural* is defined as coming from nature with no chemical manipulation before administration, conjugated equine estrogens (CEEs; Premarin), obtained from the urine of pregnant mares, is the only truly "natural" hormone. Premarin has been on the market for the longest time and has been used in more clinical studies than any other estrogen product. As a result, Premarin is prescribed for most women in the United States on postmenopausal hormone supplementation therapy.

Because of concerns about the possible (as yet unsubstantiated) adverse actions of equine estrogens within the human body or the patient's ethical concerns, a number of products now use yam or soy source plants to synthesize bio-identical compounds that are chemically identical to the hormones produced by a woman's body. Diosgenin, the precursor compound derived from the source plant, must undergo a series of chemical manipulations[3] to produce the final hormone product used by humans who do not have the chemical machinery necessary to convert the plant precursor. The claim that such hormones are natural is truly applicable only to the source; the product itself is not natural, even though it is bio-identical to the endogenous human hormone. Examples of bio-identical hormones include USP 17-beta estradiol (i.e., micronized and used to make Estrace) and USP progesterone (i.e., micronized and used to make Prometrium). These hormones are used by compounding pharmacists and large pharmaceutical companies as constituents in their more "natural" products.

10. What about synthetic hormones?

The natural-source hormones are manufactured using plant-source precursors, but synthetic hormones are produced chemically from beginning to end. An example is ethinyl estradiol, a potent synthetic estrogen used previously only in oral contraceptive formulations. Unfortunately, it is now finding its way into pharmaceutical hormone supplementation products such as in Femhrt. Ethinyl estradiol significantly increases levels of sex hormone-binding globulin (and other proteins synthesized by the liver) but is not bound by it. The result is a reduction in circulating levels of other reproductive hormones.[4] In addition, more of this synthetic hormone circulates in an unbound form protected from rapid degradation.

Other synthetic hormones, such as medroxyprogesterone acetate, add chemical moieties to the basic progesterone structure to reduce the degree of metabolism in the gastrointestinal tract, improve binding intensity to progesterone receptors, and increase resistance to degradation once the hormone is absorbed into the body. This process explains many of the adverse side effects, such as water retention and mood depression, which usually are not noted with natural progesterone use.

11. Describe the evaluation of intermenstrual bleeding or prolonged menstrual bleeding in perimenopause.

The skipping of one or a few menses does not require an evaluation unless the patient has had unprotected intercourse and does not have a reliable contraceptive method. One episode of intermenstrual bleeding in the absence of other risk factors for neoplasia is not necessarily a cause for a work-up. Perimenopause is characterized by menstrual irregularity that includes alterations in cycle length and possibly spotting immediately before or after menses. True intermenstrual bleeding (usually determined by review of a menstrual calendar) is not normal, although it may result from partial sloughing of a thick endometrium resulting from one or more missed ovulations. In addition, a small amount of mid-cycle bleeding may be due to ovulation. Any recurrence should be evaluated in perimenopausal patients.

Prolonged menstrual bleeding (> 7 days) on more than one occasion or a flow that "just won't stop" requires evaluation to determine the cause, possibly including ultrasound, endometrial sampling (not necessarily during the bleeding episode, but 1–3 weeks after it ends to allow a definitive diagnosis), and/or hysteroscopy. In addition, all patients should be evaluated for anemia to determine the need for short-term iron supplementation. Recently, hematologic dysfunction (such as clotting factor deficiencies) and thyroid disease have emerged as more frequent causes of menorrhagia in perimenopausal women than previously appreciated; thus, it may be wise to expand the differential diagnosis beyond gynecologic disease.

12. Should supplemental estrogen be used alone to treat perimenopausal or menopausal symptoms?

Because estrogen levels fluctuate so widely in perimenopausal women and newer studies[5,6] have shown that most perimenopausal women have normal or elevated estrogen levels, it is not prudent to use estrogen alone to treat symptoms in perimenopausal women. Progesterone levels, in fact, may be reduced because of intermittent anovulatory cycles. Many other, less risk-laden options, including dietary changes, progesterone, and botanical medicines, are available for treatment of symptoms in women who are not yet continually estrogen-deficient. Hormone level testing, for the reasons mentioned above, are usually unhelpful, unless they are found to be extremely outside the normal range.

In menopause, some women are unable to tolerate any form or administration route of progesterone and may have compelling risk factors that require the use of estrogen supplementation therapy. Such women must be screened periodically with ultrasound and, as needed, endometrial sampling or hysteroscopy, which should be performed to rule out pathology if the endometrium is found to be thickened or if postmenopausal bleeding occurs. If pathology is ruled out and the problems continue, a progesterone-secreting intrauterine device may be a therapeutic option for some women.

13. What herbal and supplemental alternatives may be used for treatment of "hot flushes"?

Traditional botanical treatments for hot flushes include soy, dong quai, *Vitex agnus-castus* (chaste tree berry), evening primrose seed oil, and red clover. The main botanical for which there is clinical study evidence of effectiveness for treatment of hot flushes is black cohosh (*Cimicifuga racemosa*).[7] Remifemin, an extract of black cohosh standardized to 2.5% triterpene glycosides, was used in most studies at a dose of 20–80 mg twice daily. Menopausal symptoms were reduced in up to 80% of participants. Black cohosh is also effective for sweating, headache, vertigo, and palpitations; thus, it indirectly helps treat sleep disturbance. In rare cases, black cohosh precipitates headaches, which resolve with its discontinuation. It is not known to have any direct estrogen effect on the human breast or endometrium; thus, it is probably safe for patients with breast cancer.[8]

A more recent prospective, blinded study using dong quai as a single agent showed no clinically significant benefit for hot flushes compared with placebo.[9] This study has been criticized by traditional healers because dong quai is typically used as part of multiherb combination formulas.[10] Although often helpful for menstrual irregularities, premenstrual symptoms, and mastalgia, all of which often accelerate during perimenopause, *Vitex agnus-castus* has yet to be subjected to prospective trials as a single agent to determine its efficacy for treatment of for hot flushes. However, lack of studies that confirm efficacy does not mean that a patient should be discouraged from using a particular botanical if it controls her symptoms and if she has no contraindications for its use.

14. Discuss the role of phytoestrogens during menopause.

Phytoestrogens are naturally occurring plant compounds with a steroid ring structure similar to estrogen that enables them to bind to human estrogen receptors. Studies[11,12] show that they activate these receptors weakly, presumably block estrogen hormones from binding, and thus act as competitive inhibitors. They also may have an adaptogenic effect, reversibly blocking receptors from more potent estrogens and providing more gentle stimulation periods of (or at sites of) estrogen deficiency. Soy isoflavones have been recommended at a dose of 60–100 mg/day.[13] The estrogenic effect on the breast and endometrium range from minimal to none in this dosage range. Studies are ongoing, but doses in this range may have favorable effects such as decreased cardiovascular risk, adjunctive therapy to help maintain vertebral bone mass, and improvement in vasomotor symptoms. Epidemiologically, lifetime dietary soy intake in women in Asia is linked to low incidence of menopausal symptoms as well as breast and ovarian cancers.[14,15] In fact, there is no word for "hot flash" in Asian languages because they are not commonly reported by menopausal Asian women.

Another phytoestrogen, red clover (*Trifolium pratense*), has active phytoestrogen effects, but clinical studies have found no statistically significant reduction of hot flashes or improvement in vaginal epithelial thickness compared with placebo.[16,17] Good studies of other known phytoestrogens, such as certain sunflower seeds, alfalfa, flax, and wheat, are not available.

15. How is vaginal dryness treated?

A general intravaginal lubricant such as Replens may be helpful; personal lubricants (e.g., Astroglide, KY jelly) are reserved for use as needed if lubrication after sexual stimulation is inadequate. Vitamin E oil also may be used for local dryness, but it requires frequent application. Soy intake has minimal, if any, effect at the previously mentioned dose for the prevention or treatment of vaginal atrophy. Panax ginseng, although touted as a "male tonic," has an estrogenic effect on both the vagina and the endometrium, but it is a stimulant that may disturb sleep. Panax ginseng may cause mastalgia in some women. If a patient is using Panax ginseng, it may be prudent to encourage her to use it cyclically or to add progesterone to the regimen in the same way that it is used with estrogen supplementation.

Intravaginal progesterone cream is a highly effective treatment for vaginal dryness. Several commercial preparations are available. Look for 400–600 mg progesterone/ounce, and use 1/8 to 1/4 teaspoon intravaginally each day. In addition, local compounding pharmacists can make up a custom cream or gel with a calibrated applicator. Most over-the-counter creams vary greatly in both progesterone content and quality assurance and cannot be trusted to deliver a reliable dosage without research to determine whether they contain the dosage they claim on their label.

16. What CAM treatments may be used for sleep disruption in perimenopausal and menopausal women?

Sleep disruption may have a myriad of causes, but in perimenopausal women it is most commonly due to the nighttime occurrence of hot flushes and sweating. Failure to get a good night's sleep seriously affects the patient's moods, ability to cope, and sense of well being. Education about sleep hygiene is important. Avoidance of alcohol, caffeine, and other stimulants within several hours before bedtime should be encouraged. Daily exercise improves sleep as long as it is performed more than 4 hours before bedtime. Current use of over-the-counter and prescription medications should be reviewed to rule out any precipitating or potentially exacerbating substances (which may not have created a problem in the past).

Tryptophan-containing bedtime drinks may be helpful, such as Ovaltine or warm milk and honey. Many herbs can be helpful.[18] Teas made with chamomile, catnip, and lemon balm should be taken 30–60 minutes before bedtime for their sedative and muscle relaxant properties. Magnesium, 200–600 mg at bedtime, acts as a muscle relaxant but must be titrated to avoid loose stools the next morning. Kava, most commonly used in divided doses for anxiety, may be effective in a single bed-time dose (150–240 mg of solid powdered kavalactones extract) to relax the body, but it is rarely ef-fective for sleeping difficulty due to an overactive mind. Valerian root, 160–300 mg standardized to 0.8% valeric acid (especially in combination with 80 mg of lemon balm extract) is highly effective and not associated with residual daytime sedation.

Training in self-hypnosis techniques used at bedtime may be helpful in motivated patients. Acupuncture, which reestablishes harmony among the systems, has a high success rate in the treat-ment of shorter-term insomnia. Topical progesterone supplementation also may be quite helpful for treatment of perimenopausal and menopausal insomnia. Isolated, chronic use of oral progesterone may cause fatigue[19] and therefore should be avoided for this indication.

17. What are the contraceptive options for the perimenopausal woman?

Because of the frequency of menstrual irregularities, natural family planning is particularly in-effective for perimenopausal women. Intrauterine devices often cause irregular bleeding, which may confuse the clinical picture during this time. Barrier methods, especially with concurrent use of sper-micide, are highly effective in motivated patients. Bilateral tubal ligation for a woman in whom future childbearing is not an issue is also highly effective, although it is associated with rare but sig-nificant surgical risks. Intramuscular medroxyprogesterone acetate (Depo-Provera) injections may be used but, because of the association with loss of bone mass, are not the best option for a woman who may not have the time to regain the lost mass after she discontinues use. Low-dose oral contra-ceptives (20 μg estrogen dose) provide an attractive option because of their normalization of men-strual cycles, provision of a consistent background hormone milieu (which helps minimize symptoms), and provision of reliable contraception with consistent use. Oral contraceptives are con-traindicated in perimenopausal women who smoke or have any other medical contraindication to pharmacologic dosing of estrogen (e.g., history of liver or thromboembolic disease). A contraceptive ring, placed intravaginally, recently approved by the FDA, may be an option for this group.

18. What are the benefits of hormone supplementation therapy in postmenopausal women?

Postmenopausal hormone supplementation is a preventive healthcare strategy, even though menopause is a natural, physiologic event in a woman's life. Long- and short-term benefits of estro-gen supplementation include the following[5]: prevention or treatment of hot flushes, vaginal dryness, osteoporosis, lower genitourinary atrophic changes with associated local dyspareunia, urge inconti-nence, emotional lability associated with sleep disruption, sleep disturbances, age-related macular de-generation, periodontal disease and tooth loss, dyslipidemia, hemorrhagic stroke, and colon cancer; delay in age-related cognitive decline and onset and progression of mild Alzheimer's disease; primary prevention of coronary heart disease (controversial regarding secondary prevention); reduction of symptoms in treated Parkinson's disease; decreased insulin resistance and hemoglobin A_{1C} reduction in type 2 diabetes; and possibly prevention of migraine headaches (if the continuous regimen is used).

19. What are the best choices for estrogen supplementation therapy in postmenopausal women?

The lowest dose of a bio-identical estrogen hormone product (17-beta estradiol) that controls the patient's symptoms is preferred (oral or transdermal patch). Optimally, estrogens should be taken in the morning to mimic more closely the diurnal cycling that may affect other endocrine systems. Topically applied estrogen cream is inconsistently absorbed and therefore is a poor choice to prevent or treat health concerns. Intravaginal application of estrogen cream is effective for local symptom control but achieves only 25 % of the serum estrogen levels achieved by an equivalent oral dose. However, it is enough to cause endometrial proliferation with postmenopausal bleeding in elderly women and women with extreme atrophy. Estrogen by the oral route increases levels of triglycerides, HDL cholesterol, clotting factors, and sex hormone-binding globulin but reduces levels of LDL cholesterol because of its first-pass effect on the liver.

The route of administration should be determined by the primary indications for use, medical issues, and patient preference. Unopposed estrogen therapy puts a woman at risk for neoplastic change of the endometrium and stimulation of occult abdominopelvic endometriosis. Daily dosing is recommended. There is no need to stop estrogen for 5 days each month, unless the patient is comfortable with that regimen because of long-term practice.

20. Discuss the role of tri-estrogen combinations.

Tri-estrogen compounds, which generally contain 80% estradiol (E2), 10% estrone (E1), and 10% estriol (E3), and bi-estrogen compounds, which generally contain 80–90% E3 and 10–20% estradiol in the recommended doses, provide enough estradiol for symptom control.[20] In addition, the bi-estrogens add no extra estrone, which is already the predominant circulating estrogen in postmenopausal women. Estradiol has the most potent biologic activity at any given dose because of its high affinity for estrogen receptors in target tissues. There is insufficient evidence that estrone and estriol convey any additional benefit, and Tri-Est and other compounded tri-estrogen and bi-estrogen medications are not covered by most insurance plans.

In addition, in women who do not respond to the therapies noted above, other medical issues with symptoms that mimic or exacerbate menopausal symptoms (e.g., thyroid disease) may require your attention. After they are considered, some patients may benefit from the detailed range of dosages possible with the help of a compounding pharmacist.

21. What are the best choices for progesterone therapy in postmenopausal women?

Progesterone should be used concurrently in any woman with a uterus in place or possibly a known history of significant endometriosis (usually documented in the operative report in women who have had laparoscopic surgeries of any kind or hysterectomy or oophorectomy). Oral progesterone may be used continuously or cyclically (calendar days 1–13 of each month). Intermittent bleeding may occur for up to 6–12 months, usually followed by amenorrhea with the continuous regimen. The cyclic method has the advantage of predictable withdrawal bleeding of some degree almost every month indefinitely. Most patients prefer to endure the short-term inconvenience of the continuous regimen. Progesterone should be given by a route and in a dose that reliably produces endometrial protective levels in the serum (or local levels) if one of the purposes for use is endometrial protection. For most women, standard doses are adequate for endometrial stabilization. Oral micronized progesterone (Prometrium) at 100–200 mg/day, sustained-release vaginal bioadhesive gel (Crinone) 4% or 8%, or oral troches (compounded) are more natural options to achieve this goal. Oral micronized progesterone should be taken with food to improve absorption. Skin application of progesterone cream or gel, which may be helpful for treating vasomotor and some other perimenopausal and menopausal symptoms, is not a reliable route of administration when endometrial protection is one of the objectives for its use.[21]

22. Describe the reevaluation of hormone replacement dosing.

Tailoring of the regimen for each patient is imperative. If a patient does not seem to respond to the initial regimen after 6–8 weeks, consider changing the route of administration before raising any hormone above its recommended dosage range. If the patient requires higher doses for symptom control, remember that the level of hormone needed for symptom control may be higher than what is recommended for prevention of long-term health consequences of estrogen deficiency. Reevaluation of the increased dosage after 12–24 months is prudent.

23. Does testosterone have a role in postmenopausal hormone supplementation regimens? What are the potential risks of use in women?

Testosterone production by the postmenopausal ovary slowly declines over a period of years. For women who have experienced natural menopause, lower-dose testosterone supplementation has not been shown to be effective in most cases for treatment of reduced libido.[22] Pharmacologic doses ($\geq$ 5 mg/day orally or 300 µg transdermally) have been found to be effective, but they also are associated with an increased incidence of virilization.[23,24]

Women in whom menopause is due to a surgical or ablative cause (no ovarian androgen production) have been shown to benefit from the addition of superphysiologic doses of testosterone to the regimen. Reported benefits in this group include increased sense of well-being, increased energy, and normalization of libido.[24,25] Extended use of effectively superphysiologic dosing (concomitant estrogen use reduces androgen clearance) increases the risk of other adverse androgenic effects, including hepatic damage. Currently, only oral methyltestosterone/estrogen combination pills are approved by the Food and Drug Administration for use in women; the bulk of products (pellets, patches, pills of much higher dosages) are approved only for use in men.

Compounding pharmacists can make up custom doses using USP testosterone in creams or gels for topical application. Topical testosterone is well absorbed in the proper base vehicles and may be initiated at very low doses and titrated upward or downward based on response and serum or urinary levels after several weeks of treatment. The long-term effect of supplemental androgen use in women is not yet known. If nonapproved preparations are used, the patient should be followed closely with serum or urinary levels and be fully educated about the potential for virilization and other serious side effects that depend on dose and duration of use (acne, hirsutism, reduction in HDL cholesterol, glucose level changes in diabetics, hepatic function impairment). The patient should be encouraged to keep track of her response and to report any concerns immediately.

24. Discuss other options and adjuncts for treatment of menopausal symptoms.

The perimenopausal period occurs at a time of life when many issues come to the surface for many women. Some women consider these their "golden" or wise years or refer to "power surges" rather than hot flushes. Cognitive-behavioral therapy, journals, and/or community support groups may be effective for helping the woman prioritize and examine these issues. Massage, craniosacral therapy, other energy therapies, homeopathy, ayurvedic medicine, Chinese medicine, and acupuncture[25] are helpful for many women. Exercise not only decreases frequency and severity of hot flushes but also elevates mood.[26] Meditation relaxes the body and calms the mind in the short term and is centering and consciousness-expanding in the long-term. With regular practice, it helps deepen spirituality, regardless of the patient's spiritual or religious convictions. Women who have a regular meditative practice before the onset of the perimenopause experience significantly less severe symptoms and, if they require medications at all, appear to require lower doses of botanicals or pharmaceuticals to control symptoms.

25. What sources are available for additional information?

- International Academy of Compounding Pharmacists provides referrals to compounding pharmacists in your area. The academy can be contacted by mail (P.O. Box 1365. Sugar Land, TX 77478) or telephone (800-927-4227) or on the Internet (at www.iacprx.org-).
- Christiane Northrup: The Wisdom of Menopause: Creating Physical and Emotional Health and Healing During the Change. New York, Bantam-Doubleday-Dell, 2001.
- Sadja Greenwood: Menopause Naturally: Preparing for the Second Half of Life [updated edition]. Volcano, CA, Volcano Press, 1992.
- Adriane Fugh-Berman (ed): Alternative Therapies in Women's Health. Atlanta, American Health Consultants, 1999-2001 issues.
- Robert Svoboda: Ayurveda for Women: A Guide to Vitality and Health. London, David & Charles Books, 1999.

REFERENCES

1. American College of Obstetricians and Gynecologists: Use of botanicals for management of menopausal symptoms. ACOG Practice Bulletin 28, 2001.
2. Kaufert P, et al: Women and menopause: Belief, attitudes, and behaviors. The North American Menopause Society 1997 Menopause Survey. Menopause 5:197–202, 1998.

3. Writing Group for the PEPI Trial: The effects of estrogen or estrogen/progestin regimens on heart disease risk factors in postmenopausal women. JAMA 273:199–208, 1996

4. Eskin B.: The Menopause: Comprehensive Management, 4th ed. New York, Parthenon, Pu 2000.

5. Speroff L, Glass R, Kase N: Clinical Gynecologic Endocrinology and Infertility, 6th ed. Baltimore, Lippincott Williams & Wilkins, 1999.

6. Santoro N, Brown JR, Adel T, Skurnick JH: Characterization of reproductive hormonal dynamics in the perimenopause. JClin Endocrinol Metabol 81:1495–1501, 1996.

7. Tillem J: Black cohosh for the treatment of perimenopausal and menopausal symptoms. Altern Med Alert 3:17–19, 2000.

8. Freudenstein J, Bodinet C: Influence of an isopropanolic aqueous extract of *Cimicfuga racemosa* on the proliferation of MCF-7 cells. Presented at the 23rd International Symposium on Phyto-estrogens, January 15, 1999, Ghent, Belgium.

9. Hirata JD, Swiersz LM, Zell B, et al: Does dong quai have estrogenic effects in postmenopausal women?: A double blind placebo controlled trial. Fertil Steril 68:981–986, 1997.

10. Low Dog T, Riley D, Carter T: An integrative approach to menopause. Altern Ther 7(4):45–55, 2001.

11. Rose DP: Dietary fiber, phytoestrogens, and breast cancer. Nutrition 8:47–51, 1992.

12. North American Menopause Society: The role of isoflavones in menopausal health: Consensus opinion of The North American Menopause Society. Menpoause 7:215–229, 2000.

13. Albertazzi P, et al: The effect of dietary soy supplementaion on serum lipoproteins, blood pressure, and menopausal symptoms in perimenopausal women. Menopause 6:7–13, 1999.

14. Sturdee DW: Clinical symptoms of oestrogen deficiency. Curr Obstet Gynaecol 7:190–196, 1997.

15. Punyahotra S, et al: Menopausal experiences of Thai women. Part 1: Symptoms and their correlates. Maturitas 26:1–7, 1997.

16. Baber RJ, Templeman CMT, et al: Randomized placebo-controlled trial of an isoflavone supplement and menopausal symptoms in women. Climacteric 2:85–92, 1999.

17. Knight DC, et al: The effect of Promensil, an isoflavone extract, on menopausal symptoms. Climacteric 2:79–84, 1999.

18. Pizzorno JE, Murray MT: Textbook of Natural Medicine, 2nd ed. Edinburgh, Churchill Livingstone, 1999.

19. Arafat E, et al: Sedative and hypnotic effects of oral administratrion of micronized progesterone may be mediated through its metabolites. Am J Obstet Gynecol 159:1203–1209, 1988.

20. Hudson T: Women's Encyclopedia of Natural Medicine. Lincolnwood, IL, Keats Publishing, 1999.

21. Wren BG, McFarland K, Edwards L: Micronised transdermal progesterone and endometrial response. Lancet 354:1447–1448, 1999.

22. ACOG Committee Opinion No. 244. Washington, DC, American College of Obstetricians and Gynecologists, 2000

23. Shifren JL, Braunstein GD, Simon JA, et al: Transdermal testosterone treatment in women with impaired sexual function after oophorectomy. N Engl J Med 343:682–688, 2000.

24. Sherwin BB, Gelfand MM: Role of androgen and maintenance of sexual functioning in ovariectomized women. Psychosom Med 49:397–409, 1987.

25. Wyon Y, et al: Effects of acupuncture on climacteric vasomotor symptoms, quality of life, and urinary excretion of neuropeptides among postmenopausal women. Menopause 2:3, 1995.

26. Slaven L, Lee C: Mood and symptom reporting among middle-aged women: The relationship between menopausal status, hormone replacement therapy, and exercise participation. Health Psychol 16:203–208, 1997.

39. PREMENSTRUAL SYNDROME

Alison Levitt, M.D.

1. What is premenstrual syndrome (PMS)?

PMS refers to a set of cyclical symptoms that recur during the luteal phase of the menstrual cycle, 7–14 days before menses. About 90% of women with PMS experience fatigue, irritability, and abdominal bloating; 85%, breast tenderness; about 70%, increased appetite; and about 60%, headaches.[1] Water retention, joint pain, acne, depression, nausea, tension, specific food cravings, pelvic cramping, anxiety, and low sex drive are among the other distressing symptoms that regularly plague women who suffer from PMS.

2. What makes PMS a syndrome?

PMS is a complex biomedical entity. Over 150 symptoms are associated with PMS, and the exact cause is unknown. No symptoms are unique or pathognomonic. PMS involves the interplay of culture, emotional factors, and physiologic factors, including nutritional deficiencies, endocrine system, neurotransmitters, and prostaglandin production.

3. What is the prevalence of PMS?

About 70–90% of women of reproductive age experience at least one, often more, of the symptoms characteristic of PMS; about 4 of 10 women find them severe enough to interfere with daily activities.

4. How is PMS diagnosed?

A medical diagnosis of PMS, also called premenstrual dysphoric disorder (PMDD) by the Diagnostic and Statistical Manual of Mental Disorders, 4th ed. (DSM IV), requires prospective recording of specific symptoms (as in question 1), timing of the symptoms in relation to the menstrual cycle, and symptoms of sufficient severity to impair socioeconomic functioning.

5. What other diagnoses should be ruled out when a woman complains of PMS symptoms?

Rule out major depression, mood disorders, thyroid dysfunction, early menopause, eating disorders, and substance abuse. PMS is distinguished from chronic psychological disorders by a symptom-free period less than or equal to 1 week during the follicular phase of each menstrual cycle.

6. What lifestyle factors should be considered?

Based on their own experiences, many women have intuitively understand the importance of proper exercise, healthy diet, and reduction of stress in lessening the severity of symptoms. The effects of diet, exercise, emotions, and stress must be taken into account. Exercise, especially regular aerobic exercise, has been shown to lessen both the amount and degree of premenstrual symptoms, including depression, impaired concentration, and pain. These benefits extend throughout the entire menstrual cycle.[2] The mechanism for the uplifting effects of exercise seems to be reversal of the periovulatory drop in beta-endorphins.[3]

Stress via elevated cortisol levels can cause or exacerbate many of the symptoms commonly seen in PMS, including fatigue, depression, overeating, and weight gain. Finding healthy ways to combat stress, such as meditation, yoga, gardening, taking a hot bath, or whatever the woman finds relaxing, may help decrease stress and PMS symptoms.

7. What biochemical abnormalities are commonly seen in women with PMS?

Clinical studies have uncovered a wide range of physiologic imbalances that are believed to trigger or contribute to PMS. Examples include female sex hormone imbalances, nutritional deficiencies, imbalances in fatty acid metabolism, thyroid dysfunction, glucose/insulin dysregulation, and disruptions of the body's natural circadian rhythms. Through interrelated mechanisms, nutrition, exercise, stress reduction, and hormonal therapies can help to correct these imbalances.

8. How does the female hormone cycle relate to PMS?

Because symptoms of PMS occur regularly at phases of the menstrual cycle, which in turn are modulated by changing levels of the female sex hormones estrogen and progesterone, much clinical research has focused on how imbalances of these two hormones may underlie the onset of PMS.

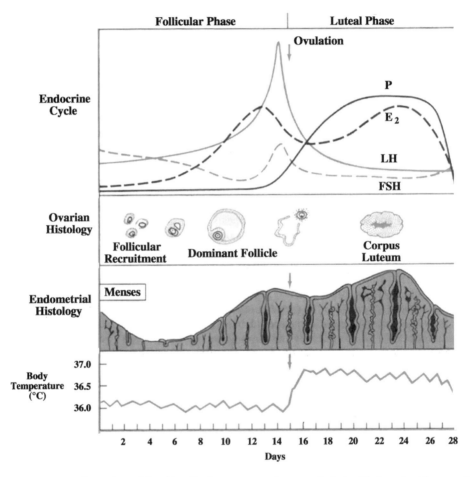

The hormonal, ovarian, endometrial, and basal body temperature changes and relationship throughout the normal menstrual cycle. P = progesterone, E_2 = prostaglandin E_2, LH = luteinizing hormone, FSH = follicle-stimulating hormone. (Adapted from Wilson JD, et al (eds): Harrison's Principles of Medicine, 12th ed. New York, McGraw-Hill. © McGraw-Hill Companies, Inc.),

PMS symptoms occur during the luteal phase of the menstrual cycle. During this phase, which is characterized by an increase in progesterone, the corpus luteum increases production of progesterone and estradiol, the body's main form of estrogen. This process occurs after the midcycle spike in luteinizing hormone (LH), theoretically on day 14 of a typical 28-day cycle. The increase of estrogen and progesterone during the first 4–5 days of the luteal phase promotes endometrial and fallopian tube secretions that allow proper nourishment and implantation of a fertilized ovum.

9. What theories may help to explain PMS?

One theory is that PMS reflects corpus luteum insufficiency, which creates a progesterone deficiency during the luteal phase of the menstrual cycle. Many women report relief of symptoms through progesterone therapy, and this finding is backed by clinical evidence suggesting that progesterone metabolites may act as antianxiety agents in reducing mood swings and anxiety associated with PMS.[4] Another possibility is that progesterone treatment improves symptoms by reducing luteal phase fluid retention.[5]

Progesterone is metabolized in the brain into a sedative-like substance called 3-alpha, 5-alpha-tetrahydropapaveroline (THP), which can reduce anxiety and promote increased activity of gamma-aminobutyric acid, an important amino acid that modulates the activity of brain neurotransmitters linked to depression and seizures. For this reason, symptoms of PMS such as anxiety and seizure susceptibility are associated with sharp declines in circulating progesterone.

10. Does deficient progesterone cause PMS?

The progesterone deficiency theory for PMS has been challenged by some researchers, because older studies have not shown consistent and significant differences in serum estrogen and progesterone levels between PMS sufferers and controls.[6] Women with PMS characterized more by anxiety and irritability may fall into a specific subset of PMS, of which lower progesterone levels are a possible cause.[7] Further research is needed. Some studies have observed a positive correlation between low progesterone levels and PMS symptoms but found a negligible effect—or even a worsening of symptoms—after initiation of progesterone therapy.[8]

One possible explanation for these conflicting results may lie in the biochemical individuality of each woman, which underscores the importance of considering multiple factors in PMS rather than singling out one hormone.

11. What role does estrogen play in PMS?

Both high and low levels of estrogen have been implicated in the etiology of PMS. A common finding in women with PMS is excessive estradiol during the luteal phase. A recent study by Swedish researchers reveals that the severity of PMS symptoms correlates with levels of estradiol during the luteal phase of the menstrual cycle.[9] In addition to an increase in negative mood symptoms such as depression, anxiety, tension, and irritability, this study showed that higher luteal-phase estradiol levels are associated with increased headaches, swelling and breast tenderness.

On the other hand, because optimal levels of estrogen are crucial for the healthy function of important brain neurotransmitters that guard against depression, extreme deficiencies of estrogen during the luteal phase are associated with a relatively rare type of PMS characterized primarily by marked depression.[10]

Many experts believe, however, that the relative balance between progesterone and estradiol over the entire menstrual cycle, rather than isolated imbalances of either hormone alone, is the most important factor to evaluate in women with PMS. Some experts have linked the combination of low progesterone and high estradiol, for example, with a form of PMS characterized by anxiety, irritability, mood swings, and nervousness.[11] Other researchers point to the combination of elevated estrogen with elevated progesterone in the luteal phase as a possible synergistic cause of PMS symptoms.

12. What are some common causes of high levels of estrogen and lower levels of progesterone?

Higher estrogen levels are due to endogenous overproduction (from excessive adipose tissue), exogenous sources, or poor elimination via the liver. There also may be a relative increase in estrogen levels secondary to low progesterone secretion from an improperly functioning corpus luteum. Higher estrogen levels also are associated with vitamin B_6 and B_{12} deficiencies. The liver requires these vitamins for the breakdown and deactivation of estrogen. In addition, the liver requires adequate amounts of vitamins C and E, magnesium and selenium.[12] Good nutrition and optimal hepatic function may help regulate hormone levels naturally without the need for supplemental hormone therapy.

13. What factors can help decrease excess estrogen levels?[13,14]

• Maintenance of ideal weight. Excessive body weight, specifically excessive body fat, leads to increased conversion of circulating hormones into estrogen.

• Adequate fiber. Women with high-fiber diets excrete more estrogen in the feces. Supplementing the diet with high fiber (20 gm wheat bran) can significantly reduce the amount of serum estrogens, thus decreasing the overbalance of estrogen in relation to progesterone.

14. How does inflammation contribute to PMS?

Studies have shown that women with PMS have abnormal serum levels of prostaglandins (PGs) and their precursors.[15] PGs are hormone-like substances that function as mediators in the inflammatory response as well as in vascular dilation and immunity. Prostaglandins can be either pro- or anti-inflammatory. Lower levels of the beneficial, anti-inflammatory prostaglandins (PGE_1 type) are seen in women with PMS. Imbalances in the PG series can produce inflammation in tissues, thus stimulating PMS.[16] For this reason, medications such as nonsteroidal anti-inflammatory drugs (NSAIDs) work better than other analgesics for PMS pain. NSAIDs directly inhibit this part of the inflammatory cascade.

15. Can we alter the production of prostaglandins to favor the anti-inflammatory mediators?

Supplements with essential fatty acids, mainly in the form of gamma linolenic acid (found in evening primrose oil and borage seed oil) should raise PGE_1-type prostaglandins. Studies using these oils, however, show mixed results. Four double-blind, crossover, controlled trials with evening primrose oil showed improvement in most PMS symptoms, mainly in headaches and clumsiness. Treatment doses of gamma-linolenic acid (GLA) ranged from 3 to 4 gm/day.[17]

On the other hand, a diet rich in saturated fats, red meat, eggs, and alcohol has been shown to increase proinflammatory prostaglandins. Poor insulin regulation and stress-mediated release of catecholamines also tip the balance toward inflammation.[18]

16. How do nutritional imbalances affect women with PMS?

Nutritional imbalances can play a profound role in PMS symptoms. Certain foods can directly trigger pathophysiologic mechanisms, whereas lack of others can predispose to PMS. Specific foods that should be avoided in women with PMS include:

• Caffeine, which increases the effects of adrenaline and aggravates stress related symptoms.[19]
• Refined sugar, which depletes the body of chromium, manganese, zinc, magnesium, and most B vitamins. Sugar also increases the tendency for hyperinsulinemia, which in turn increases the tendency for hypoglycemia, giving rise to mood swings, irritability, and headaches.[20]
• Limit intake of dairy and red meat, which tend to promote inflammation.
• Reduce salt intake, especially if susceptible to edema.

17. What other nutrients have been shown to be effective in the treatment of PMS?

Nutritional supplementation has been shown to be effective in controlling PMS symptoms.[21–23] Examples include magnesium, vitamin B_6, zinc, niacin, and vitamin C. Magnesium and B vitamins play an integral role in many biochemical functions related to the development of symptoms involved in PMS. Magnesium, for example, is involved in the conversion of linolenic acid to GLA, a rate-limiting step in anti-inflammatory series 1-type prostaglandins. It is important in the synthesis of dopamine and estrogen conjugation in the liver. Magnesium is also involved in the activation of vitamin B_6. The recommended dose of magnesium is 300 mg 1–3 times/day.

Vitamin B_6 (pyridoxine) is another important cofactor for enzymes involved in estrogen conjugation in the liver. It is essential for the synthesis of several neurotransmitters, including dopamine, serotonin, and norepinephrine, and plays an integral role in prostaglandin synthesis. Vitamin B_6 also stimulates cell membrane transfer of magnesium along with the amino acid taurine. The recommended dose of B_6 is 50–100 mg/day. Pyridoxine can be neurotoxic when taken in dosages greater than 2000 mg/day; in some cases, lower dosages also have neurotoxic effects.

Additional nutrients include:

• Vitamin E (may help to relieve breast tenderness)
• Vitamin B_1 (thiamine; shown to be an effective treatment for dysmenorrhea)[24]
• Calcium carbonate (improves smooth muscle responsiveness)

18. Which herbs are used to treat PMS?[18,27]

- Chaste tree berry (*Vitex agnus-castus*) relieves cramps, water retention, weight gain, and mood swings. Vitex targets the hypothalamic-pituitary axis, which regulates hormone synthesis.
- Cramp bark (*Vibrium opulus*) acts as an antispasmodic, relaxing the uterus.
- Ginger root (*Zingiber officinale*) has been used as an anti-inflammatory herb. It inhibits PG and leukotriene synthesis.
- Don quai root (*Angelica sinensis*) is used to regulate menses and aid in smooth muscle relaxation.
- Licorice root (*Glycerrhiza uralensis*) minimizes the effects of stress by supporting the adrenal glands and aiding digestion. One caution: the rhizome component of true licorice contains substances that can raise blood pressure.

These herbs should be used with the guidance of a trained herbalist practitioner.

19. Discuss the role of hormone testing in women with PMS.

Hormone testing is not essential in evaluating and treating a patient with PMS. Diagnosis of PMS is usually made by observation of symptoms and their occurrence during the luteal phase of the menstrual cycle. Because most women with PMS show no difference in absolute level of hormones, assessment of hormone levels appears to have limited value. However, in the small portion of women who in fact have notable hormonal imbalances, testing can be helpful and also can be used as a guide for the practitioner in deciding whether to use hormones as a form of treatment.

Urine and serum levels of progesterone may be helpful in determining corpus luteum insufficiency. These samples measure one level of the hormone progesterone, on day 21 or 3 weeks after the onset of menstruation. Levels below normal indicate possible luteal dysfunction. Salivary testing, which measures the bioavailable protion of progesterone, also can be beneficial.[25] The advantage of salivary testing is that it is noninvasive, making it easier for women to sample hormone levels throughout the entire menstrual cycle. Serial samples reveal patterns of deficiencies or excesses that do not show up on a single sample. Because scientific research has associated so many different patterns of female hormone imbalances with PMS, a comprehensive evaluation of sex hormone activity over the complete menstrual cycle may be helpful in establishing the specific needs of each woman.

20. Do natural hormones have a role in the treatment of PMS?

Hormone therapy is often considered for PMS when the woman does not respond to lifestyle and nutritional therapies. Synthetic oral contraceptives have not been documented as effective treatment of PMS.[26] Natural progesterone (see Chapter 38) is becoming more popular and is widely used to treat PMS.[4,5,27] Many holistic practitioners believe that it is important to document baseline progesterone levels via laboratory testing before embarking on replacement therapy. Natural progesterone creams can be used topically or orally.

Oral micronized: 300 mg/day (100 mg in the morning and 200 mg in the evening). Use for approximately 10 days, starting 3 days after ovulation and discontinuing 1 day before menses.

Cream: Apply one-fourth teaspoon (400 mg per ounce of cream) twice daily, starting at mid cycle and stopping on the day before menses.

21. What about use of antidepressants for PMS?

Although allopathic medicine has been slow to recognize PMS as a true medical entity, some antidepressant medications are specifically marketed for its treatment. Sarafem is the same as fluoxetine, also sold as Prozac. Although selective serotonin reuptake inhibitors (SSRIs) may be effective in treating true depressive symptoms associated with PMS, the underlying hormonal, nutritional, and inflammatory components as well as the underlying cause of PMS itself may not be fully addressed. Use of an SSRI requires a physician's supervision to monitor for efficacy and adverse side effects.

22. How do you summarize an integrated approach to PMS?

First it is important to determine whether in fact you are dealing with PMS or perhaps another type of pathology (e.g., hypothyroidism or depression; see question 4). Once the diagnosis of PMS is established, individualizing the treatment begins with the patient's self-awareness of her unique cyclic behavioral and body changes. It is important, therefore, to take a thorough history, including a record of daily diet, exercise routine, life stressors, and techniques for stress management. Nutrition and exercise therapies are the first steps in PMS management and often result in significant improvement. Nutritional therapies include avoidance of exacerbating factors (e.g., refined sugar, caffeine, saturated fats) and incorporation of beneficial foods and nutrients (e.g., high fiber, magnesium, B vitamins, calcium). Diet and lifestyle changes are not only challenging to achieve but also can take time to show effects. In addition, because every woman has unique contributing factors, the physician's support and patience help dramatically. Botanical, pharmacologic, and hormonal therapies can be considered if lifestyle changes alone are not effective in controlling PMS symptoms.

REFERENCES

1. Mortola JF, Girton L, Beck L, Yen SS: Diagnosis of premenstrual syndrome by a simple prospective reliable instrument. Obstet Gynecol 76:302, 1990.
2. Aganoff J, Boyle GJ: Aerobic exercise, mood states, and menstrual cycle symptoms. J Psychosom Res 38(3): 83–92, 1994.
3. Chuong CJ, Hsi BP, Gibbons WE: Periovulatory β-endorphin levels in premenstrual syndrome. Obstet Gynec 83(5 Pt 1):755–760, 1994.
4. Baker ER, Best RG, Manfredi RL, et al: Efficacy of progesterone vaginal suppositories in alleviation of nervous symptoms in patients with premenstrual syndrome. J Assist Reprod Genet 12:205–209, 1995.
5. Watanabe H, Lau DC, Guyn HL, Wong NL: Effect of progesterone therapy on arginine vasopressin and atrial natriuretic factor in premenstrual syndrome. Clin Invest Med 20(4):211–223, 1997.
6. Andersch B, Abrahamsson L, et al: Hormone profile in premenstrual tension: Effects of bromocriptine and diuretics. Clin Endocrinol 11:657–664, 1979.
7. Abraham GE: Nutritional factors in the etiology of PMS. J Reprod Med 28 446–464, 1983.
8. Tiemstra JD, Patel K: Hormonal therapy in the management of premenstrual syndrome. J Am Board Fam Pract 11(5):378–381, 1998.
9. Seippel L, Backstrom T: Luteal -phase estradiol relates to symptom severity in patients with premenstrual syndrome. J Clin Endocrinol Metab 83:1988–1993, 1998.]
10. Hammarback S, Damber JE, Backstrom T: Relationship between symptom severity and hormone changes in women with premenstrual syndrome. J Clin Endocrinol Metab 68:125–130, 1989.
11. Fink G, Sumner BE, Rosie R, et al: Estrogen control of central neurotransmission: Effect on mood, mental state, and memory. Cell Mol Neurobiol 16:325–344, 1996.
12. Kleijnen J, ter Jtiet G, Knipschild P: Vitamin B6 in the treatment of PMS: A review. Br J Obstet Gynaec 97:847–852, 1990.
13. Goldin BR, Aldercruetz H, et al: Estrogen excretion patterns and plasma levels in vegetarian and omnivorous women. N Engl J Med 307:1542–1547, 1982.
14. Rose DP, et al : Effects of diet supplementation with wheat bran on serum estrogen levels in the follicular and luteal phases of the menstrual cycle. Nutrition. 13:535–539,1997.
15. Koshikawa N, Tatsunuma T, Furuya K, Seki K: Prostaglandins and premenstrual syndrome. Prostaglandin Leukot Essent Fatty Acids 45:33–36, 1992.
16. Brush MG, Watson SJ, Horrobin DF, Manku MS: Abnormal essential fatty acid levels in plasma of women with premenstrual syndrome. Am J Obstet Gynecol 150:363–366, 1984.
17. Severino SK, Moline ML: Premenstrual Syndrome: A Clinician's Guide. New York, Guilford Press, 1989.
18. Pizzorno J, Murray MT. Premenstrual syndrome. In Encyclopedia of Natural Medicine, 2nd ed. Rocklin, CA, Prima Publishing, 1998, pp 730–752.
19. Rossignol AM: Caffeine containing beverages, total fluid consumption and PMS. Am J Public Health 80: 1106–1110, 1990.
20. Rossignol AM, Bonnlander H: Prevalence and severity of PMS symptoms: Effects of food and beverages that are sweet or high in sugar content. J reproduct Med 36(2): 131–136, 1991.
21. Werbach M: Textbook of Nutritional Medicine. Tarzana, CA, Third Line Press, 1999.
22. Mayo JL: Premenstrual syndrome: A natural approach to management. Appl Nutr Sci Rep 5:1–8, 1999.
23. Facchinetti F, Borella P, Sances G, et al: Oral magneisum successfully relieves premenstrual mood changes. Obstet Gynecol 78(2):177–181, 1991.
24. Wilson ML, Murphy PA: Herbal and dietary therapies for primary and secondary dysmenorrhoea. Cochrane Library, vol. 3, Oxford, Update Software, 2001.
25. Lu Y, Bentley GR, et al: Salivary estradiol and progesterone levels in conception and nonconception cycles in women: evaluation of a new assay for salivary estradiol. Fertil Steril 71:863–8,1999.
26. Smith S, Schiff I: The premenstrual syndrome diagnosis and management. Fertil Steril 4:54–59, 1989.
27. Hudson T: Women's Encyclopedia of Natural Medicine. CITY, Keats, 1999.

40. PREGNANCY

Aviva Romm, CPM, AHG

1. Should alternative and complementary medicine (CAM) therapies be used during pregnancy?

Because of physiologic changes in the mother and unknown effects on the fetus, care should be exercised in using many CAM therapies during pregnancy. Routine prenatal visits with an appropriately trained professional is of paramount importance. Some CAM techniques, such as massage therapy, have been well-studied, and pregnant women can seek a qualified professional for care. Other therapies, such as the use of herbal medicines, have not been as well studied for safety and efficacy during pregnancy, largely because of ethical constraints in testing pregnant women. Furthermore, controls over manufacturing of dietary supplements in the United States, including herbal medicines, homeopathic preparations, and essential oils, do not always prevent adulteration or contamination of products, leading to additional potential problems. However, when such therapies are used carefully and appropriately, they can provide great benefits in relieving common discomforts associated with the childbearing cycle, and in many cases they may be safer than comparable pharmaceutical preparations. Expert consultation should be sought about the use of natural therapies during pregnancy.

2. Are homeopathic remedies safe and effective for use during pregnancy?

Homeopathic remedies are infinitesimally reduced quantities of herbal, mineral, and animal-derived substances given to treat symptoms similar to those that would be caused by ingestion of large amounts of the remedy. Hence, the fundamental principle of homeopathy is "like cures like" (see Chapter 13). Homeopathic preparations contain no chemical trace of the original substance from which the remedy was prepared, nonetheless, caution should be used when administering homeopathics that are derived from substances known to be toxic or otherwise contraindicated during pregnancy.

3. Should essential oils be used during pregnancy?

Essential oils are highly concentrated extracts of the volatile oil component of plants, capable of crossing the placenta and reaching the developing fetus. Many also cross the blood-brain barrier, and most essential oils, taken internally in even moderate quantities, are toxic and can even be fatal. Used externally in small quantities—diluted in a neutral carrier oil (such as almond or avocado oil, which is easily absorbed) for massage; added to the bath (7–10 drops); or placed in an aromatherapy diffuser—essential oils can be quite safe and beneficial in relieving many common complaints of pregnancy, including nausea, stress, fatigue, and headache. They should never be used internally during pregnancy.

4. Can herbal medicines be used safely during pregnancy?

Yes. Herbs and spices are consumed daily around the world by pregnant women as a natural part of the diet. By taking small amounts and using only herbs that are known to be safe during pregnancy, women can obtain relief for many minor pregnancy complaints; in expert hands, herbs also can be used for more complex pregnancy-related problems. However, herbs are also potent medicinal agents; therefore, great care and precaution are advised during pregnancy.

Whenever possible, avoid the use of herbs during the first trimester. If it is necessary to use herbs during this time, use only herbs with no known teratogenic or abortifacient properties under the supervision of a professional knowledgeable about the use of herbs during pregnancy and in the lowest possible doses. Carefully follow guidelines for avoiding herbs that are contraindicated during pregnancy, and use only herbs that are considered safe when necessary.

5. What are the key points to remember in using herbal therapies during pregnancy?

Although many herbal remedies are gentle and safe, they are also pharmacologically active agents that should be administered with care. Consider the following key points:

- Natural is not synonymous with harmless or safe. Many botanical medicines contain potent pharmacological substances.
- Most herbal constituents are capable of passing through the placenta and can therefore directly affect the fetus.
- Physiologic and metabolic changes during pregnancy may influence pharmacokinetics.
- Unless they are medically indicated, avoid use of herbs (and drugs) during the first trimester.
- Preventive treatment and early intervention with herbs are safer and more effective than treating advanced problems.
- Know your herbs, work simply and gently whenever possible, and clearly understand side-effects and contraindications for herbs in pregnant women.

6. Which forms of administration can be used for herbal therapies during pregnancy.

Botanical medicines can be administered in a variety of forms. Those most commonly used methods during pregnancy are internal (teas, infusions, syrups, tinctures [alcohol- and glycerol-based], capsules, enemas) and external (oils, baths, compresses, periwashes [teas put into a squeeze bottle and used to lavage the perianal area], creams).

Each of the internal forms offers specific advantages and disadvantages. For example, infusions are mild, effective, and generally safe. However, because of the volume required for an effective dose, the amount of liquid or taste may be prohibitive to pregnant women. Tinctures provide small, concentrated doses but contain alcohol. Therefore, one must choose the method most appropriate to the patient's needs. Convenience to the patient is always important. Many herbal preparations can be absorbed transdermally, making baths an effective mode of administration when used correctly.

7. What herbs should be avoided during pregnancy?

The following list is a composite of some of the herbs most commonly contraindicated for use during pregnancy. Some herbs on this list may be used in small quantities for certain conditions, under expert guidance. In addition, certain herbs that are contraindicated by western scientific research for use during pregnancy are regularly used in other countries. For example, tang gui (*Angelica sinensis*) is prescribed as a blood tonic for pregnant women in China. However, it is wise to use such herbs cautiously if at all during pregnancy. For more information about herbs contraindicated during pregnancy see McGuffin et al., *The Botanical Safety Handbook*: "Class 2b . . . herbs not to be used during pregnancy unless otherwise directed by an expert qualified in the appropriate use of this substance."[1]

A few basic groups of herbs are contraindicated for use during pregnancy, such as those containing pyrrolizidine alkaloids (PAs), which are known to cause liver damage in fetuses. Comfrey, coltsfoot, and borage are the main suspects because they contain varying amounts of PAs. They should be avoided for internal use, and topical use should be avoided in patients with broken skin.

Herbs with strong hormonal properties and those that are known to promote menstruation (emmenagogues) should be used with caution. Stimulating laxatives, as well as anthelmintics and vermifuges are contraindicated, as is the internal use of all essential oils.

Aloe *(Aloe vera)*	Licorice *(Glycyrrhiza glabra)*
Barberry *(Berberis vulgaris)*	Lily of the valley *(Convallaria majalis)*
Blood root *(Sanguinaria canadensis)*	Lobelia *(Lobelia inflata)*
Blue Cohosh *(Caulophyllum thalyctroides)*	Mistletoe *(Viscum album)*
Coltsfoot *(Tussilago farfara)*	Mugwort *(Artemisia vulgaris)*
Comfrey *(Symphytum officinale)*	Osha *(Ligusticum porten)*
Damiana *(Turnera diffusa)*	Pennyroyal *(Mentha pulegium)*
Dong quai *(Angelica sinensis)*	Rhubarb *(Rheum palmatum)*
Ephedra, ma huang *(Ephedra vulgaris)*	Sage *(Salvia officinalis)*
Feverfew *(Tanacetum parthenium)*	Senna *(Cassia senna)*
Goldenseal *(Hydrastis canadensis)*	Thuja *(Thuja occidentalis)*
Ipecac *(Cephalis ipecacuanha)*	Wormwood *(Artemisia absinthium)*
Juniper berries *(Juniperus communis)*	Yarrow *(Achillea millefolium)*

Romm A: The Natural Pregnancy Book. Freedom, CA, Crossing Press, 1997.

8. **Should herbal laxatives be used during pregnancy?**

Herbs, such as cascara sagrada and senna, that strongly promote bowel peristalsis and act as laxatives should be avoided during pregnancy because they can promote uterine contractions as well as bowel evacuation. Other methods of promoting bowel functioning should be used, such as dietary changes, exercises, and bulk or nutritive laxatives (e.g., flax, psyllium seeds).

9. **Can herbs and supplements be used safely to reduce morning sickness?**

In one double-blind, randomized, cross-over, placebo-controlled study,[2] **ginger** was found to be significantly more effective than placebo for relieving the symptoms of morning sickness. Although no reports of teratogenicity or mutagenicity due to ginger are found in the literature, some concern has arisen over its ability to inhibit platelet function. Ginger is considered safe to use in small amounts for the reduction of nausea and vomiting of pregnancy but should be used carefully, and dosage should not exceed the quantity used in the clinical trial (1 gm/day). For best results, ginger is taken as a tea or capsule.

Vitamin B$_6$ (pyridoxine) has been used since at least the 1940s to treat morning sickness. In a recent double-blind, randomized trial[3] in pregnant women at less than 17 weeks' gestation, vitamin B$_6$ was shown to have a statistically significant effect in reducing nausea and vomiting. The dose used was 30 mg, but some experts postulate that slightly higher doses may be more effective.

10. **What are the basic guidelines for nutrition during pregnancy?**

Expectant mothers should eat a well-balanced diet, with 70–90 gm/day of protein and a variety of fresh fruits, vegetables and whole grains. Supplemental prenatal vitamins should include 400 μg of folic acid to prevent neural tube defects, 1500 mg of calcium, and appropriate amounts of B vitamins, vitamin E, and minerals. Megavitamin therapy should be strictly avoided during pregnancy. Excessive vitamin A can lead to teratogenesis, although daily doses less than 5000 IU have been reported as safe.[4] Excessive vitamin C also can be hazardous. One case report series found that infants born to women taking more than 5000 mg/day of vitamin C during pregnancy developed rebound scurvy from the relative lack of vitamin C after delivery.[5] Of course, avoid alcohol completely, and limit caffeine consumption to less than 300 mg/day (greater amounts have been associated with intrauterine growth retardation).[6]

11. **Are herbs effective for the treatment of urinary tract infections during pregnancy?**

Numerous studies[7] demonstrate the safety and efficacy of cranberry juice (*Vaccinium macrocarpon*) for the treatment of urinary tract infection (UTI), a common problem of pregnancy due to the physiologic displacement of the growing uterus onto the ureters and increased urinary stasis due to bladder compression. Cranberry prevents the adherence of bacterial organisms to the bladder wall, thus reducing infection. Daily intake of cranberry juice as a dietary beverage is advisable for women with a history of chronic UTI. For the treatment of acute UTI, a woman may consume up to 6 glasses of cranberry juice per day. Unremitting or worsening symptoms require medical treatment. Cranberry juice and reconstituted cranberry concentrate are considered completely safe during pregnancy; however, concentrated cranberry products should be avoided, because they have not been evaluated for use during pregnancy.

12. **Define partus preparators. Are they are safe and effective during pregnancy?**

Partus preparators are herbs used during the last weeks of pregnancy to tone and prepare the uterus for labor. Historically they have been used to ensure a speedy delivery. Typical partus preparators include blue cohosh (*Caulophyllum thalictroides*), black cohosh (*Cimicifuga racemosa*), partridge berry (*Mitchella repens*), and spikenard (*Aralia racemosa*). The use of such herbs to prepare women for labor begs the question of why one would use an herbal preparation to prepare the body for something it naturally knows how to do. Furthermore, the safety of these herbs before the onset of labor is questionable. At least one recent report[8–10] implicates the use of blue cohosh in late pregnancy as a cause of myocardial infarction in the neonate. This herb contains a number of potent alkaloids, including methylcystine and anagyrine. Anagyrine is known to have an effect on cardiac muscle activity. It is therefore prudent to avoid the use of partus preparators, particularly those containing blue cohosh.

13. Is moxibustion effective for breech presentation?

Traditional Chinese medicine has long used moxibustion for the treatment of breech presentation during pregnancy (see Chapter 12). Moxibustion is the indirect application of the heated herb *Artmesia vulgaris*, usually in the form of a cigar-like roll, to acupuncture point bladder 67 (located on the outside corner of the small toe), which for unknown reasons may result in spontaneous turning of the fetus to a vertex position. A randomized, control trial[11] concluded that, when performed for 1–2 weeks from the 33rd week of pregnancy, moxibustion is an effective method for turning a breech infant.

However, a significant number of breech infants turn spontaneously between 33 and 37 weeks of pregnancy, regardless of intervention. In fact, conventional obstetric efforts to rectify a breech presentation to a vertex presentation are not begun until between 36 and 38 weeks for this reason. Therefore, although moxibustion treatment appears to be safe and may be effective, the study cannot be considered conclusive evidence of its efficacy.

14. How safe is home birth with a midwife?

Fortunately, this question is also being asked by researchers, physicians, and midwives world-wide, and a wealth of statistical evidence helps to answer this safety question. Although no method of care can guarantee any specific "safe" outcomes in child-bearing, statistical evidence based on numerous studies of midwifery care and out-of-hospital birth sites, including freestanding birthing centers and domicilliary sites (homes), is exceptionally encouraging about the safety of child-bearing when care is provided in an out-of-hospital setting. In general, midwifery care has been shown to improve general outcomes for women and infants from a large variety of socioeconomic backgrounds and to reduce difficult outcomes even in situations of moderately high risk.

15. How does midwifery care compare with obstetric care in terms of safety?

The World Health Organization (WHO), which has closely evaluated the safety of midwifery care, has recommended midwives as the ideal care providers for child-bearing women worldwide. It cannot be overstated that conventional obstetrics is essential for women with high-risk pregnancies and for obstetrical emergencies. Although 90% of all births are normal and uncomplicated, in the United States, where 96% of babies are born in the hospital with obstetricians in attendance, the infant mortality rate ranks 23rd in the world. In stark contrast, in the Netherlands, where midwives deliver 50% of infants, and Sweden, where midwives deliver nearly 100%, the infant mortality rates rank fourth and seventh, respectively.[12]

Numerous studies, some of which have been controlled, have shown that maternity care provided by nurse-midwives and other midwives in hospitals, birth centers, and homes results in birth-weights, infant mortality rates, and other health indicators similar to or better than those obtained by specialists in acute medical settings.[13]

16. Can having a doula during labor make a difference?

Yes, significantly so. The word *doula* refers to an experienced woman who provides support for a new mother in her infant care duties. Precedent in Guatemala shows that the continuous presence of a female companion during labor and delivery results in fewer obstetric interventions, shorter labor, and fewer perinatal complications in newborns. A well-conducted study in the U.S.[14] used doulas to provide continuous emotional support to first-time mothers during labor. The doula stayed by the mother's bedside during the entire hospitalized period, soothing and touching the mother, and provided a layperson's description of what was occurring and likely to happen next. Impressive reductions were seen in the use of epidural anesthesia (about 8% in doula group compared with 55% in controls) as well as the rate of cesarean section (8% compared with 18%). This simple behavioral intervention seems to be a win-win situation for new mothers and their infants, and, if implemented more broadly, could result in significant savings in hospital labor and delivery care.

17. Do herbal therapies have a role in the treatment of postpartum perineal discomfort?

Astringent herbs (e.g., witch hazel, white oak bark), vulnerary herbs (e.g., calendula), and antiseptic herbs (e.g., sage, myrrh) can be made into a tea that can be applied to the perineum via a periwash (see question 6) or sitz-bath. These herbs can accelerate the healing process for superficial perineal tears and episiotomy, reduce swelling and bruising, and reduce pain and soreness. Use 7 gm of each herb, and steep in 2 liters of water for 30 minutes. Strain and place in the peribottle or sitz bath. Use once or twice daily for up to 5 days postnatally.

18. How can herbs be used successfully to support lactation?

Herbs have been used for centuries to improve the quantity and quality of breast milk. Warm drinks in general may be beneficial, because adequate fluids are essential for proper breast milk production. Fenugreek is commonly used to promote increased lactation. It is generally recommended as safe by the Food and Drug Administration, and the American Herbal Products Association does not consider it contraindicated for breast-feeding mothers.[1,15]

19. What herbs should be avoided during lactation?

As during pregnancy, a number of herbs should not be consumed during lactation because of possible harmful effects on the newborn (see partial list below). These herbs may be different than those not to be consumed during pregnancy. For more information about herbs contraindicated during lactation, see *The Botanical Safety Handbook,* "Class 2c . . . not to be used while nursing unless otherwise directed by an expert qualified in the appropriate use of this substance":

Alkanet	Bladderwrack	Coltsfoot	Garlic	Purging buckthorn
Aloe vera	Borage	Comfrey	Joe pye	Senna
Aloes	Bugleweed	Elecampane	Licorice	Stillingia
Basil	Cascara sagrada	Ephedra	Male fern	Wormwood
Black cohosh	Chinese rhubarb			

20. Is fatty acid supplementation necessary during pregnancy and breast-feeding?

Essential fatty acids are considered crucial for optimal human development and wellness, yet they cannot be synthesized by the human body. According to recent research,[16] the maternal diet should contain adequate essential fatty acids not only for the mother's nutritional needs but also for the developing fetus. Furthermore, breast milk may be a poor source of essential fatty acids if maternal intake is inadequate. Essential fatty acids consumption may be optimized by the regular consumption of cold water fish such as salmon in the maternal diet, or they may be supplemented by the addition of DHA in the form of fish oil (to be used under medical direction during pregnancy to avoid excessive vitamin A intake), alginate-based DHA, evening primrose oil, or flax seed oil.

REFERENCES

1. McGuffin M, et al: Botanical Safety Handbook. New York, CRC Press, 1997.
2. Fischer-Rasmussen W, Kjaer WK, Dah C, Asping U: Ginger treatment of hyperemesis gravidarum. Eur J Obstet Gynecol Reprod Biol 38:19–24, 1990.
3. Vutyananich T, et al: Pyridoxine for nausea and vomiting of pregnancy: A randomized, double-blind, placebo-controlled trial. Am J Obstet Gynecol 173:881–884, 1995.
4. Werback MR: Pregnancy-related illness. Nutritional Influences on Illness, 2nd ed. Tarzana CA, Third Line Press, 1996, p 526.
5. Rhead WJ, Schrauzer GN: Risks of long-term ascorbic acid overdosage. Nutr Rev 29(11):262–223,1971.
6. Berger A: Effects of caffeine consumption on pregnancy outcome. A review. J Reprod Med 33:945–956, 1988.
7. Upton R: Cranberry. In Upton R (ed): American Herbal Pharmacopoeia and Therapeutic Compendium, Santa Cruz, CA, American Herbal Pharmacopoeia, 2002, p 28.
8. Wright IM: Neonatal effects of maternal consumption of blue cohosh. J Pediatrics 134:384–385, 1999.
9. Brinker F: Blue cohosh. J Am Herb Guild 2(2):4–8, 2001.
10. LowDog T: Blue cohosh and myocardial infarction in a newborn. J Am Herb Guild 2(2):9–10, 2001.
11. Cardini F, Huang Weixin: Moxabustion for correction of breech presentation: A randomized controlled trial. JAMA 280:1580–1584, 1998.
12. World Population Data Sheet. Washington, DC, Population Reference Bureau, 1988.
13. Women's Institute for Childbearing Policy, 1994, Roxbury, VT.
14. Kennell J, Klaus M, et al: Continuous emotional support during labor in a U.S. hospital: A randomized controlled trial. JAMA 265:2197-2201,1991.
15. LowDog T: An Integrative Approach to Women's Health. Integrative Medical Education Association, 2001.
16. Hornstra G: Essential fatty acids in mothers and their neonates. Am J Clin Nutr 71(5):126–129, 2000.

41. BENIGN PROSTATIC HYPERTROPHY

David Rakel, M.D.

1. Describe the presentation of benign prostatic hypertrophy (BPH).

Symptoms usually begin in men in their late 50s or early 60s, and the condition tends to be progressive over time. Classical symptoms include nocturia, urinary frequency, difficulty with urinating, dribbling of urine, reduction of urinary stream, incomplete emptying of the bladder, and, when symptoms become severe, urinary retention. Mild symptoms should be treated if they are being disruptive to the patient's lifestyle. Severe symptoms can lead to incomplete emptying that result in urinary tract infections and a back-pressure of urine causing kidney damage and uremia.

2. Describe the underlying pathophysiology of BPH.

Although BPH is one of the most common diseases of aging men, its etiology remains relatively unknown. From our current understanding, it appears to be related to age, androgens, estrogens, and detrusor dysfunction of the bladder neck. An accumulation of dihydrotestosterone (DHT) inhibits prostatic cell death and promotes cell proliferation that increases the size of the gland.

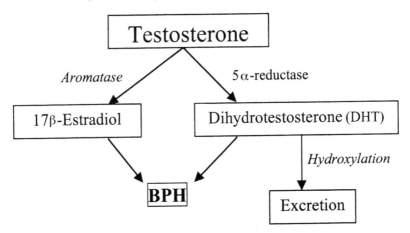

Proposed pathophysiology of benign prostatic hypertrophy.

As men pass the fifth decade, serum testosterone levels decrease and serum levels of estrogen (as well as prolactin, luteinizing hormone, and follicle-stimulating hormone) increase. Estrogen increases the number of androgen (DHT) receptors in the prostate and inhibits its metabolism by interfering with hydroxylation. As urinary outflow obstruction develops, the detrusor muscles of the bladder try to compensate by increasing pressure to expel urine, which leads to instability of the muscle and worsening symptoms. In summary, factors that promote the accumulation of DHT and estrogens lead to symptoms of BPH and obstruction of the lower urinary tract that leads to detrusor muscle dysfunction. Stimulation of the alpha-adrenergic system leads to contraction of the smooth muscle fiber, resulting in further flow restriction in an enlarged gland. Finally, prostaglandins and leukotrienes also play a role in the inflammatory process of the prostate.

3. What are xenobiotics? How do they affect the prostate?

A xenobiotic is any chemical or toxin that is foreign to the body. Many herbicides, pesticides, and plastics fall into this category and can worsen BPH by altering hormone metabolism and mimicking estrogen's effect on the body. Meat, poultry, and dairy products often contain residues of estrogenic hormones (xenoestrogens, or foreign estrogens), which are used to increase meat and milk production and can stimulate prostate cell growth and increase the risk of BPH as well as prostate cancer. Xenobiotic exposure should be reduced by limiting the intake of meat, poultry, and dairy or by consuming organic, hormone-free products. Eating organic produce and using a water-purifying system also reduce exposure to these chemicals.[1]

4. What role does soy play in the treatment and prevention of BPH?

Soy is thought to work in two ways. It is an inhibitor of 5α-reductase, which reduces DHT build-up. Soy is also a low-potency estrogen that may block the receptor sites that stronger estrogens use to increase the accumulation of DHT. Epidemiologic studies show an association with a lower incidence of prostate cancer in Asian men who consume soy products in their diet, and there are supporting in vitro data as well.[2]

Beta-sitosterol (a major phytosterol found in soy), at a dose of 20 mg/day, was found to increase urinary flow and decrease residual volume in the bladder in a double-blind, placebo-controlled study.[3] A 3.5-ounce serving of soybeans, tofu, or other soy food preparation provides approximately 90 mg of beta-sitosterol.[4] A 1-ounce preparation (which is a portion about the size of the palm of the hand) equals approximately 25 mg.

5. Does reducing serum cholesterol help BPH?

Cholesterol has been associated not only with BPH but also with prostate cancer. Its metabolites (epoxychoesterols) have been found to accumulate in the hyperplastic and cancerous prostate gland. For this reason hypocholesterolemic drugs (HMG-CoA reductase inhibitors or "statins") have been associated with a lower risk of BPH and prostate cancer.[5] Limited evidence supports this indication, but a diet low in cholesterol is beneficial not only for the prostate, but also for general health.

6. How can diet and nutrition influence the symptoms of BPH?

Prostaglandins and leukotrienes are inflammatory mediators that promote inflammation of the prostate gland. There are different types of prostaglandins: those that promote inflammation (PGE-2 family) and those with anti-inflammatory properties (PGE-1 and 3). The proinflammatory prostaglandins (PGE-2) and leukotrienes arise from arachidonic acid, which is consumed in the diet mainly in the form of animal foods, including meat and dairy. The anti-inflammatory prostaglandins (PGE-1 and 3) arise from the consumption of omega-3 fatty acids. A diet rich in omega-3 fatty acids helps reduce the influence of prostaglandins and leukotrienes on the inflammatory component of BPH. Recommend foods rich in omega-3 fatty acids, such as cold-water fish (salmon, mackerel and sardines), green vegetables, and ground flax seed. Encourage patients to limit red meat, dairy, and fried foods.

7. Should omega-3 rich oils be recommended for the treatment of BPH?

It is always best to improve the beneficial influences of omega-3 fatty acids via whole foods. Limited research recommends supplementing omega-3 for BPH, but if the patient is unable to change his diet, appropriate doses of omega-3 rich oils may provide benefit. These oils, which include fish, flax seed, and hemp oils, have been found beneficial for many inflammatory conditions. But if taken in too high of a dose, they may do more harm than good. When the body breaks these fatty acids down into energy, free radicals are produced. If excessive amounts are consumed, these pro-oxidants worsen inflammation by mobilizing arachidonic acid into inflammatory mediators. Doses should be limited to less than 4 gm/day to prevent this side effect, and 1–2 gm/day is the recommended starting dose. Flaxseed oil or fish oil is used at a dose of 500 mg, 2–4 capsules twice daily. Flaxseed has twice the amount of omega-3 fatty acids as fish oil and is much cheaper. Ground flax seeds may be better than using the oil because they contain more of the fiber compound called lignan. Lignan binds to testosterone, resulting in lower levels—beneficial for both BPH and prostate cancer prevention.

8. What herbs, supplements, or pharmaceuticals can worsen symptoms of BPH?

Over-the-counter cold remedies or diet aids often contain substances that stimulate the sympathetic nervous system. This stimulation leads to increased tone of the detrusor muscles of the bladder and of the smooth muscle of the prostate, resulting in urinary retention. Over-the-counter hormonal products also should be avoided because of their influence on prostatic cell growth, as should pharmaceuticals with anticholinergic properties that can lead to urinary retention.

Products that Worsen Symptoms of Benign Prostatic Hypertrophy

Over-the-counter cold remedies	Hormonal products	
Pseudoephedrine	Dehydroepiandrosterone (DHEA)	Human growth hormone
Phenylpropanolamine (PPA)	Androstenedione	Estrogens and testosterone
Herbs	**Pharmaceuticals**	
Ma huang (ephedra)	Antihistamines	Tricyclic antidepressants
	Bowel antispasmodics	Antipsychotics
Caffeine	Bladder antispasmodics	

9. How does zinc influence BPH?

Intestinal uptake of zinc is inhibited by estrogen. Because estrogen levels increase in aging men, zinc levels may be low. In fact, marginal zinc deficiency is common in the elderly and may worsen the symptoms of BPH. Research in the 1970s showed that zinc supplementation reduces the size of the prostate gland and symptoms of BPH.[6] Further research has shown that zinc inhibits 5α-reductase[7] and inhibits the binding of androgens to their receptors in the prostate.[8] This latter effect is thought to result from the ability of zinc to inhibit prolactin, which, like estrogen, increases the receptors for DHT in the prostate. Zinc not only decreases the production of DHT; it also inhibits binding to its receptors. Unfortunately, recent studies showing therapeutic benefit are limited.

Prescription drugs that can result in low serum zinc levels include thiazide diuretics, steroids, and methotrexate. Consider zinc supplementation in patients with BPH taking these medications. But do not give zinc to men taking tetracycline or flouroquinalone antibiotics because zinc can affect their absorption.

The dose of zinc is 30 mg/day, best taken with food. Caution should be used in men taking more than 50 mg/day, which can lead to malabsorption of copper, iron, and calcium.

10. What are plant sterols? What role do they play in BPH?

A sterol is a plant steroid that is found in many herbs used in the treatment of BPH, including saw palmetto, soy products, pygeum bark, stinging nettle root, and pumpkin seed extract. Beta-sitosterol is one of the main sterols and is thought to be an active agent in improving BPH symptoms. The exact mechanism of action remains unknown, but the underlying properties of sterols may provide some clues. First of all, sterols block the absorption of cholesterol from the intestinal tract. In fact, sterols from vegetable oils are the active ingredient in cholesterol-lowering margarines such as Benecol and Take Control. As discussed above, lowering cholesterol has been shown to have a beneficial effect on BPH, in part because the prostate synthesizes testosterone from cholesterol. Sterols also may improve the hormonal influence on BPH because they cannot be converted into testosterone in the human body. These compounds seem to be a recurring theme in the herbal treatment of BPH.

11. Which herbs are used most commonly for the treatment of BPH?

The most commonly used and best-studied herbal therapy for BPH is saw palmetto (*Serenoa repens*). Other herbs that have shown benefit include rye grass pollen (*Secale cereale*), pygeum (*Prunus africana*), stinging nettles (*Urtica dioica*), and pumpkin seed extract (*Cucurbita pepo*).

12. What is known about the role of saw palmetto in the treatment of BPH?

Saw palmetto is a small palm tree found along the coastal Southeastern United States and West Indies. The exact mechanism of action in relieving BPH symptoms remains elusive. It has been found to be a weak inhibitor of 5α-reductase but may have a more active role in reducing the number of estrogen and androgen (DHT) receptors. In addition, saw palmetto may have an anti-inflammatory effect on the prostate by inhibiting the metabolism of inflammatory mediators from arachidonic acid. Saw palmetto decreases the inner prostatic epithelium but does not shrink the size of the gland. Nonetheless, it has been found to improve symptom scores, nocturia, residual urine, and urinary flow in patients with BPH. It was found to be as effective as finasteride (Proscar) without the side effects[9] (finasteride is not considered first-line therapy in the treatment of BPH.)

Saw palmetto does not effect levels of prostate-specific antigen (PSA)[10] and is indicated for mild-to-moderate symptoms of BPH. The most beneficial extract is standardized to at least 85% fatty acids and 0.2% sterols. For example, a 160-mg pill should have a minimum of 136 mg fatty acids and 0.32 mg sterols. The usual dose is 160 mg 2 times/day. Allow 8 weeks for therapeutic benefit to be seen.

13. How can rye grass pollen be of help in BPH?

Rye grass pollen is also known as grass pollen and grass pollen extract. Clinical studies used a form called Cernilton (flower pollen), a brand manufactured by Cernitin. This extract has been used in Europe for BPH for more than 35 years. Double-blind clinical studies have found it to be effective with an overall response rate near 70%.[11] Rye grass contains a substance that has been found to inhibit prostatic cell growth[12] as well as reduce inflammation of the prostate by inhibiting prostaglandins and leukotrienes.[13]

Studies have shown the greatest improvements in nocturia, urinary frequency, and residual urine volume.[14] Rye grass and flower pollen also are used for symptomatic relief of prostatitis and prostatodynia. The typical dose of rye grass pollen is 126 mg 3 times/day. A product called Cernilton TS (TS for triple strength) was used in the original studies and has 180 mg of pollen extract. It is taken 1–2 times a day.

14. How does pygeum work?

Pygeum is obtained from the bark of the African plum tree. Like saw palmetto, its benefits are thought to come from fatty acids and sterols that reduce inflammation through the inhibition of prostaglandins and prostatic cholesterol levels. It also increases prostatic and seminal fluid secretions.

A meta-analysis revealed that men taking pygeum had a 19% reduction in nocturia with a 24% reduction in residual urine volume. Peak urine flow was increased by 23%, and side effects were similar to placebo.[15] Pygeum is more expensive than saw palmetto, and overharvesting of the bark is threatening the survival of the species. Typical dosage is 100–200 mg/day.

15. Are botanical products used for BPH more frequently in other parts of the world?

Plant-based medicines are much more popular in Europe than in the United States. In Austria and Germany, botanical products are the treatment of choice and account for more than 90% of all drugs prescribed for BPH. In Italy, herbs account for approximately 50% of all medications given for BPH, and alpha blockers are prescribed for only 5%.[16]

16. When should herbal products be used in the treatment of BPH?

If a patient presents with severe symptoms (American Urologic Association [AUA] score > 19), it is beneficial to begin with more aggressive pharmaceutical therapy with an alpha blocker or referral to a urologist for surgical evaluation. But if the patient has mild-to-moderate symptoms, herbal therapy should be considered as a safe, cost-effective approach.

17. Can herbs be useful for prostate cancer?

Because BPH and prostate cancer have similar hormonal triggers, it makes sense that herbal products useful in treating BPH also may have benefit in treating prostate cancer. Saw palmetto has been found to induce cell death and apoptosis of prostate cancer cells in vitro.[17]

Saw palmetto is also part of an herbal regimen, PC-SPES, that has been found to benefit patients with prostate cancer. PC stands for prostate cancer, and *spes* is Latin for hope. This combination contains eight different herbs: *Isatis indigotica* (da quing ye), *Glychyrrhiza glabra* and *uralensis* (gan cao), *Panax pseudoginseng* (san qi), *Ganoderma lucidum* (ling zhi, reishi), *Scutellaria baicalensis* (huang qin), *Denodrantherma (Chrysanthemum) morifolium*, *Rhabdosia rubescens*, and *Serenoa repens* (saw palmetto).[18] Although the exact mechanism of PC-SPES is unclear, researchers theorize that, by working synergistically, the herbs within PC-SPES inhibit angiogenesis, stimulate the immune system, induce an estrogenic effect, and inhibit 5-α reductase.[19] PC-SPES prevents the promotion and progression of both androgen-sensitive and androgen-insensitive prostate cancer.[20] The treatment is not without side effects. Adverse reactions may include skin rash, nausea, impotence, breast tenderness, fluid retention, and blood clots, including pulmonary embolus. Monthly out-of-pocket cost ranges from $300 to $400.

REFERENCES

1. Welshams WV, Nagel SC, Thayer KA, et al: Low-dose bioactivity of xenoestrogens in animals: fetal exposure to low doses of methoxychlor and other xenoestrogens increases adult prostate size in mice. Toxicol Industr Health 15 (1–2):12–25, 1999.
2. Geller J, Sionit L, Partido G, et al: Genistein inhibits the growth of human-patient BPH and prostate cancer in histoculture. Prostate 34(2):75–79, 1998.
3. Berges RR, et al: Randomized, placebo-controlled, double-blind clinical trial of beta-sitosterol in patients with benign prostatic hyperplasia. Lancet 345:1529–1532, 1995.
4. Pizzorno JE, Murray MT: Benign prostatic hyperplasia. In Pizzorno JE, Murry MT (eds): Textbook of Natural Medicine, 2nd ed. Edinburgh, Churchill Livingstone, 1999, pp 1147–1152.
5. Padayatty SJ, Marcelli M, Shao TC, Cunningham GR: Lovastatin-induced apoptosis in prostate stromal cells. J Clin Endocrinol Metab 82:1434–143-9, 1997.
6. Fahim M, Fahim Z, Der R, et al: Zinc treatment for the reduction of hyperplasia of the prostate. Fed Proc 35:36, 1976.
7. Leake A, Chisholm GD, Habib FK: The effect of zinc on the 5-alpha-reduction of testosterone by the hyperplastic human prostate gland. J Steroid Biochem 20:651–655, 1984.
8. Leake A, Chisholm GD, Busuttil A, et al: Subdellular distribution of zinc in the benign and malignant human prostate : Evidence for direct zinc androgen interaction. Act Endocrinol 105:281–288, 1984.
9. Carraro JC, et al: Comparison of phytotherapy with finasteride in the treatment of benign prostate hyperplasia: A randomized international study of 1098 patients. Prostate 29:231, 1996.
10. Gerber GS, et al: Saw plametto in men with lower urinary tract symptoms: Effects on urodynamic parameters and voiding symptoms. Urology 51:1003–1007, 1998.
11. Buck AC, et al: Treatment of outflow tract obstruction due to benign prostatic hyperplasia with the pollen extract, Cernilton: A double-blind, placebo-controlled study. Br J Urol 66:398–404, 1990.
12. Habib FK, et al: Identification of a prostate inhibitory substance in a pollen extract. Prostate 26:133–139, 1995.
13. Loschen G, Ebeling L: Inhibition of arachidonic acid cacade by extract of rye pollen [in German]. Arzneimittelforschung 41(2):162–167, 1991.
14. Becker H, Ebeling L: Conservative therapy for benign prostatic hyperplasia (BPH) with Cernilton. Br J Urol 66:398–404, 1988.
15. Ishani, A, MacDonald R, Nelson D, et al: *Pygeum africanum* for the treatment of patients with benign prostatic hyperplasia: A systematic review and quantitative meta-analysis. Am J Med 109:654–664, 2000.
16. Buck AC: Phytotherapy for the prostate. Br J Urol 78:325–336,1996.
17. Iguchi K, Okumaura N, Usui S, et al: Myristoleic acid, a ctyotoxic component in the extract from *Serona repens*, induces apoptosis and necrosis in human prostatic LNCaP cells. Prostate 47:59–65, 2001.
18. Lewis, J: The Herbal Remedy for Prostate Cancer. Westbury, NY, Health Education Literary Publisher, 1999, pp 34–37.
19. Darzynkiewicz Z, Traganos F, Wu JM, Chen S: Chinese herbal mixture PC SPES in treatment of prostate cancer (review). Int J Oncol 17(4):729–736, 2000.
20. Small EJ, et al: Prospective trial of the herbal supplement PC-SPES in patients with progressive prostate cancer. J Clin Oncol 18:3595–3603, 2000.

42. HIV/AIDS

Benjamin Kligler, M.D., M.P.H.

1. How does the complementary/alternative medicine (CAM) approach to HIV differ from the conventional approach?

The conventional approach emphasizes therapies directed at inhibiting or preventing replication of the human immunodeficiency virus (HIV). The CAM approach relies primarily on the concept that a healthier immune system in a healthier person will be in a stronger position to fight the effects of HIV. Both approaches are critical to the health of the HIV-positive person; combining conventional and CAM approaches is clearly the most sensible way to approach HIV disease.

2. What is the prevalence of use of CAM among HIV positive people?

Depending on the study, 27–100% of HIV-positive people may be using CAM approaches.[1] Vitamins, acupuncture, relaxation/mind-body therapies, and massage are the most commonly used alternative therapies among HIV-positive patients. Most patients cite a wish to supplement conventional therapies as their major reason for pursuing alternatives rather than a feeling of disillusionment with conventional medicine

3. Why are HIV positive patients using CAM?

People with HIV typically use alternative approaches for several reasons. First is to promote healthier functioning of the immune system; this approach can apply both to patients early in the course of HIV infection who do not yet take antiretroviral medications and to patients with more advanced disease who take conventional medications. Second is the claimed antiviral effect of the alternative therapy, as in the use of intravenous vitamin C infusions. Third is to treat an HIV-associated symptom or condition; pursuing acupuncture for peripheral neuropathy of HIV is an example. Fourth is to mitigate one or more of the side effects of conventional antiretroviral medications, as in the use of glutamine supplements for protease inhibitor-associated diarrhea.

4. What general nutritional recommendations are appropriate for HIV-positive patients?

Weight loss and decreases in body mass index and percent body fat may take place even during the asymptomatic phase of HIV infection and may be the first signs of declining nutritional status. Many patients with HIV/AIDS undergo wasting and lose body weight with nutrition that should be adequate for body height and weight. Studies have shown a significant relationship between low serum cholesterol, a marker for poor nutrition, and adverse patient outcome.[2]

Nutritional counseling early in the course of HIV disease is a critical component of the prevention-oriented treatment plan and may help prevent the adverse nutritional changes described above. The use of small, frequent meals is often recommended to ensure adequate calories and reduce the likelihood of malabsorption. Many nutritionists recommend a diet high in omega-3 essential fatty acids, such as flaxseed and fish oils, for their anti-inflammatory properties. Avoiding simple sugars, which, according to some studies, may inhibit proper immune function on a short-term basis and avoiding large amounts of alcohol and caffeine, are also common, though unproven, recommendations.

5. Describe the role for vitamin supplements in patients with HIV.

There is certainly a role for nutritional supplementation in HIV disease, although the benefits of specific nutrients have been difficult to demonstrate conclusively. Vitamin A deficiency initially appeared to be associated with lower CD4 counts and higher risk of progression to AIDS[3] as well as with increased maternal-fetal transmission of HIV in African women.[4] However, prospective trials have demonstrated no significant difference in risk of AIDS progression or maternal-fetal transmission rates with vitamin A levels,[5] and trials of vitamin A supplementation have failed to show an effect on CD4 or CD8 counts or progression of disease.[6]

Vitamin B_{12} supplementation has been a common practice for HIV-infected patients, based on prospective studies in which lower vitamin B_{12} levels were associated with HIV progression and shorter time to development of AIDS.[7] However, as with vitamin A, trials of B_{12} supplementation have not conclusively shown a benefit. Nevertheless, vitamin B_{12} supplementation continues to be widely used in HIV disease.

Because of the widespread belief that wasting and other complications of HIV disease may be due in part to excessive oxidative processes in the body as a consequence of HIV infection, a number of supplements with antioxidant properties—including vitamins C and E, selenium, and alpha-lipoic acid—have been examined for a role in treatment of HIV disease. Although the antioxidant theory is appealing, none of these substances to date have been shown to have an effect on the course of disease. Vitamins E and C are certainly safe at standard doses and may decrease lipid peroxidation and enhance immune function; however, conclusive evidence on the effects of these vitamins in HIV disease is still lacking.

In addition to its antioxidant effects, vitamin C has been shown in vitro to inhibit viral replication at high doses.[8] Based on this in vitro effect, many patients have sought out intravenous vitamin C therapy as a way to achieve the high serum levels necessary for the proposed antiviral activity. No trials support the use of high-dose intravenous vitamin C. However, this practice also has not proved to be as dangerous as initially feared, and there are no reports of serious adverse outcomes in HIV-positive patients resulting from intravenous vitamin C therapy.

Despite the lack of definitive effect of any single vitamin on disease progression, many providers recommend a daily multivitamin to prevent the development of the subclinical vitamin deficiencies that are clearly a hallmark of both early and late HIV disease.

6. What about other nutritional supplements?

Glutathione is an amino acid critical to the function of superoxide dismutase, one of the body's most potent antioxidant enzymes. Depletion of intracellular glutathione levels has been shown to correlate with progression from asymptomatic HIV to AIDS.[9] Because glutathione is not well absorbed orally, attention has focused on use of N-acetyl-cysteine (NAC), a supplement that is converted to glutathione, as a means to replete intracellular glutathione levels. However, trials to date have not shown an impact of NAC supplementation on disease progression. There are no reported adverse effects of NAC supplementation.

L-carnitine, at a dose of 2000 mg/day, may help relieve the peripheral neuropathy associated with certain antiretroviral medications and also may lower triglyceride levels. HIV-positive people have been found to have decreased levels of carnitine compared with HIV-negative people. In addition, AIDS patients taking AZT (zidovudine) or ddI (didanosine) who experienced peripheral neuropathy were found to have significantly lower levels of acetyl-carnitine than patients without neuropathy.[10] Increased proliferation of peripheral blood mononuclear cells in vitro also was found after oral supplementation with L-carnitine. Another study found a significant decrease in triglyceride levels in patients treated with L-carnitine.[11] No significant adverse effects or interactions of L-carnitine have been demonstrated to date; further study is needed to substantiate possible benefits. Acetyl-carnitine plays an important role in the transport of essential fatty acids across cell membranes; this action may explain its possible effect on intracellular lipid metabolism and peripheral nerve function and regeneration.

L-glutamine supplementation, also at 2000 mg/day, may help to mitigate protease inhibitor-associated chronic diarrhea. Animal models have shown that this supplement speeds proliferation of colonocytes. Glutamine deficiency also may play a role in the process of HIV-associated wasting.[12]

Another supplement commonly recommended to HIV-positive people, particularly if symptoms of gastrointestinal dysfunction are present, are the **probiotics** or **friendly bacteria**, including *Lactobacillus* and *Bifidobacterium* species. These bacteria may help restore and maintain the proper balance of intestinal flora needed for healthy digestive function, particularly in patients whose intestinal flora have been significantly altered by repeated courses of antibiotics.

7. Can any CAM options replace antiretroviral medications?

No evidence suggests that any of the CAM approaches has significant antiretroviral activity. It is possible that early evidence of the efficacy of some Chinese herbal preparations may be due in part to an antiviral effect of one or more of the herbs in the formula; this area requires a great deal of further study before any such conclusions can be drawn. At this point, CAM approaches should be used *in combination* with antiretroviral medications for the treatment of HIV—not as a stand-alone approach.

8. Do herbal medicines have a role in the treatment of HIV?

Herbal medicines are used for immune support, potential (but unproven) antiretroviral activity, and treatment of HIV-related and medication-induced symptoms. Chinese herbal preparations, in particular, may have promise for the first two uses (see question 11); several Western herbals can be very useful for the third.

Two Western herbs have been studied for a role in slowing progression of HIV disease: **boxwood** and **mistletoe**. Based on one small trial, it appears that SPV-30, an extract derived from the boxwood plant, may delay progression in asymptomatic HIV-positive subjects compared with placebo.[13] The data are only preliminary; thus, the only appropriate application of boxwood at this point may be in the patient with a low viral load for whom antiretroviral medications are not yet clearly indicated. Another herb that may have a role in early HIV is mistletoe (*Viscum album*), which has been investigated as a potential immunomodulator in patients with cancer. In HIV disease, mistletoe has been shown to cause proliferation of granulocytes, natural killer cells, and CD4 cells and to stimulate T-cell activity. Some studies have found improved appetite, decreased pain, and weight gain in HIV-positive patients. Mistletoe is administered subcutaneously and may cause swelling or induration at the site of injection. Other potential adverse effects include fever, flu-like symptoms, fatigue, and headache. In the studies, 1–2 mg *Viscum Album* extract was delivered subcutaneously every other week, starting gradually with 0.01 mg for the first week and escalating to 1–2 mg by week 4.[14,15]

Milk thistle extract (standardized to the silymarin fraction), usually given at a dose of 240 mg of standardized extract twice daily, may help restore normal liver function in patients experiencing liver function abnormalities due to antiretroviral therapies. In vitro studies have shown that milk thistle extract can speed regeneration of hepatocytes after chemical injury.[16] Other studies have found a significant improvement in liver function in patients with alcoholic hepatitis after treatment with milk thistle extract.[17] No study to date has investigated whether this hepatoprotective function will be borne out in the specific case of liver damage due to antiretrovirals. In clinical practice, however, milk thistle in fact has proved to be useful, particularly in patients who are coinfected with hepatitis C. There are no reported contraindications or adverse effects. There is a common misconception among patients with HIV and many practitioners that milk thistle may have an antiviral effect; this has *not* been shown to be the case in either HIV or hepatitis C.

Many patients taking protease inhibitors develop hyperlipidemia as a side effect and require additional medications. A standardized extract of **Chinese red rice yeast**, at a dose of 1200 mg twice daily, can reduce cholesterol levels up to 20% in certain patients.[18] As with milk thistle and its hepatoprotective function, red rice yeast extract has not been tested specifically in protease inhibitor-related hyperlipidemia. No significant adverse effects have been reported to date. However, because this supplement contains statin-like compounds, it is probably prudent to monitor liver function periodically with long-term use.

9. What about interactions between herbal treatments and conventional medicines?

Interaction with antiretroviral agents is a major concern for both patients and health care providers and are one of the primary reasons that providers must include discussion of CAM practices on a regular basis in their conversations with HIV-positive patients. For example, St. John's wort, a popular antidepressant herbal treatment, is an activator of the cytochrome P450 system and lowers serum levels of indinavir by 57%; it may have the same effect on other protease inhibitors.[19] The question of interactions is particularly difficult in dealing with Chinese herbal preparations, which typically can contain 15–20 different herbs.

10. Is massage helpful for people with HIV?

Massage therapy has great benefits in terms of improved mood and decreased anxiety; psychoneuroimmunology has found mood states to be intimately linked with immune function. Some evidence indicates that in HIV-positive people regular massage therapy improves natural killer cell function and increases CD8 counts; to date no connection has been made between massage and CD4 counts or other markers of disease progression.[20] One study of HIV-exposed neonates showed a significant benefit of massage.[21] Because massage therapy has almost no potential for significant adverse effects and significant potential for benefit in terms of mood and decreased anxiety, it is a reasonable modality to include in the prevention-oriented treatment plan of HIV-positive patients.

11. What mind-body approaches should be recommended for HIV-positive patients?
Mind-body strategies play a vital role in the prevention-oriented treatment plan for HIV. Extensive research in psychoneuroimmunology (PNI) has shown a clear connection between psychological stress and impaired immune function. Some studies of these approaches in HIV disease have found a trend toward increased T-cell count in patients practicing a mind-body approach, and others have found improvement in natural killer cell function and other immune parameters.[22,23] Many studies have demonstrated improvement in quality-of-life ratings and emotional well-being. Studies to date have examined biofeedback, meditation, systematic relaxation, hypnosis, and cognitive-behavioral stress management training in HIV-positive patients. Future studies should examine whether any one of these approaches to stress reduction is more effective than the others in patients with HIV. Generally these strategies are considered extremely safe.

12. Does any evidence support the use of Chinese medicine approaches in HIV disease?
In traditional Chinese practice, **herbal medicines** are prescribed as individualized combinations to treat a particular person's condition. In the U.S. in recent years, standardized formulas for certain diseases have become popular. Clinical trials of two such formulas, Enhance and Clear Heat (marketed by Health Concerns), showed a nonsignificant trend toward reduced symptoms and improved quality of life in the treatment group compared with placebo.[24] Larger and longer-term studies of Chinese herbal preparations are needed. Many practitioners remain extremely concerned about possible herb–drug interactions, given the large number of herbs in most Chinese formulas. This is a challenging issue, especially in patients taking antiretroviral medications.

Acupuncture has been widely used both to enhance immune function and general well-being in HIV-positive patients and to treat specific HIV- or medication-related symptoms. One randomized, controlled trial that examined amitriptyline plus acupuncture found no benefit of true standardized acupuncture over sham (placebo) acupuncture[25] in the treatment of HIV-related peripheral neuropathy.

A final point about this study is that in practice acupuncture is much more effective in treating peripheral neuropathy if treatment is initiated as soon as possible after onset of symptoms. Perhaps future HIV/acupuncture trials should focus on efficacy specifically in treating new-onset neuropathies.

13. Discuss the controversy among some CAM providers about whether HIV is actually the cause of AIDS. Is there legitimate cause to question the relationship between HIV and AIDS?
There has been discussion over the past several years of a theory that HIV is not in fact the cause of AIDS and that it is merely one of many cofactors that influence the development of the illness. The proponents of this theory believe that if lifestyle issues are addressed thoroughly enough, a person can become infected with HIV and be at no risk of developing AIDS.

This theory is completely unfounded and in fact quite dangerous. The vast numbers of HIV-infected patients who have been able to reverse completely the progression of AIDS by starting antiretroviral medications stand as indisputable proof of the causative role of HIV in AIDS. The direct link between viral load and progression of disease is further evidence. The danger of the theory described above is that some people with HIV have taken it as license not to practice safe sex, believing that host factors are more important than the virus itself in developing AIDS. Providers must be aware of this misguided belief to reinforce the need for HIV-positive patients to continue safe-sex practices.

14. What sources are available for additional information:
• Jon Kaiser: *Immune Power: The Comprehensive Healing Program for HIV*. New York, St. Martin's Press, 1995.

• www.DAAIR.org: Direct Access Alternative Information Resources, a members-only, not-for-profit buyers' club to promote self-empowered healing.

REFERENCES

1. Ernst E: Complementary AIDS therapies: the good, the bad and the ugly. Int J STD AIDS 8:281–285, 1997
2. Guenter P, Muurahainen N, Simons G, et al: Relationships among nutritional status, disease progression, and survival in HIV infection. J Acq Immune Defic Syndr 6:1130–1138, 1993.
3. Beach R, Mantero-Atienza E, Shor-Posner G, et al: Specific nutrient abnormalities in asymptomatic HIV-1 infection. AIDS 6:701–708, 1992.
4. Semba R, Miotti P, Chiphangwi J, et al: Maternal vitamin A deficiency and mother-to-child transmission of HIV-1. Lancet 172:1461–1468, 1994.
5. Tang A, Graham N, Semba R, et al: Association between serum vitamin A and E levels and HIV-1 disease progression. AIDS 11:613–620, 1997.
6. Humphrey J, Quinn T, Fine D, et al: Short-term effects of large-dose vitamin A supplementation on viral load and immune response in HIV-infected women. J Acq Immune Defic Syndr Hum Retrovirol 20:44–51, 1999.
7. Tang A, Graham N, Chandra R, et al: Low serum vitamin B-12 concentrations are associated with faster human immunodeficiency virus type 1 (HIV-1) disease progression. J Nutr 127:345–351, 1997.
8. Jariwalla RJ, et al: HIV suppression by ascorbate and its enhancement by glutathione precursor. Proceedings of the Eighth International Conference on AIDS, 1992, Amsterdam, 2:B207.
9. Buhl R, et al: Systemic glutathione deficiency in symptom-free HIV seropositive individuals. Lancet 2:1294–1298, 1989.
10. Famularo G, Moretti S, Marcellini S, et al: Acetyl-carnitine deficiency in AIDS patients with neurotoxicity on treatment with antiretroviral nucleoside analogues. AIDS 11:185–190, 1997.
11. De Simone C, Tzantzoglou S, Famularo G, et al: High dose L-carnitine improves immunologic and metabolic parameters in AIDS patients. Immunopharmacol Immunotoxicol 15:1–12, 1993.
12. Shabert JK, Wilmore DW: Glutamine deficiency as a cause of human immunodeficiency virus wasting. Med Hypoth 46:252–256, 1996.
13. Durant J, et al: A multicenter, randomized , double-blind, placebo-controlled trial of efficacy and safety of *Buxus sempervirens* L. preparations (SPV-30) in HIV-infected asymptomatic patients. Proceedings of the Eleventh International Conference on AIDS 1996, abstract B6040.
14. Stoss M, Van Wely M, Musielsky H, et al: Study on local inflammatory reactions and other parameters during subcutaneous mistletoe application in HIV-positive patients and HIV-negative subjects over a period of eighteen weeks. Drug Res 49:366–373, 1999.
15. Gorter R, Van Wely M, Reif M, et al: Tolerability of an extract of European mistletoe among immunocompromised and healthy individuals. Altern Ther 5:37–48, 1999.
16. Blumenthal M, et al (eds): Milk thistle fruit. Herbal Medicine: Expanded Commission E Monographs. Newton, MA, Integrative Medicine Communications, 2000, pp 257–263.
17. Flora K., et al: Milk thistle for the therapy of liver disease. Am J Gastroenterol 93:139–143, 1998.
18. Heber D, et al: Cholesterol-lowering effects of a proprietary Chinese red-yeast-rice dietary supplement. Am J Clin Nutr 69:231–236, 1999.
19 Piscitelli SC, Burstein AH, Chaitt D, et al: Indinavir concentrations and St. John's wort. Lancet 355:547–548, 2000.
20. Ironsen G, Field T: Massage therapy is associated with enhancement of the immune system's cytotoxic capacity. Int J Neurosci 84:205–217, 1996.
21. Scafidi F, Field T: Massage therapy improves behavior in neonates born to HIV-positive mothers. J Pediatr Psychol 21:889–897, 1996.
22. McCain NL, et al: The influence of stress management training in HIV disease. Nurs Res 45:246–253, 1996.
23. Robinson F, Mathews H, Witek-Janusek L: Stress reduction and HIV disease: A review of intervention studies using a psychoneuroimmunology framework. J Assoc Nurses AIDS Care 11(2):87–96, 2000.
24. Burack J, et al: Pilot randomized controlled trials of Chinese herbal treatments for HIV-associated symptoms. J AIDS 12:386–393, 1996.
25. Shlay CJ, et al: Acupuncture and amitriptyline for pain due to HIV-related peripheral neuropathy. JAMA 280:1590–1595, 1998.

43. COMMON COLD

Jeffrey Jump, M.D.

1. What is an upper respiratory tract infection (URI)?

URI, also known as the common cold, is characterized by inflammation of the respiratory mucosa from the nose to the lower respiratory tree, not including the alveoli. Symptoms are self-limited and include nasal congestion, sore throat, rhinorrhea, malaise, cough, and low-grade fever. Symptoms generally peak within 1–3 days and resolve within 1 week, although cough may persist.

2. What causes URIs?

Approximately 200 viruses are capable of infecting the upper respiratory tract. Transmission is primarily through hand-to-hand contact, not via air-borne droplets. Most respiratory viruses are hardy and can survive on the hand up to 4 hours.[1] Therefore, avoidance of contact with infected people and frequent hand washing are defenses from the common cold. Of course, not everyone who is exposed to a cold virus becomes infected. As Pasteur is often quoted as saying, "The environment is everything, the germ is nothing." Integrative treatment of the common cold not only aims at eliminating pathogens but also emphasizes the importance of enhancing the immune system to prevent illness in the first place.

3. Who is susceptible to catching a cold?

On average adults suffer 2–4 colds per year, whereas children have 6–8. Seasonal peaks in incidence are early fall and mid to late spring, which implicates schoolchildren as carriers who introduce colds into the family. Controversy surrounds the influence of environmental exposure on susceptibility to infection with a cold virus. Common folk wisdom holds that exposure to cold, damp, and windy conditions is a direct cause of colds. However, in a classic study a few volunteers exposed to wet, cold conditions were no more likely to become infected with a respiratory virus after direct nasal inoculation than normal volunteers.[2] The transmission vector in this study can be questioned, however, and the debate is far from complete.

4. What role does stress play?

Good clinical evidence links stress to susceptibility to the common cold. Cohen et al. concluded that psychological stress was associated with an increased risk of infection rather than merely an increased reporting of symptoms in subjects under greater stress.[3] In a prospective trial involving 1,149 people, subjects with the most negative stress were 3.7 times more likely to suffer from URI than subjects under little stress.[4] Mechanisms of exactly how stress weakens immunity are still being explored, but we know there are strong biologic links between the autonomic nervous system and the immune system.

5. What role does diet play?

Diet influences immune response, especially simple sugars. Oral administration of 100 gm of simple sugar significantly reduces neutrophil phagocytosis. The effect is seen within 30 minutes and lasts for over 5 hours. Peak response is seen about 2 hours after ingestion and amounts to a 50% reduction in phagocytic activity. Oral intake of 75 gm of glucose also has been shown to reduce lymphocytic response to mitogens. Considering that the average American consumes 125 gm of sucrose and 75 gm of other simple sugars per day, we would do well to consider diet in the evaluation of susceptibly to the common cold.[5]

6. Why consider complementary therapies for the common cold?

One primary reason is the fact that no conventional treatment has been found effective in reducing the duration or severity of a cold. Decongestants have shown minimal symptom relief after a single dose, but no benefit with longer use. Antihistamines have shown small clinical benefit for runny nose and sneezing.

Secondly, despite a lack of evidence documenting their benefit, antibiotics continue to be prescribed in 30–75% of all office visits for URIs.[6,7] Doctors site patient expectation as the primary reason for prescribing antibiotics. A recent survey[8] showed that 50% of patients believed that bacteria played a causal role in URIs, and 44% believed that antibiotics are helpful in treating a cold, even though 85% of the same people believed that URIs were self-limiting. The widespread practice of prescribing antibiotics does harm by contributing to bacterial resistance and is associated with significant side effects.[9] Therefore, any complementary approach that may provide benefit without causing harm would be a welcome addition to the treatment of URIs.

7. Can vitamin C be used to prevent or treat a cold?

Few remedies elicit more controversy than the use of vitamin C for the common cold. The role of vitamin C remains contentious despite many controlled trials. The results of treatment trials vary greatly. However, modest benefit was seen with relatively high doses (> 1 gm/day) of vitamin C. No consistent benefit in prevention was seen with doses as high as 1gm/day for several months.[10]

Although dosage regimens need further exploration, some practitioners recommend as much as 1–2 gm every 4–6 hours for the first 24 hours on first recognition of the symptoms of a cold. Side effects of excessive vitamin C intake include primarily diarrhea, which is reversible by lowering the dose. A recent study[11] concluded that the human body does not seem to absorb more than 200 mg/day of vitamin C; thus, higher doses are wasteful. High doses for acute use were not assessed. Further studies need to be done to clarify the vitamin C controversy.

8. Is zinc helpful?

Use of zinc lozenges is a popular complementary/alternative medicine (CAM) treatment for the common cold and associated sore throat. Of the 10 published randomized trials of zinc, only half have shown a reduction in duration of cold symptoms. Some studies are confounded by blinding and randomization problems.[12] Studies also differ in the use of zinc acetate or gluconate lozenges. The formulation of the zinc gluconate lozenges may be a key factor; zinc ionization in saliva may be a critical factor to effectiveness.[13] Dosage is usually 15–25 mg elemental zinc, best taken with food. Zinc lozenges with the amino acid glycine and without citric acid, sorbitol, or mannitol are recommended.[14]

9. What about echinacea?

The use of echinacea in preventing and treating the common cold has a rich history among herbal practitioners in the United States and Europe. Popular use is also high: 45% of people enrolled in a controlled trial had already used echinacea at least once before participation in the study.[15] According to the Cochrane Review, most available studies report positive effects.[16] However, the use of different products and preparations of echinacea confounds these studies. Three species of echinacea are used medicinally: *Echinacea angustifolia, E. purpurea,* and *E. pallida. E. purpurea* has become the most widely used species because the whole plant (root, leaf, flowers, and seed) may be used, and it is the easiest to cultivate. Only the root and rhizome of *E. pallida* and *E. angustifolia* are used medicinally.

Echinacea is an immunostimulant. In vitro studies have demonstrated increased production of lymphokines by lymphocytes, and elevated cytokine levels (tumor necrosis factor-alpha, interleukins 1, 6, and 10) produced by macrophages. Echinacea also increases the number of granular leukocytes, segmented granulocytes and macrophages in vitro. In vivo tests demonstrate nonspecific enhancement of phagocytic activity.[17]

10. Is echinacea safe?

There are no reports of the toxic effects of echinacea. According to the German Commission E, echinacea is contraindicated in "progressive systemic disease conditions" such as multiple sclerosis and autoimmune processes because the immunostimulant activity of echinacea may worsen these conditions. Currently there are no reports in the medical literature about worsening of any autoimmune conditions, but the theoretical possibility is still documented.

11. Can echinacea be used safely for extended periods?

An oft-repeated caution for echinacea is that use for extended periods (continuously for over 2 weeks) may make the immune system less responsive. No evidence supports caution, and it has been extensively criticized as a misinterpretation of the literature.[18] On the other hand, because echinacea seems to be most effective in shortening the duration of a viral URI when it is started early, it is probably better used as a short-term agent for acute URIs instead of a longer-term prophylactic agent.[19] In healthy people no evidence indicates the need for prolonged use of echinacea. It is prudent, at least in theory, not to overdo any botanical medicine.

12. How should echinacea be prescribed?

Determining which echinacea preparation is most efficacious is difficult. Arguments among naturopathic physicians and herbalists about preparations and species of echinacea are unresolved. In general, dried powdered extracts of *E. purpura*, 150–300 mg 3 times/day, or fresh freeze-dried root of *E. angustifolia* or *E. pallida*, 325–650 mg 3 times/day, is preferred. Standardization is to 4% echinacosides (*E. angustifolia*) or 4% sesquiterpene esters (*E. purpurea*). Some prefer to use the fresh pressed juice of the aerial parts of *E. purpurea*, 2 tsp 3 times/day. These botanicals are thought to be most effective if started at the earliest onset of symptoms.

13. Is chicken soup beneficial?

Chicken soup, a mainstay of home remedies for the common cold, has actually been studied clinically. Rennard et al. found that chicken soup has mild anti-inflammatory activity in vitro. Extracts of chicken soup inhibited neutrophil chemotaxis. This finding may explain some of the seemingly beneficial effects of chicken soup on the symptoms of the common cold.[20]

14. Should associated fever be treated?

Fever has been shown to have a beneficial effect on the course of most viral illnesses, despite the persistent belief among the public and many physicians that fevers should be treated.[21] Elevated temperature inhibits viral shedding. Antipyretic medication use, especially salicylates with their link to Reye syndrome in children, should be discouraged.

15. What about rest and hydration?

Although studies on the benefits of rest and proper hydration on the course of the common cold are limited, these common sense recommendations should not be discarded. In one study of influenza, proper hydration was found to be important in loosening secretions.[22] Fever and viral damage to ciliated epithelium also increase the importance of proper rest and hydration.

16. How does osteopathic medicine view URIs?

Certainly most osteopathic physicians agree with the view that the common cold is triggered by a virus. However, osteopathic theories about contributing factors are interesting and should not be discarded. Of importance is the influence of the autonomic nervous system, specifically the superior cervical ganglion, on the vasomotor stability of the nasal mucous membranes. Osteopathic treatment for URI symptoms emphasizes restoring vasomotor integrity as well as facilitating lymphatic drainage of the head and neck region.

17. How does traditional Chinese medicine (TCM) explain a cold?

TCM, an ancient medical tradition, uses a different paradigm for viral infection. However, certain aspects may be valuable to consider. First, TCM places much importance on the person's ability to defend against attacks by pathogens. In modern TCM, distinctions are made between the classic pathogens, particularly cold and wind in the case of a URI, and pathogens as considered by Western medicine (e.g., rhinoviruses). People who are weak in constitution, especially in what is referred to as defensive qi, are unable to defend the body from attack by pathogens. Secondly, not all colds are viewed in the same way. For every patient, the particular circumstances leading to invasion by the pathogen must be evaluated. We would do well to remember these bits of wisdom when we evaluate patients for cold symptoms.

18. What is Sambucol? Is it effective against respiratory viruses?

Sambucol is a patented extract of the berries of the black elder (*Sambucus nigra*). It has been reported to inhibit the replication of several strains of influenza virus. In one well-conduced trial,

Sambucol reduced the symptoms of influenza infection, including fever, from 6 to 4 days. A complete cure was seen in 2 –3 days in 90% of treated patients.[23] In healthy volunteers, Sambucol significantly increased production of inflammatory cytokines (interleukins 1 beta, 6, and 8, tumor necrosis factor alpha), which may explain its immune-stimulating properties.

19. Is Sambucol safe?

There are no reports of adverse effects with the short-term use of black elderberry. Sambucol has mild diuretic properties; theoretically, long-term use or concomitant use with diuretics may prove harmful. Considering its reported efficacy in inhibiting viral replication in vitro and in treating influenza as well as the absence of side effects, it should be considered as a treatment of influenza and possibly the common cold..

REFERENCES

1. Lauber B: The common cold. J Gen Intern Med 11:229–236,1996
2. Douglas RC Jr, Couch RB, Lindgren KM: Cold doesn't affect the "common cold" in study of rhinovirus infections. JAMA 199:29–30, 1967
3. Cohen S, Tyrill DA, Smith AP: Psychological stress and susceptibility to the common cold. N Engl J Med 325:606–612, 1991
4. Takkouche B, et. al: A cohort of stress and the common cold. Epidemiology 12:345–349, 2001.
5. Pizzorno J, Murray M: Immune support. In Textbook of Natural Medicine. Edinburgh, Churchill Livingstone, 1999, p 481.
6. Gonzales R, Steiner JF, Sandle MA: Antibiotic prescribing for adults with colds, upper respiratory tract infections, and bronchitis by ambulatory care physicians. JAMA 278:90–904, 1997.
7. Mainous III AG, Hueston WJ, Clark JR: Antibiotics and upper respiratory tract infection: Do some folks think there is a cure for the common cold? J Fam Pract 42:357–361, 1996.
8. Braun BL et al: Patient beliefs about the characteristics, causes, and care of the common cold. J Fam Pract 49:153–156, 2000
9. Cochran Review: Antibiotics for the common cold. Cochran Library, vol. 2, 2001.
10. Douglas RM, Chalker EB, Treacy B: Vitamin C for preventing and treating the common cold. Cochran Library, vol. 2, 2001
11. Levine M, Rumsey SC, Daruwala R, t al: Criteria and recommendations for vitamin C intake. JAMA 281:1415–1423, 1999.
12. Jackson EA: Are zinc acetate lozenges effective in decreasing the duration of symptoms of the common cold? J Fam Pract 49:1153, 2000.
13. Zarembo JE, et al.: Zinc (II) in saliva: Determination of concentration produced by different formulations of zinc gluconate lozenges containing common excipients. J Pharm Sci 81:128–130, 1992.
14. Pizzorno JE, Murray JT: Common cold. In Encyclopedia of Natural Medicine, 2nd ed, pp 373–376, 1998.
15. Melchart D, Walther E, Linde K, et al: Echinacea root extracts for the prevention of upper respiratory tract infections. A double-blind, placebo-controlled randomized trial. Arch Fam Med 7:541–545,1998.
16. Melchart D, Linde K, Fisher P: Echinacea for preventing and treating the common cold. Cochrane Library, vol. 2, 2001.
17. Bone K, Mills S: Principles and Practice of Phytotherapy. Edinburgh, Churchill Livingstone, 2000, pp 354–357.
18. Bone K: Modern Phytother 3(3):17–21, 1997.
19. Hoheisel O, et al: Echinacea treatment shortens the course of the common cold: A double-blind, placebo-controlled clinical trial. Eur J Clin Res 9:261–269, 1997.
20. Rennard BO, et a:. Chicken soup inhibits neutrophil chemotaxis in vitro. Chest 118:887–888, 2000.
21. Mackowiak P: Benefits versus risk of the febrile response. In Mackowiak P (ed): Fever: Basic Mechanisms and Management, vol 58. Philadelphia, Lippincott-Raven, 1997, pp 444–458.
22. Ramphal R, Fischlschweiger W, Shands JW Jr, et al: Murine influenzal tracheitis: A model for the study of influenza and tracheal epithelial repair. Am Respir Dis; 120:1313–1324, 1979.
23. Zakay-Rones Z, et al: Inhibition of several strains of influenza virus in vitro and reduction of symptoms by an elderberry extract (Sambucus nigra L.) during an outbreak of influenza B in Panama. J Altern Complement Med 1:361–369, 1995.

44. SINUSITIS

Robert S. Ivker, D.O.

1. What are sinuses? What is their primary function?
The sinuses are air-filled cavities located behind and around the nose and eyes. In anatomy texts they are called air sinuses or paranasal sinuses. There are usually four sets, roughly divided in half for each side of the head. The halves can be asymmetrical in size and shape.

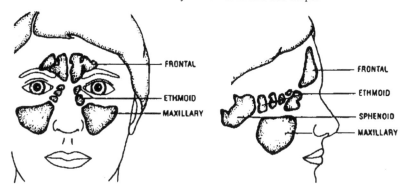

Location of sinuses. (From Ivker RS: Sinus Survival: The Holistic Medical Treatment for Sinusitis, Allergies, and Colds, 4th ed. New York, Tarcher/Putnam/Penguin, 2000, with permission.)

To make mucus drainage and air exchange possible, each sinus is connected to the nasal passage by a thin duct about the size of pencil lead. The openings of the ducts, called ostia, average about two millimeters in diameter. The ducts of the maxillaries are located at the top of the sinus, making drainage difficult. Although most of the human body seems to have been created perfectly, the maxillary sinuses are a distinct exception. They appear to be better suited to four-legged animals, particularly in regard to the position of the ostia. As upright posture evolved, ease of sinus drainage diminished.

The outermost lining of the entire respiratory tract is one continuous tissue, the respiratory epithelium. This mucous membrane serves as the first line of defense against bacteria, viruses, pollen, animal dander, cigarette smoke, dust, chemicals, automobile exhaust, and any other potentially harmful air pollutants. With a protective capability and breathability far beyond that of Gore-Tex or any similar high-tech material, it also has the job of humidifying dry air and warming cold or cooling hot air. The bulk of the job of filtering, humidifying, and regulating temperature occurs in the nose and sinuses—the entrance and vestibule of the respiratory tract.

2. Define sinusitis, both acute and chronic.
Acute sinusitis, or sinus infection, is an inflammation and infection of one or more of the paranasal sinuses. It is usually preceded by the common cold and is most often accompanied by the symptoms of: head congestion, headache and facial pain, fatigue, and purulent (yellow-green) postnasal drainage or rhinorrhea. The cold that persists beyond 7–10 days is most symptomatic of acute sinusitis.

Chronic sinusitis is defined as persistent or recurrent episodes of infection and/or inflammation of one or more sinus cavities. It has been categorized by Jafek and Ivker into three types[1]:

Type 1: a persistent low-grade infection with periodic flare-ups of acute sinusitis. People with type 1 chronic sinusitis are always sick to some degree. It may have been many months or, in most cases, years, since they have been healthy. Chronic illness takes the form of an ongoing sinus infection with any or all of the symptoms previously described for acute sinusitis. Extreme fatigue, headaches, and persistent yellow-green postnasal mucus drainage top the list of a multitude of systemic symptoms.

Type 2: recurrent or repeated sinus infections (acute sinusitis). People with type 2 chronic sinusitis suffer at least three or more infections within a 6-month period. They usually have most of the symptoms described above for acute sinusitis.

Type 3: chronic inflammation with little or no infection. People with type 3 chronic sinusitis are not nearly as sick or uncomfortable as those with types 1 and 2. They have chronic inflammation of the mucous membranes lining the nose and sinuses with infrequent (one or two per year) or no infections. Inflammation involves pain, swelling, and increased secretions from the mucous membrane, but without the causative agents of infection (bacteria, viruses, or fungi).

3. How prevalent is sinusitis?

In 1993, Gwaltney performed a landmark study of students and university employees who thought that they had the common cold. CT scans revealed that 87% had sinus infections.[2] According to the most recent National Health Interview Survey,[3] administered jointly by the Centers for Disease Control and Prevention and the National Center for Health Statistics, chronic sinusitis is the most common chronic disease in the United States. It afflicts nearly 15% of people of all ages, or 1 of every 7 people in the population.

4. What are the causes and risk factors of sinusitis?

The primary reason that sinusitis has been the most common chronic condition in the U.S since 1981 is the growing plague of air pollution—both indoor and outdoor.[4] Air pollution is also responsible for the dramatic increase in both allergic rhinitis (fourth most common chronic ailment) and asthma (eighth most common chronic ailment). Together these three conditions afflict nearly 1 of every 3 people in the population, making respiratory disease the first environmental epidemic in the U.S.. Other important risk factors include the following:
- Emotional stress (especially repressed anger)
- Common cold and cigarettes (both can paralyze the cilia)
- Fungal and candidal organisms
- Allergies and sensitivities: pollen, animal dander, mold, food (dairy and wheat are most common)
- Dry air and cold air
- Gastroesophageal reflux disease (GERD)
- Occupational hazards (e.g., auto mechanics, construction workers, painters, beauticians)
- Dental infection
- Immunodeficiency
- Malformations(e.g., polyps, cysts, deviated septum)

5. What role does fungus play in chronic sinusitis?

In 1999 a Mayo Clinic study[5] reported that an immune system response to fungal rather than bacterial infection is the cause of most cases of chronic sinusitis. The investigators studied 210 patients with chronic sinusitis and discovered 40 different kinds of fungus, including *Candida* sp., in the mucus of 96%. They found similar organisms in a control group of normal healthy volunteers. They concluded that the immune system response to fungi is markedly different in patients with chronic sinusitis and healthy people. This unusual immune reaction is responsible for the chronic inflammation, pain, and swelling of the mucous membrane associated with sinusitis. The investigators call the condition **allergic fungal sinusitis**.

The investigators, however, failed to speculate about the effect of multiple courses of broad-spectrum antibiotics on the immune response to fungal organisms in patients with chronic sinusitis. Many practitioners now believe that the vast majority of patients with type 1 chronic sinusitis (the people who are most debilitated with sinus disease) suffer from sinus infections caused by fungus and/or candidal organisms. This yeast overgrowth is most often a result of multiple courses of antibiotics.

6. How is sinusitis diagnosed?

Although most otolaryngologists rely on the CT scan for a definitive diagnosis of sinusitis, in the primary care setting a good history and the presence of most or all of the above symptoms can provide a reliable diagnosis of both acute and chronic sinusitis.

7. Describe the conventional medical treatment for sinusitis.

A 10-day or 2-week course of broad-spectrum antibiotics is typically the first choice for treating acute sinusitis. Multiple courses are often prescribed for more resistant cases. If they, too, fail to resolve the problem, referral to an otolaryngologist is the next step, and endoscopic sinus surgery is the usual outcome. Well over 200,000 of these procedures are performed each year.[6] Most patients who undergo sinus surgery experience temporary relief (for 6 months to 1 year) and then often begin to repeat the cycle of infection and antibiotics. Unfortunately, many also return for additional surgeries.

To an increasing extent conventional medical treatment offers only temporary relief, and recent evidence suggests it may not help at all. In a study of 161 children with acute sinusitis, researchers concluded that "antimicrobial treatment offered no benefit in overall symptom resolution, duration of symptoms, recovery to usual functional status, days missed from school or child care, or relapse and recurrence of sinus symptoms."[7]

8. Who can most benefit from a holistic medical treatment program for sinusitis?

1. People who have not responded to antibiotics or surgery.
2. People who are not candidates for surgery or who see surgery only as a last resort after all other options have been tried.
3. Postoperative patients who would like to prevent recurrence of sinusitis or polyps.
4. People who are committed to addressing the underlying causes of sinus disease, experiencing a greater level of health, and potentially curing chronic sinusitis.

9. What are the primary objectives of the holistic approach to chronic sinusitis?

1. To heal the chronically inflamed mucous membrane lining the nose and sinuses
2. To strengthen and/or restore balance to a dysfunctional immune system
3. To reduce greatly the candidal or fungal organisms in the mucous membranes (if applicable)

10. What is considered optimal air? How do you create it indoors?

Ideal air quality is rated by clarity (freedom from pollutants), humidity (35–55%), temperature (65–85°F), oxygen content (21% of total volume and 100% saturation), and negative ion content (3,000–6,000 0.001-micron ions per cubic centimeter). Air that is clean, moist, warm, oxygen-rich, and high in negative ions[8–10] is the healthiest air that humans can breathe. To create optimal indoor air, experts recommend:

- Negative ion generator: used as an air cleaner, it should be placed in the room(s) in which the person spends the bulk of his or herr time, especially the bedroom and office.
- Furnace filter: an electrostatic or pleated filter (Filtrete by 3M is excellent).
- Furnace cleaning
- Carpet cleaning
- Humidifier: a warm-mist room unit, especially during the winter months.
- Plants, especially those that can remove formaldehyde (Boston fern, chrysanthemums, striped dracaena, dwarf date palm) and carbon monoxide (spider plants).

11. Describe the basic methods used to heal the mucous membranes.

Because we breathe, on average, about 23,000 times /day, healthy air (see question 10) instead of pollutant-laden, dry, oxygen- and ion-depleted air can heal rather than irritate the mucosa. In addition to the recommendations in question 10, other helpful suggestions include the following:

- Bottled or filtered water: drink ½ oz/lb of body weight on days without exercise and ⅔ oz/lb on days when you exercise for at least 20–30 minutes aerobically.
- Saline nasal spray: use daily every 2–3 hours. A spray with medicinal herbs (aloe vera, goldenseal, and grapefruit seed extract) is especially helpful.
- Steam inhaler[11]: use 15–20 minutes 2–3 times daily. It is even more therapeutic when a few drops of medicinal eucalyptus oil are added to the steam.
- Nasal irrigation[12–14]: several methods are available, including Neti pot or SinuCleanse device, Grossan nasal irrigator (attaches to WaterPik), or ear bulb syringe. Perform 2–3 times daily. Nasal irrigation works best after steam inhalation. Irrigation with hypertonic saline (½ teaspoon

of noniodized salt in 8 oz of filtered water with a pinch of baking soda) is probably the most effective method for nasal hygiene and maintenance of healthy mucous membranes as well as for treatment of sinusitis.

12. How does diet affect the sinuses?

Many sinus sufferers have food allergies or food sensitivities. The foods most likely to trigger inflammation of the mucous membrane are cow's milk and all other dairy products[15] (which tend to produce more mucus), wheat,[16] chocolate, oranges, eggs, and artificial food coloring. Sugar,[17] caffeine, and alcohol also should be avoided. People with sinusitis are encouraged to increase consumption of fresh organic vegetables and fruits, whole grains, fiber, and protein.

If candidiasis is suspected (history of multiple antibiotics), patients are instructed to adhere closely to a candidal control diet, which is quite restrictive. No sugar, bread, alcohol, or refined carbohydrates are allowed.[1]

13. What are the most important antioxidants for treatment of sinusitis?

One of the key objectives of the holistic approach to sinusitis is to strengthen and/or restore balance to the immune system. The antioxidant vitamins, minerals, and herbs assist in the healing of the immune system and can be taken in pill or capsule form or through the diet. The most therapeutic for treating sinusitis are as follows:

1. **Vitamin C:** a natural antihistamine and anti-inflammatory agent that enhances immune response and white blood cell activity. Foods highest in vitamin C include guavas, oranges, cantaloupe, strawberries, red chili peppers, red and green sweet peppers, kale, parsley, broccoli, and cauliflower.[18]

2. **Vitamin E:** strong antioxidant that helps to minimize effects of air pollution. Foods highest in vitamin E include crude and unrefined soybean oil and wheat germ oil, fresh wheat germ, whole grains, raw nuts (most varieties), and all green, leafy vegetables.[19]

3. **Grape seed extract (proanthocyanidin):** a type of bioflavonoid that, according to multiple studies, is an extremely potent antioxidant (50 times more powerful than vitamin E and 20 times more powerful than vitamin C). It has been used for prevention of infections, as an anti-inflammatory agent, and for anti-aging. In Europe it is widely used for treating allergic rhinitis and asthma.[20]

4. **Selenium:** an antioxidant that breaks down leukotrienes, an allergy-related inflammatory compound. Foods highest in selenium include whole-wheat products, fish, whole grains, mushrooms, beans, garlic, and liver.

14. What other medicinal herbs and supplements can be used for acute sinusitis?

1. **Garlic:** an antibacterial, antiviral, antifungal, and anti-inflammatory agent.[21]
2. **Echinacea:** a powerful immunostimulator and anti-inflammatory agent.[22]
3. **Grapefruit seed extract:** an excellent antifungal herb.
4. **Essential fatty acids (EFAs):** as a supplement, EFAs both nourish the mucous membranes and act as a potent anti-inflammatory. They should be taken in the form of omega-3 oils, eicosapentaenoic acid (EPA), and dehydroacetic acid (DHA). Sources include cold-water fish (e.g., salmon, sardines, tuna, sole, mackerel), flaxseed oil (which contains almost twice as much omega-3 fatty acid as fish oils), wild game, canola oil, walnuts, pumpkin seeds, soybeans, fresh sea vegetables, and leafy greens.[23]

15. Should people with chronic sinusitis exercise?

Although exercise can be an effective immunostimulator, people with chronic sinusitis should begin exercising at a heart rate below the mild level and work their way up gradually. For sufferers from chronic sinusitis air quality is a critical factor in determining where and when to exercise. Ozone, a harmful air pollutant, is created by the combination of nitrogen oxides, hydrocarbons, and sunlight. A bright sunny day in the downtown area of most large cities produces high concentrations of ozone. In the summer, ozone builds up during the morning, reaches its maximum late in the afternoon, and then ebbs in the evening. In the winter ozone is less of a problem, but cold night air can trap a layer of carbon monoxide, nitrogen dioxide, sulfur dioxide, and particulates that may linger into the early morning. A good general practice is to do outdoor exercise in the morning during the summer and in the evening during the winter.

16. What role does sleep play in treating sinusitis?

Although diet, supplements, and exercise can benefit physical health and improve immune function, perhaps the most powerful and overlooked key to overall physical well-being is sleep. Lack of sleep and the resultant depression of the immune system can be factors in many chronic health conditions and are a common cause of colds and sinus infections. Additional sleep is an essential component in the holistic treatment of such conditions. As a general rule of thumb, if you wake up to an alarm clock, you are not getting enough sleep.

17. What are the key mental and emotional health components of the holistic medical treatment program?

The most limiting belief held by most chronic sinus sufferers is, "I'm going to have to live with this for the rest of my life." This thought can generate a great deal of anger, along with sadness. To change limiting beliefs and attitudes and to express or release the painful emotions responsible for the depressed immunity contributing to chronic sinusitis, the essential mental and emotional components are to practice affirmations and visualizations; to create a goal list and an ideal life vision (develop clarity about personal and professional objectives); to undergo counseling or psychotherapy or practice biofeedback; to learn safe release of anger, grief, and fear; journal ; and to find more humor, optimism, and play in life.

18. How do you begin the holistic treatment program for sinusitis?

It is helpful for patients to read Ivker's *Sinus Survival* to become familiar with the holistic approach. Because the treatment is based on self-care, this orientation helps patients to make the necessary commitment for successful treatment of chronic sinusitis. Patients also are advised to take the Candida Questionnaire and Scoresheet in Sinus Survival or in Crook's *The Yeast Connection* and/or the Comprehensive Diagnostic Stool Analysis (CDSA; Great Smokies Lab) to determine whether they are a candidate for the candidal treatment program as well. At the first office visit, the physical and environmental health components of the Sinus Survival Program are introduced (see tables below).

Physical and Environmental Health Components of the Sinus Survival Program for Preventing and Treating Sinusitis

	PREVENTIVE MAINTENANCE	TREATMENT OF INFECTION
* Sleep	7–9 hr; no alarm clock	8–10+ hr/day
* Negative ions or air cleaner	Continuous operation; use ions especially with air conditioning	Continuous operation
** Room humidifier, warm mist; and *** central humidifier	Use during dry conditions, especially in winter if heat is on and in summer in summer if air conditioner is on	Continuous operation
* Saline nasal spray (SS spray)	Use daily, especially with dirty and/or dry air.	Use daily, every 2–3 hr
* Steam inhaler	Use as needed with dirty and/or dry air	Use 2–4 times/day; add eucalyptus oil (VVAX)
* Nasal irrigation	Use as needed with dirty and/or dry air	Use 2–4 times/day after steam
* Water, bottled or filtered	Drink ½ oz/lb body weight; with exercise, drink ⅔ oz/lb	½ to ⅓ oz/lb body weight
* Diet	More fresh fruit, vegetables, whole grains, fiber; less sugar, dairy, caffeine, alcohol	No sugar, dairy products
* Exercise, preferably aerobic	Minimum: 20–30 min 3–5 times/wk; avoid outdoors in presence of high pollution or pollen, extremely cold temperatures	No aerobic; moderate walking okay. Avoid outdoors in presence of high pollution or pollen, cold temperatures

* Stage one: use to begin the program.
** Stage two: start after 3 weeks into the program or earlier if desired.
*** Stage three: start 6 weeks into the program or sooner if patient and practitioner are comfortable doing so.

Vitamins and Supplements for Preventing and Treating Sinusitis

	ADULTS		CHILDREN (> 3 YR OLD)		PREGNANCY	
	Prevention[1]	Treatment	Prevention	Treatment	Prevention	Treatment
Antioxidant vitamins and supplements						
* Vitamin C (polyascorbate or ester C)	1000–2000 mg 3 ×/d	3000–5000 mg 3 ×/d	100–200 mg 3 ×/d	500–1000 mg 3 ×/d	1000 mg 2 ×/d	1,000 mg 4 ×/d
** Beta carotene	25,000 IU 1 or 2 ×/d	25,000 IU[2] 3 ×/d	5,000 IU 1 or 2 ×/d	10,000 IU 2 ×/d	25,000 IU 1 ×/d	25,000 IU 2 ×/d
* Vitamin E	400 IU 1 or or 2 ×/d	400 IU 2 ×/d	50 IU 1 or 2 ×/d	200 IU 2 ×/d	200 IU 1 ×/d	200 IU 2 ×/d
* Proanthocyanidin (grape seed extract)	100 mg 1 or 2 ×/d (on empty stomach)	100 mg 3 ×/d (on empty stomach)	-	100 mg 1 ×/d	-	100 mg 1 ×/day
*** Vitamin B$_6$	50 mg 2 ×/d	200 mg 2¥/d 2 ×/d	10 mg 1¥/d 1 ×/d	25 mg 1 ×/d	25 mg 1 ×/d	25 mg 2 ×/d
Other supplements						
* Multivitamin[3]	1–3 ×/d	1–3 ×/d	Pediatric multivitamin		Prenatal multivitamin with 800 mg folic acid	
** Selenium	100–200 µg/d	200 µg/d	-	100 µg/d	25 µg/d	100 µg 2 ×/d
** Zinc picolinate	20–40 mg/d	40–60 mg/d	10 mg/d	10 mg 2 ×/d	25 mg/d	40 mg/d
** Magnesium citrate, aspartate, or glycinate	500 mg/d	500 mg/d	150–250 mg/d	300 mg/d	500 mg/d	500 mg/d
** Calcium (citrate or hydroxyapatite)	1000 mg/d Menopause: 1500 mg/d	1000 mg/d Menopause: 1500 mg/d	600–800 mg/d from diet		1200 mg/d	1200 mg/d
*** Chromium picolinate	200 µg/d	200 µg/d			In prenatal multivitamin vitamin	
Botanicals/herbs						
* Garlic	1200 mg/d	1200–2000 mg 3 ×/d		1000 mg 3 ×/d	-	1200 mg 3 ×/d
* Echinacea	200 mg 2 ×/d or 25 drops 2–3 ×/d (allergy prevention)	200 mg 3 ×/d or 25 drops 4–5 ×/d	-	100 mg 3 ×/d or 7–10 drops 3 ×/d	-	200 µg 3 ×/d or 25 drops 4 ×/d
** Berberis or goldenseal[4]		200 mg 3 ×/d or 20 drops 5 ×/d		100 mg 3 ×/d or 7–10 drops 3 ×/d		
*** Bee propolis	-	500 mg 3 ×/d	-	200 mg 3 ×/d or 500 mg 1 ×/d	-	500 mg 3 ×/d
* Grapefruit (citrus) seed extract	-	100 mg 3 ×/d or 10 drops in water 3 ×/d	-	4 drops in water 2 ×/d	-	100 mg 3 ×/d or 10 drops in water 3 ×/d

Continued on following page

Vitamins and Supplements for Preventing and Treating Sinusitis (Continued)

	ADULTS		CHILDREN (> 3 YR OLD)		PREGNANCY	
	Prevention[1]	Treatment	Prevention	Treatment	Prevention	Treatment
Essential fatty acids						
** Flaxseed oil or omega-3 fatty acids in fish oil	2 tbsp/d	2 tbsp/d	1 tbsp/d	1 tbsp/d	2 tbsp/d	2 tbsp/d
* Antibiotics[5]						

* Stage one: use to begin the program.
** Stage two: start after 3 weeks into the program or earlier if desired.
*** Stage three: start t6 weeks into the program or sooner if patient and practitioner are comfortable doing so.
[1]Use the higher dosage on days of higher stress, less sleep, and increased air pollution.
[2]Use this dosage for a maximum of 1 month.
[3]Dosage depends on brand.
[4]Some people with ragweed allergy are sensitive to goldenseal.
[5]Antibiotics are an option for sinusitis if taken infrequently (i.e., 1 or 2 ×/year) or if no improvement is seen with this program after 2 weeks.

19. How well does this program work for sinusitis?

According to a questionnaire to which nearly 200 patients responded, 92% of those who made at least a 2-month commitment to follow the program closely experienced either cure or significant improvement in chronic sinusitis. After suffering with the problem for 10 years, the author has been free of chronic sinusitis since 1987.

20. Should antifungal medication be used in treating the more severe cases of chronic sinusitis that are unresponsive to conventional treatment?

It appears so. In 2000, in collaboration with William Silvers, a Denver allergist, the first Sinus Survival Study was completed. Each of the participants was a patient of Dr. Silvers with a long-term history of moderate-to-severe chronic sinusitis. All had been treated with multiple courses of broad-spectrum antibiotics for several years. Each was treated with fluconazole (200 mg/day for 1 month, then every other day for another 2 weeks) in addition to the entire Sinus Survival Program as outlined above. After four months in the program, including 6 weeks on fluconazole, 9 of 10 participants experienced statistically significant improvement. One patient with severe asthma had to take a course of antibiotic and prednisone during the study. The recently completed statistical analysis of the 1-year follow-up revealed persistence of significant improvement (statistically and clinically). Publication of the study is anticipated in 2002.

REFERENCES

1. Ivker RS: Sinus Survival: The Holistic Medical Treatment for Sinusitis, Allergies, and Colds, 4th ed. New York, Tarcher/Putnam/Penguin, 2000.
2. Gwaltney JM, Phillips CD, et al: Computed tomographic study of the common cold. N Engl J Med 330:25–30, 1994.
3. Centers for Disease Control and Prevention/National Center for Health Statistics: Current Estimates from the National Health Interview Survey. Washington, DC, U.S. Government Printing Office, 1995.
4. Dockery DW, Pope CA, et al: An association between air pollution and mortality in six U.S. cities. N Engl J Med 329:1753–1759, 1993.
5. Ponikau JV, Sherris DA, Kern EB, et al: The diagnosis and incidence of allergic fungal sinusitis. Mayo Clinic Proc 74:877–884, 1999.
6. Terris M, Davidson T: Review of published results for endoscopic sinus surgery. Ear Nose Throat J 73:574–580, 1994.
7. Garbutt JM, Goldstein M, Gellman E, et al: A randomized, placebo-controlled trial of antimicrobial treatment for children with clinically diagnosed acute sinusitis. Pediatrics 107:619–625, 2001.
8. Ben-Dov, et al: Effect of negative ionization of inspired air on the response of asthmatic children to exercise and inhaled histamine. Thorax 38:584–88, 1983.
9. Warner JA, Marchant JL, Warner JO: Double-blind trial of ionizers in children with asthma sensitive to the house dust mite. Thorax 48:330–33, 1993.

10. Kornblueh I: Artificial ionization of the air and its biological significance. Clin Med 68: 467–470, 1962.

11. Ophir D, Elad Y: Effects of steam inhalation nasal patency and nasal symptoms in patients with the common cold. Am J Otolaryngol 8(3):149–153, 1987.

12. Talbot AR, Herr TM, Parsons DS: Mucociliary clearance and buffered hypertonic saline solution. Laryngoscope 107:500–503, 1997.

13. Georgitis JW: Nasal hyperthermia and simple saline irrigation for perennial rhinitis, changes in inflammatory mediators. Chest 106:1487–1482, 1994.

14. Heatley DG, McConnell KE et al: Nasal irrigation for the alleviation of sinonasal symptoms. Otolaryngol Head Neck Surg 125:44–48, 2001.

15. Ogle KA, Bullock JD: Children with allergic rhinitis and/or bronchial asthma treated with elimination diet. Ann Allergy 39:8–11, 1977.

16. Bell IR, Schwartz GE, Peterson JM, et al: Symptom and personality profiles of young adults from a college student population with self-reported illness from foods and chemicals. J Am Coll Nutr Dec:693–702, 1993.

17. Sanchez A: Role of sugars in human neutrophilic phagocytosis. Am J Clin Nutr 26:1180–1184, 1973.

18. Vojdani A, Ghoneum M: In vivo effect of ascorbic acid on enhancement of human natural killer cell activity. Nutr Res 13:753–764, 1993.

19. Meydani SN, Barklund MP, Liu S, et al: Vitamin E supplementation enhances cell-mediated immunity in healthy elderly subjects. Am J Clin Nutr 52:557–563, 1990.

20. Agache P: Mise en Evidence d'un Effet-Dose l'Antagonisme Vis à Vis de la Papule Histaminique. Vie Med 16:1153–1154, 1979.

21. Garlic in cryptococcal meningitis: A preliminary report of 21 cases. Chinese Med J 93:123–126, 1980.

22. Bauer VR, Juric K, Puhlmann J, et al: Immunologic in vivo and in vitro studies on echinacea extracts. Arzneimittelforschung 38:276–281, 1988.

23. Meydani SN, Lichtenstein AH, White PJ, et al: Food use and health effects of soybean and sunflower oils. J Am Coll Nutr Oct:406–428, 1991.

45. URINARY TRACT INFECTION

Bhaswati Bhattacharya, M.P.H., M.D.

1. Who gets urinary tract infections (UTIs)?

Because most infections are thought to arise from organisms ascending from the perineum to the sterile bladder, cystitis (bladder inflammation) is very common in adult women, whose urethra is short compared with that of men. In fact, 90% of UTIs are found in women.

Statistics show that 10–20% of all women have UTIs at least once a year; 37.5% of women with no history of UTIs will have one within 10 years. In random samples, 2–4% of healthy women have elevated levels of bacteria in the urine. Recurrent bladder infections can be a significant problem for some women, and some infections eventually involve the kidneys. Recurrent kidney infection is associated with progressive damage of tissue, resulting in scarring and, rarely, kidney failure.

2. Describe the clinical symptoms of UTIs.

Clinical symptoms of UTIs in adults include urinary frequency, dysuria (burning pain on urination), nocturia, lower abdominal pain, and turbid, foul-smelling, or dark urine. Physical examination may also reveal mucosal edema, redness, and occasionally, ulcerations around the urethra. Urinalysis should be done and often shows significant pyuria and bacteriuria. Conventionally, the presence of more than 100,000 microorganisms per ml of clean-catch urine is considered to be definitive for UTI.

However, the diagnosis of UTIs has been somewhat empirical because clinical symptoms and presence of significant amount of bacteria in the urine do not correlate well in many scientific studies. Only 60% of women with classic symptoms actually had significant level of bacteriuria.[1]

3. What is the role of pH in urinary infections? Is acid or alkaline pH more helpful for preventing UTIs?

Much debate has occurred about the level of pH that predisposes to UTIs. Theories exist for either acidifying or alkalinizing urine. Alkaline urinary pH in the range of 7.5–9 is seen in chronic UTIs caused by microorganisms that produce urease, such as *Proteus* and *Klebsiella* spp. Urine that has a low pH inhibits bacterial growth.[2] Attempts to acidify the urine have been difficult because so many buffers in the kidney prevent acidification, and many researchers discuss the improbability of maintaining acidified urine as a protective measure. Yet some doctors believe that periods of acidified urine protect from overgrowth of species such as *Proteus*, which favors alkaline environments.

On the flip side, alkalinization for prophylaxis has also been used for treating some types of UTIs. Citrate salts, such as potassium citrate or sodium citrate, work without affecting gastric pH or producing laxative effects. They are excreted partly as carbonate, thus raising the pH of the urine, and long have been used in the treatment of lower UTIs.[3] In addition, many of the herbs used to treat UTIs, such as goldenseal and *Arctostaphylos uva ursi*, work best in an alkaline environment; therefore, alkalization is promoted. Currently, there is no consensus about alkaline vs acidified urine for protection against UTIs.

4. Which dietary elements can predispose to UTIs?

Many naturopaths believe that food allergies can produce cystitis in some patients and therefore use food elimination diets to cure or prevent UTIs. Excessive sugar consumption and nutritional deficiencies can contribute to the development of UTIs.

It is recommended that patients predisposed to UTIs should avoid all simple sugars and refined carbohydrates and drink only diluted fruit juices, because bacteria tend to thrive in high-sugar environments. Eating plenty of watermelon is also recommended because it acts as a natural diuretic. Eating liberal amounts of garlic and onion, which have antimicrobial properties, is also highly recommended.

5. What is the relationship between chronic cystitis and UTIs?

Cystitis is defined as inflammation of the transitional epithelium of the urinary tract due to microbial invasion. Chronic interstitial cystitis (IC) is a severe bladder disorder of at least 12 months' duration that causes chronic suprapubic pain, urinary frequency, and nocturia. Routine urine cultures are negative, and symptoms do not respond to antibiotics. Other causes of cystitis must first be ruled out, including tumors, bladder calculi, and medication side effects. Possible causes include autoimmune reaction against bladder antigens, deficiency in the glycosaminoglycan mucosal layer, and mast cell infiltration. Food allergies have been implicated as a cause of chronic cystitis,[4] and a trial elimination diet may be useful. Chronic interstitial cystitis can predispose patients to UTIs and is frequently responsible for persistent, subclinical symptoms. Acupuncture has been reported to be useful for IC, but clinical studies have not confirmed this finding.

6. What risk factors are associated with UTIs?

Factors associated with UTIs include pregnancy (during which UTIs are twice as frequent), sexual intercourse, homosexual activity, diabetes, mechanical trauma or irritation, and structural abnormalities of the urinary tract that block the free flow of urine, such as enlarged prostates, kidney stones, or catheters. Complicated UTIs are more likely among men, immunosuppressed patients, people with diabetes, and pregnant women.

7. What anatomic factors are related to development of UTIs?

Because urine from the kidneys remains sterile until it reaches the urethral opening, infection requires introduction of bacteria by ascension from the urethra or, less commonly, through the bloodstream (< 5%). Usually fecal contamination or vaginal secretions are factors in creating ascending infections. In addition, anatomic or functional obstructions to flow, such as indwelling catheters, and immune system dysfunction are thought to play a role. Free flow, complete emptying of the bladder, and good hygiene are also important, as is maintenance of optimal immune defense.

Pooling of urine in bladders of men with enlarged prostates also contributes to UTIs. In pregnant women, both bladder compression from the gravid uterus and physiologic dilatation of the ureters increases the risk of UTIs. For older women, loss of the integrity of the pelvic floor muscles can lead to bladder prolapse and loss of normal sphincter protection. Pessaries can be a useful and comforting nonpharmacologic tool to help approximate normal genitourinary anatomy in older women to prevent UTIs.

8. What defenses in the host's immune system enhance protection against UTIs?

The healthy body has several defenses to prevent bacterial growth in the urinary tract. In addition to urine flow that washes away bacteria, the surface of the bladder has antimicrobial properties via its smooth epithelial cell structure and mucosal coating. which make it less amenable to adhesion by bacteria. In addition, the slightly acidic pH of most people's urine inhibits the growth of many organisms. Moreover, it has been found that prostatic fluid has antimicrobial substances. The body also quickly secretes white cells in the pelvis at the first sign of bacterial invasion. Adequate estrogenization and maintenance of normal vaginal flora in postmenopausal women also aids in reducing incidence of UTIs.[5]

9. What is the most common error in screening asymptomatic patients for UTIs?

Failure to teach patients how to provide a clean-catch sample of urine may result in false-positive results of urinalysis and urine cultures, leading to unneeded antibiotic treatment.

10. What is the difference between the conventional and holistic approach to UTIs?

Whereas most conventional methods of treating UTIs consist of antibiotics to combat the bacterial infection or surgical intervention to correct an anatomic abnormality, the holistic approach involves prevention through enhancing normal host protective measures and giving the damaged uroepithelium a chance to heal. Emphasis is placed on enhancing the flow of urine through proper hydration and urine production; promoting alkaline or acidic urinary pH (depending on the type of bacteria and infection) , which inhibits growth of the microorganism; preventing bacterial adherence to the endothelial cell of the bladder; and enhancing the immune system. Botanical medicines with antimicrobial properties are used only when needed. Antibiotic medications are prescribed only when the risk-to-benefit ratio of not using antibiotics is too high.

Providers should inquire into contributory factors, including access to toiletry; mobility; age; financial access to herbs, drugs, or hygiene products; cultural issues; sexual practices; and personal preferences for self-care. If a patient has recurrent UTIs or is at high risk, a prophylactic regimen of herbs, supplements. and homeopathy may be useful. In addition, health education is essential, so that the patient understands the importance of exercise, a healthy immune system, and good hygiene.

11. How does exercise help to prevent UTIs?

Generally, exercise keeps muscles toned and improves lymphatic flow. Pelvic floor muscles (sphincter urethrae muscle, deep transverse perineal muscles, levator ani) and associated fascia help to maintain the anatomy of the urinary tract. Kegel exercises are designed to improve the tone of this muscular sling in women and to prevent bladder prolapse and urethral obstruction. Patients are instructed to tighten and release the vaginopelvic muscles for 10 second intervals in a series of 10 contractions and to repeat the exercise at least 3 times/day for optimal conditioning. During acute infections, it is best to avoid activities such as prolonged motorcycle rides, horseback riding, and bicycling.

12. Why is hydration helpful for UTIs?

Increasing urine flow is an important, safe, natural, and inexpensive intervention. Drinking more fluids, especially cranberry juice, green tea, herbal teas, and clean, filtered water, promotes good flow through the kidneys. Patients should drink diluted unsweetened juices and avoid juices high in fructose corn syrup. They also should avoid soft drinks and concentrated fruit drinks because of the high sugar content. Coffee and alcohol may overstimulate or irritate the bladder. Care obviously must be taken in patients with compromised renal function or prerenal abnormalities, such as congestive heart failure, edematous tendencies due to hypoosmotic states, and hypertension.

13. What types of hygiene are important for preventing UTIs?

1. Personal hygiene is difficult to counsel and address with adult patients, most of whom were taught toilet habits at young ages. Second-nature behaviors are conditioned and difficult to alter. Care and tact must be taken to cover the basics of cleaning after bowel movements and how to wash the perineum. A helpful tool is a diagram of the perineal area, with review of how to wipe from front to back, the detailed anatomy of the labia in females and scrotum in males, and the basics of where flora tend to reside in the perineal area. A compassionate but not pedantic approach is of utmost importance.

2. Handwashing is another basic type of hygiene that must be emphasized. Washing before exiting the bathroom is important because fixtures are often contaminated with *Escherichia coli* and *Staphylococcus aureus*. Soap is useful only if lathered for 20–30 seconds before rinsing. Otherwise, mechanical rubbing of the hands and clean water are essential.

3. Sexual hygiene is important for preventing UTIs and is discussed in question 14.

4. Good hygiene also consists of complete emptying of the bladder and not holding urine for prolonged periods (e.g., during travel), with free flow to wash away bacteria.

5. Avoid perfumed bath products, toilet papers, sanitary napkins and douches, and strong washing detergents, because they may add unneeded chemical irritation to the area.

6. Change underclothing daily, avoiding thongs or tight underpants or leotards made of nylon or synthetic fabrics. Cotton and silk are the best fabrics for people with a predisposition to UTIs.

14. What issues of sexual hygiene should be discussed with patients with frequent UTIs?

Sexual hygiene is another difficult topic to address with patients and may cause even more discomfort for patients of certain ethnic backgrounds. A portion of the world's population has culture-based values regarding touch and discussions about sex, which may be difficult for doctors to appreciate. Periods of increased sexual intercourse resulting in "honeymoon cystitis" are caused by inflammation of the bladder due to infections arising as bacterial flora move from the perineum and vagina into the urethral canal. This problem can often be prevented with effective hygiene techniques.

Basic issues include the importance of urinating before and after intercourse, hand-washing, avoiding genital intercourse immediately after anal intercourse, techniques for safe anal-genital contact, washing the perineum carefully after mechanical trauma, and techniques for clean oral-genital contact. Patients should be advised that the use of spermicides with or without a diaphragm increases the frequency of vaginal colonization with uropathogens and UTIs because of the change in pH and the change in epithelial lining due to the cell-damaging chemicals in spermicides. In postmenopausal women who use lubricants during intercourse, it is important to emphasize that lubricants can also alter the vaginal flora. Perhaps the details of some of these topics are not immediately relevant for each sexually active patient with predisposition to UTIs, but a physician should be prepared to explore and discuss such issues.

15. What is the role of cranberry juice in UTI treatment and prevention?

Much attention has been given to cranberries and cranberry juice because clinical trials showed their effectiveness in resolving active UTIs and preventing recurrence of bladder infection.[6] The action of cranberry juice was previously thought to occur by its acidification of the urine and through the antibacterial effects of hippuric acid. Subsequent studies have focused on components in cranberry juice that reduce the ability of bacteria to adhere to the lining of the bladder and urethra, and this mechanism is now considered the most likely explanation. A study of nursing home patients showed that drinking 4–6 ounces of cranberry juice almost daily for 7 weeks prevented UTIs in two-thirds of patients.[7] Unfortunately, some studies have shown an increased recurrence rate once regular prophylaxis is discontinued.

The recommended dosage of unsweetened cranberry juice is of 0.5 L/day (approximately 2 glasses, 8 ounces each) for prophylaxis. However, care must be taken to avoid juice products, most of which have added sugar and are diluted to as little as 10% cranberry juice. Because many clinical studies used commercial products containing concentrated sugars, it is difficult to compare unsweetened products. Sweetening is advised only with apple or grape juice. Simultaneous consumption of citrus and other acidic juices is not recommended. Lastly, the cranberry extracts now available in pill form are not highly recommended, because scientific evidence has not yet shown that they contain all of the elements necessary to reproduce the beneficial medicinal effects of the juice.

16. What other juices may help prevent UTIs?

It appears that the juice of blueberries, which belong to the same botanical *Vaccinium* genus and Ericaceae family as cranberries, has similar effects. Both contain a specific high-molecular-weight polymeric compound that potently inhibits *E. coli* fimbrial adhesion and thus prevents colonization in both gut and bladder. Other juices (e.g., grapefruit, mango, pineapple, orange juice) do not contain this inhibitor.[8] Cranberry juice is often recommended because it is more widely available.

17. Does scientific evidence support the efficacy of the traditional herb gotu kola?

In chronic interstitial cystitis, the integrity of the bladder wall interstitium has been interrupted. Extracts of *Centella asiatica*, or gotu kola, have been shown to have strong wound-healing activity through triterpene compounds (asiatic acid, madecassic acid, asiaticoside, and madecassoside), which stimulate collagen synthesis and normal connective tissue matrix when taken orally.[9] Historically, gotu kola is well documented in the ancient ayurvedic surgical texts and was used internally and externally by surgeons and people of Java and other islands of Polynesia to aid in wound healing of the female genitourinary tract.

Clinically, *C. asiatica* also has been used for burns, cellulite, cirrhosis of the liver, keloids, scleroderma, and perineal lesions. For preventing UTIs, it can improve the integrity of the interstitium as well as heal ulcerations of the bladder,[10] especially in patients with chronic cystitis. Standardized extract of gotu kola contain 30–40% asiaticosides and 2–4% triterpenes per dose. Gotu kola has been shown to be abortifacient in animal studies and is strictly contraindicated during pregnancy.

18. How is goldenseal useful in UTIs?

Goldenseal (*Hydrastis canadensis*), although endangered and thus discouraged for general use, has long been regarded as a powerful antimicrobial, working especially against *E. coli, Klebsiella* spp.,

Proteus spp., *Staphylococcus* spp., E*nterobacter aerogenses*, and *Pseudomonas* spp. Goldenseal's active component, berberine, works better in alkaline urine. Women who tend to develop bladder infections should wash the labia and urethra with a strong, tepid tea of goldenseal (2 tsp/cup) before and after intercourse, if possible. The dosage is 4–6 ml of 1:5 tincture or 250–500 mg of powdered solid extract standardized to 8% alkaloid.

19. What is the basis for the action of uva ursi?

Research related to *Arctostaphylos uva ursi*, also known as bearberry or upland cranberry, has shown that 7–9% of the leaves is composed of arbutin, a powerful antiseptic. Arbutin is hydrolyzed to hydroquinone, which alkalinizes the urine. Because crude plant extracts have been shown to be more effective than isolated arbutin, recent clinical trials have focused on the use of standardized ura ursi extract and found that it was effective for recurrent cystitis. Care must be taken to avoid toxicity. Pure uva ursi has a narrow therapeutic window. Toxic signs include tinnitus, nausea, vomiting, shortness of breath, and, later, convulsions. Dosage for uva ursi is standardized to 10–5% arbutin.[11]

20. Next to antibiotics when they are needed, what can be used to enhance the restoration of natural balance?

Probiotics, or "friendly" bacteria, live in the human body and have a protective effect on the tissues in which they reside, such as the gut, vagina, and bladder. *Lactobacillus* species are the most commonly known probiotics. Replacing friendly flora killed by antibiotic usage helps to prevent settlement and proliferation of pathogenic bacteria and to maintain the bladder epithelium. The recommended dosage is a capsule form of live *Lactobacillus acidophilus* in the morning and immediately before bedtime. Vaginal suppositories, in addition to oral therapy, are especially helpful immediately after a course of antibiotic is completed.

21. When is homeopathy an appropriate treatment for UTIs?

Homeopathic remedies, although they do not fit within the theories of the scientific analysis, have been shown to be among the most effective treatments for diseases involving inflammation or infection. Although remedies are specifically tailored to individual symptoms of illness, staphysagria 6C is especially useful for honeymoon cystitis and recurrent infections, and cantharis 6C can be used for the first days of burning pain during urination Typically, 3–5 pellets are taken under the tongue 3–4 times/day when the symptoms first appear.

22. When do holistic practitioners use conventional treatments such as antibiotics?

Patients with persistently positive urine cultures or recurrent untreated UTIs should consider a course of 4–6 weeks of antibiotics for cure. Men may have an upper tract or prostatic source of infection and benefit greatly from 4–6 weeks of systemic antibiotic treatment. Trimethoprim/sulfamethoxazole or ciprofloxacin is the usual agent of choice; both cover *E. coli, Staphylococcus saprophyticus, Klebsiella* spp., and *Enterococcus* spp. UTIs acquired systemically often require stronger agents because of the development of resistant organisms.

23. What food supplements are useful for UTIs?

Nutritional supplements are generally used for enhancing immune stimulation and increasing antioxidant protection. A typical regimen includes vitamin C, 500 mg every 2 hours for the first day of infection; bioflavonoids,1 gm/day; vitamin A, 25,000 IU/day; zinc, 30 mg/day; and choline, 1gm/day.[12]

24. What resources are available for more information?

- www.garynull.com (online reports of Gary Null, Ph.D., and excerpts from the Clinician's Handbook of Natural Healing)
- www.healthy.net (articles on UTIs written by well-known naturopaths)

REFERENCES

1. Pizzorno JE, Murray MT: Cystitis. In Pizzorno JE and Murray MT (eds.): Textbook of Natural Medicine. New York, Churchill Livingstone, 1999, pp1183–1188.
2. Gupta K, Rubin RH: Infections of the urinary tract, In Dale DC (ed): Scientific American Medicine. New York , Scientific American, 1999.
3. Spooner JB. Alkalinization in the management of cystitis. J Int Med Res, 1984;12:30-34.
4. Palicios AS, Quintera de Juana A, Sagarra JM, et al: Eosinophilic food-induced cystitis. Allergol Immunopathol 12(6):463–469, 1984.
5. Raz R, Stamm WE: A controlled trial of intravaginal estriol in post menopausal women with recurrent urinary tract infections. N Engl J Med 329:753, 1993.
6. Kontiokari T, Sundqvist K, Nuutinen M, et al: Randomized trial of cranberry-lingonberry juice and *Lactobacillus* GG drink for the prevention of urinary tract infections in women. BMJ 322: 1-5, 2001.
7. Gibson L, et al: Effectiveness of cranberry juice in preventing urinary tract infections in long-term Care Facility Patients. J Naturopathic Medicine, 1991; 2(10):45-47.
8. Ofek I, Goldhar J, Zafriri D, et al: Anti-*Escherichia coli* adhesion activity of cranberry and blueberry juices. N Engl J Med 324:1599, 1991.
9. Bonte F, Dumas M, et al: Influence of asiatic acid, madecassic acid, and asiaticoside on human collagen I synthesis. Planta Med 60:683–688, 1994.
10. Etrebi A, Ibrahim A, Zaki K: Treatment of bladder ulcer with asiaticoside. J Egypt Med Assoc 58:324, 1975.
11. La Valle JB, et al: Uva ursi. In Natural Therapeutics Pocket Guide. Hudson, OH, Lexi-Comp, 2001, p 515.
12. Pizzorno JE, Murray MT (eds): Textbook of Natural Medicine. New York, Churchill Livingstone, 1999.

46. CHRONIC PAIN SYNDROME

Reid Blackwelder, M.D.

Pain ... is the breaking of the shell that encloses your understanding.

Kahlil Gibran

1. How prevalent is pain as a medical diagnosis?

Pain is an extremely intricate series of signs and symptoms. It is considered primarily a symptom in the acute state; pain, however, becomes a disease when it becomes more chronic. In the general United States population, the prevalence of chronic pain is estimated at 20–40%; in nursing home patients, at 80%; and in patients with cancer, at 75%.[1]

Because chronic pain affects the whole person, the holistic approach is ideal. In this sense, pain is definitely "psychosomatic" because it involves the psyche as well as the body—independently as well as interdependently.

2. Why is pain management becoming such an issue?

An estimated 50% of patients with chronic pain in ambulatory practice settings receive inadequate relief.[2] For this reason, it is becoming a major public health problem. For hospitalized patients, new standards for pain management were issued by the Joint Commission on Accreditation of Healthcare Organizations (JCAHO) in 2001. These standards state the following[3]:

- The patient has the right to appropriate assessment and management of pain.
- Health care providers must assess the existence, nature, and intensity of pain.
- Staff competency in both addressing and managing pain must be ensured.
- Policies must be in place to support appropriate prescription of effective medications.
- Patients and families must be educated about their rights concerning effective pain management.
- At the time of discharge, patient needs for symptomatic management of pain must be assessed.

These standards apply to hospitalized patients and are not legally formalized for outpatient management of pain. However, they can be generalized, and outpatient standards can be expected eventually.

3. What are the key components of the approach to pain treatment?

Pain management creates a number of challenges in diagnosis as well as treatment. It is important to learn to diagnose and deal with both objective and subjective issues of chronic pain. The patient's perception of pain is a subjective but fundamental component that must be addressed in the treatment plan. Most important, the treatment of chronic pain involves a long-term commitment between provider and patient. Pain is a dynamic rather than static process. Certain pain conditions change over time; for example, as the pain of degenerative arthritis progresses, patients' ability to cope with pain may change. In addition, the relationship between patient and provider also changes over time, affecting the adequacy of pain management.

4. What constitutes "alternative approaches" to pain management?

In general, complementary and alternative medicine (CAM) approaches are constantly being reevaluated and even redefined. As more information is obtained from experiential use as well as research studies, some approaches initially considered CAM modalities become mainstream. Examples include hypnosis, acupuncture, and manual medicine.

Traditional allopathic approaches, such as how pharmaceutical medications are prescribed, also are undergoing significant reevaluation. For example, the use of narcotics in nonmalignant chronic pain is in transition as a therapeutic approach. Not long ago, the medical literature suggested that narcotic prescriptions had no role in the treatment of chronic pain. Now a number of professional pain management organizations, and an increasing number of articles in medical journals suggest that narcotic medications indeed have a role in the management of both malignant and nonmalignant chronic pain.[4] Data support both sides of this ongoing argument. Of note, California recently passed a law requiring doctors to complete courses in pain management to retain medical licensure.

5. Why do patients seek alternative approaches for pain management?

As documented extensively by some of the ground-breaking authors in CAM research, such as Eisenberg and Adler, alternative approaches are much more commonly sought for conditions that Western biomedicine does not treat well. As stated above, "traditional" approaches to pain management are seen with increasing frequency as inadequate. Chronic pain includes such conditions as fibromyalgia, diabetic peripheral neuropathy, and osteoarthritis. In fact, pain is often a separate subset of these diagnoses. Such areas that are not easily or effectively managed by traditional biomedicine. Patients who continue to suffer will seek other treatment options.

In addition, awareness of adverse reactions and deaths related to traditional pharmaceutical approaches has increased. Although the published numbers have generated some controversy, deaths due to the right prescription for the right patient with the appropriate diagnosis have been called either the fourth or sixth leading cause of mortality in the U.S.[5] As patients become more aware of adverse consequences of traditional approaches, they begin to seek alternatives that they hope are safer.

6. Discuss the role of communication skills in pain management.

Although not included in the traditional definition of alternative approaches, communication skills easily meet the definition of CAM offered by the National Institutes of Health (NIH). In general, good communication skills are not routinely taught in U.S. medical schools, available in U.S. hospitals, or reimbursed by third-party payers. Moreover, as opposed to other integrative approaches, communication skills are readily available for learning as well as for practice by any health care professional. Accordingly, they should play a prominent role in the management of chronic pain.

Communication skills are key to the more difficult aspects of pain management. Patients dealing with chronic pain often have a great deal of fear about their problem and treatment options. This fear often manifests as anger or frustration, directed at the provider or other aspects of the "system." Excellent communication skills can help identify these issues early in the therapeutic relationship and create a collaborative rather than antagonistic partnership. In this way, communication skills alone become a potentially healing technique; they are at the heart of the art of medicine and good bedside manner.

7. What are the components of communication skills?

Although, unfortunately, the change is not universal, a number of medical schools are beginning to emphasize core communication skills, which include the following:
- Rapport-building techniques
- Agenda setting for both patient and provider (e.g., the patient desires pain-free walking; the provider wants to maximize lifestyle changes)
- Use of open-ended instead of closed-ended questions, especially early in the interview (e.g., "How would you describe your knee pain?" vs. "Is it a sharp pain?")
- Active listening for cues and clues to elicit the patient's perspective of illness (e.g., What impact does the problem have on the patient's life?)
  Recognizing and responding to emotions
- Negotiating common ground (agreeing on an exercise routine with proper use of medications)
When used well, these skills are time-efficient as well as therapeutic. They ensure that the topics that need to be covered are quickly identified and facilitate efficient gathering of the necessary medical information for diagnostic and therapeutic purposes.

8. To address pain treatment appropriately, what medical information needs to be collected?

As with any medical problem, a number of basic pieces of information must be obtained to make an appropriate diagnosis and to direct therapeutic recommendations. Even for chronic pain, the nature of the original injury or onset of the problem should be elicited. Symptoms should be noted, along with exacerbating and relieving factors. The best way to document objectively the strongly subjective components of pain is not certain. In general, some form of visual analog scale (VAS) should be used, especially in children. Perhaps such visual scales are more useful than the traditional verbal pain scale that rates paint from 0 to 10.

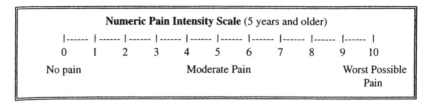

Traditional verbal pain scale.

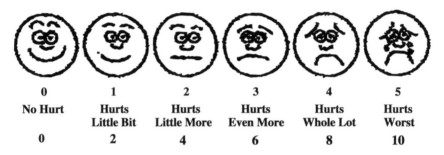

Wong-Baker FACES Pain Rating Scale for assessment of pain. (From Wong DL, Hockenberry-Eaton M, Wilson D, Winkelstein ML, Schwartz P: Wong's Essentials of Pediatric Nursing, 6/e. St. Louis, 2001, p 1301. Copyrighted by Mosby, Inc. Reprinted by permission.)

Chronic pain and acute pain often are conceptualized differently. Even when making progress, patients may describe chronic pain as 7 on a scale of 10. Using similar evaluations not only of pain but also of sleep, emotions, and mood may help create objective measurements that can be readily and consistently obtained at each visit.

In addition, previous attempts at pain treatment should be clearly documented to ensure that all options are explored. A review of records often reveals that some therapeutic attempts or even medications were given an inadequate trial. Finally, it is critically important to explore whether the patient has had problems with drugs of potential abuse in the past. Such drugs should include not only narcotics,but also nicotine, alcohol, and caffeine.

9. What additional information is needed but often omitted from a typical medical history?

Chronic pain affects the whole patient, including family, friends, and activities. Such effects must be part of of an effective treatment plan. Medical schools now routinely refer to this method of history-taking as the "bio-psycho-social model," which should be broadened to include spiritual components as well. How patients deal with stress, what coping skills they implement, and their support systems should be clearly identified.

More and more evidence emphasizes that isolation and control play a key role in how medical problems are seen and handled. The less isolated and the more in control a patient feels, the greater the benefit of various treatment approaches. Exploring ways to address these issues specifically in terms of chronic pain is important.

It is also important to identify specific activities that are limited by the pain (e.g., mopping the floor, walking up a flight of stairs, sitting for more than 10 minutes) and to avoid broad generalities. These factors must be followed to identify progress. Moreover, it is important to ask patients about their expectations from the treatment approach and from the provider to clarify boundaries.

10. What is meant by "boundary setting" in pain management?

Clear identification of the patient's expectations is crucial to setting goals and boundaries. In the absence of functional goal setting, patients' expectations may be unrealistic and impossible to meet. Unrealistic expectations can create frustration, anxiety, and a conflictual therapeutic relationship. For example, patients with chronic pain who expect the provider to "fix" them or to have complete pain relief from a medication may have unreasonable goals.

In addition, providers are obligated to be clear about their own boundaries in terms of what medical management they are willing to provide. Examples include whether the provider is willing to use opioids or is comfortable with integrating CAM therapies (e.g., acupuncture, botanicals) that the patient may desire. Such issues should be settled at the beginning of the patient-provider relationship to avoid frustrations on both sides. In addition, the provider's personal availability to the patient should be clearly identified. Important factors include kind of practice and willingness to "gray" some of the boundaries.

Most important, both patient and provider should be clear about the patient's own responsibility for health and healing. It is not the provider's job to "make" the patient better. The patient must agree to be actively involved in his or her own care plan. In many ways, this approach helps to create a personal sense of empowerment and involvement for patients who are willing to make such a commitment.

11. What clues help identify patients whose pain has a strong behavioral component?

Chronic pain has significant behavioral components, which have been studied by a number of investigators, most notably Waddell. In 1980, he studied 26 clinical signs in 350 patients.[6] Eight behavioral signs were consistently found to be reliable as well as reproducible indicators of nonstructural pain:

1. Superficial tenderness of skin
2. Nonanatomic tenderness
3. Axial loading (pushing on the top of the head)
4. Simulated rotation
5. Distracted straight leg raise
6. Regional sensory change (nondermatomal)
7. Regional weakness
8. Overreaction

It is important to recognize that "nonorganic" pain does not necessarily mean no pain. Moreover, patients with back problems, for example, can demonstrate additional behavioral signs because of fear or desire to please the provider. The predictive value of behavioral signs is improved if three or more indicators are present in any one patient. A number of other signs can be explored as well. For example, looking at shoe wear patterns in people who limp; wear patterns on canes, braces. and support; and callous patterns on hands. Most importantly, diagnosis and management decisions are based on individual patients and circumstances—not the presence or absence of any one sign or finding.

12. How can recognizing behavioral components affect pain management?

Identification of behavioral components creates the often uncomfortable challenge of discussing them with the patient. For example, the patient may complain of 9/10 back pain, but your exam reveals few objective findings. How to discuss these differences of perspective is challenging. Solid communication skills are critical, as a number of emotions inevitably surface on both sides. Good communication skills can allow exploration of the behavioral components of pain in a nonthreatening manner. Ultimately, they decrease fear and most likely how the pain is perceived as well.

Communication skills can help avoid one of the most important pitfalls in pain management: the inappropriate placement of labels. Inevitably, pain is often managed with medications that have potential for abuse and addiction. Behavioral aspects of a patient's response to pain, as well as the way in which the provider and patient interact, can lead to inappropriate labeling.

13. What is the difference between use, dependence, and addiction?

Clear understanding of certain definitions is important. **Use** of a drug (e.g., caffeine, alcohol, nicotine, marijuana, narcotics) does not automatically imply addiction. Even though some drugs that a patient may use are illegal, legality does not determine addiction. **Physical dependence** is the development of withdrawal symptoms when the medication is withheld. In and of itself, dependence occurrence does not imply addiction. Physical dependence on some medications even may result when the focus is appropriately on symptom relief and reaching functional goals. Moreover, dependence can occur with many classes of drugs, such as hypertensive agents (e.g., clonidine, beta blockers). **Addiction** is characterized by loss of control over use of the drug, compulsive use, preoccupation with getting and using the drug, and continued use despite objective harm.

14. What is pseudoaddiction?

Incomplete pain treatment can create pseudoaddictive behavior. Patients may make strong or aggressive demands for the medication, may demonstrate strong emotions such as anger, and may even focus on the medication itself as opposed to functional goals. However, they do not display loss of control, continued use despite harm, or other defining characteristics of addiction. Once the pain is better controlled, the demanding behavior subsides, and the escalating and self-abusive traits of addiction are not present. Because traditional approaches to pain management are often inadequate, the potential for generating such behaviors often exists. In this case, if the patient is labeled an "addict," a vicious cycle is created.

15. What lifestyle choices are important to address with a diagnosis of chronic pain?

Several important lifestyle issues affect any treatment protocol for chronic pain. The most obvious include diet, exercise, and personal habits. In addition, coping skills and support systems have a major effect on positive behavioral choices.

Dietary changes are critical in the treatment of such conditions as rheumatoid arthritis and other inflammatory processes. Reducing the intake of red meat results in emphasizing omega-3 over omega-6 oils. This shift leads to a biochemical pathway that produces less inflammatory chemicals. Although no current review exists for generalized chronic pain, it would make sense that in any condition with some inflammatory component, making such a change could be beneficial.

Similarly, **exercise** has been shown to be therapeutic for depression,[7] which often accompanies chronic pain. Exercise has been shown to release natural endorphins, which directly treats pain, as long as the exercise is not overly taxing which may cause further damage and pain. Weight loss is often important in patients with pain issues. It's important to remember that the best exercise for a patient is the exercise the patient will do.

Personal habits play an important role as well. The role of alcohol is particularly important to clarify. It may be used as a sleep aid or as a coping skill; neither is particularly helpful over time. The most important personal choice is probably the role of nicotine. Nicotine starves the body of oxygen, impairs blood flow, and has other bad effects. It is becoming common practice for orthopedic surgeons to contract with patients to stop smoking for 2 weeks before and after surgery before agreeing to do back surgery because of nicotine's effect on wound healing. Patients who choose to continue to use nicotine in any form during treatment of chronic pain are working against the integrated treatment plan. Smoking cessation should be cornerstone of the integrated treatment plan for chronic pain.

16. How should sleep be addressed in an integrated fashion?

More and more evidence demonstrates the critical importance of sleep for good health. In managing chronic pain and its sequelae, adequate sleep becomes even more important. Unfortunately, alcohol and a number of prescription medications often decrease rapid-eye-movement (REM) sleep. A number of integrative approaches can be utilized to improve the patient's sleep. Practical advice on sleep hygiene includes:

- The bed and bedroom are for sleep and sex only. This means no television watching or book reading in bed.
- Stimulants(e.g., caffeine, nicotine) should be avoided for several hours before bedtime.
- People should not attempt to go to bed until they are sleepy.
- People who are unable to fall asleep after 20 minutes should get out of bed and do something until they feel tired again.
- Daytime naps should be avoided.

- Some form of meditative practice (e.g., modulating breathing patterns) should be considered as part of a sleep ritual
- Several botanical agents and supplements (e.g., melatonin, B vitamins) may improve sleep patterns without many of the consequences of prescription medications. However, botanicals do have possible adverse consequences; their use should be discussed with a trained professional.

17. Discuss the role of a multidisciplinary approach to management of chronic pain.

A number of studies have demonstrated that tapping into treatment approaches from a variety of different providers can dramatically improve success rates in managing chronic pain. Psychological support (e.g., individual counseling, with behavioral and cognitive approaches) may be a key factor in the patient's success. Indeed, many chronic pain clinics include psychological counseling or cognitive therapy as a critical part of the multidisciplinary plan. Good patient education is another factor that can decrease fear and anxiety about pain as well as about treatment plans.

Group processes can also be helpful. Bringing together a number of patients with chronic pain, regardless of its cause, allows sharing of fears as well as successes. The group process can improve coping skills and reframe pain issues for individual members. Such work can reduce Beck depression inventory scores as well as pain index scores.[8]

18. How does evidence-based medicine affect CAM approaches to pain treatment?

The National Center for Complementary and Alternative Medicine (NCCAM) has issued a number of grants to asses different types of pain, including acute pain (e.g., acupuncture for dental pain), fibromyalgia (acupuncture), and different approaches to low back pain. Many new studies are being sponsored and will play a key role in providing evidence on which to base treatment protocols.

The U.S. Department of Health and Human Services (DHHS) recently published "Clinical Practice Guidelines for Acute Pain Management," which can be somewhat generalized for exploring information about types of treatment for chronic pain and the evidence that supports each option. In general, look for randomized controlled trials and meta-analyses, which are the strongest type of evidence (types Ia and Ib, respectively). Type II evidence involves well-designed but nonrandomized studies. Type III evidence includes case studies, and type IV consists of expert opinions.

19. Give examples of evidence that may support CAM techniques.

Based on information published by DHHS,[9] a number of different techniques were reviewed for the management of acute pain. For example, simple imagery, progressive muscle relaxation, and simple jaw relaxation are supported by strong evidence (type Ia). These techniques require a limited amount of time and no special training. Simple relaxation using music is supported by type Ib evidence.

Complex relaxation involving biofeedback is supported by type Ib evidence. Although this technique requires more time, skilled personnel, and special equipment, it is often included in different aspects of medical training. In fact, several articles[10,11] have discussed nonpharmacologic approaches to successful treatment of hypertension. Unfortunately, for different reasons, this noninvasive, low-risk process is rarely implemented in treating hypertension, much less chronic pain, despite strong supporting evidence. In addition, guided imagery is supported by type Ib evidence. Although it requires some training or skilled personnel, it is readily accessible and easily implemented.

Patient education is strongly supported by evidence-based data. It takes 5–15 minutes and can be done by other support staff as well as the physician or practitioner

20. Which techniques for treating chronic pain are well accepted by evidence-based medicine?

Some of the more readily accepted and more frequently used techniques include mind-body approaches, hypnosis, acupuncture, and manipulative therapy. Moreover, the emerging field of psychoneuroimmunology is gaining increased acceptance. This field may allow understanding of how many of these techniques achieve their effect.

21. What is meant by mind-body medicine?

Mind-body medicine can be defined in various ways. In the simplest definition, illness and health are considered as a psychosomatic (mind-body) process. In terms of approaches for chronic pain management, a number of different techniques should be considered. Simple (e.g.,. listening to music, progressive muscle relaxation) and complex relaxation techniques (e.g., biofeedback, imagery) fit this definition.

Another powerful technique for management of pain includes ground-breaking work by Kabat-Zinn,[12] who demonstrated a significant improvement in the McGill-Melzack pain rating index after 4 years of mindfulness meditation in 225 patients. Another study,[13] published almost 20 years ago, demonstrated that a number of different pain syndromes that had not improved with traditional medical care responded to an integrated outpatient program based on the practice of mindfulness meditation. Although this study was uncontrolled, it raises a number of interesting questions about which useful CAM therapies may be helpful in patients with this difficult-to-treat diagnosis .

22. How is hypnosis used in the treatment of pain syndromes?

A number of studies[14] have documented the use of hypnosis in acute situations. Several involved pediatric patients and hypnosis in the management of fractures and suturing. In addition, a number of surgeries have been performed using hypnosis as the sole anesthetic with positive results. For chronic pain, less evidence is available. Because hypnosis is another means of altering perception, it makes sense that it can be incorporated as a means of reframing chronic pain issues. A number of sources offer formal training in hypnosis (see Chapter 6).

23. For what types of pain is acupuncture a reasonable approach?

The NIH has published a consensus statement about acupuncture and pain management.[15] Several areas are designated as appropriate for the use of acupuncture, including postoperative dental pain, headaches, fibromyalgia, and myofascial pain. In addition, acupuncture may be used alone or as part of a comprehensive program for treatment of osteoarthritis as well as low back pain. Unfortunately, studies of acupuncture for treatment of osteoarthritis have reported conflicting results. The meta-analyses for chronic pain have been similarly conflicting. Currently, there is no strong recommendation for acupuncture in generic pain syndromes. Its exact role is best left to the practitioner, the patient, and the clinical setting.

24. Is manual medicine acceptable for chronic pain management?

A number of studies demonstrate that chiropractic manipulation or physical therapy produces significant improvements in patients with low back pain compared with minimal intervention. As a result of these studies, the Agency for Health Care Policy and Research recommends manipulative approaches as first-line treatment for acute uncomplicated back pain. Similar studies of chronic back pain produced less certain results; however, manual techniques may still be considered acceptable Other manual approaches include physical therapy and massage. Some studies suggest that massage may be as effective or even more effective than acupuncture for low back pain[16] and fibromyalgia.[17]

24. Can keeping a diary help with pain?

A recent article[18] examined the technique of journaling for treating the pain of patients with rheumatoid arthritis as well as other symptoms in patients with asthma. Patients were asked to write about emotionally traumatic experiences on a regular basis. Over time, the symptom scores of pain in patients with rheumatoid arthritis and the respiratory symptoms of patients with asthma were noted to decrease. This finding suggests that patients who keep a journal or diary as a regular part of their daily activities may tap into another technique for managing symptoms (e.g., by increasing coping skills through reshaping the cognitive representation of the stressful event).

25. Is the use of magnets safe?

In general, magnetic therapy includes a number of different approaches. Several techniques take advantage of bioelectromagnetic fields for diagnostic as well as treatment purposes. The most readily recognized technique is transcutaneous electrical nerve stimulation (TENS), which is generally well accepted in managing several chronic pain syndromes, particularly orthopedic injuries or muscle spasm. Other modalities use pulsatile electromagnetic fields.

On the other hand, the use of magnets is less well accepted. Lack of acceptance, however, does not mean that studies have not been done. A number of animal models have shown that magnetic therapy can block the activity of dorsal root ganglion neurons. Vallbona and Richards[19] reviewed a number of research projects, and the Agency for Health Care Policy and Research reviewed 33 double-blinded studies.[20] Twenty-six reported some beneficial effects. Bone pain, neurogenic pain, and sleep disorders were targets of the studies. Perhaps the most exciting research involves the use of magnet therapy in treating diabetic neuropathy, which is notoriously poorly treated by conventional approaches.

Unfortunately, despite such positive work, the use of magnets creates a number of challenges. Much of the information available to patients and practitioners is anecdotal or testimonial rather than based on more acceptable research. In addition, the large cottage industry currently in operation should make patients and practitioners wary of pursuing expensive treatment approaches without looking for more solid evidence.

26. How does aromatherapy work in reducing pain?

Aromatherapy is not well understood by medical practitioners. Most do not know that at least one state board of nursing has accepted it as part of holistic nursing care. Aromatherapy is the use of essential oils, either topical or inhaled, for therapeutic purposes. It is used for a number of different problems, including skin and wound care, stress reduction, and pain management. Early clinical trials in a number of these areas are currently under way. In the meantime, a lot of evidence comes from the experiences of various practitioners. Currently, its mode of action is uncertain and probably varied. Potential mechanisms of action include the placebo response, a parasympathetic response to touch or smell, a pharmacokinetic process of the oil itself, or pharmacologically active ingredients in the substances. Because health care practitioners are exposed to the concept of pheromones in their training, appreciation of aromatherapy should not be too unrealistic.

27. How do I put all of the options outlined above into practice?

Chronic pain is an ideal problem for an integrative treatment approach in the ambulatory setting. It requires a team effort by practitioner and patient, individualized for specific diagnoses. The usual pieces of medical history should be obtained, such as origins of the pain, past treatment, and use of nontraditional methods. Moreover, clear goal-setting by the patient is required, and objective and functional measures should be identified. The patient's coping skills and support systems need to be identified and mobilized. The patient needs to be involved at each step in his or her care plan and must take responsibility for personal health and healing.

A number of integrative approaches are readily adopted and should be examined in terms of anecdotal as well as evidence-based support. Patient education, and a therapeutic physician-patient relationship are key in any treatment plan. Lifestyle choices of the patient are also foundation pieces. Sleep cannot be overemphasized as a necessary healing tool in the management of chronic pain.

In terms of the different approaches described above, the most important requirements are an open mind and communication skills that allow calm and supportive negotiation of common ground in terms of the patient's preferences. Resources such as practitioners, insurance reimbursement, and safety are also important to address.

In many ways, patients are the provider's best resources, particularly in regard to nontraditional treatment approaches.Patients can introduce providers to alternative health care practitioners within the medical community and inform them of what supplies and modalities are readily accessible. The journey begins with being open to what patients have used or are considering.

REFERENCES

1. Verhaak PF, et al: Prevalence of chronic benign pain disorder among adults: A review of the literature. Pain 77:231–239, 1998.
2. Glajchen M: Chronic pain: treatment barriers and strategies for clinical practice. J Am Board Fam Pract 143:178–183, 2001.
3. Joint Commission of Accreditation of Healthcare Organizations: Pain Standards for 2001. Available at http://www.jcaho.org/standart/pm.html; accessed 3/21/2002.

4. Aronoff GM: Opiods in chronic pain management: Current review of pain. Pain News 4:112–211, 2000.
5. White TJ, Arakelian A, Rho JP: Counting the cost of drug related adverse events. Pharmacoeconomics 15:445–458, 1999.
6. Waddell G, McCulloch JA, et al: Nonorganic physical signs in low back pain. Spine 5:117–125, 1980.
7. Weyerer S, Kupfer B: Physical exercise and psychological health. Sports Med 17:108–116, 1994.
8. Buyck D, Blackwelder R: unpublished data from a pain group study at University Family Physicians of Kingsport. Kingsport, TN, 2000–2002.
9. U.S. Department of Health and Human Services: Quick Reference Guide for Clinicians: Acute Pain Management in Adults: Operative Procedures. Washington, DC, U.S. Department of Health and Human Services, 1992.
10. Beilin LJ, Burke V, et al: Non pharmacologic therapy and lifestyle factors in hypertension. Blood Pressure 10(5-6):352–365, 2001.
11. Thakkar RB, Oporil S: What do international guidelines say about therapy? J Hypertens (Suppl):S23–S31, 2001.
12. Kabat-Zinn J, et al: Four-year follow-up of a meditation-based program for the self-regulation of chronic pain: Treatment outcomes and compliance. Clin J Pain 2:159–173, 1987.
13. Kabat-Zinn J: An outpatient program in behavioral medicine for chronic pain patient based on the practice of mindfulness meditation: Theoretical considerations and preliminary results. Gen Hosp Psychiatry 4:33–47,1982.
14. Holroyd J. Hypnosis treatment of clinical pain: Understanding why hypnosis is useful. Intl J Clin Exp Hypnosis 44:33–51, 1996.
15. Acupuncture. National Institutes of Health Consensus Statement. Nov 3–5, 15(5):1–34, 1997.
16. Cherkin DC, Eisenberg D, et al: Randomized trial comparing traditional Chinese medical acupuncture, therapeutic massage and self-care education for chronic low back pain. Arch Intern Med 161:1081, 2001.
17. Berman BM, Swyers JP: Complementary medicine treatments for fibromyalgia syndrome. Baillieres Best Pract Res Clin Rheumatol Sep 13(3):487–492, 1999.
18. Smyth JM, Stone AA, Hurewitz A, Kaell A: Effects of writing about stressful experiences on symptom reduction in patients with asthma or rheumatoid arthritis: A randomized trial. JAMA 281:1304–1309, 1999.
19. Vallbona C, Richards T: Evolution of magnetic therapy from alternative to traditional medicine. In Kraft GH (ed): Complementary Therapies in Physical Medicine and Rehabilitation. Philadelphia, W.B. Saunders, 1999, pp 729–754.
20. U.S. Department of Health and Human Services: Quick Reference Guide for Clinicians. Acute Pain Management in Adults: Pperative Procedures. Washington, DC, U.S. Department of Health and Human Services, 1992.

47. LOW BACK PAIN

Wendy Kohatsu, M.D.

1. How prevalent is low back pain?

Low back pain (LBP) is one of the most common reasons that people seek medical care. An estimated 70–80% of the population is affected by LBP at some time in their lives; 30–50% of adults have low back pain each year at an annual cost of approximately $60 billion.[1] Complementary and alternative medicine (CAM) is used for LBP more frequently than for any other indication, although data for efficacy are fragmentary.[2]

2. What causes LBP?

The body is a dynamic, interconnected system of which the back is a vital part. Orthopedic injuries to other parts of the body (e.g., knee, hip) can lead to muscular spasms and imbalances that trigger pain in the low back. Poor posture and gait can cause LBP. Lifestyle factors—under- or over-exercising, working to exhaustion, obesity—can have a profound effect on what we feel in our backs. The mind's influence on chronic, debilitating problems such as LBP must not be underestimated. Part of the dilemma of diagnosing LBP stems from the fact that the back is a complex system that includes the spinal column and sacrum, spinal cord and nerves, intervertebral discs, layers of muscles, and deep investing fascia. Pain can arise from any of these structures.

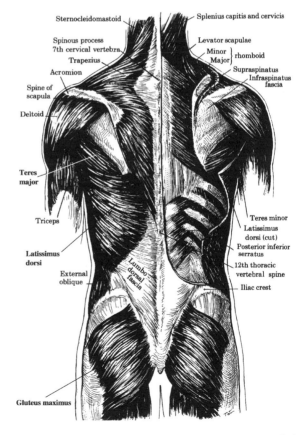

Muscles of the back. (From Dorland's Illustrated Dictionary, 28th ed. Philadelphia, W.B. Saunders, 1994, p 1069, with permission.)

313

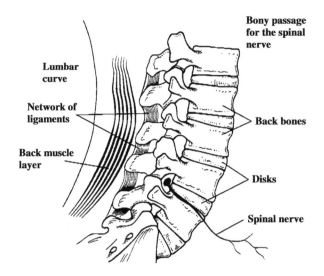

Side view of the vertebral column. (From Anderson BC: Office Orthopedics for Primary Care—Diagnosis and Treatment, 2nd ed. Philadelphia, WB Saundeers, 1999, p 264, with permission.)

3. How is LBP typically classified?

LBP is diagnosed as acute (< 6 weeks' duration), subacute (6–12 weeks), or chronic (> 12 weeks). Some therapies, allopathic or CAM, have been shown to work for acute but not chronic LBP. LBP is also classified as simple or complex. Patients with simple LBP have no risk factors or signs of underlying pathology, whereas in patients with complex LBP risk factors may include age > 50 years, history of cancer or intravenous drug abuse, signs or symptoms of systemic disease (weight loss, fever, lymphadenopathy), sciatica, and/or neurologic deficit on examination.

4. What are "red flags" in the work-up for low back pain?

One needs to rule out infection, tumor, fracture, cauda equina syndrome, and referred pain from other diseases (e.g., pyelonephritis, pancreatitis). A good history followed by a thorough exam elucidates nearly all of these conditions. The Agency for Health Care Policy and Research[3] recommends awareness of the following "red flags" in the history and presentation of low back pain:

- Radiation below the knee
- History of trauma
- Atypical pain (nocturnal pain, unrelenting pain)
- Pain that is worse with sitting (suggestive of herniation)
- Pain relieved with forward flexion (suggestive of spinal stenosis)
- Neurologic symptoms (e.g., bowel or bladder incontinence, weakness, gait impairment)
- History of cancer, especially prostate, breast, lung, thyroid, kidney, multiple myeloma, and lymphomas

These factors may require further evaluation, including radiographic studies and/or surgical referral. Basic lab tests, if indicated, should include complete blood count, erythrocyte sedimentation rate, and urinalysis.. Serious pathology such as fracture, tumor, infection, and cauda equina syndrome must be ruled out before a diagnosis of simple, mechanical LBP is made. Only 3% of patients with sciatica present with true radiculopathy, and only one-third of these (1% total) have urgent neurologic symptoms requiring immediate surgical consultation.[4] The presence of sciatica does not automatically mean that conservative measures should be bypassed in favor of more aggressive treatment. Many patients with LBP plus sciatica do well with conservative treatment, including manipulation.

5. How can I conduct a thorough, but time-efficient exam for LBP?

The exam should be history-focused and include a full neurologic exam. Because the psychosocial nature of LBP can be befuddling, taking note of nonorganic clues (Waddell signs)[5] can signal a need for greater psychological interventions such as counseling. Biewen outlines some of the major examination techniques that can be completed in a time-efficient manner.[6]

Physical Examination for Low Back Pain

PATIENT POSITION	TEST PERFORMED OR FEATURE OBSERVED	TIME REQUIRED (SEC)	POSSIBLE FINDINGS
All positions	Observation	Ongoing	Behavioral factors, physical limitation
Standing	Posture and gait	15	Poor postural habits, alteration due to pain
	Toe and heel walking	10	L5 or S1 weakness
	Symmetry, asymmetry	5	Scoliosis, atrophy
	Range of motion	15	Pain response, physical limitation
Sitting	Straight-leg raise	10	Radicular pain
	Neurologic testing	40	Neurologic deficit
Supine	Leg length	5	Mechanical contribution
	Straight-leg raise	10	Radicular pain
	Patrick's test (fabere* sign)	10	Hip involvement
Prone	Palpation	20	Muscle dysfunction
	Hip extension (5–20°)	10	Radicular pain (L2–L4 nerve roots)
	Prone prop†	10	Facet joint dysfunction
Total time		2 min, 40 sec	

* Fabere sign: a mnemonic for the movements required to elicit pain due to the hip: **f**lexion, **a**bduction, **e**xternal **r**otation, and **e**xtension. Place the lateral malleolus of the side to be tested over the top of the other knee, applying gentle downward pressure on the flexed knee to cause external rotation of the hip.

† Prone prop: in the prone position, have the patient prop him- or herself on the elbows, allowing passive extension of the lumbar spine. This maneuver reduces compression on the intervertebral disk; it may relieve pain that originates at the nerve roots but may worsen facet joint pain.

From Biewen PC: A structured approach to low back pain. Postgrad Med 106(6):102–114, 1999.

6. How important is imaging?

Surgery for LBP is more prevalent in the U.S. than any other country. Often physicians order radiographic studies to prove or disprove the existence of LBP. But 64% of 45-year-old people have silent disc herniation on magnetic resonance imaging (MRI) and walk around pain-free. Likewise, other studies show that anatomic evidence of a herniated disc is found in 20–30% of imaging tests of normal persons,[7] and the extent of protrusion does not often correlate with severity of symptoms. Contrary to popular belief, jobs involving lifting, pulling, pushing, or carrying have *not* been associated with an increased risk for prolapsed disc.[8]

Radiologic studies have *not* been proved to help diagnose uncomplicated LBP. A review of observational studies of spinal radiographic findings concluded that "There is no firm evidence for the presence or absence of a causal relationship between radiographic findings and nonspecific low back pain."[9] Likewise, patients in whom computed tomography (CT) scans showed spinal stenosis, disc bulging, protrusion, or extrusion had similar clinical exams compared with patients with normal findings. Experts conclude that obtaining CT scans of the spine to evaluate chronic, nonprogressive back pain "does not seem to be important."[10] Unfortunately, radiographic studies often do not help clinicians diagnose the root cause of chronic back pain.

7. Why is an integrative approach to LBP important?

An approach that truly integrates the best of allopathic medicine and CAM therapies offers a comprehensive, yet practical way to help patients with LBP more effectively. Physicians tend to "overmedicalize" LBP with excessive and expensive testing; patients often compartmentalize their pain, and thus a whole-person approach becomes lost. An integrative approach begins with the history and physical exam and is directed toward understanding the patient as well as the disease. Questions should address daily habits, life situations, and stressors. The history may reveal chemical dependency, insomnia, occupational issues, or other contributing factors. It is important simply to *ask* patients about what they believe causes their pain. This inquiry often yields valuable clues that facilitate understanding of the person's disease process.

Successful resolution of LBP requires that the patient take an active role in his or her own care. With the vast array of CAM therapies available for LBP (from acupuncture to manipulation and homeopathy), it is just as easy to get lost trying to find suitable CAM therapies as it is dealing with the frustration that patients often experience with allopathic treatments. An integrative practitioner may help guide therapeutic choices.

8. How can physicians improve their exam of the low back?

Most physicians need to learn how to perform more precise physical exams of the low back. The term *low back pain* is a catch-all phrase that is neither precise nor clinically useful. Eighty-five percent of patients with LBP do not receive a more definitive diagnosis. LBP may be due to fascial strain, sacral torsion, disc herniation, muscle spasms, trigger points, or some combination of these or other factors. Most allopathic physicians have inadequate training in conducting a thorough physical examination of the structures and functions of the low back. Although most physicians may not need to distinguish between an L4 versus an L3 subluxation, it is helpful to be able to palpate differences in tissue texture and asymmetry of the lower body frame. Greater understanding of the multiple causes of LBP and the skill to differentiate among them may lead to more precise therapy. For example, back pain arising primarily from sacroiliac joint somatic dysfunction may be best approached through osteopathic manipulation, whereas muscular strain of the erector spinae may respond simply to stretching exercises at home. Improved examination skills may expedite appropriate therapy and mitigate the need for excessive testing.

9. What are trigger points?

Janet Travell, M.D., pioneered the practice of trigger point therapy in the U.S. in the 1930s. Because trigger points can cause significant pain and even mimic neurologic symptoms, it is important to be able to distinguish them. Various manual therapies or direct intramuscular injection with anesthetic and anti-inflammatory agents can be used to treat trigger points.

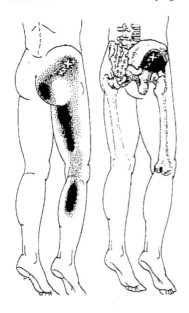

Trigger points in the gluteus medius muscle. Note the stippled areas of referred pain mimicking sciatica. (From Travell and Simons' Myofascial Pain and Dysfunction: The Trigger Point Manual, Vol. 2: The Lower Extremities, 2nd ed. Baltimore, Williams & Wilkins, 1999, p 169, with permission.)

10. What is the first step in the treatment plan for LBP? What is the second step?

Reassuring the patient about the benign nature of uncomplicated LBP and the high rate of favorable outcomes with treatment is the essential first step. A positive attitude and confidence can reduce pain and pave the path for treatment adherence. Restoration of function—not necessarily eradication of pain—is the first major goal. The long-term goal for patients with LBP is to minimize dependence on any outside provider, CAM or allopathic. Self-reliance can be taught through self-care and a coordinated partnership with a primary physician.

The second step is to work with the patient to create a **therapeutic game plan** that incorporates exercise, judicious use of medications, and a defined follow-up plan if complications arise. Involving patients in the decision-making process can increase adherence to the therapy and avoid inactivity because of pain and fear. The physician may want to include a written prescription that includes not only medications but also timing and amount of exercises to perform at home. With an integrative approach, it is also important to ask patients about their specific goals are for the visit (e.g., pain-free walking, returning to work, reducing reliance on pain medicines) so that progress can be monitored in a way that is meaningful to the patient.

11. What is the role pharmacotherapy in the treatment of LBP?

An evidence-based review of the conservative treatment of LBP by van Tulder et al.[11] evaluated the pharmaceutical agents commonly used for LBP:

Nonsteroidal anti-inflammatory drugs (NSAIDs). Strong evidence indicates that NSAIDs are no more effective than analgesics and that the various types of NSAIDs (ibuprofen, diclofenac, piroxicam, felbinac) are equally effective in comparison with each other. NSAIDs were more effective than placebo in patients with simple, acute LBP. Optimal treatment with NSAIDS should last no longer than 12 weeks. Data about the use of COX II inhibitors for LBP are still pending.

Analgesics (acetaminophen, opioids) were found to be as effective as NSAIDs. Opioids should be considered a third line of treatment and limited to 1–3 days for a maximum 3 weeks. Patients should be informed of the potential addictive properties.

Muscle relaxants. Strong evidence indicates that muscle relaxants are more effective than placebo for acute LBP but less effective for chronic LBP. The different types of muscle relaxants were found to be equally effective. Optimal use is for 1 week, with a maximum of 4 weeks.

Antidepressants. Compared with placebo, antidepressants (amitriptyline, imipramine, trazodone) were not found to be effective for chronic LBP.

12. Are botanicals useful for low back pain?

Not really, especially compared with other treatment options. Botanicals are not considered a mainstay of treatment for LBP, and few relevant data are available. A few that have been used include:

Arnica (*Arnica montana*) is widely known as a homeopathic medicine for acute trauma, especially of musculoskeletal origin. It is the number-one ingredient in many topical homeopathic preparation (6x to 30C dilution) for bruises and muscle strain. Arnica contains sesquiterpenes and lactones, which have active antioxidant properties. However, no sound studies support its routine use for treatment of LBP.

White willow bark (*Salix alba*). The precursor for aspirin (acetylsalicylic acid) was first isolated from white willow bark in the late 1800s. The crude extract of white willow is still popular among European herbalists, although the low concentration of salicin, its most active component, limits its effectiveness. One study reported that concentrated extract of white willow is effective in relieving LBP exacerbation at high doses (240 mg salicin, which is about same as 3 baby aspirin).[12]

Tumeric, **ginger**, and **boswellia** are other botanicals used for their anti-inflammatory effects, but they have not been studied for LBP.

13. How can exercise help patients with LBP?

Strong evidence supports the use of exercise for chronic LBP; typically, the sooner it is begun, the better the results.[13] Exercise modalities include stretching, McKenzie exercises, strengthening exercises, and intensive dynamic training. The ultimate goal of exercise therapy is to allow patients to have greater control and to feel more at ease with their bodies. Aerobic exercise has been shown to increase blood flow, improve mood, and increase pain tolerance. The optimal plan incorporates aerobic exercise 2–3 times/week (20–30 minutes), strength training to help build weak muscles 2–3 time/week on alternate days, and daily mild stretching. Small, achievable incremental goals help the patient to gain confidence. Even if the pain was still reported as the same, exercise increased coping skills and resulted in less disability and fewer days lost from work.[14]

14. What are McKenzie exercises for back pain?

Robin McKenzie, a physiotherapist from New Zealand, developed a highly evolved system of treatment that emphasizes frequent self-exercise (2–3 minutes every 2 hours), slight end-range stretching, and centralization of pain.[15] He states that "the most common cause of low back pain is postural stress. . . especially poor sitting posture." McKenzie exercises also proved to be of significant benefit for acute LBP. A recent randomized, controlled trial showed that McKenzie exercises were just as effective as chiropractic care provided at the same cost.[16] Responders require an average of only 6 or fewer visits to achieve closure. The McKenzie Institute works directly with physicians to individualize self-treatment programs; (800) 635-8380 is the U.S. referral telephone number.

15. How can mind-body approaches be helpful for patients with LBP?

Some evidence indicates that behavioral therapy in the form of operant conditioning, cognitive treatment, or progressive muscle relaxation is an effective short-term treatment for chronic LBP. Referral to a clinic specializing in care of chronic pain may include an evaluation from a therapist trained to address the psychosocial issues of chronic pain. Music therapy, hypnosis, and imagery have been suggested as other helpful mind-body therapies.

John Sarno, M.D., at the New York University School of Medicine developed a novel program that has helped thousands of people overcome back pain—without drugs or surgery. He states that the primary tissue involved is muscle and describes tension myositis syndrome (TMS) as a painful change of state in the muscle. Sarno's program takes a mind-body approach with reported high rates of success. As Sarno observes, "TMS is characterized by physical pain but acute discomfort is induced by psychological phenomena rather than structural abnormalities or muscle deficiency."[17] Sarno advocates shifting attention from physical pain to underlying psychological pain (e.g., family stress, financial concerns), resuming normal activity, talking to your brain, and discontinuing all physical treatment, including manipulation, heat, exercise, acupuncture, and massage. This all-or-none psychological approach to LBP seems to be radical but works well for some people.

16. How helpful is massage for low back pain?

Older studies of massage for back pain have shown no consistent benefit, in large part due to poor study design and the type of massage used. Of note, two more recent randomized, controlled trials[18,19] using deep tissue techniques reported short-term benefit. More studies need to be conducted using massage techniques specifically targeting the fascia and deep anatomical structures of the low back, with longer follow-up. Massage can be a useful adjunct and helps alleviate stress associated with LBP.

17. Does acupuncture provide relief for LBP?

Yes, but both a systematic review[20] and meta-analysis[21] of acupuncture in LBP report that there are not enough data to prove efficacy above placebo. This finding may point to the inherent methodologic difficulties in conducting acupuncture research. Acupuncture also may not work as well when isolated from the whole system of oriental medicine, which may include herbs, dietary changes, and moxibustion. The skill of the acupuncturist may be highly variable; treatment outcome may depend on the particular method as well as the expertise of the practitioner. Of interest, patients with high expectations for acupuncture or massage were five times more likely to report substantial relief compared with patients with average expectations.[22] The power of belief may serve as a potent catalyst for healing.

18. How can osteopathic principles improve treatment of patients with LBP?

In addition to the wide variety of soft tissue manipulations that are available, a distinct advantage to an osteopathic approach is the holistic philosophy of treating the whole person and the interrelatedness of body functions. Two techniques commonly used by osteopathic physicians for LBP are muscle energy technique and counterstrain:

In **muscle energy**, the operator positions the patient to localize precisely the problem area (e.g., malrotated vertebra, overtight hamstring). The goal is to reset the length of the culprit muscle by a series of isometric contractions, thus changing golgi tendon organ and extrafusal fiber inhibitory input to the alpha motorneuron. All of the active motion, held for 5- to 6-second intervals, is applied by the patient.

Counterstrain is a passive technique wherein the goal is to reset the gamma gain (intrafusal fibers) of a tightened muscle to allow it to reset to a more relaxed state. Tightness in specific muscles can cause sufficient referred pain to mimic neurologic back pain.

A recent randomized trial in patients with LBP found no statistical difference between osteopathic manipulative therapy (OMT) and standard care consisting of physical therapy, transcutaneous electrical nerve stimulation (TENS), ultrasound, and hot/cold packs. The OMT group, however, used significantly less medication (NSAIDs, analgesics, muscle relaxants).[23]

19. What are the "dirty half-dozen" diagnoses of LBP?

Phil Greenman, D.O., compiled the "dirty half-dozen" osteopathic diagnoses of LBP that were refractory to conservative therapy or surgery[24]:

1. Muscle imbalance between the trunk and thighs	100%
2. Non-neutral lumbar dysfunction	88%
3. Pubic dysfunction	76%
4. Short leg/pelvic tilt syndrome (> 6 mm difference)	65%
5. Posterior sacral base (and loss of lumbar lordosis)	60%
6. Innominate shear	24%

Terms such as *non-neutral, pubic dysfunction,* and *posterior sacral base* refer to specific musculoskeletal mechanical diagnoses based on careful osteopathic evaluation. Ninety-eight percent of these "untreatable" patients fell into one or more of the treatable diagnostic categories above. Patients were treated 6 times over 12 weeks, with an additional 15–25 visits to a physical therapist. Seventy-five percent of this disability-bound population returned to work or prior functional status. As mentioned before, better training in the basic biomechanics of the low back can enable physicians to identify treatable causes of LBP.

20. Can chiropractic treatment help?

Spinal manipulation is of short-term benefit in some patients, particularly those with uncomplicated, acute LBP. A recent meta-analysis confirms that manipulation is more effective than placebo for acute LBP, and strong evidence also supports its use in chronic LBP.[25,26] A major concern, however, is the high rate (29%) of inappropriate use.[27] Patients should note positive effects (if any are likely to occur) after about 4–6 chiropractic treatments; if no positive effects are noted, treatment should be discontinued.

Complications of spinal manipulation have been thoroughly reviewed.[28] Most worrisome are vertebrobasilar accidents. which have been associated only with cervical manipulation. For the lumbar area, 62 cases were described in which spinal manipulation was associated with disc herniation or cauda equina syndrome (CES). About half of these lumbar complications occurred during manipulation under anesthesia, now an obsolete technique. Manipulation does not appear to be contraindicated for patients with bulging discs or herniation.[29] Shekelle et al. estimate that the rate of occurrence of CES as a complication of spinal manipulation is about 1 per 100 million manipulations.

21. What is the utility of TENS and PENS as adjunctive treatments

Transcutaneous electric nerve stimulation (TENS) is often applied as an adjunct to physical therapy. A handful of good studies have been conducted, but the results are contradictory. More studies may be able to uncover a true therapeutic trend.[30] Percutaneous electric nerve stimulation (PENS) is essentially equivalent to electroacupuncture. A small current is run at various Hz levels through needles inserted into specific points in the low back and may be more efficacious than TENS.

22. What is the bottom-line message for an integrative approach to low back pain?

Eighty percent of episodes of acute uncomplicated LBP resolve within 6 weeks regardless of the treatment approach.[31] Unfortunately, widespread acceptance of this finding tends to allow a period of "benign neglect" during which function is still limited, pain is acutely felt, and management could be more easily implemented. The recurrence rate of LBP is very high—up to 75%of patients have one or more relapses, and 72% continue to have pain after 1 year.[32] Many patients report persistent limitations of activity. Therefore, it is important to take action early, tailor an integrative plan to enable the patient to recover and maintain a healthy back.

Learning about trigger points and examining patients for the "dirty half-dozen" may increase diagnostic acuity and lead to more directed therapies. Awareness of mind-body interactions and how they influence LBP is critical. Prevention of LBP involves maintenance of good posture and regular exercise. Stretching for a few minutes daily can be useful as a treatment for acute LBP or as primary prevention.[33]

Reassurance, judicious use of medications, and awareness of the variety of CAM therapies for LBP can enable practitioners to partner with their patients for optimal outcomes.

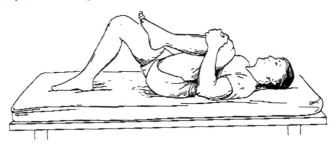

Low back stretches. (From Mayo Clinic Health Letter 18(2), 2000, p 5. By permission. of Mayo Foundation for Medical Education and Research.)

REFERENCES

1. Wipf J, Deyo R: Low back pain. Med Clin North Am 79:231–245, 1995.
2. Ernst E, Pittler MH: Experts' opinion on complementary/alternative therapies for low back pain. J Manip Physiol Ther 22(2):87–90,1999.
3. Agency for Health Care Policy and Research, Public Health Service, Department of Health and Human Services: Clinical Practice Guideline for Acute Low Back Problems in Adults (AHCPR publication no 95-0642). Rockville, MD, Agency for Health Care Policy and Research, 1994.
4. Wipf J, Deyo R: Low back pain. Med Clin of North Am 79:231–245, 1995.
5. Waddell G, Mc Culloch JA, Kummel E, et al: Nonorganic physical signs in low back pain. Spine 5(2):117–125, 1980.
6. Biewen PC: A structured approach to low back pain. Postgrad Med 106:102–114, 1999.
7. Boden SD, et al: Abnormal magnetic resonance scans of the lumbar spine in asymptomatic subjects. J Bone Joint Surg 72A:403–408, 1990.
8. Kelsey JL: An epidemiological study of the relationship between occupation and acute herniated lumbar intervertebral discs Int J Epidemiol 4:197–205, 1975.
9. van Tulder MW, et al: Spinal radiographic findings and nonspecific low back pain: A systematic review of observtional studies. Spine 22:427–434, 1997.
10. Elkayam O, et al: The lack of prognostic value of computerized tomography imaging examinations in patients with chronic non-progressive back pain. Rheumatol Int 16:19–21, 1996.
11. Van Tulder MW, Koes BW, Bouter LM: Conservative treatment of acute and chronic nonspecific low back pain: A systematic review of randomized controlled trials of the most common interventions. Spine 22:2128–2156, 1997.
12. Chrubasik S, Eisenberg E, Balan E, et al: Treatment of low back pain exacerbations with willow bark extract: A randomized double-blind study. Am J Med 109:9–14, 2000.
13. Carter IR: How effective are exercise and physical therapy for chronic low back pain? J Fam Pract 51:209, 2002.

14. Moffett JK, Torgerson D, Bell-Syer S, et al: Randomized controlled trial of exercise for low back pain: Clinical outcomes, costs, and preferences. Br Med J 319:279–283, 1999.
15. Simonsen RJ: Principle-centered spine care: McKenzie principles. Occup Med State Art Rev 13:167–183, 1998.
16. Cherkin DC, Deyo RA, Battie M, et al: A comparison of physical therapy, chiropractic manipulation, and provision of an educational booklet for the treatment of patients with low back pain. N Engl J M ed 339:1021–1029, 1998.
17. Sarno JM: Healing Back Pain: The Mind-Body Connection. New York, Warner Books, 1991.
18. Cherkin DC, Eisenberg D, Sherman KJ, et al: Randomized trial comparing traditional Chinese medical acupuncture, therapeutic massage and self-care education for chronic low back pain. Arch Intern Med 161:1081–1088, 2001.
19. Preyde, M: Effectiveness of massage therapy for subacute low-back pain: A randomized controlled trial. Can Med Assoc J 162:1815–1820, 2000.
20. Van Tulder MW, Cherkin DC, Berman B, et al: The effectiveness of acupuncture in the management of acute and chronic low back pain: A systematic review within the framework of the Cochrane collaboration back review group. Spine 24:1113–1123, 1999.
21. Ernst E, White AR: Acupuncture for back pain: A meta-analysis of randomized controlled trials. Arch Intern Med 158:2235–2241, 1998.
22. Kalauokalani D, Cherkin DC, et al: Lessons learned from a trial of acupuncture and massage for low back pain. Spine 26:1418–1424, 2001.
23. Andersson GBJ, et al: A comparison of osteopathic spinal manipulation with standard care for patients with low back pain. N Engl J Med 341:1426–1431, 1999.
24. Greenman P: Syndromes of the lumbar spine, pelvis, and sacrum. Phys Med Rehabil Clin North Am 7(4):773–785, 1996.
25. Koes BW, Bouter LM, van Mameren H, et al: A randomized clinical trial of manual therapy: Results of one year followup. Br Med J 304:606, 1992.
26. Koes BW, Bouter LM, van Mameren H, et al: A randomized clinical trial of manual therapy and physiotherapy for persistent back and neck complaints. J Manip Physiol Ther 16:211–219, 1993.
27. Shekelle PG, Coulter I, Hurwitz EL et al: Congruence between decisions to intiate chiropractic spinal manipulation for low back pain and appropriateness criteria in North America. Ann Intern Med 129:9–17, 1998.
28. Assendelft WJJ, Bouter LM, Knipschild PG: Complications of spinal manipulation: A comprehensive review of the literature. J Fam Pract 42:475–480, 1996.
29. Haldeman S, Rubinstein SM: Cauda equina syndrome following lumbar spine manipulation. Spine 17:1469–1473, 1992.
30. Van Tulder MW, Koes BW, Bouter LM: Conservative treatment of acute and chronic nonspecific low back pain: A systematic review of randomized controlled trials of the most common interventions. Spine 22:2128–2156, 1997.
31. Cherkin DC: Primary care research on low back pain: The state of the science. Spine 23:1997–2002, 1998.
32. Van der Hoogen HJ, Koes BW, van Eijk JT, et al: On the course of low back pain in general practice: A one year follow up study. Ann Rheum Dis 57:13–19, 1998.
33. Carpenter DM, Nelson W: Low back strengthening for the prevention and treatment of low back pain. Med Sci Sports Exerc 31:18–24, 1999.

48. OSTEOARTHRITIS

Stefanie L. Shaver, M.D.

I don't deserve this award, but I have arthritis, and I don't deserve that either!

Jack Benny

1. Define osteoarthritis (OA).

Osteoarthritis, also called degenerative joint disease (DJD), is the most common form of arthritis. It is defined as a chronic, progressive degenerative process involving the loss of hyaline cartilage, development of irregularities in the articular surface, and ultimately damage to subchondral bone. Impairment to the joint and eventually the surrounding tissue leads to increased pain and decreased functioning.

2. Summarize the incidence and impact of OA in the United States.

- OA is found in 6% of people over 30 years old.
- More than 50% of people over 60 years old have significant symptoms from degeneration of at least one joint
- Pain and loss of function due to OA accounts for 2% of all office visits to family physicians.
- OA is the 10th leading diagnosis in primary care and the most common cause of disability.

3. What are the risk factors for accelerated OA?

Obesity, joint injury, previous inflammatory disease of joints, age > 40 years, family history, occupation involving repetitive stress to joints, and female gender. A genetic component is implicated in evolving OA research. Whether OA is an eventual result of aging remains controversial. However, animal studies suggest that degenerative joint change occurs in virtually all vertebrates.

4. What happens to the joint in OA?

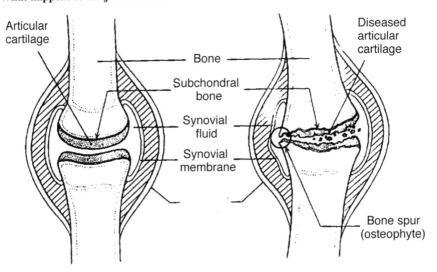

Normal (left) and osteoarthritic (right) joint. (From Arthritis Rheumatism 33:160–172, 1990. Reprinted by permission of Wiley-Liss, Inc., a subsidiary of John Wiley & Sons, Inc.)

The degenerative process in OA potentially involves a complex mechanism with mechanical, biochemical, and immunological components. Mechanical factors include abnormal load and excessive repetitive motions. Biochemical and immunological damage appears to be secondary to cytokines, enzymes, and release of nitric oxide. Eventually the smooth surface of hyaline cartilage develops irregularities secondary to a loss of proteoglycan. As OA progresses, the nearby bone remodels abnormally and may develop osteophytes. These changes progressively lead to asymmetric narrowing of the joint spaces and potentially subchondral sclerosis. Inflammation may also be a factor in OA, but its role is controversial.

5. What are the clinical manifestations in OA?
- Pain that worsens with joint use and is relieved by rest
- Local tenderness
- Mild early morning stiffness and stiffness after inactivity
- Restricted movement and mobility
- Periarticular muscle wasting
- Most affected joints are weight-bearing (ankle, knee, hip, cervical and lumbosacral spine)
- The following hand joints are also commonly involved: distal interphalangeal (DIP) joint (Heberden nodes), proximal interphalangeal (PIP) joint (Bouchard nodes), and the first carpometacarpal joint.

6. How is OA diagnosed?
The diagnosis of OA relies predominantly on clinical evaluation. No sound data support the use of specific history or physical exam findings, but bony enlargement of the interphlangeal joints, flexion contractures, and varus deformities of the knee are common. Radiographic findings suggestive of degenerative changes include joint space narrowing, osteophytes, irregular joint surfaces, sclerosis of subchondral bone, and bone cysts. However, clinical correlation is necessary because epidemiologic surveys show that 50% of patients with radiographic findings have no symptoms.

7. Describe the conventional treatments for OA.
Current conventional therapies include analgesics, nonsteroidal anti-inflammatory drugs (NSAIDs), joint injections, and, ultimately, joint replacement. Acetaminophen is considered the conventional first-line agent. However, long-term use has been associated with chronic renal failure.[1] Nonselective NSAIDs and acetaminophen result in comparable reductions in pain. Some experts suggest that a combination of acetaminophen and an NSAID is superior to either alone. However, chronic use of oral NSAIDs is associated with increased morbidity and mortality from GI bleeds. In addition, studies suggest that NSAIDs may inhibit cartilage repair and/or accelerate cartilage destruction with chronic use. Potential advantages in using the newer COX-2 inhibitors may be increased safety benefits in patients with multiple risk factors of adverse GI events (> 65 years old, history of GI bleeding, use of oral glucocorticoids or anticoagulants, or comorbid medical conditions). Meta-analysis shows no difference in efficacy of the COX-2 agents compared with nonselective NSAIDs. Opioids are also often used for the relief of severe pain associated with OA, but studies indicate no greater efficacy than acetaminophen. Topical NSAIDs (e.g., capsaicin cream) applied twice per day are more effective than placebo in small trials, but more studies are needed.[2]

8. How useful are joint injections in OA?
Steroid/analgesic injections are commonly used for OA but have a short term effect. Newer injectable agents include glycosaminoglycans such as hyaluronic acid. However, studies found that a 3- to 5-week course of injections of the knee with hyaluronate sodium (Hyalgan) or hylan G-F 20 (Synvisc) was no more effective than NSAIDs. Injection of a 10% dextrose solution has also been used, with the intention of stimulating the release of growth factors into the joint space secondary to an inflammatory reaction.[3] Several small studies have suggested that dextrose "prolotherapy" may be clinically effective in the treatment of OA pain with respect to joint movement and range of motion in the hand and knee.

9. Does exercise improve joint function and reduce pain in OA?

Yes. An optimal exercise program for the patient with OA to relieve pain and increase function includes flexibility movements, strengthening exercises, and aerobic exercise or fitness walking. Flexibility movements include range-of-motion exercises to help maintain normal joint movement and relieve stiffness. Yoga and tai chi are excellent alternative choices that are becoming more mainstream. Strengthening exercises, such as weight training, help stabilize joints and protect them from injury. Moderate aerobic exercise has been shown to improve symptoms, maintain weight loss, and contribute to a general sense of well-being.[4] Weight loss is particularly important in reducing the risk of developing OA.[5] In general, exercise is important for maintaining muscle strength and joint stability and mobility but initially should be closely monitored for optimal long-term efficacy. Pool exercise/therapy in comfortably warm water has been shown to be especially useful. Adjunctive physical therapy modalities often used include manual physical therapy, heat/hydrotherapy, and transcutaneous electrical nerve stimulation (TENS).[6]

10. What is the advantage to an integrative approach to treating OA?

Conventional OA treatments provide only symptomatic relief with respect to pain and function and do not alter the progression of the disease. Unfortunately, the mainstays of conventional pharmaceutical treatment for OA have significant systemic toxicities with chronic use. In chronic conditions with complex etiologies such as OA, a multifaceted, integrative approach is likely to yield the greatest benefit.[7]

11. What complementary and alternative medicine (CAM) treatments are used for OA?

Fairly good evidence supports the use of supplemental nutraceuticals, manual therapies, and electromagnetic/laser therapies. Homeopathy, relaxation therapy, therapeutic touch, and other such modalites may also prove to be useful.

12. Is there a "best" CAM treatment for OA?

Currently the best evidence supports the efficacy of glucosamine sulfate. Glucosamine is found in almost every tissue in the body as an essential substrate for glycosaminoglycans (GAGs), which compose the extracellular matrix of connective tissue. GAGs are acetylated to become hyaluronan, keratan sulfate, and heparan sulfate. They comprise 50% of hyaluronic acid, a major component in joint synovial fluid. Glucosamine sulfate may be the rate-limiting step in the synthesis of GAGs. Some evidence indicates that, as people age, the body produces less glucosamine; therefore, supplemental glucosamine may enable the body to maintain a certain level of repair for cartilage, disc, and connective tissue.[8]

13. How does glucosamine work in OA?

Glucosamine inhibits pain, increases function, and may have a chondroprotective role.[9,10] Its efficacy is probably mediated by several mechanisms. In animal studies, glucosamine has been shown to stabilize cell membranes, reduce the generation of free radicals by macrophages, and inhibit proinflammatory mediators and lysosomal enzymes, which are crucial to cartilage repair.[11] Several in vitro studies have shown that the addition of glucosamine to chondrocyte culture affects chondrocyte expression and leads to a dose-dependent increase in proteoglycan synthesis.[12]

14. What is the most effective form and dose of glucosamine?

Most studies have used glucosamine sulfate, but the hydrochloride form is much more bioavailable. However, it is not known whether the sulfur moiety contributes to glucosamine's efficacy. Comparative trials are needed to assess which form is superior. Both forms are cost-effective (about $15–20 per month). The most effective dose of glucosamine is 500 mg 3 times/day for a total of 1500 mg. Generally a trial of at least 6 weeks is needed before symptoms improve.

Numerous studies, including meta-analyses, demonstrate glucosamine's efficacy with respect to improving pain and functioning.[13] Efficacy was comparable or better than that of NSAIDs. Most trials used the dosage described above and assessed the knee.

15. Does glucosamine have potential adverse reactions or side effects?

Glucosamine has been used to treat OA in Europe for over 30 years, and is generally well tolerated. It has the potential to affect blood sugar levels via its ability to enter the hexosamine biosynthetic pathway. However, the longest glucosamine study to date demonstrated no change in yearly fasting blood sugar levels. In clinical trials, glucosamine generally has a side-effect profile similar to that of placebo; gastrointestinal (GI) intolerances predominate. People with seafood allergies should avoid glucosamine, which is derived from chitin in crustacean shells.

16. Is chondroitin useful in the treatment of OA?

Chondroitin is the most abundant GAG in cartilage. Supplements are produced from hydrolyzed cartilage extracts. How it is absorbed and utilized from the GI tract and its ultimate mechanism remain unclear. As with glucosamine, in vitro and animal studies suggest that chondroitin stimulates collagen synthesis, may have chondroprotective properties, and may inhibit proinflammatory mediators, which compromise cartilage repair.[14] Meta-analysis of clinical trials has demonstrated some effectiveness at a dose of 800–1200 mg/day.[13] In comparative trials, preliminary data suggest that chondroitin may prove to be even more effective than glucosamine.[17] However, the benefit of combining glucosamine with chondroitin remains controversial. A few studies in animal models suggest a possible synergy, but no studies to date support additional efficacy in humans.[18] The National Institutes of Health (NIH) is supporting a multicenter, randomized, double-blind, placebo-controlled study of patients taking glucosamine sulfate alone, chondroitin sulfate alone, glucosamine and chondroitin sulfate together, a COX-2 inhibitor alone, or placebo. Results are expected in 2004.

17. Is methylsulfonylmethane (MSM) useful in the treatment of OA?

MSM supplies a biologically active form of sulfur, which is essential in the repair and maintenance of bone, cartilage, and connective tissue. It is a nontoxic metabolite of dimethyl sulfoxide (DMSO), which substantial data indicate is effective in pain management.[19] But no large, well-controlled clinical trials have assessed the role of MSM in OA. However, some physicians have used 3000 mg of MSM clinically for the treatment of OA for many years, and are strong advocates of its therapeutic efficacy.[20] A few small studies suggest that MSM may indeed have promise.[21]

18. Discuss the role of s-adenosyl methionine (SAMe) in the treatment of OA.

SAMe is a modified amino acid that serves as a cofactor in may diverse biosynthetic pathways. Evolving data suggest that it may have a beneficial role in the treatment of depression, cardiovascular disease, and arthritis. In one double-blind trial, 1200 mg of SAMe was as effective as naproxen in 676 patients with osteooarthritis of the hip and knee.[22] SAMe has a slower onset of action than NSAIDS, but its benefits appear to last longer.

19. What supplements are useful in treating OA?

Published data suggest that the antioxidant vitamins A, C, and E and the mineral selenium may be particularly useful.[23,24] Vitamins A, C, D, and E play key roles in modulating oxidative stress, immune response, and cell differentiation and are potentially synergistic. Although fewer studies support the use of vitamin A and the carotenoids in OA, they play a fundamental role in cell differentiation, bone development, and maintenance of epithelial tissue, and future studies may demonstrate a significant role in the treatment of OA.

Vitamin C is required for collagen synthesis and tissue repair. It is an electron donor involved in hydroxylation of proline in the synthesis of type II collagen. It also serves as a sulfate carrier in the formation of GAGs. The Framingham Osteoarthritis Cohort Study found that groups with a higher than average intake of vitamin C (1000–3000 mg/day) had a threefold decrease in osteoarthritis.[24]

Studies indicate that **vitamin E** may play a role in the prevention of arthritis, and several clinical trials using 600 IU of vitamin E have shown efficacy with respect to OA of the knee.[25] In vitro studies suggest that chondrocyte lipid peroxidation may play a role in the pathogenesis of cartilage aging and osteoarthritis, and that vitamin E may protect against this oxidation via stabilization of lysosomal membranes.[26]

Selenium is a component of the antioxidant enzyme glutathione peroxidase and may mediate the OA process via an antioxidant effect.[27] It is postulated that selenium may downregulate cytokine signaling in the inflammatory response. Selenium may be beneficial, but further studies are needed.

20. What is the role of vitamin D in treating OA?

In the Framingham study, both low dietary intake and low serum levels of vitamin D were associated with increased radiographic progression of OA of the knee but not with the incidence of newly diagnosed OA.[28] Similar benefit has been shown in a longitudinal study involving OA of the hip.[29] This benefit may relate to vitamin D's ability to modulate the immune response to inflammatory products. However, published trials point to vitamin D activity involving polymorphism of the vitamin D receptor (VDR) gene.[30] Experimental antibodies against vitamin D and retinoic acid receptors showed that these nuclear receptors are involved in the regulation of decorin gene expression in articular chondrocytes. Decorin, a small leucine-rich proteoglycan, has the ability to bind collagen fibrils and growth factors such as transforming growth factor-beta (TGF-β), which is secreted by chondrocytes in cartilage regeneration. Decorin may play an important role in the attempt at cartilage repair initiated by chondrocytes in early stages of OA. Therefore, vitamin D may have a direct effect on cartilage repair via its potential regulation of decorin gene expression.

21. Discuss the role of niacinamide in the treatment of OA.

In 1953, Kaufman reported that high-dose niacinamide was beneficial in OA. Recent controlled trials have confirmed the potential benefit of frequent, divided doses.[31] Niacinamide, 250–500 mg 6 times/day, improved joint flexibility, reduced inflammation, and reduced the need for anti-inflammatory medications compared with placebo. The mechanism of action seems to be related to the ability to inhibit adenosine diphosphate ribosylation and thereby suppress interleukin-1 (IL-1)-mediated induction of nitric oxide (NO) synthase in various types of cells.[32] As stated previously, it is thought that the pathogenesis of OA may be related to the synovium generating IL-1 and inducing NO synthase, which subsequently inhibits chondrocytes. The need for frequent dosing is presumably related to the short half-life of niacinamide, but it is available in a sustained-release formula. Niacinamide in this high dosing range can cause glucose intolerance and liver damage; liver function tests are recommended every 3 months. In general, niacinamide is well tolerated and appears to be fairly safe for long-term use.

22. Are supplemental minerals useful in the treatment of OA?

Minerals that have been used for the treatment of OA include manganese, zinc, copper, and boron. No published evidence either recommends or discourages their use.

23. Are certain foods useful in treating OA?

Avocado/soybean unsaponifiables (ASUs) have shown benefit in several multicenter, double-blind clinical trials.[33,34] The ASU compound (Piascledine, manufactured in France) consists of one-third avocado oil and two-thirds soybean unsaponifiables. A comparison of a daily intake of 300 or 600 mg vs. placebo suggested that ASUs may provide long-term symptomatic relief for chronic OA. In vitro studies show that ASU has an inhibitory effect on inflammatory cytokines and prostaglandins and activates TGF-β. Other foods that may have a therapeutic effect but are not well studied. Examples include blueberries, cherries, and hawthorn berries, which may enhance collagen structure. It is also postulated that sulfur-containing foods such as garlic, onions, eggs, and asparagus may be helpful in OA.

24. Should people with OA avoid the nightshades?

A group of plants called nightshades (e.g., tomatoes, potatoes, eggplant, peppers, tobacco) have received considerable comment in the popular press as potential aggravants of OA secondary to an alkaloid that they contain, but this effect is not well studied in any clinical trails. It is estimated that about 10% of people with OA may have food sensitivities. If the patient is motivated, an elimination diet of these particular foods may be done to determine adverse sensitivity to the nightshades.

25. Discuss the role of botanicals in the treatment of OA.

One of the challenges of using botanicals as a specific treatment is that, in general, they are used in combination rather than individually. There may be benefit in the singular use of certain botanicals demonstrated to be helpful in inflammatory conditions such as rheumatoid arthritis. OA may include an inflammatory component that responds to their use.[35] Ginger has known anti-inflammatory properties and is often used for OA. One of the mechanisms for a therapeutic effect may be related to inhibition of prostaglandin and leukotriene biosynthesis. However, the few studies of ginger in people with OA have not shown a significant benefit. Other botanicals that have been used for the treatment of OA include nettle leaves, white willow bark, turmeric, Devil's claw, feverfew, various Chinese and ayurvedic preparations, and combination preparations such as Reumalex and Phytodolor.[36] No evidence either recommends or discourages their use.

26. How is acupuncture useful in the treatment of OA?

Meta-analysis has shown that acupuncture improves pain and overall function in the knee.[37,38] Yet evidence that real acupuncture is more effective than sham acupuncture is controversial. One controlled German study showed marked improvement regardless of where the needles were placed in the hip.[39] The most rigorous studies suggest that acupuncture is not superior to sham-needling in reducing the pain of osteoarthritis; both alleviate symptoms to roughly the same degree.[38] This observation supports basic science research, which suggests that acupuncture relieves pain through activation of the gate-control system, in which large nerve fibers are stimulated and suppress small fibers that transmit signals in the dorsal horn of the spinal cord. Alternatively, the effect may be mediated through the release of neurochemicals in the central nervous system. However, larger, more recent trials support the efficacy of acupuncture under sham controlled conditions. This finding raises the possibility that the equivocal results obtained previously were a function of small samples. The NIH is supporting two large multicenter clinical trials to evaluate the long-term efficacy, safety, and cost-effectiveness of acupuncture for osteoarthritis of the knee.

27. Is bodywork (e.g., chiropractic adjustment, osteopathic manipulation, massage) useful in OA?

Despite the widespread use of bodywork modalities in both acute and chronic pain syndromes, including OA, few studies validate their effectiveness in OA. Theoretically, manipulation and massage can increase blood flow or relieve potential nerve impingement at the joint and thereby optimize function. In addition, muscle pain and spasms secondary to OA may be helped by manual manipulation. Furthermore, by correcting chronic postural or structure imbalance, bodywork may help prevent undue wear and tear on the joints. Considering the high utilization of chiropractic and other forms of bodywork worldwide for musculoskeletal pain, including that related to OA, more clinical trials to assess efficacy are long overdue.

28. How are electromagnetic modalities used in treating OA?

Collagen, like bone, is considered piezoelectric. It is capable of converting electromagnetic oscillations to mechanical vibrations. Certain pulsed electromagnetic fields (PEMFs) affect the growth of bone and cartilage in vitro. PEMF stimulation is already a proven remedy for delayed union fractures and has potential clinical application for OA. Several double-blind, randomized controlled studies have shown benefit from low-frequency magnetic field therapy in relieving chronic knee pain secondary to OA (31–46 % relief compared with 8% for sham magnetic therapy).[39,40] Static magnets may provide temporary pain relief under certain circumstances, but data are limited. Overall, the use of magnets and electromagnetic fields is a potentially promising area for future therapeutics.

29. Discuss the role of low-level laser therapy (LLLT) in treating OA.

LLLT is a nonthermal, single wavelength light source with an effect based on photochemical reactions in cells. It has been used as an alternative noninvasive treatment for OA for approximately 10 years, but its effectiveness remains controversial. One randomized, controlled trial demonstrated a decrease in pain and paravertebral muscle spasm, with an increase in the range of neck motion and in the LLLT group compared with placebo.[41] However, despite positive findings, meta-analysis failed to show how LLLT effectiveness is affected by four important factors: wavelength, treatment duration, dosage and application over nerves vs. joints.[42] Further studies are needed with a laser standard.

30. Describe an integrative approach to OA.

In summary, the health practitioner looking for an integrative approach to OA may find a combination of the above modalities useful. Along with the general mind/body approach described in initial chapters, it is reasonable to start with a foundation of moderate exercise, physical therapy, healthy diet, and a nutraceutical such as glucosamine. Initially pain can be controlled with NSAIDs and/or analgesics, especially at the onset of an exercise program, then potentially discontinued with improvement. Manual modalities such as acupuncture may be added, along with other agents such as chondroitin, niacinamide, and vitamins C, D, and E, until the desired therapeutic response is achieved.

REFERENCES

1. Sheild MJ: Anti-inflammatory drugs and their effects of cartilage synthesis and renal function. Eur J Rheum Inflamm 13:7–16, 1993.
2. Zhang WY, et al: The effectiveness of topically applied capsaicin. A meta-analysis. Eur J Clin Pharmacol 46:517–522, 1994.
3. Reeves KD, et al... Randomized, prospective, placebo-controlled double-blind study of dextrose prolotherapy for osteoarthritic thumb and finger (DIP, PIP, and trapeziometacarpal) joints: Evidence of clinical efficacy. J Altern Compl Med 6:311–320, 2000.
4. Clyman B: Exercise in the treatment of osteoarthritis. Curr Rheumatol Rep. 2001 Dec;3(6):520-3.
5. Felson DT, et al: Weight loss reduces the risk for sympromatic knee osteoarthritis in women. The Framingham Study. Ann Intern Med 116:535-539, 1992.
6. Osiri M, et al: Transcutaneous electrical nerve stimulation for knee osteoarthritis. Cochrane Database Syst Rev 2000.
7. Felson DT, et al: Osteoarthritis: New insights. Part 2: Treatment approaches. Ann Intern Med 133:726–737, 2000.
8. Deal CL, et al: Nutraceuticals as therapeutic agents in osteoarthritis: The role of glucosamine, chondroitin sulfate, and collagen hydrolysate. Rheum Dis Clin North Am 25:379–395, 1999.
9. Reginster JY, et al: Long-term effects of glucosamine sulfate on osteoarthritis progression: A randomized, placebo controlled clinical trail. Lancet 357:251–156, 2001.
10. Conrozier T, et al: Glucosamine sulfate significantly reduced cartilage destruction in a rabbit model of osteoarthritis. Arthritis Rheumatol 41:S147, 1998.
11. Shikhaman AR, et al: N-acetylglucosamine prevents IL-1-mediated activation of chondrocytes Arthritis Rheum 42(Suppl):S381, 1999.
12. Bassleer C, et al: Stimulation of proteoglycan production by glucosamine sulfate in chondrocytes isolated from human osteoarthritic articular cartilage in vitro. Osteoarthr Cart 6:427–434, 1998.
13. McAlindon TE, et al: Glucosamine and chondroitin for treatment of osteoarthritis: A systematic quality assessment and meta-analysis. JAMA 238:1469–1475, 2000.
14. Uebelhart D, et al: Protective effect of exogenous chondroitin 4,6-sulfate in the acute degredation of articular cartilage in the rabbit. Osteoarthr Cart 6(Suppl A):6–13, 1998.
15. Uebelhart D, et al: Effects of oral chondroitin sulfate on the progression of knee osteoarthrtis: a pilot study. Osteoarthr Cart 6(Suppl A):37–38, 1998.
16. Mazieres B, et al: Chondroitin sulfate in osteoarthritis of the knee: A prospective, double blind, placebo controlled multicenter clinical study. J Rheumatol 28:173–181, 2001.
17. Kreder HJ, et al: Glucosamine and chondroitin were found to improve outcomes in patients with osteoarthritis. J Bone Joint Surg 82A:1323, 2000.
18. Lippiello L, et al: In vivo chondroprotection and metabolic synergy of glucosamine and chondroitin sulfate. Clin Orthop 381:229–240, 2000.
19. Evans MS: Dimethyl sulfoxide (DMSO) blocks conduction in peripheral nerve C fibers: A possible mechanism of analgesia. Neurosci Lett 150:145–148, 1993.
20. Jacob SW, Lawrence RM: The Miracle of MSM—the Natural Solution for Pain. New York, G.P. Putnam's Sons, 1999.
21. Lawrence RM: Methylsulfonylmethane (MSM): A double-blind study of its use in degenerative arthritis. Int J Anti-aging Med (1):50, 1998.
22. Marcolongo R, et al: Double-blind multicenter study of the activity of S-adenylmethionine in hip osteoarthritis. Curr Ther Res 37:82–94, 1985.
23. Sowers M, et al: Vitamins and arthritis: The roles of vitamins A, C, D, and E. Rheum Dis Clin North Am 25:315–332, 1999.

24. McAlindon TE, et al: Do antioxidant micronutrients protect against the development and progression of knee osteoarthritis? Arthritis Rheum 39:648–656, 1996.
25. Machtey I, Ouaknine L: Tocopherol in osteoarthritis: A controlled pilot study. J Am Geriatr Soc 26:328–330, 1978.
26. Tiku ML: Evidence linking chondrocyte lipid peroxidation to cartilage matrix protein degradation: Possible role in cartilage aging and the pathogenesis of osteoarthritis. J Biol Chem 275:20069–20076, 2000.
27. Darlington LG, et al: Antioxidants and fatty acids in the amelioration of rheumatoid arthritis and related disorders. Br J Nutr 85:251–269, 2001.
28. McAlindon TE, et al: Relation of dietary intake and serum levels of vitamin D to progression of osteoarthritis of the knee among participants in the Framingham Study. Ann Intern Med 125:353–359, 1996.
29. Lane NE, et al: Serum vitamin D levels and incident changes of radiographic hip osteoarthritis: A longitudinal study. Study of Osteoporotic Fractures Research Group. Arthritis Rheum 42:854–860, 1999.
30. Demoor-Fossard M, et al: A composite element binding the vitamin D receptor and the retinoic X receptor alpha mediates the transforming growth factor-beta inhibition of decorin gene expression in articular chondrocytes. J Biol Chem 276:36983–36992, 2001.
31. Jonas WB, et al: The effect of niacinamide on osteoarthritis: A pilot study. Inflamm Res 45:330–334, 1996.
32. McCarty MF, et al: Niacinamide therapy for osteoarthritis—does it inhibit nitric oxide synthase induction by interleukin 1 in chondrocytes? Med Hypoth 53(4):350–360, 1999.
33. Meheu E, et al: Symptomatic efficacy of avocado/soybean unsaponifiables in the treatment of osteoarthritis of the knee and hip: A prospective, randomized, double-blind, placebo-controlled, multicenter clinical trial with a six-month treatment period and a two-month followup demonstrating a persistent effect. Arthritis Rheum 41:81–91, 1998.
34. Blotman F, et al: Efficacy and safety of avocado/soybean unsaponifiables in the treatment of symptomatic osteoarthritis of the knee and hip: A prospective, multicenter, three-month, randomized, double-blind, placebo-controlled trial. Rev Rheum (English edition) 64:825–834, 1997.
35. Long L, et al: Herbal medicines for the treatment of osteoarthritis: A systematic review. Rheumatology (Oxford) 40:779–793, 2001.
36. Little CV, et al: Herbal therapy for treating osteoarthritis. Cochrane Database Syst Rev. 2001.
37. Puett DW, et al: Published trials of nonmedicinal and noninvasive therapies for hip and knee osteoarthritis. Ann Intern Med 121:133–140, 1994.
38. Ezzo J, et al: Acupuncture for osteoarthritis of the knee: A systematic review. Arthritis Rheum 44:819–825, 2001.
39. Trock DH: Electromagnetic fields and magnets. Investigational treatment for musculoskeletal disorders. Rheum Dis Clin North Am 26:51–62, 2000.
40. Zizic TM, et al: The treatment of osteoarthritis of the knee with pulsed electrical stimulation. J Rheumatol 22:1757–1761, 1995.
41. Brasseau L, et al: Low level laser therapy (classes I, II and III) for the treatment of osteoarthritis. Cochrane Database Syst Rev 2000.
42. Brasseau L, et al: Low level laser therapy for osteoarthritis and rheumatoid arthritis: A metaanalysis. J Rheumatol 27:1961–1969, 2000.

49. FIBROMYALGIA

Betsy B. Singh, Ph.D., S. P. Vinjamury, M.D., and V. J. Singh, B.A.

1. Define fibromyalgia and fibromyalgia syndrome.

Fibromyalgia is made up of three Latin words: *fibro* = fibrous tissue such as ligaments, tendons, or fascia; *myo* = muscle tissue; and *algia* = pain. In simple terms, it is the pain that emanates from tendons, ligaments, bursae, and muscle tissue. The pain of fibromyalgia is usually a diffuse aching or burning, described as "head to toe." It is often associated with muscle spasms. **Fibromyalgia syndrome** (FMS) is defined as more than one disease (syndrome) rather than a single disease because the symptoms vary from person to person and may include more generalized discomfort beyond chronic pain.

2. Describe the symptoms of fibromyalgia.

Fibromyalgia is characterized by widespread, persistent, nonarticular musculoskeletal pain; sleep disturbance; fatigue; and the presence of multiple discrete tender points on physical examination. These symptoms are usually associated with chronic anxiety or tension, chronic headaches, subjective soft tissue swelling, and pain modulated by physical activity, weather, anxiety, or stress. Fibromyalgia has been called "the invisible disability" or the "irritable everything" syndrome, because it has few symptoms that are outwardly noticeable. Unlike other chronic musculoskeletal ailments that may be crippling, the good news is that fibromyalgia is neither crippling nor fatal. Nonetheless, work disability is a serious concern in FMS, and the ability to work is limited in most women with FMS.

3. What other diseases are associated with fibromyalgia?

An interesting and important aspect of fibromyalgia is that it is often associated with a variety of other disorders of both musculoskeletal and nonmusculoskeletal origin. Examples include myofacial pain, irritable bowel, migraine headache, chronic fatigue syndrome, carpal tunnel syndrome, sleep disorders, dysmenorrhea and urinary tract symptoms, nonallergic rhinitis, nasal congestion, lower respiratory symptoms, recurrent noncardiac chest pain, heart burn, palpitations, irritable bowel symptoms and multiple chemical sensitivities. It is still not clear whether these disorders are precursors to or secondary to fibromyalgia.

4. Who gets FMS?

Fibromyalgia occurs worldwide and does not have a predisposition to a specific ethnic population. It is the second most common rheumatic disorder, affecting approximately 8–10 million persons in the U.S. Fibromyalgia is more common in women than men (female-to-male ratio: 9:1).[1] Wolfe and colleagues found a worldwide prevalence of 2% for both sexes, 3.4% for women, and 0.5% for men.[2] Prevalence of the syndrome increases with age and is highest between the ages 60 and 79 years. It is estimated that 15–20% of patients seen by rheumatologists have FMS. Although most cases of FMS are reported in middle-aged women, it also has been diagnosed in children, though much less frequently.

Although recent findings discount a hereditary link in the development of FMS, Yunus et al. confirmed the existence of a possible gene for FMS that is associated with the HLA region in a 1999 study. The authors of this study encourage further investigation.[3]

5. How is FMS diagnosed?

In 1990, the American College of Rheumatology (ACR) adopted the recommendations of a national panel convened to review the diagnostic criteria of FMS for statistical and epidemiologic purposes. The criteria to establish a diagnosis include widespread pain in all four body quadrants of at least 3 months' duration and mild or greater tenderness at 11 of the 18 tender points (see figure in question 8.)

Because there are no specific biologic markers FMS, the above criteria currently are considered the most appropriate for diagnosis. However, they are not without drawbacks. It is reported that more and more people with fibromyalgia are sensitive to painful stimuli throughout the body, not merely at the ACR-identified locations. In addition, patient-reported tenderness may vary from day to day and month to month. This variance in reported pain may result in an increase or decrease in the tender point count essential to the standardized diagnostic criteria. But in the absence of any diagnostic laboratory tests or x-rays, the ACR criteria are widely used in the diagnosis of FMS.

6. What causes fibromyalgia?

The exact causes of fibromyalgia are still not clear after 30 years and over 500 publications on cause alone. Proposed etiologies include the following:

Neurological factors
- Altered responsiveness of the stress system responsiveness, most notably in the hypothalamic-pituitary-adrenal axis.[3]
- Although alpha intrusion during sleep can demonstrate different patterns in people with chronic pain, the polyphasic alpha sleep activity of patients with FMS is correlated more closely with clinical manifestations.[4]
- The pathophysiologic significance of the reduction in the blood flow to the pontine tegmentum and thalami in women with FMS, as evidenced through single-photon-emission computed tomography (radioimaging) is also under study.[5]

Circulatory factors
- Vasoconstriction occurs in the skin above tender points, supporting the hypothesis that FMS is related to hypoxia in the skin above tender points.[6]

Hormonal factors
- Altered synthesis of the growth hormone somatomedin C as well as substance P, a pain modulator,[7] may cause fibromyalgia.
- The decreased nocturnal levels of both growth hormone and prolactin in women with FMS during sleep support the hypothesis that a dysregulated neuroendocrine system during sleep may play a role in the pathophysiology.[8]

Viral infections
- An increased prevalence of the IgM antibodies against enterovirus in patients with acute onset of FMS duplicates a viral infection.[9]
- An association between FMS and infections with hepatitis virus has been suggested, but studies have found no such correlation.[10]

Psychological factors
- Studies show that depression, generalized psychological distress, and other psychological factors have an associative, but not causal, relationship with the onset and persistence of fibromyalgia symptoms in adults.[11]

7. Is fibromyalgia synonymous with chronic fatigue immune dysfunction syndrome (CFIDS)?

No. Although symptoms of the two disorders overlap, they are two separate entities. The pathologic nature of the concomitant sleep disturbances in fibromyalgia correlates with a secondary diagnosis of CFIDS, particularly in patients with a suspected infectious onset. However, no common connection has been found. Some of the following aspects differentiate the two diseases. Fibromyalgia seems to be associated with more localized musculoskeletal pain and trigger points, which are areas on the body that the examiner can typically push and elicit pain. FMS often follows a stressful situation such as a car accident, divorce, or financial losses. CFIDS may be identified after some type of infection. The onset of CFIDS is typically more rapid, whereas FMS usually has a gradual onset.

A relatively new blood test may be a potential biochemical marker for CFIDS.[12] This test looks for a specific polypeptide in the blood, which has been found in 88% of patients who met the strict case definition for CFIDS but only in 28% of controls. The control group included not only healthy people but also but people who suffered from depression and/or fibromyalgia. This test may be a new useful diagnostic tool for further distinguishing patients suffering from CFIDS. There is no such single decisive marker to diagnose fibromyalgia.

8. Is fibromyalgia a form of somatoform disorder?

The literature is conflicting. The belief that FMS is a form of somatoform disorder remains unproven. No definitive evidence indicates that FMS develops as a result of posttraumatic stress or abuse. However, the clinical hallmarks of fibromyalgia suggest, to many doctors, that the syndrome is a biopsychosocial phenomenon—not merely a medical or psychiatric phenomenon. Increased rates of psychiatric disorders, such as depressive, anxiety, and somatoform disorders, are apparent in populations diagnosed with clinical FMS.

As a pervasive and debilitating rheumatic disorder with an unknown etiology, fibromyalgia is often dismissed in Western medicine as a factitious or somatoform disorder. The level of diffuse, severe pain, the descriptions of the "typical" narrative from patients with fibromyalgia, and the frustrating resistance to treatment have made FMS synonymous with a disease that begins in the mind and ends in the body. In addition, it has been suggested that patients with fibromyalgia are more susceptible to psychological exacerbation and disruptions of daily functioning and are much more vigilant about pain phenomenalism. Indeed, patients with fibromyalgia have higher objective anger and depression scores than patients with rheumatoid arthritis. To some experts, the syndrome becomes a functional, self-validating way of life, which is perpetuated to the point of abnormality.[13]

9. List the anatomic tender points commonly seen in patients with FMS.

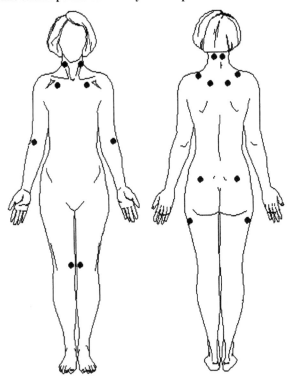

Tender points according to the criteria of the American College of Rheumatology.

To qualify for a diagnosis of fibromyalgia, patients must ache all over and have tenderness in at least 11 of the following 18 spots when 4 kg of pressure is applied[14]:

1. Occiput: suboccipital muscle insertions. (attachment of neck muscles at the base of the skull)
2. Trapezius: midpoint of the upper border (midway between neck and shoulder)
3. Supraspinatus: above the medial border of the scapular spine (muscle over upper inner shoulder blade)

4. Lateral epicondyle: 2 cm distal to the epicondyles (2 cm below side bone at elbow)
5. Gluteal: upper outer quadrant of buttocks (upper outer buttock)
6. Greater trochanter: posterior to the trochanteric prominence (hip bone)
7. Knee: medial fat pad proximal to the joint line (just above the knee on the inside)
8. Low cervical: anterior aspects of the intertransverse spaces at C5–C7 (lower neck in front)
9. Second rib: second costochondral junctions (edge of upper breastbone)

The ACR's 1990 diagnostic criteria do not specify hat the aching must be continuous—just chronic. Patients with FMS can hurt almost anywhere, not just at the 18 diagnostic tender points, which were chosen because they are the most consistent from patient to patient. People who ache all over, particularly if they have some of the other commonly associated symptoms, should try to find a doctor who is knowledgeable about FMS and can perform a standardized tender point examination.

10. How is FMS treated?

Treatment is mostly palliative and often consists of patient education, physical therapy, and counseling. Most people with FMS have difficulty in attaining restorative sleep. Therefore, a multifaceted approach for treating fibromyalgia involves exercise to reduce pain and strengthen muscles, regular sleep routines, drug therapies to improve sleep and other symptoms, and psychological tools for coping with the emotional distress caused by the disease and for reducing stress that can exacerbate pain. Studies support the efficacy of the following treatments

- Aerobic exercise, such as swimming and walking, improves muscle fitness and reduces muscle pain and tenderness.[15]
- Heat and massage may give short-term relief.
- Tricyclic antidepressants may help elevate mood, improve quality of sleep, and relax muscles.[16] Low doses have been considered useful for pain and standard doses for antidepressive effects.
- Data also suggest that smoking cessation programs, support groups, and available medications can modify symptom perception and improve coping.[17]

11. What pharmacologic agents have been used to treat fibromyalgia?

Drugs used in the treatment of FMS have included antidepressants, nonsteroidal anti-inflammatory drugs (NSAIDs), and neuroleptics. The most commonly prescribed antidepressants are tricyclics such as amitriptyline, cyclobenzapine, and dotheipin, which provide short-term benefit, generally in combination with selective serotonin reuptake inhibitors (SSRIs). Various trials of tricyclics and SSRIs have shown inconsistent benefit to patients.[18] The negative aspects of pharmacologic therapy are adverse events and short-term action in FMS. Amitriptyline often produces dry mouth and sedation and may produce hypotension and tachycardia. Therefore, its use must be considered in the context of the side-effect potential. For example, adverse reactions have been found in 56% of patients who use NSAIDs, 51% who use antidepressants, 31% who use muscle relaxants, and 18% who use analgesics.[19]

Due to the complexity of the disease, FMS is better managed with a combination of pharmacological and nonpharmacologic therapies. The nonpharmacologic therapies have provided, though not curative, some improvement in perception of pain, mood state, function, sleeplessness, fatigue by introducing new mechanisms of coping with this chronic disorder.

12. Describe the complementary and alternative medicine (CAM) approaches to FMS.

Despite scant knowledge about the efficacy and tolerance of CAM therapies, interest in their use for fibromyalgia is widespread. This interest may be due to the short term or ineffective action of pharmacologic treatments. The clinical trials in CAM therapies are often criticized for poor designs in terms of sample size, controls, compliance, and follow-up. However, research in CAM is becoming increasingly rigorous. Indeed, funds from the National Institutes of Health have been awarded to investigate the efficacy of CAM therapies for FMS.

According to the Center for Evidence-Based Medicine (CEBM), CAM therapies that for FMS that have been studied so far can be categorized under three headings: no definitive benefit, some benefit, and clear benefit.[20]

NO DEFINITIVE BENEFIT	SOME BENEFIT	CLEAR BENEFIT
Bright light treatment	Biofeedback	Acupuncture
Low-output helium neon laser	S-adenosyl methionine (SAMe)	
Maltic acid, 200 mg	Balneotherapy (spa treatment)	
Magnesium, 50 mg orally 3 times/day	Hypnotherapy	
Rheumajecta and Vasolastine injections	Meditation	
Selenium 100 mg/day orally (daily in low-selenium soil areas)	Massage	
Musical vibrations, 60–300 Hz		
Chiropratic		

13. Does exercise moderate symptoms of fibromyalgia?

Exercise therapy has received a moderate degree of support from the literature and has been subjected to more randomized studies than any other intervention. A study designed to determine whether there is any difference between land exercise and pool exercise found that physical capacity increased in both groups almost equally except for grip strength, which showed greater improvement with land exercise.[22]

An outcome study by Hakkinen et al. showed that progressive strength training decreased the impact of the syndrome on the neuromuscular system, perceived symptoms, and functional capacity.[23] Low-intensity walking 2–3 times/week has also made a positive impact on daily activities.[24]

Because every patient with fibromyalgia is unique, stretching, strength maintenance, and aerobic conditioning should be modified to meet individual needs. Too intense a level of training can actually trigger a stress response; it is wise to ease into exercise gradually but persistently.

14. Is acupuncture useful in the treatment of FMS?

Acupuncture is the only CAM modality that is recognized to have a clear benefit in patients with FMS. The popularity of acupuncture has grown tremendously in recent years. Many people use acupuncture for chronic pain. Comparison of the adverse event rate for acupuncture and conventional treatment for pain suggests that acupuncture is relatively safe. Although laboratory evidence documents a biochemical basis of acupuncture analgesia, the effectiveness of acupuncture for chronic pain relief remains in question.

A study in patients with FMS showed that acupuncture decreased pain levels and tender point index (TPI), as measured by visual analog scale (VAS) and dolorimetry, and also showed changes in the serum concentrations of pain-modulating substances such as serotonin and substance P.[13] Electroacupuncture also has been found to be effective in reducing the pain, sleep quality, and morning stiffness. Currently three trials are under way at various sites to study the efficacy of acupuncture in FMS.

15. Can chiropractic treatment help fibromyalgia patients?

Not many studies address the role of chiropractic treatment in FMS. However, the few that are available suggest improvement in cervical and lumbar ranges of motion, straight leg raise, and reported pain levels. Recent studies of chiropractic treatment show that spinal manipulative therapy, soft tissue therapy, and lifestyle and ergonomic advice resulted in optimal improvement only after approximately 12 treatments within a 5-week period. Further improvement was only marginal.[21]

16. Can dietary change and supplements modify fibromyalgia symptoms?

A vegan diet rich in antioxidants, lactobacilli, and fiber produced a decrease in joint stiffness and pain as well as improvement in self-reported health state.[25] Another study with a strict, low-salt, uncooked vegan diet rich in lactobacteria showed beneficial effects on FMS symptoms at least in the short term.[26]

Nutritional supplements such as freeze-dried aloe vera gel extract, a combination of freeze-dried aloe vera gel extract and additional plant-derived saccharides, and a formulation of dioscorea complex containing the saccharides and a vitamin/mineral complex reduced initial symptom severity with continued improvement in the period between initial symptom severity and the follow-up. [27]

In another interesting study, four female patients who had tried multiple treatment modalities in the past were asked to eliminate monosodium glutamate (MSG) and other excitotoxins such as aspartate from their diets. The investigators reported that all patients had complete or nearly complete resolution of symptoms within months after elimination of MSG or MSG plus aspartates. All had recurrence of symptoms whenever MSG was ingested.[28] Even though the numbers are small, a trial of MSG elimination diet will cause no harm and may benefit the patient.

17. What does cognitive/behavioral therapy have to offer the patient with fibromyalgia?

Relaxation-based techniques are commonly used to manage pain and stress by decreasing muscle tension. The type of coping strategies used by the patient can influence pain perception. The methods may include relaxation, hypnosis, guided imagery, biofeedback, and cognitive behavioral therapy. A current concept of optimal management uses a blend of multidisciplinary therapies and individualized clinician-based treatment. A study of combined therapy or a multidisciplinary approach showed a better effect on the FMS symptoms. The combination of biofeedback/relaxation training, exercise training, and an educational/attention control program had a very good effect on tender point index scores and physical activity in patients with FMS.[29]

A mind-body intervention, including patient education, meditation techniques, and movement therapy, was found effective as an adjunctive therapy in FMS.[30] This study followed ACR criteria for diagnosis of FMS and used standardized outcome measures. Patients continued to improve for 3 months even after treatment was ended as opposed to returning to baseline scores of pain, stiffness, and dissatisfaction. This study indicates that cognitive/behavioral therapy may have a role in the long-term treatment of FMS.

Meditation is under investigation as another promising method to reduce stress and relax the muscles for relief from FMS symptoms.[31] It is also believed that cognitive/behavioral interventions in combination with physiotherapy can be effective.[30]

18. What evidence is there for homeopathy to treat fibromyalgia?

Although homeopathy is one of the most frequently used complementary therapies worldwide, little research evidence addresses its effect in FMS. In a double-blind, placebo-controlled, crossover trial with *Rhus toxicodendron* 6c (tincture of poison oak diluted in ethanol), the treatment group did better in all variables compared with the placebo group. The number of tender spots was reduced by one-fourth, and significant improvement in pain and sleep was reported.[32] However, *R. toxicodendron* was not effective in three patients with FMS when administered in a lower, 6X potency using a time-series design. The authors added that the study may be flawed by design issues or sample selection. Further studies of *R. toxicodendron* are ongoing.

19. What other therapeutic modalities may be considered?

Ayurveda, the traditional system of health care of India, and yoga also have been shown to be effective in FMS. Detoxification methods, oil massages, herbal concoctions prepared according to Ayurvedic Formulary of India, and yoga release the blocked wind (vata) and reduce pain. Although no published data address the use of these modalities in FMS, some studies support their efficacy in rheumatic disorders.

Static magnetic fields have shown little promise for treatment of FMS.

In an open prospective study, tender point injections (0.5 ml of 1% lidocaine and 0.25 ml intralesional triamcinolone diacetate suspension) were demonstrated as a safe adjunctive form of therapy for pain in FMS. Further investigations are under way.[33]

20. What studies of treatment for FMS are under way?

- Acupuncture in fibromyalgia (Georgetown University)
- Randomized, controlled trial of mind-body intervention (University of Maryland)
- Effectiveness of acupuncture in fibromyalgia as an adjuvant therapy (South California University of Health Sciences)

- Effectiveness of combination therapy with amitriptyline and fluoxetine (National Institute of Arthritis and Musculoskeletal and Skin Diseases [NIAMS])
- Matching treatments to people with FMS on the basis of psychosocial and behavioral characteristics (NIAMS)

21. What resources are available for more information about FMS?

- Fibromyalgia Network
P.O. Box 31750
Tucson, AZ 85751-1750
Tel: 1-800-853-2929
- Fibromyalgia Partnership
140 Zinn Way
Linden, VA 22642-5609
Tel: 1-866-725-4404 (toll-free)
Internet: www.fmpartnership.org
- National Fibromyalgia Awareness Campaign (NFAC)
2415 N. River Trail Road, Suite 200
Orange, CA 92865
Tel: 714-921-0150
- Arthritis Foundation
National Headquarters
P.O. Box 7669
Atlanta, GA 30357-0669
Tel: 1-800-283-7800
Internet: www.arthritis.org

REFERENCE

1. Yunus MB: The role of gender in fibromyalgia syndrome. Curr Rheumatol Rep 3(2):128–134, 2001.
2. Wolfe F, Ross K, Anderson J, et al: The prevalence and characteristics of fibromyalgia in the general population. Arthritis Rheum 38:19–28, 1995.
3. Yunus MB, Khan MA, Rawlings KK, et al: Genetic linkage of multianalysis of multicase families with fibromyalgia syndrome. J Rheumatol 26 :408–412, 1999.
4. Roizenblatt S, Moldofsky H, Benedito-Silva AA, Tufik S: Alpha sleep characteristics in fibromyalgia. Arthritis Rheum 44:222–230, 2001.
5. Kwiatek R, Barnden L, Tedman R, et al: Regional cerebral blood flow in fibromyalgia: Single-photon emission computed tomography evidence of reduction in the pontine tegmentum and thalami. Arthritis Rheum 43:2823–2833,2000.
6. Jeschonneck M, Grohmann G, Hein G, Sprott H: Abnormal microcirculation and temperature in skin above tender points in patients with fibromyalgia. Rheumatology 39:917–921, 2000.
7. Clauw DJ: Fibromyalgia: Musculoskeletal pain and evaluation. In EDITOR: Textbook of Rheumatology, CITY, PUBLISHER, 2000, pp 417–427.
8. Landis CA, Lentz MJ, Rothermel J, et al: Decreased nocturnal levels of prolactin and growth hormone in women with fibromyalgia. J Clin Endocrinol Metab 86:1672–1678, 2001.
9. Wittrup IH, Jensen B, Bliddal H, et al: Comparison of viral antbodies in 2 groups of patients with fibromyalgia. J Rheumatol 8:601–603, 2001.
10. Wittrup IH, Jensen B, Bliddal H, et al: Lack of correlation between hepatitis markers and fibromyalgia in Danish patients. J Musculoskel Pain 9:57–65, 2001.
11. Anthony KK, Schanberg L: Juvenile primary fibromyalgia syndrome. Curr Rheumatol Rep 3:165–171, 2001.
12. De Meirleir K, Bisbal CA, Campine L, et al: A 37 kDa 2-5A binding protein as a potential biochemical marker for chronic fatigue syndrome. Am. J Med 108(2):99–105, 2000.
13. Sprott H, Franke S, Kluge H, Hein G: Pain treatment of fibromyalgia by acupuncture. Rheumatol Int 18:35–36, 1998.
14. Wolfe F, Smythe HA, Yunus MB, et al: The American College of Rheumatology 1990 criteria for the classification of fibromyalgia: Report of the multicenter criteria committee. Arthritis Rheum 33:160–172, 1990.

15. Wigers SH, Stiles TC, Vogel PA: Effects of aerobic exercise versus stress management treatment in fibromyalgia: A 4.5 year prospective study. Scand J Rheumatol 25:77–86. 1996.
16. Arnold LM, Keck PE, Welge JA: Antidepressant treatment of fibromyalgia: A meta analysis and review. Psychosomatics 41:104–113, 2000.
17. Bailey A, Starr L, Alderson M, Moreland J: A comparative evaluation of a fibromyalgia rehabilitation program. Arthritis Care Res 12:336–340, 1999.
18. Jung AC, Staiger T, Sullivan M: The efficacy of selective serotonin reuptake inhibitors for the management of chronic pain. J Gen Intern Med 12:384–389, 1997.
19. Skeith KJ, et al: Adverse drug reactions and debrisoquine/sparteine (P450IID6) polymorphism in patients with fibromyalgia. Clin Rheumatol 16:291–295, 1997.
20. Ebell MH, Beck E: How effective are complementary/alternative medicine (CAM) therapies for fibromyalgia? J Fam Pract 50:400–401, 2001.
21. Schneider M: The effectiveness of chiropractic management of fibromyalgia patients. J Manip Physiol Ther 21(4):307, 1998.
22. Jentoft ES, Kvalik AG, Mengshoel AM: Effects of pool-based and land-based aerobic exercise on women with fibromyalgia/chronic widespread muscle pain. Arthritis Rheum 45:42–47, 2001.
23. Hakkinen A, Hakkinen K, Hannonen P, Alen M: Strength training induced adaptations in neuromuscular function of premenopausal women with fibromyalgia: Comparison with healthy women. Ann Rheum Dis 60:21–26, 2001.
24. Meyer BB, Lemley KJ: Utilizing exercise to affect the symptomatology of fibromyalgia: A pilot study. Med Sci Sports Exerc 32:1691–1697, 2000.
25. Hanninen A, Kaartinen K, Rauma AL, et al: TITLE OF ARTICLE Toxicology 155(1–3):45–53, 2000.
26. Kaartinen K, Lammi K, Hypen M, et al: Vegan diet alleviates fibromyalgia symptoms. Scand J Rheumatol 29(5):308–313, 2000.
27. Dykman KD, Tone C, Ford C, Dykman RA: The effects of nutritional supplements on the symptoms of fibromyalgia and chronic fatigue syndrome. Integr Physiol Behav Sci 33:66–71, 1998.
28. Smith JD, Terpening CM, Schmidt SO, Gums JG: Relief of fibromyalgia symptoms following discontinuation of dietary excitotoxins. Ann Pharmacother 35:702–706, 2001.
29. Bucklew SP, Conway R, Parker J, et al: Biofeedback/relaxation training and exercise interventions for fibromyalgia: A prospective trial. Arthritis Care Res 11:196–209, 1998.
30. Singh BB, Berman BM, Hadazhy VA, Creamer P: A pilot study of cognitive behavioral therapy in fibromyalgia. Altern Ther Health Med 4(2):67–70, 1998.
31. Kaplan KH, Goldenberg DL, Galvin-Nadeau M: The impact of a meditation-based stress reduction program on fibromyalgia. Gen Hosp Psychiatry. 15(5):284–289, 1993.
32. Fisher P, Greenwood A, Huskisson EC, et al: Effect of homoeopathic treatment on fibrositis (prmary fibromyalgia). Br Med J 299:365--336, 1989.
33. Reddy SS, Yunus MB, Inanci F, Aldag JC: Tender point injections are beneficial in fibromyalgia syndrome: A descriptive open study. JOURNAL VOL. PAGES YEAR

50. ALZHEIMER'S DEMENTIA

Raffaele Filice, M.D., FRCPC

1. What is Alzheimer's disease?

Alzheimer's disease (AD) is the most common cause of dementia in the elderly in Western countries. It was first described in 1907 by Professor Alois Alzheimer in Germany. Alzheimer discovered the amyloid neuritic plaques and intraneuronal neurofibrillary tangles that are the hallmarks of AD in the brain of a demented patient .

2. Define dementia.

Dementia is defined as memory loss with a least one other impaired cognitive function, such as language ability, orientation, attention and concentration, frontal executive function (self-monitoring, judgment, problem solving), praxis (ability to perform previously acquired motor skills), or activities of daily living (e.g., finances, using appliances, bathing, toileting).[1]

3. Describe the clinical features of AD.

Clinically, AD most often presents with subtle onset of memory loss followed by a slowly progressive dementia that has a variable course of several years. In the early stages, the memory loss may seem trivial, forgetting information or misplacing objects. Although such lapses may occur in normal people, they become a pattern in patients with AD. Patients, families, and physicians often miss the early symptoms of AD because they do not necessarily interfere with the carrying out of everyday tasks. However, as AD progresses, the person becomes less able to carry out daily activities, such as keeping track of finances, following instructions on the job, shopping, driving, and keeping appointments. As the disease progresses the ability to perform previously familiar tasks continues to deteriorate. Many patients experience behavioral changes, such as apathy, anxiety, depression, agitation, or even psychosis. In the later stages patients are unable to function independently.

4. List the ten warning signs of AD, according to the Alzheimer's Association.

1. Recent memory loss that affects job skills
2. Difficulty in performing familiar tasks
3. Problems with language
4. Disorientation to time and space
5. Poor or decreased judgment
6. Problems with abstract thinking
7. Misplacing objects of importance
8. Changes in mood or behavior
9. Changes in personality
10. Loss of initiative

5. What is MCI?

MCI stands for mild cognitive impairment.[2,3] It is a term used to differentiate incipient dementia from age-associated memory impairment (AAMI) and age-associated cognitive decline (AACD). MCI refers to a transitional but progressively degenerative cognitive phase that precedes the onset of dementia or AD. Longitudinal studies indicate that persons with MCI progress to dementia at a rate of approximately 10–15% per year compared with control subjects, who progress at a rate of only 1–2%. Predictors of progression include apolipoprotein E -4 allele carrier status, certain features of memory function, and volume of the hippocampus (as determined by magnetic resonance imaging) at the time of diagnosis. Progression occurs gradually over the course of several years.

6. What causes AD?

The exact cause of AD is not known. It appears to be a complex disease with both inherited and acquired factors. In *Brain Longevity*, Dharma S. Khalsa reminds us that the brain is a flesh-and-blood organ, subject to the same physiologic stresses as the rest of the body—specifically the heart. Numerous studies have found correlation between AD and coronary artery disease, hypertension, and cerebrovascular disease. Furthermore, people with coronary artery disease may develop similar pathologic findings in the brain as those with AD.[4,5] Even Alzheimer, in his original paper, described atherosclerotic changes and endothelial proliferation with neovascularization along with the findings of plaques and tangles.

7. Discuss some of the current working theories about the pathogenesis of AD.

In the conventional world there are basically two camps: the so-called **BAP-tists** (working on **b**eta **a**myloid **p**roteins in the neuritic plaques) and the **tauists** (working on the *tau* protein of the neurofibrillary tangle). Considerable progress has been made in understanding pathologic states found in the brains of patients with AD. Whether the plaques and tangles are causative or simply pathologic end-points of the disease remains a controversial issue. Recent animal studies have generated some evidence that if amyloid plaque formation can be interrupted, memory loss can be prevented. In fact, a beta-peptide vaccine has been successfully used in an animal model. Human trials are planned if not already under way.[6]

8. What are the risk factors for developing AD?

- Age
- Family history (4-fold increase with an affected first-degree relative)
- Genetic factors
- History of moderate or severe head injury
- Gender (women more often than men)
- Educational level (inversely related)
- Mild cognitive impairment
- Cardiovascular disease
- Chronic stress

9. Is exposure to aluminum a risk factor?

The answer is at best controversial. Although the causal role of aluminum in dialysis-associated dementia is widely accepted, the role of aluminum exposure from food and water in AD is not so clear. A recent epidemiologic study reaffirmed increased risk of AD in a cohort of people in southwestern France exposed to relatively high levels of aluminum in the drinking water.[7] This study also found that increased levels of silicates in the water lowered the risk of AD.

A recent preliminary study of the effects of dietary intake of aluminum was also suggestive of increased risk.[8] The authors point out that aluminum is prevalent in the food supply, particularly in processed foods. Aluminum is used in anticaking agents, leaveners, and thickeners. For example, 1 ounce of American cheese or one baking-powder biscuit yields approximately 20 mg of aluminum. Many over the counter medicines (e.g., Bufferin, Amphojel, Mylanta, Maalox, Rolaids) also contain significant amounts of aluminum. In some cases, food sources of aluminum may be substantially higher than water sources. An interesting study in the early 1990s showed a reduced rate of decline in patients with AD who were treated with aluminum ion-specific chelation therapy for a 2-year period.[9] It is safe to say that aluminum has some relationship to AD, but the nature of the relationship is unclear.

10. Is the aluminum used in antiperspirants a concern?

Virtually no hard data address this question. One experiment in mice published in 1997 demonstrated the possibility of transcutaneous absorption of aluminum. However, the skin of the mouse lacks functional sweat glands and therefore cannot be considered an adequate model to study aluminum chemistry at the human skin surface. The possibility of significant accumulation of aluminum in the body from antiperspirants is theoretical at best.

It is possible to produce aluminum salts that are less bioavailable than the commonly used chloro-hydrate salts. Much of the aluminum applied topically is likely to be sloughed off with the skin. Aerosolizing antiperspirants, however, results in ingestion of aluminum through the nose and lung. The amount is quite small, particularly in relation to the amount that most people ingest in food and water. Although aluminum in antiperspirants is unlikely to cause significant systemic exposures, questions surrounding the bioaccumulation of aluminum should not be ignored. Aluminum absorption studies in humans are necessary to determine the role of antiperspirants in total aluminum exposure.[10]

11. What is the differential diagnosis for AD?

Several reversible disorders should be considered in the face of cognitive impairment: hypothyroidism, delirium from taking too many medications in combination, drug or other substance abuse, environmental toxins (e.g., carbon monoxide, organophosphates, solvents), vitamin deficiencies (e.g., B_{12}), brain tumor, multi-infarct dementia, liver or kidney failure and severe depression. Depression tends to be underdiagnosed and undertreated in the elderly.

12. How should one approach the treatment of persons with AD?

The treatment approach varies with the severity of the patient's symptoms. The goal should be early intervention. Complaints of declining cognitive function should never be taken lightly. Preventative measures such as a nutritious low-fat diet, regular exercise, adequate rest, and remaining intellectually and socially active are applicable to everyone. Meditation is also recommended as both a preventative and therapeutic measure. Most complementary and alternative therapies have the greatest impact in patients with MCI or mild-to-moderate AD. Although most of these measures can be adopted in more advanced cases, the focus should be on symptomatic allopathic treatment and supportive measures for both patients and families.

13. What dietary recommendations should you make to people with AD? Why?

Epidemiologic studies have demonstrated significant dietary links to AD. Countries with high amounts of fat in the diet (U.S. United Kingdom, Canada) have the highest incidence of AD. The countries with the lowest intake of fat (Japan, Nigeria, China) show the lowest incidence. These findings have been corroborated in ethnic groups within the United States that have differing amounts of fat and total calorie consumption in their respective diets.[11] Genetic and cultural differences, therefore, may be contributing factors.

The type and quality of fats also have a bearing on the incidence of many diseases, both cerebrovascular and cardiovascular. Furthermore, pathologic evidence indicates that AD is, at least in part, an inflammatory process. The recommended diet, therefore, is low-fat (15–25%), favoring monounsaturated fats (olive oil), including omega-3 essential fatty acids (e.g., salmon or flaxseed), and completely eliminating partially hydrogenated oils that contain trans-fatty acids. (See Chapter 19). Increased intake of vegetables and fruits is strongly recommended if not a frank shift toward a vegetarian diet.

14. Does exercise improve the lives of patients with AD?

Regular physical exercise has been found to slow the development of AD.[12] A retrospective study of adults aged 40–60 years who exercised regularly were found to have a reduced incidence of AD. Exercise programs for nursing home residents also have been found to have considerable benefit. Regular exercise, such as daily walking, is particularly important for people with MCI or milder forms of AD. Cognitive exercises, such as news headline discussion, crossword puzzles, and participating in music or art, help to maintain cognitive ability.

15. Why is meditation a recommended therapy for AD?

Meditation, like some other measures, has the greatest potential for benefit if implemented early, before cognitive functioning has deteriorated beyond the point of being able to follow simple directions. Stress is a major contributing factor to memory and cognitive dysfunction. Cortisol has a direct toxic effect on cells of the hippocampus, which are critical in normal memory function.[13] Regular meditation practice reduces stress and serum cortisol levels and improves cognitive functioning.

Furthermore, more advanced yoga techniques (called kriyas), which engage the breath, intonations, movement, and mind, have been found to increase cerebral blood flow and glucose utilization.[14]

16. Which alternative healing systems should be considered?

As with many illnesses, early intervention in AD is most likely to yield beneficial effects. This finding seems to be almost universal in the clinical trials of both drug and nutraceutical therapies. Of course there is a wide spectrum of severity in AD, and therapies need to be tailored to the clinical scenario. Two somewhat more mainstream approaches are music therapy and art therapy. A systematic review of music therapy for dementia symptoms concluded that, despite insufficient empirical evidence to justify its use to treat dementia symptoms, the available evidence strongly suggests benefit. More adequately designed studies need to be undertaken.[15]

The same probably can be said for many other healing systems, including art therapy, traditional Chinese medicine, ayurvedic medicine, energy medicine, yoga, tai chi, healing touch, and massage therapy. These systems should be considered for symptomatic or generalized treatment; they have shown efficacy in other contexts and can be incorporated safely into treatment protocols.

17. Which supplemental vitamins are recommended?

Mounting evidence supports the theory of oxygen free radical damage as a cause of cellular degeneration and aging. Oxidative damage in neuronal systems is being investigated, specifically as it relates to AD.[16] A good case can be made for the complementary use of antioxidants. Of the antioxidants vitamins (vitamins E, A, and C), vitamin E has been the most extensively studied. In vitro and animal studies have shown that antioxidant vitamins have neuronal protective effects. Similarly, the B vitamins (thiamine, niacin, B_6, B_{12}, and folate) have neuroprotective properties. Although vitamins in isolation cannot be considered as efficacious in the treatment of AD, they certainly have a role in minimizing progression and optimizing neuronal function.

Suggested daily intakes

Vitamin E.	400 IU bid	B_1	50–100 mg/day
Vitamin C	250–500 mg bid	B_3	100–200 mg/day
Vitamin A	10,000 IU	B_6	Up to 50 mg/day
Folate	400 µg/day	B_{12}	Up to 1000 µg/day

18. Should other nutritional supplements be considered?

Vitamin and mineral supplementation is an ancillary treatment. A select spectrum of minerals is most appropriate. Magnesium, selenium, and zinc have strong antioxidant properties and are commonly included in high-quality multivitamin formulas. **Amino acids** such as phenylalanine, glutamine, methionine, arginine, and tryptophan are important in neurotransmitter production and functioning. Usually they can be acquired in a balanced diet. However, because adequate nutrition is often at issue in patients with AD, protein supplementation should be considered (25–50 gm/day) to supply amino acids.

19. What is gingko biloba? Does it really work?

Ginkgo biloba is the name of a tree of the Ginkgoaceae family. The distinctive fan-shaped leaves are used in herbal preparations. Most of the bulk herb comes from China, Japan, Korea, and plantations in Europe and North America. The most often quoted study of the use of ginkgo for dementia was reported by LeBars et al. in 1997.[17] In this multicenter trial, a particular extract of gingko biloba (EGb 761) was found to have a modest but significant benefit compared with placebo therapy in improving the cognitive performance and social functioning of patients with dementia, as noted by standardized scales as well as by caretakers. No significant adverse events were noted. A systematic review published in 1998 essentially concurred with the findings of the LeBars study.[18] The dosage range is 120–240 mg/day. In more severe cases, the higher dose is advised. The greatest benefit seems to be in the earlier stages of mental dysfunction.

20. How is ginkgo biloba thought to work?

Numerous active substances are found in the ginkgo leaves. The extract used in the LeBars study is standardized for some 60 constituents, although there are many more. The flavanoids are free radical scavengers (antioxidants). Several different terpenes, named ginkgolides A, B, C, and so on, are antagonists of platelet-activating factor. Both classes of compounds have neuroprotective properties. Numerous studies also demonstrated efficacy in treating peripheral vascular disease.[19]

The incidence of side effects from using ginkgo biloba is low. There is, however, a theoretical possibility of interaction with antiplatelet medications (e.g., aspirin) to induce bleeding. Caution also is advised for patients who concurrently take anticoagulants or have bleeding diatheses. Such patients should be questioned specifically about gingko biloba use, and closer-than-usual monitoring of the international normalized ratio (INR) and bleeding time is recommended.

21. Numerous Ginkgo biloba products are available. Which should I recommend?

As with any natural product, quality is an issue. A number of standardized ginkgo biloba products use the flavonone glycosides and terpenes as marker compounds. The products aim for 22–27% flavonone glycosides and 5–7% terpenes. The product used in most clinical trials (EGb 761), however, was standardized for approximately 60 compounds. This identical form is marketed in North America as Ginkgold by Nature's Way. An extrapolation to other products is speculative at best. In fact, electroencephalographic (EEG) studies confirm different activation patterns with various ginkgo extracts that may well translate into varying degrees of clinical efficacy.[20]

22. Some natural products for optimizing brain function also contain phosphatidyl serine and acetyl-L carnitine. Does any evidence support the efficacy of these compounds?

Phosphatidyl serine (PS) is a naturally occurring phospholipid that forms part of the structural matrix of cell membranes. PS is the most abundant phospholipid in the brain and contributes to maintenance of cell membrane fluidity, cell-to-cell communication, and function of neurotransmitter receptors. Historically, the source of PS was bovine brain. Today however, PS is derived from soy. Numerous studies have been done in both animal and plant models, in vitro and in vivo. PS facilitates regrowth of damaged nerve networks, enhances neuronal metabolism, and maintains nerve cell numbers and size in aging rats. Clinical trials, although not numerous, have demonstrated improved memory and cognitive functioning of patients with AD.[21] PS seems to be particularly helpful in the early phases of the dementia. The therapeutic dose of PS is 100 mg orally 3 times/day. The preventive dose is 100 mg/day orally.

Acetyl-l-carnitine (ALC) is an ester of the amino acid L-carnitine and is synthesized in the human brain, liver, and kidney by the enzyme ALC-transferase. It facilitates the uptake of acetyl CoA into mitochondria for fatty acid oxidation, enhances acetylcholine production, and stimulates protein and membrane phospholipid synthesis. It also may have a cholinomimetic effect. Results of using ALC to improve cognitive functioning in patients with AD have been variable. A recent 1-year, multicenter, randomized, controlled trial failed to demonstrate significant effect.[22] An earlier study, however, showed a slowing of deterioration in treated patients.[23] An interesting study combining both clinical and in vivo spectroscopic neurochemical assessment found positive effects from 3 gm/day.[24] This finding also raises the possibility of a synergistic effect with PS. Although clinical results are variable, there seems to be little doubt that ALC has neurocognitive effects. The usual therapeutic dose is 1–3 gm/day in 3–4 divided doses.

23. What other herbal products have been found to be of value in the treatment of AD?

Huperzine-A, an alkaloid isolated from Chinese club moss (*Huperzia serrata*), has potent reversible cholinesterase-inhibiting properties. In a comparative animal study, huperzine-A was found to be more potent, more selective, and longer lasting and to have fewer side effects than tacrine.[25] In two small clinical trials, memory enhancement was found in both normal subjects[26] and patients with AD.[27] This alkaloid has the potential to be a safe and effective treatment. The recommended dose is 50–100 μg once or twice daily.

24. What are the main conventional therapies for AD?
Cognition enhancement
- Rivastigmine (Exelon), 1.5 mg orally 2 times/day for 2–4 weeks; then increase to 3 mg orally 2 times/day for several weeks. If well tolerated, the dose may be increased by 1.5-mg increments to a maximum of 6 mg orally 2 times/day.

- Donepezil (Aricept), 5 mg/day orally for 1 month; then 10 mg/day orally.
- Tacrine (Cognex), 10 mg orally 4 times/day; increase by 10 mg/dose every 6weeks. Check liver enzymes every 2 weeks until dose is stable—then every 3 months.

Agitation/psychosis suppression
- Thioridazine (Mellaril), 10–25 mg orally 3 times/day
- Respiridone (Resperdal), 0.5–2 mg orally once or twice daily
- Haloperidol (Haldol), 0.5–2 mg orally 2 times/day

Adapted from Smith DR: Alzheimer's disease. In Rakel RE (ed): Conn's Current Therapy. Philadelphia, W.B Saunders, 1999.

25. What lies on the horizon for treatment of AD?

Hormone replacement therapy. There is a growing interest in more extensive hormone replacement therapy in both men and women. Emerging evidence supports the role of human growth hormone, testosterone, dehydroepiandrosterone (DHEA), and pregnenelone replacement as an anti-aging measure that clearly has ramifications for the treatment and prevention of physical and cognitive decline as well as dementia. Female hormone replacement therapy is already beginning to show evidence of efficacy. A recent review of the effect of estrogen replacement therapy on memory concluded that estrogen specifically maintains verbal memory, may prevent deterioration in short- and long-term memory, and also decreases the incidence of AD.[28]

DHEA is widely available in health food stores and is in widespread use. A systematic review published in the Cochrane Database in 2000 identified a need for more study. In short-term studies (2 weeks or less), no significant improvement in cognition was found. An excellent 3-month trial at the University of California, San Deigo, in 1994 studied the effects of DHEA supplementation. The investigators found a remarkable increase in perceived physical and psychological well-being in both men and women. However, they did not specifically assess cognitive function. No studies of chronic use are available.[29] In summary, DHEA may prove to be beneficial. Until more is known, supplementation may be considered for short periods (3–6 months) with the dose (5–50 mg/day for men and 5–25 mg/day for women) titrated against serum levels to correct to a young adult range of normal.

Beta-amyloid vaccine. Several recent articles in *Nature* describe reduction in plaques and prevention of behavioral and cognitive impairment in a transgenic mouse model of AD.[31,32] Look for human trials of the vaccine in the future.

Beta-secretase inhibitors inhibit the formation of beta-amyloid from amyloid precursor protein in the brain.

REFERENCES

1. Smith D: Alzheimer's disease. In Rakel RE (ed): Conn's Current Therapy. Philadelphia, W.B. Saunders, 1999.
2. Shah Y, et al: Mild cognitive impairment. Geriatrics 55(9):62–68, 2000.
3. Petersen RC, et al: Mild cognitive impairment: Clinical characterization and outcome. Arch Neurol 56:303–308, 1999.
4. Sonaria S, Scott P: The cognitve status of non-AD subjects with CAD. Clin Anat 9:118–127, 1996.
5. Sparks LD: The link between AD and heart disease. Neurobiol Aging 11:601–607, 1990.
6. Morgan D, et al: A beta-peptide vaccination prevents memory loss in an animal model of Alzheimer's disease. Nature 408:982–985, 2000.
7. Rondeau V, Commenges D, Jacquim-Gadda H, Dartigues J: Relation between aluminum concentrations in drinking water and Alzheimer's disease: An 8-year follow-up study. Am J Epidemiol 152:59–66, 2000.
8. Rogers AM, Simon DG: A preliminary study of dietary aluminum intake and risk of Alzheimer's disease. Age Aging 28:205–209, 1999.
9. Crapper McLachlan DR, Smith WL, Kruck TP: Ther Drug Monit 15:602–607, 1993.
10. Exley C: Mol Med Today 4(3):107–109, 1998.
11. Grant WB: Dietary links to Alzheimer's siseaose. Alzheim Dis Rev 2:42–45, 1997.
12. Smith AL, et al: The protective effects of physical exercise on the development of Alzheimer's disease. Neurology 50:A89–A90, 1998.
13. Sapolsky RM: Why Zebras Don't Get Ulcers. New York, W.H. Freeman, 1998.
14. Khalsa DS, Stauth C: Brain Longevity. NewYork, Warner Books, 1997.
15. Koger SM, Brotons M: Music therapy for dementia symptoms. Cochrane Database of Sytematic Reviews 2000.

16. Markesbery WR: Oxidative stress hypothesis in Alzheimer's disease. Free Rad Biol Med 23:134–147,1997.
17. LeBars PL, Katz MM, Berman N, et al: A placebo-controlled, double-blind randomized trial of an extract of ginkgo biloba for dementia. JAMA 278:1327–1332, 1997.
18. Oken BS, Storzbach DM, Kaye JA: The efficacy of ginkgo biloba on cognitive function in Alzheimer disease. Arch Neurol 55:1409–1415, 1985
19. Blumenthal M, Goldberg A, Brinckmann J: Herbal Medicine: Expanded Commission E Monographs. Newton, MA, American Botanical Council, Integrative Medicine Communications, 2000.
20. Itil TM, Erlap E, Ahmed I, et al: The pharmacological effects of ginkgo biloba, a plant extract, on the brain of dementia patients in comparison with tacrine. Psychopharmacol Bull 34:391–397, 1998.
21. Crook T, Petrie W, Wells C, Massari DC: Effects of phosphatidylserine in Alzheimer's disease. Psychopharm Bull 28:61–66,1992.
22. Thal LJ, Calvani M, Amato A, Carta A: A 1-year controlled trial of acetyl-l-carnitine in early onset AD. Neurology 55(6):805–810, 2000.
23. Spagnoli A, Lucca U, Menasce G et al: Long-term acetyl-L-carnitine treatment in Alzheimer's disease. Neurology 41:1726–1732, 1991.
24. Pettegrew JW, Klunk WE, Panchalingam K, et al: Clinical and neurochemical effects of acetyl-L-carnitine in Alzheimer's disease. Neurobiol Aging 16:1–4, 1995.
25. Cheng DH, Tang XC: Comparative studies of huperzine A, E2020 and tacrine on behavior and cholinesterase activities. Pharm Biochem Behav 60(2):377–386, 1998.
26. Sun QQ, Xu SS, Pan JL, et al: Huperzine A capsules enhance memory and learning performance in 34 pairs of matched adolescent students. Acta Pharm Sinica 20(7):601–603, 1999.
27. Mazurek A: An open label trial of huperzine A in the treatment of Alzheimer's disease. Altern Ther 5(2):97–98, 1999.
28. Sherwin BB: Can Estrogen keep you smart? Evidence from clinical studies. J Psychiatry Neurosci 24:315–321, 1999.
29. Huppert FA, Van Niekerk JK, Herbert J: DHEA supplementation for cognition and well-being. Cochrane Database of Systematic Reviews, 2000.
30. Janus C, Pearson J, McLaurin J, Mathews PM, et al: A beta peptide immunization reduces behavioral impairment and plaques in a model of Alzheimer's disease. Nature 408:979–982, 2000.
31. Morgan D, Diamond DM, Gottschall PE, et al: A beta peptide vaccination prevents memory loss in an animal model of Alzheimer's disease. Nature 408:982–985, 2000.

51. HEADACHE

Ken Peters, M.D.

1. What symptoms characterize a migraine?

The most common symptoms are a debilitating unilateral headache that is throbbing, associated with nausea, vomiting, sensitivity to light (photophobia), sensitivity to sound (phonophobia), and pain that worsens with exertion. Forty percent of migraines may be bilateral. The pain usually lasts from 4 to 48 hours. Approximately 25% of patients experience an aura, or focal neurologic sensation that precedes the pain by no more than 1 hour and lasts from several minutes to 1 hour. The most common symptoms are visual, including flashing lights (photopsia) and partial vision loss (scotomata).

Many migraineurs also experience a prodrome of various symptoms (e.g., yawning, lethargy, fatigue, nasal congestion) up to 24 hours before the aura or pain phase. Many patients also experience a postdrome after the pain phase consisting of fatigue, lethargy, neck pain, and cognitive impairment. The postdrome can last up to 24 hours.

A chronic disabling headache that is stable over time is usually a migraine.

2. Are headaches a major problem?

Twelve percent of the population suffers from migraine. Headaches account for 18 million outpatient visits per year. Approximately 6% of men and 18% of women suffer from migraines. Most migraineurs are disabled to some degree by their headaches. Low work productivity and absenteeism due to headache cost employers from $5.6 to 7.2 billion annually.[1]

3. How can a headache diary be helpful?

A headache diary is extremely helpful not only for the headache sufferer but also for the health care provider (see figure on following page). It allows the provider to review quickly the frequency of headaches as well as headache triggers. The provider also learns what medications and nonmedication approaches have been used and which ones are effective. The diary helps the patient to determine individual headache triggers and keep track of medication use. The diary can also be used to determine whether migraines are related to phase of menstrual cycle or use of oral contraceptives. Triggers may be environmental, nutritional, psychological, hormonal, or musculoskeletal (e.g., referred from the neck [cervicogenic] or jaw [temporomandibular joint dysfunction]).

4. What types of foods can trigger a migraine?

Many foods can trigger migraines. The most common examples are alcoholic beverages; red wine, beer, and sherry are more likely to be potential triggers for migraine than white wine or vodka.[2] Aged cheeses and other fermented foods can induce migraines because of high levels of tyramine. Chocolate, dairy products, wheat, citrus fruits, and eggs are also possible food triggers.[3] Patients should eat regularly and not skip meals.

5. What about food additives?

Monosodium glutamate (MSG) can dilate the blood vessels and precipitate a vascular headache. MSG is found not only in Chinese food but also in most frozen, packaged, and canned foods (often labeled as "hydrolyzed vegetable protein," "natural flavor," or "natural seasoning"). Another common trigger is aspartame (Nutrasweet).[4] Other triggers include nitrites in hot dogs, turkey or chicken dogs, bacon, and other processed luncheon meats.

Caffeine is a double-edged sword. Most migraineurs find that caffeine can help reduce pain if taken during an acute attack. However, patients who consumes caffeine on a near daily basis can experience caffeine rebound, which can cause chronic daily headaches.

NORTHERN CALIFORNIA HEADACHE CLINIC
Your Headache Diary

(*1) Severity Scale   Headache Keys   (*4) Relief Scale

1	5	10
None	Mild Moderate	Severe

1	5	10
Complete	Mild Moderate	No Relief

Date	Time Onset/Ending (Insert Hour and a.m./p.m.)	(*1) Severity of Head-ache	(*2) Psych. & physical factors	(*3) Food and drink	Medication taken and dosage	Non-medication approach	(*4) Relief of head-ache

(*2) Psychological and physical factors
1. Emotional upset/family or friends
2. Emotional upset/occupation
3. Business/reversal
4. Pushing self too hard
5. Vacation days
6. Weekends
7. Strenuous exercise
8. Strenuous labor
9. High-altitude location
10. Anticipation anxiety
11. Crisis/serious
12. Post-crisis period

13. New job/position
14. New move
15. Menstrual days
16. Physical illness
17. Oversleeping
18. Too little sleep
19. Weather
20. Skipping meal
21. Insufficient rest and relaxation
22. Bright light or loud noise
23. Other

(*3) Food and drink
1. Ripened cheese (pizza)
2. Herring
3. Chocolate
4. Vinegar
5. Fermented foods (pickled or marinated) (sour cream/yogurt)
6. Freshly baked yeast products
7. Nuts (peanut butter)
8. Monosodiumglutamate (Chinese foods)
9. Pods of broad beans
10. Raw onions or garlic

11. Canned figs
12. Citrus foods
13. Bananas
14. Pork
15. Caffeinated drinks
16. Avocados
17. Fermented sausage (cured cold cuts)
18. Chicken livers
19. Wine
20. Alcohol
21. Beer

6. What role does stress play in migraines?

Stress is a major factor and is probably the most common trigger for migraines and tension headaches. Often migraines occur not at the time of stress but during a letdown period after a stressful time is over (e.g., on a weekend or during vacation). Depression, bipolar disorder, panic attacks, and generalized anxiety are comorbid psychological conditions often associated with migraine. Tension headaches usually occur at the time of stress.

7. Describe the pathophysiology of migraines.

The pathophysiology of migraines is not completely understood. Four inter-related hypotheses include (1) intracranial vasomotor instability, (2) abnormal central nervous system modulation, (3) platelet dysfunction, and (4) serotonin depletion.[5] When the activation/accumulation of headache triggers exceeds a certain threshold, the migraine generator in the brainstem initiates a wave of spreading cortical depression in the occipital cortex, which may manifest as a visual aura. Activation of the trigeminal system causes vasodilation of the meningeal blood vessels and release of inflammatory peptides, which in turn cause neurovascular inflammation. Activation of the autonomic centers can cause nausea and vomiting as well as photophobia, phonophobia, nasal congestion, and rhinorrhea.

8. What is the rebound phenomenon?

The rebound phenomenon is the triggering of headache by the overuse of headache medications. Drug-rebound causes the majority of chronic daily headaches (70%).[6] Usually patients take excessive amounts of over-the-counter or prescription medications, which may be helpful if used sparingly.If used more than twice weekly, however, they can trigger transformation of headaches to a chronic daily type. Abortive medications—aspirin, acetaminophen, and short-acting nonsteroidal anti-inflammatory drugs (NSAIDs) such as ibuprofen—can cause rebound.

The most common over-the-counter medicines that trigger rebound are caffeine-containing analgesics such as Excedrin Migraine, Excedrin (which is exactly the same as Excedrin Migraine), and Anacin. The most common prescribed drugs causing rebound are barbiturate-containing medications, such as butalbital combinations (Fiorinal and Esgic), and opiate-containing medications, such as codeine or hydrocodone (Vicodin). Even the newer and highly effective triptans can cause rebound if used more than twice weekly. Treatment includes tapering patients off medications, teaching them behavioral modalities, and using prophylactic medicines.

9. What medications are commonly used to treat migraines?

The most specific effective medicines for migraines are the triptans (e.g., sumatriptan [Imitrex]). The triptans are serotonin agonists and work by activating the serotonin 1B and 1D receptors in the blood vessel walls and trigeminal nerve endplates, respectively. They constrict the dilated meningeal arteries to their normal diameter and inhibit the release of inflammatory peptides, thereby reducing neurovascular inflammation. They also may turn off the migraine generator in the brainstem. Triptans are highly effective and have greatly improved the quality of life of millions of migraineurs since their release approximately 10 years ago.

Triptans are more effective if taken early and should be considered as first-line treatment for disabled migraineurs. For milder migraines, NSAIDs or isometheptene/dichloralphenazone/acetaminophen (Midrin) can be used. Opiates or barbiturate-containing medications can be used as an occasional rescue agent, but close monitoring is necessary because they are addictive and commonly trigger rebound if used more than two days per week. Prophylactic medicines include beta blockers, tricyclic antidepressants, calcium channel blockers, long-acting NSAIDs, and antiepileptic medicines such as divalproex acid (Depakote), gabapentin (Neurontin), and topirimate (Topamax). Selective serotonin reuptake inhibitors are effective if the patient is depressed.

10. Which botanical is helpful for treating migraine?

Two double-blind, controlled studies in England indicate that feverfew is effective for preventing migraines.[7,8] The usual dose is approximately 100 mg of feverfew extract, standardized to 0.7% parthenolide. Feverfew probably works by inhibiting platelet aggregation and release of serotonin from platelets and neutrophils. It also inhibits inflammatory prostaglandin synthesis and release of arachidonic acid, therefore reducing vascular inflammation.

11. Which supplement is helpful for migraines?

The supplement with the most supporting evidence is magnesium., which inhibits platelet aggregation and the synthesis, release, and action of inflammatory mediators. Magnesium also directly alters cerebrovascular tone by inhibiting vasospasm and stabilizing cell membranes.[9] The recommended dosage is 400–600 mg/day of magnesium citrate or oxide. It has been shown to benefit menstrual as well as common migraine.[10-14] Some centers use intravenous magnesium for acute abortive treatment of migraine.

12. Which vitamin helps reduce migraines?

Sound data indicate that riboflavin (vitamin B_2) can be quite effective in reducing migraine frequency.[15,16] It is a coenzyme in the electron transport chain and is thought to improve cerebrovascular tone by enhancing mitochondrial energy reserves. The recommended dose is 400 mg/day.

13. Do fatty acids play a role in headache treatment?

Synaptic terminals are rich in essential fatty acids (EFAs). Because omega-3 fatty acids mediate anti-inflammatory pathways, it makes sense that a diet rich in EFAs would benefit migraine sufferers. One study showed that linoleic acids may be effective in preventing migraines.[17] However, a conflicting study[18] reported this year found no benefit from supplemental EFA. More evidence is needed.

14. What behavioral techniques have been proven beneficial for migraine treatment?

Behavioral techniques are highly beneficial for migraine treatment. Biofeedback is quite effective.[19-22] A simple relaxation technique to warm the hands can be learned by holding a small thermometer. Patients find this method easy to master with home practice. It seems to work well in reducing migraine frequency. Meditation techniques, such as mindfulness meditation, yoga, and t'ai chi. can also be used, as well as cognitive therapy and other types of psychotherapy.

15. What symptoms characterize tension headaches?

Tension headaches are a much less debilitating type of headache than migraine. Usually they are characterized by bilateral pressure or a vise-like sensation in the forehead, temples, or back of the head. Tension headaches may be associated with neck pain, but they are not associated with nausea, vomiting, or sensitivity to light or sound. Exertion does not worsen the headache; in fact, exercise may even help reduce its intensity.

16. What factors are associated with tension headaches?

Several factors are associated with tension headaches. A key factor is poor ergonomics. A common cause of tension headaches is neck and shoulder strain, which is often seen in people who work at a computer (see figure on following page).

Neck and shoulder exercises can be taught to patients with tension headaches. Temporomandibular joint (TMJ) dysfunction can sometimes be a trigger for tension headaches. Inquire into nocturnal grinding of the teeth (bruxism); a mouth splint may reduce pressure from TMJ-associated headaches. As with migraines, stress reduction techniques such as mindfulness meditation, yoga, biofeedback, and regular aerobic exercise program (with appropriate stretching) can be of benefit.

17. Does bodywork help to treat tension headaches?

Neck exercises can be highly effective for alleviating tension headaches. Passive interventions such as massage and osteopathic manipulation also can help, especially if the headache is triggered by a problem with neck muscle spasm (cervicogenic headache).

18. Give examples of alternative therapies for tension headache.

Biofeedback, especially electromyographic (EMG) biofeedback, in which the state of muscle can be monitored, or galvanic stimulus response (GSR), which allows overall monitoring of stress reactivity.

Ergonomics Quick Tips

1. Avoid overextending your body - keep frequently used items such as binders, telephone, or 10-key within easy reach.
2. Maintain the natural curve of the spine with correct posture and lumbar support.
3. Consider ergonomics on and off the job - use tools and techniques that reduce force, repetition, and awkward postures.
4. Make the most of scheduled breaks. Rest tired eyes, stretch and exercise muscles.
5. Remember that your comfort at work is related to your overall health, fitness and lifestyle.

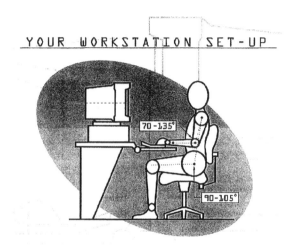

From the Idaho Department of Health and Welfare.

Acupuncture and acupressure also can be effective.[23,24] Specific acupoints include gallbladder 20 (behind the occipital area) for tension headaches and large intestine 4 (in the muscular web between the thumb and forefinger) for migraine headaches.

Stress reduction (via exercise, meditation) may be enhanced with use of an antidepressant.[25]

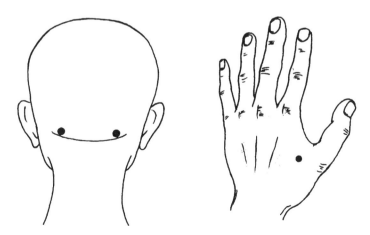

Effective acupoints for headache treatment include gallbladder 20 (left) and large intestine 4 (right).

19. What symptoms characterize cluster headaches?

A cluster headache is an excruciating pain syndrome seen predominantly in middle-aged men, whereas migraines are seen more commonly in young women (3:1 ratio of females to males). The cluster headache is always on the same side for the individual patient. The pain is usually located behind the eye and is associated with unilateral rhinorrhea, lacrimation, and conjunctival redness. The headaches last approximately 45 minutes and usually begin during the night an hour or two after the patient falls asleep. They are called cluster headaches because of their cyclical nature. The cycles of daily headaches usually last for weeks, followed by completely pain-free states for months to years. They are more common in the autumn and spring. Alcohol is a common trigger when a patient is in the midst of a cluster cycle.

20. Is the treatment for cluster headaches the same as for other types of headache?

The treatment is quite different. For acute treatment sumatriptan is used subcutaneously. Onset of relief is rapid. The traditional use of an oxygen mask (100% O_2 at 7 L/min for 15 minutes) can be highly effective for stopping cluster headache. For prevention of cluster headaches, avoidance of alcohol is strongly recommended during the cluster cycle. Dietary nitrites and nitrates also should be avoided. Prophylactic medicines, such as prednisone, calcium channel blockers (e.g, verapamil), and lithium carbonate can be helpful. If patients with cluster headache smoke, they are encouraged to stop.

21. What factors constitute "red flags" during the evaluation of headache?

Take a careful history. Usually you can make the correct diagnosis of headache by listening closely to the history and performing a careful general and neurologic exam. Red flags that suggest a life-threatening cause of headache and warrant further investigation include the following:

- New onset of a headache after the age of 40
- Change in the quality of a chronic headache (suggests a new cause)
- Complaint that this is the worst headache that the patient has ever had (rule out subarachnoid hemorrhage)
- Abnormal vital signs (e.g., hypertension, fever)
- Progressive neurologic abnormalities
- Comorbid medical illness
- Progressive headache pattern
- Presence of fever with a stiff neck associated with headache (suggests meningitis)

22. How should a holistic/integrative practitioner approach patients with headache?

The holistic practitioner allows patients to communicate their history in a relaxed, supportive atmosphere that promotes a feeling of attentiveness and caring. A therapeutic alliance is crucial for effective healing. Perform a careful general and neurologic exam. Usually no further diagnostic tests are necessary. However, appropriate tests should be ordered if a red flag is present or if the diagnosis is in doubt. Once the proper diagnosis is made, practitioner and patient should develop a therapeutic plan based on the patient's goals. This plan should include education, lifestyle changes, psychological-behavioral interventions, medications, and appropriate alternative therapies. The headache diary should be used to delineate triggers and monitor therapy.

REFERENCES

1. Kumar KL, Cooney TG: Headaches. Med Clin North Am 79:261–285, 1995.
2. Jarisch R, Wantke F: Wine and headache. Int Arch Allergy Immunol 110:7–12, 1996.
3. Egger J, et al: Is migraine food allergy? A double-blind controlled trial of oligoantigenic diet treatment. Lancet ii:865-868, 1983.
4. Koehler SM, Glaros A: The effect of aspartame on migraine headache. Headache 28:10–13, 1988.
5. Pizzorno JE, Murrary MT (eds): Textbook of Natural Medicine, vol. 2. Edinburgh, Churchill Livingstone, 1999, pp 1402–1404.
6. Mathew NT: Chronic refractory headache. Neurology 43:S26–S33, 1993.
7. Johnson ES, et al: Efficacy of feverfew as prophylactic treatment ofmigraine. Br Med J 29:569–573, 1985.

8. Murphy J, et al: Randomized double-blind placebo-controlled trial of feverfew in migraine prevention. Lancet ii:189–192, 1988.
9. Weaver K: Magnesium and its role in vascular reactivity and coagulation. Contemp Nutr 12(3):1–2, 1987.
10. Ramdan N, et al: Low brain magnesium in migraine. Headache 29:590–593, 1989.
11. Weaver K: Magnesium in migraine. Headache 30:168, 1990.
12. Faccinetti F, et al: Magnesium prophylaxis of menstrual migraine: Effects on intracellular magnesium. Headache 31:298–304, 1991.
13. Peikert A: Prophylactic of migraine with oral magnesium: Results from a prospective, multi-center, placebo-controlled and double-blind randomized study. Cephalalgia 16: 257–263, 1996.
14. Pfaffenrath V, et al: Magnesium in the prophylaxis of migraine: A double-blind, placebo-controlled study. Cephalalgia 16:436–440, 1996.
15. Schoenen J, et al: Effectiveness of high dose riboflavin in migraine prophylaxis: A randomized, controlled trial. Neurology 50:466-470, 1998.
16. Schoenen J, et al: High dose riboflavin as a prophylactic treatment of migraine: Results of an open pilot study. Cephalalgia 14:328–329, 1994.
17. Wagner W, Nootbarr-Wagner U: Prophylactic treatment of migraine with gamma-linolenic and alpha-linolenic acids. Cephalalgia 17:127–130, 1997.
18. Pradalier A, et al: Failure of omega 3- polyunsaturated fatty acids in prevention of migraine: A double-blind study versus placebo. Cephalgia 21:818–823, 2001.
19. Diamond S, Montrose M: The value of biofeedback in the treatment of chronic headache: A four year retrospective study. Headache 24:5–18, 1984.
20. Blanchard E, et al: Five year prospective follow-up on the treatment of chronic headache with biofeedback and /or relaxation. Headache 27:580–583, 1987.
21. Wauquier A, et al: Changes in cerebral blood flow velocity associated with biofeedback-assisted relaxation treatment of migraine headaches are specific for the middle cerebral artery. Headache 35:358–362, 1995.
22. McGrady A, et al: Effect of biofeedback-assisted relaxation on migraine headache and changes in cerebral blood flow velocity in the middle cerebral artery. Headache 34:424–428, 1994.
23. Melchart D, Linde, et al: Acupuncture for recurrent headaches: A systematic review of randomized controlled trial Cephalalgia 19:779–786, 1999.
24. Lundeberg T: Acupuncture in headache. Cephalalgia 19(Suppl 25):65–68, 1999.
25. Holroyd KA, O'Donnell FJ, Stensland M, et al: Management of chronic tension-type headache with tricyclic antidepressant medication, stress management, and their combination: A randomized controlled trial. JAMA 285:2208–2215, 2001

52. MULTIPLE SCLEROSIS

Patricia Ammon, M.D.

1. What is multiple sclerosis (MS)? What causes it?

MS, the most common cause of chronic neurologic disability in young adults, is characterized by demyelination of the central nervous system with subsequent plaque formation. Despite decades of research, the cause of MS remains unknown. Presently there are four major theories: immunologic, environmental, infectious agent, and genetic. The theory that MS is an organ-specific autoimmune disease, although unproved, is widely accepted.

For at least 30 years it has been documented that the incidence of MS increases with increasing distance from the equator. The dietary influence on MS was first reported by Roy Swank in 1952. Swank noted that people living in colder climates tended to consume diets higher in fat compared with those living in more tropical regions. At least 16 different infectious agents have been identified as possible causes of MS, but none of them has been definitely proven to cause MS. Although most cases of MS are sporadic, susceptibility to develop MS is substantially affected by genetic factors.

Given the wide variability in presenting symptoms, response to therapies, and course of disease, MS is probably not a single disease but is more accurately defined as a syndrome, the cause of which is a combination of genetics, infectious agents, environmental agents, and a dysfunctional immune system.

2. Describe the pathophysiology of MS.

Increased free radical formation and/or decreased antioxidant defense in the central nervous system leads to an unregulated immune reaction, inflammation, and damage to the myelin sheath.[1,2] Demyelination causes slowed conduction in individual nerve fibers, prolongation of the relative refractory period, or conduction block. Many symptoms of MS may be explained by the effects of demyelination.

3. How is MS diagnosed?

The hallmark for the clinical diagnosis of MS is neurologic dysfunction that is disseminated in space and time. Objective evaluation includes magnetic resonance imaging (MRI), evaluation of the cerebrospinal fluid (CSF), and evoked potentials. The pathologic hallmark of MS is the presence of demyelinated plaques involving the periventricular white matter, optic nerves, brainstem, cerebellum, or spinal cord white matter. Although not specific to MS, the detection of oligoclonal bands in the CSF also supports the clinical diagnosis, as does increased latency with visual evoked potentials.

4. Why not just use the conventional pharmaceuticals to treat MS?

All three of the so-called ABC drugs—interferon beta 1A (Avonex), interferon beta 1B (Betaseron), and glatiramer (Copaxone)—are quite expensive, have significant side effects, and despite modest short-term benefits, have a relatively limited impact on overall disease course. No information about long-term use is available. Studies so far have not provided solid evidence for improvement in quality of life with the ABC drugs; in fact, studies have demonstrated that treatment with interferon beta has a high cost per quality-adjusted life years gained.[3]

5. What is the advantage to taking an integrative approach to treating MS?

MS affects all aspects of the patient's life, and all aspects of the patient's life affect the course of MS. MS may damage quality of life substantially. The neurologic symptoms, including numbness, tingling, weakness, and spasticity, are unpredictable and highly variable and can progress to complete disability. Visual symptoms can be particularly disturbing, ranging from blurring of vision to blindness. Measurable difficulties in mental functioning are seen in approximately 43% of patients, possibly leading to job loss and awkward interpersonal relationships. Depression is common, and death by suicide occurs seven times more frequently than in the general population.[4] MS is chronic and, at present, without cure.

By addressing the patient's dietary habits, physical activity, interpersonal relationships, support system, life stressors, and coping mechanisms, an integrative approach offers a more individualized treatment plan that can facilitate symptom-free, long-term stabilization of the disease with good quality of life.

6. What role does diet play in MS?

Although the concept that diet plays a role in MS has not been widely accepted by conventional medicine, contemporary research continues to show a direct relationship between dietary saturated fat, animal fat, and MS.[5]

Swank's research added significantly to the understanding of the role of diet in MS. The Swank diet, as outlined in *The Multiple Sclerosis Diet Book*, is highly restrictive. Saturated fat intake is very low, and polyunsaturated fat intake is high.[6] A word of caution in considering the Swank diet: recognize the different effects of the different polyunsaturated fats.

Dietary fats are converted to prostaglandins (PG-1, PG-2, and PG-3) by a pathway of chemical reactions. The PG-1 and PG-3 series modulate the immune response to decrease inflammation, and the PG-2 series signals the lymphocytes to become more active in the immune response and thus increases inflammation.[7] PG-2 production is triggered by dietary saturated fat, dairy, cholesterol, and alcohol.

7. How can PG-1 and PG-3 be increased?

Dietary intake of essential fatty acids such as omega-3 and specific omega-6 fatty acids, can help shift prostaglandin production. Omega-3 fatty acids (flax or fish oil) increase production of PG-3, and omega-6 fatty acids (evening primrose oil, borage oil, or black currant oil) increase production of PG-1. Deficiency of omega-3 fatty acids is thought to permanently impair formation of normal myelin.[8]

Omega-3 fatty acids must be converted to docosahexanoic acid (DHA) to increase PG-3. The optimal dose of DHA to increase PG-3 production is 500 mg/day. Omega-6 fatty acids must be converted to gamma-linolenic acid (GLA) to increase PG-1. The optimal dose of GLA to increase PG-1 production is 300 mg/day. PG-3 also can be increased by eating walnuts, flax seed, or cold-water fish (e.g., salmon, tuna, sardines).

8. What role do antioxidants play in treating MS?

Because decreased antioxidant activity has been implicated as a causal factor of MS, supplying antioxidants to the central nervous system (CNS) is a good idea. Not all antioxidants, however, readily cross the blood-brain barrier.

9. Which antioxidants cross the blood-brain barrier?

Alpha-lipoic acid is rapidly absorbed from the gut, crosses the blood-brain barrier, and has powerful antioxidant activity. The usual dose varies from 100 to 250 mg/day. Glutathione is the primary cellular defense against free radicals, but it has been questioned whether glutathione levels increase with oral administration.[9] Some qualified complementary/alternative medicine (CAM) providers give glutathione intravenously at a dose of 600–800 mg diluted in 10 ml of normal saline, but this dosage must be delivered 2–3 times/week for optimal results. An alternative to intravenous methods of raising glutathione levels is N-acetyl-cysteine (NAC). Oral NAC in a dose of 200 mg/day produces an increase in blood glutathione levels.

10. What about vitamin B_{12} and MS?

Deficiency of vitamin B_{12} and errors in B_{12} metabolism are known to cause demyelination of the CNS.[10] During an MS attack, B_{12} deficiency can enhance the destruction of myelin and compromise the body's ability to repair the myelin sheath after the attack has subsided. Because serum B_{12} levels do not always correspond to CSF levels of B_{12}, it is not sufficient simply to measure serum B_{12} level in evaluating for a B_{12} deficiency.[11] Although there are no controlled reports of neurologic benefit from B_{12} injections, teaching patients self-injection of B_{12} can be a cost-effective way of improving overall well being.

11. Are the other B vitamins important?

Yes. Vitamins B_3 (as niacinamide or inositol hexaniacinate) and B_6 (pyridoxine) can reduce the production of PG-2, thereby potentially reducing inflammation. The usual dose of both B_3 and B_6 is 50 mg/day.

12. What other supplements may play a role in treating MS?

- **Vitamin D**, in the mouse model, has been shown to prevent the development of an MS-like disease.[12] Decreased formation of the active form of vitamin D from decreased sun exposure may be one reason why MS is more prevalent in northern latitudes.
- **Gingko biloba** acts as an antioxidant and enhances neurotransmission.[13]
- **Phosphatidylserine** is a phospholipid that plays a major role in determining the integrity and fluidity of cell membranes. Phospholipids make up more than 50% of the cell membrane's lipid barrier, which restricts the transport of potentially harmful molecules into the cell.[14]
- **Coenzyme Q10** (CoQ10) is an essential component of the electron transport chain and functions as a fat-soluble antioxidant.
- **Vitamin C** and the minerals **zinc** and **magnesium** also can reduce the production of PG-2.

13. What about using sex hormones to treat MS?

Evidence for the role of sex hormones is observed in the alteration of MS symptoms with alterations of sex hormones during pregnancy, menopause, or use of hormone replacement therapy and oral contraceptives. In most patients, symptoms of MS disappear with pregnancy. Estriol, the form of estrogen formed by the fetal-placental unit, is significantly elevated in the last trimester of pregnancy and has been shown in animal models to ameliorate symptoms of cell-mediated autoimmune disease.[15] Progesterone at concentrations consistent with late pregnancy also has been shown to decrease activation of proinflammatory cytokines.

Dehydroepiandrosterone (DHEA) is a steroid hormone that has been studied in numerous autoimmune diseases.[16] Although DHEA has been shown to be beneficial in systemic lupus erythematosus, little specific evidence supports its use in MS. An exception is the person whose serum DHEA-sulfate (DHEA-S) level is low. Before recommending DHEA, ascertain that the patient has no predisposition to develop hormone-driven cancers and obtain laboratory evaluation of serum DHEA-S. If DHEA-S is low, consider prescribing DHEA in physiologic doses (5–15 mg for women and 10–30 mg for men).

14. Are antibiotics used to treat MS?

The two infectious agents receiving the most attention at present are human herpesvirus 6 (HHV-6) and *Chlamydia pneumoniae*. Recent research describing the possible relationship between MS and *C. pneumoniae* is quite compelling.[17] Based on this research, it is not unreasonable for patients with MS to be treated with a course of doxycycline.

Epstein-Barr virus (EBV) also has been suggested to play a role in the etiology of MS. Until recently individual epidemiologic studies have been inconclusive because of the high prevalence of previous infection among people without MS. The strongest evidence for a role of EBV in MS was reported in a 2001 study.[18] Although this study is intriguing, there is no effective treatment for EBV.

15. What about exercise and MS?

Because symptoms can temporarily worsen with exposure to heat, patients with MS have traditionally been advised to avoid exercise. However, with the proper exercise environment and appropriate consideration of balance and coordination issues, exercise training can improve fitness and quality of life. Petajan and White developed a physical activity pyramid structure, with the most basic functions forming the base and the most integrated functions on top. By individualizing the exercise program, beginning with passive range of motion and progressing with active resistance and specific strengthening, physical activity can be optimized.[19]

16. What is the relationship between mercury from dental fillings and MS?

This relationship is extremely controversial. Some studies found a clear relationship between mercury and MS,[20] whereas other studies show a relationship between the extent of dental caries and

MS, but no association between MS and the number of mercury fillings.[21] At present there are too many similarities between mercury toxicity and MS to be ignored. Further research may clarify this relationship.

17. How is acupuncture used to treat MS?

A recent survey evaluating acupuncture use by patients with MS showed that approximately two-thirds of people reported beneficial effects on pain, spasticity, bowel and bladder difficulties, tingling, weakness, walking difficulties, incoordination, and sleep disorders.[22] More studies exploring the role acupuncture in MS need to be done to assess these encouraging findings.

18. Which mind-body therapies are used in the treatment of MS?

Craniosacral manipulation, Feldenkrais therapy, massage, Pilates method, reflexology, and Tragerwork all have been shown to reduce anxiety, improve self-image and self-esteem, possibly reduce spasticity, and relieve different types of pain. Combining counseling with bodywork therapies is a highly effective way to counter the major depression that affects about 50% of all patients with MS. Encouraging patients to learn some form of stress reduction (e.g., meditation, relaxation exercises, breathing techniques) is imperative in the overall treatment plan. Yoga can be a highly effective form of relaxation while providing exercise and stretching.

19. What other therapies may be considered?

- **4-Aminopyridine** is a potassium channel blocker that improves nerve conduction.[23] The dose must be increased gradually to reduce side effects, which include seizure, dizziness, nausea and vomiting, and nervousness. The beneficial effects are short-lived, and the medication must be taken frequently (i.e., 3 times/day).
- **Beesting therapy (apitherapy)** was first advocated for treating MS in the 1930s. Bee venom contains a large mixture of substances. Despite numerous reports of benefit, it is not yet understood exactly how the venom interacts with the body. One component of the venom, melittin, may have anti-inflammatory activity. No studies document benefits of apitherapy for people with MS. On the other hand, there are potentially serious adverse effects.[24]
- **Hyperbaric oxygen therapy** (HBO) can enhance oxygen levels in plasma, CSF, and intracellular fluids. Although this treatment is FDA-approved, its use in MS is quite controversial. Some studies show mild improvement,[25] but most studies conclude that HBO has no long-term benefit.[26]
- **Transdermal histamine and caffeine (Procarin)** is a novel treatment developed by a nurse with MS to control her own symptoms. No studies have used Procarin, but reports of improvement include better balance and bladder control, less fatigue, greater heat tolerance, improved cognitive function, and increased extremity strength.

20. What source is available for more information?

www.ms-cam.org

REFERENCES

1. Karg E, Klivenyi P, Nemeth I, et al: Nonenzymatic antioxidants of blood in multiple sclerosis. J Neurol 6(7):533–539, 1999.
2. Hunter MIS, Nlemadim BC, Davidson DLW: Lipid peroxidation products and antioxidant proteins in plasma and cerebrospinal fluid from multiple sclerosis patients. J Neurochem Res 10:1645–1652, 1985.
3. Parkin D, Jacoby A, McNamee P, et al: Treatment of multiple sclerosis with interferon beta: An appraisal of cost-effectiveness and quality of life. J Neurol Neurosurg Psychiatry 68:144–149, 2000.
4. Weinshenker BG: The natural history of multiple sclerosis. Neurol Clin 1:119–46, 1995.
5. Esparza ML, Sasaki S, Kesteloot H: Nutrition, latitude and multiple sclerosis mortality: An ecologic study. Am J Epidemiol 142:733–777, 1995.
6. Swank RL, Dugan BB: The Multiple Sclerosis Diet Book. New York, Doubleday, 1987.
7. Mayer M: Essential fatty acids and related molecular and cellular mechanisms in multiple sclerosis: New looks at old concepts. Folia Biologica (Praha) 45:133–141, 1999.

8. Murray MT, Pizzorno JE: Multiple sclerosis. In Murray MT, Pizzorno JE (eds): Textbook of Natural Medicine, 2nd ed. Edinburgh, Churchill Livingstone, 1999, pp 1415–1423.

9. David Perlmutter, M.D., personal communication, December, 2000.

10. Kira J, Tobimatsu, Goto I: Vitamin B-12 metabolism and massive-dose methyl vitamin B-12 therapy in Japanese patients with multiple sclerosis. Intern Med33(2):82–86, 1994.

11. Reynolds EH: Multiple sclerosis and vitamin B-12 metabolism. J Neuroimmunol 40(2–3):225–230, 1992.

12. Hayes CE, Cantorna MT, DeLuca HF: Vitamin D and multiple sclerosis. Proc Soc Exp Biol Med 216:121–127, 1997.

13. Yoshikawa T, Naito Y, Kondo M: Gingko biloba leaf extract: Review of biological actions and clinical applications. Antioxid Redox Signal 1:469–80, 1999.

14. Mahan LK, Escott-Stump S (eds): Krause's Food, Nutrition, and Diet Therapy, 10th ed. Philadelphia, W.B. Saunders, 2000, pp 48–49.

15. Kim S, Liva SM, Dala MA,et al: Estriol ameliorates autoimmune demyelinating disease: Implications for multiple sclerosis. Neurology 52:1230–1238, 1999.

16. DHEA. Altern Med Rev Jun (3):314–318, 2001.

17. Sriram S, Stratton CW, Yao S, et al: *Chlamydia pneumoniae* infection of the central nervous system in multiple sclerosis. Ann Neurol July 46:6–14, 1999.

18. Ascherio A, et al: Epstein-Barr virus antibodies and risk of multiple sclerosis: A prospective study. JAMA 286:3127–3129, 2001.

19. Petajan JH, White AT: Recommendations for physical activity in patients with multiple sclerosis. Sports Med 27(3):179–191, 1999.

20. Huggins HA, Levy TL: Cerebrospinal fluid protein changes in multiple sclerosis after dental amalgam removal. Altern Med Rev 3(4):295–300, 1998.

21. McGrother CW, Dugmore C, Phillips MJ, et al: Multiple sclerosis, dental carries and fillings: A case-control study. Br Dent J 187:261–264, 1999.

22. Wang Y, Hashimoto S, Ramsum D, et al: A pilot study of the use of alternative medicine in multiple sclerosis patients with special focus on acupuncture. Neurology 52(6 Supple 2): A550, 1999.

23. Stefoski D, Davis FA, Fitzsimmons WE, et al: 4-Aminopyridine in multiple sclerosis: Prolonged administration. Neurology 41:1344–1348, 1991.

24. Bowling AC: Alternative Medicine and Multiple Sclerosis. New York, Demos Medical Publishing, 2001.

25. Fischer BH, Marks M, Reich T: Hyperbaric-oxygen treatment of multiple sclerosis: A randomized placebo-controlled, double blind study. N Engl J Med 308:181–186, 1983.

26. Kindwall EP, McQuillen MP, Khatri BO, et al: Treatment of multiple sclerosis with hyperbaric oxygen: Results of a national registry. Arch Neurol 48(2):195–199, 1991.

53. PERIPHERAL NEUROPATHY

Sunil Pai, M.D.

1. What is peripheral neuropathy? What causes it?

Peripheral neuropathy, or peripheral neuritis, is a common neurologic disorder resulting from damage to the peripheral nerves. It may be caused by diseases of the nerves or systemic illnesses. The various causes include toxic trauma, certain medications, and chemotherapeutic agents (see tables below) or mechanical injury resulting in compression or entrapment (e.g., carpal tunnel syndrome). Even simple pressure on superficial nerves, such as prolonged use of crutches or even sitting in the same position for too long, can be a cause. Nutritional causes include vitamin B deficiency (e.g., alcoholism, pernicious anemia, isoniazid-induced pyridoxine deficiency, malabsorption syndromes). Other causes include viral and bacterial infections (e.g., HIV infection, Lyme disease), autoimmune reactions (e.g., Guillain-Barré syndrome), cancer (lymphoma, multiple myeloma), collagen vascular disorders (systemic lupus erythematosus, rheumatoid arthritis, polyarteritis nodosa, Sjögren's syndrome), endocrinopathies (hypothyroidism, acromegaly), and rare inherited genetic abnormalities. Finally, metabolic disorders such as diabetes and uremia can cause peripheral neuropathy.[1]

Agents Causing Symptoms Associated with Toxic Neuropathy

Acrylamide (truncal ataxia)
Allyl chloride
Arsenic (sensory abnormalities, brown skin, Mee's lines)
Buckthorn toxin
Carbon disulfide
Cyanide
Dimethylaminopropionitrile (urinary complaints)
Biologic toxin in diphtheritic neuropathy (pharyngeal neuropathy)
Ethylene oxide
n-Hexane
Lead (wrist drop, abdominal colic)
Lucel-7 (cataracts)
Mercury
Methyl bromide
Organophosphates (cholinergic symptoms, delayed onset of neuropathy)
Thallium (pain, alopecia, Mee's lines)
Trichloroethylene (facial numbness)
Vacor

From Hamberg H: Diseases of the peripheral nervous system. In Wyngaarden JB, Smith LH Jr, Bennett JC (eds): Cecil Textbook of Medicine, 19th ed. Philadelphia, W.B. Saunders, 1992, pp 2240–2247, with permission.

Pharmaceutical Agents Associated with Generalized Neuropathy

Chloramphenicol	Isoniazid[†]	Platinum (cisplatin)[†]
Dapsone*	Metronidazole-misonidazole	Pyroxidine[†]
Disulfiram	Nitrofurantoin*	Sodium cyanate
Ethionamide	Nitrous oxide	Taxol
Gold	Nucleosides (ddC, ddI)	Thalidomide
Glutethimide	Phenytoin	Vincristine
Hydralazine		

* Predominantly motor.   † Predominantly sensory.
From Hamberg H: Diseases of the peripheral nervous system. In Wyngaarden JB, Smith LH Jr, Bennett JC (eds): Cecil Textbook of Medicine, 19th ed. Philadelphia, W.B. Saunders, 1992, pp 2240–2247, with permission.

2. What is the most common cause of peripheral neuropathy?

The most common cause of peripheral neuropathy is diabetes. An estimated 40–60% of people with diabetes for 25 years[1] have peripheral neuropathy, and it is now thought to be the most common form of peripheral neuropathy in humans.[2] Although the exact pathophysiology of diabetic neuropathy has not yet been clearly identified, multiple factors, such as persistent hyperglycemia and autoimmune and microvascular mechanisms, play important roles.

3. How do autoimmune and microvascular mechanisms contribute to diabetic neuropathy?

In addition to accumulation of intraneural fructose and sorbitol,[3] in some patients immunologic mechanisms play a role in the development of diabetic neuropathy. Damage is caused by antineural autoantibodies that circulate in the serum of some diabetic patients. Antiphospholipid antibodies also may be present in some patients and may contribute to nerve damage in combination with vascular abnormalities.[4]

Endoneural vascular insufficiency also has been implicated as a primary cause of diabetic neuropathy.[4] It is postulated that ischemia due to endoneural and epineural vascular changes thickens the blood vessel wall and results in ischemic nerve damage. Eventually occlusion of the vessel may occur, affecting permeability and compromising endoneural blood flow.

4. Describe the presentation and common symptoms of peripheral neuropathy.

The sensory, autonomic, and motor nerves are affected, typically in the distal lower extremities first. As the condition worsens (from diabetes, the most common cause), the neuropathy begins to involve the upper extremities.[3] A stocking-and-glove distribution of diabetic neuropathy usually presents with sensory loss, dysesthesias, and painful paresthesias, most commonly in the lower extremities. Common symptoms include tingling, prickling, or numbness; burning or freezing pain; sharp, jabbing, or electric pain; extreme sensitivity to touch; muscle weakness; and loss of balance and coordination. Because diabetic neuropathy is the most common peripheral neuropathy and often is accompanied by pain, management includes not only prevention of diabetes (see Chapter 31) but also treatment of the painful symptoms.

5. What roles do lifestyle and nutrition play in preventing peripheral neuropathy?

Lifestyle and nutrition play important roles. Strict glycemic control between 70 and 120 mg/dl reduces the incidence of neuropathy by up to 64%.[5] Healthy eating habits should be followed (see Chapters 19 and 31). Because a lean body habitus can play an important role in control of glycemia, regular daily exercise (walking a minimum of 30 minutes/day 3 times/week) should be implemented. An optimal regimen is to walk daily for 30 minutes to 1 hour, if tolerated. Other factors that can contribute to peripheral neuropathy include heavy metals, cigarettes, alcohol, and pollution. Thus, the most important factors are prevention of uncontrolled diabetes and avoidance of environmental toxins.

6. How is biofeedback used in treating peripheral neuropathy?

Biofeedback may reduce stress and improve coping skills, which in turn may improve compliance, thus attaining better glycemic control and reducing pain associated with diabetic neuropathy.[6,7] Patients can be referred to a behavioral therapist or psychologist who teaches biofeedback therapies. The recommendation is a minimum six 1-hour biofeedback sessions at approximately 1-week intervals. Usually treatments include sessions of guided imagery or relaxation techniques that are taught to patients while they are attached to devices that measure physiologic parameters such as electromyographic response, electrodermal response, and vital signs (blood pressure, pulse, oxygen saturation). The monitoring enables the patient to see directly how emotions, anxiety, stress, and pain can affect physiologic states. Once patients learn how to alter their physiologic state, they are taught to perform the relaxation biofeedback techniques at home with the use of audiotapes or guided imagery exercises (10–20 minutes each day) to attain the same result without the monitoring equipment. Thus, patients gain tools that they can use to control certain physiologic conditions during time of stress or pain to help alleviate their own symptoms.

7. Many people use magnet therapy (i.e., belts, straps) for aches and pains. Can it be used for peripheral neuropathy?

Yes. Preliminary research demonstrates benefits. A recent study reported positive outcome for 90% of patients suffering from diabetic neuropathy.[8] Magnetic footpad insole devices (Magstep) with a 475-gauss steep field gradient were worn for 24 hours for as long as 4 months. This study speculates that magnets may lessen the sensation of pain by altering C-fiber firing frequency, possibly stimulating the potassium internal rectifying channels to repolarize and/or hyperpolarize. Thus, magnets can be a safe alternative to pain control of peripheral neuropathy, especially at the soles of the feet.

8. Has acupuncture been useful in treating neuropathic pain?

Acupuncture and electroacupuncture have been found to be useful in treating neuropathic pain through their well-known effect in stimulating the production of endorphins in the central nervous system.[9,10] Acupuncture may reduce primary and/or secondary symptoms of peripheral neuropathy up to 77%, in some cases (67%), enabling patients to reduce or stop pain medications.[11] Patients can receive six courses of classical acupuncture analgesia[12,13] to both lower limbs over a 10-week period at the traditional Chinese acupuncture points.

In addition to classic acupuncture, electroacupuncture may have positive influences on conduction nerve velocities and also neuropathic pain.[12] Before recommending the therapies in the above articles, a constitutional evaluation by a qualified acupuncturist should be considered because each prescription is based on the patient's unique symptoms and physical examination.

9. Is the antioxidant alpha-lipoic acid an effective treatment for peripheral neuropathy?

Alpha-lipoic acid (thiotic acid) serves as a coenzyme in the Krebs cycle and in the production of cellular energy. The method by which alpha-lipoic acid is synthesized within the body has not yet been fully characterized, but both alpha-lipoic acid and its reduced form have potent antioxidant properties. Alpha-lipoic acid increases muscle cell glucose uptake and insulin sensitivity.[14] Deficiency of alpha-lipoic acid causes a limitation of energy for the cells, cell damage, and far-reaching disturbances in the metabolism of sugar. This process has a particularly chronic effect on the peripheral nerve cells. Alpha-lipoic acid increases neuronal blood flow, reduces oxidative stress, and improves distal nerve conduction.[15] It is thought to act by chelating copper ions[16]; thus, it works as an antioxidant.

Reduction in chief symptoms with a dosage of 600 mg 3 times/day takes at least 3 weeks, but research has not tested the effects beyond that point.[17] Administration of 800 mg (divided into 4 daily doses) for 4–7 months appears to ameliorate neuropathic deficits and cardiac autonomic neuropathy and to improve motor and sensory nerve conduction over the long term.[18] No toxicity was reported in human studies (800 mg/day for 4 months and 600 mg 3 times/day for 3 weeks), but excessive amounts may cause problems not yet identified.[19] Alpha-lipoic acid also has a favorable side-effect profile. It protects vitamins E, vitamin C, glutathione, and coenzyme Q10, therefore reducing the consequences of a deficiencies in these nutrients.

10. Can patients with peripheral neuropathy benefit from taking B vitamins?

Yes. Vitamins B_1 (thiamine), B_6 (pyridoxine), and B_{12} (cobalamine) play an important role in peripheral neuropathy in deficiency syndromes such as alcoholism, pernicious anemia, isoniazid-induced pyridoxine deficiency, and malabsorption syndromes. The recommended supplement is a B-100 vitamin complex (a multivitamin that usually contains 100 μg or 100 mg of each B vitamin and also may include other vitamins such as folate) for ease of administration and intake of all B vitamins. Benfothiamine (Millgamma), 100 mg, is a lipid-soluble vitamin B_1 analog. Its lipid solubility is thought to make it better able to penetrate the nerves. It has been found to give higher bioavailability of thiamine than its water-soluble counterparts[20] and to reduce neuropathy scores significantly.[21,22] In prescribing a B-100 complex vitamin, make sure that the patient is not already taking another supplement that contains B vitamins.

11. What side effects may result from excessive B vitamins?

All B vitamins can be safe in high doses except vitamin for B_3 and B_6. Vitamin B_3 (niacin) at doses greater than 300 mg/day may cause headache, nausea, skin tingling, and flushing. Vitamin B_6

(pyridoxine) at doses greater than 250 mg/day may cause reversible nerve damage. One should counsel patients about taking megadoses of vitamins or a B-100 complex along with a multivitamin supplement that contains high doses of B vitamins.

12. Do vitamin C and vitamin E help with peripheral neuropathy?

Unlike vitamin C, which has not been shown to help with peripheral neuropathy, vitamin E improves nerve conduction velocity measurements.[23] The effects of vitamin E may be a result of antioxidant activity.[23] In general, d-alpha tocopherol (natural type) has better antioxidant effects than dl-alpha tocopheryl (synthetic type). The recommended dose is 400–800 IU daily.

13. What relative contraindications or warnings are associated with the use of vitamin E for peripheral neuropathy?

The dosage should be stopped 1 week before surgical and/or dental procedures because vitamin E can result in an impairment of hemostasis. Toxicity may occur if vitamin E (> 200 IU) is taken with anticoagulants, and prothrombin time may be prolonged.

14. What topical agent can be used for neuropathic pain?

Capsaicin cream, an extract of chili peppers, is thought to relieve neuropathic pain by depleting substance P.[24] Capsaicin does not reverse, stabilize, or improve neuropathy but can decrease the pain. Remind patients that burning occurs in more than 30 percent of users but diminishes with continued use. Pain more commonly occurs when the cream is applied less than 3 times/day; thus, application is recommended 3–4 times/day. Wash hands immediately after application.

15. What is thought to be the mechanism of action of antidepressants in the treatment of neuropathic pain?

Tricyclic antidepressants (TCAs) such as amitriptyline, nortriptyline, and desipramine have been the mainstay in the palliation of pain secondary to diabetic neuropathy.[25] TCAs work by increasing the postsynaptic concentration of norepinephrine (NE). Because the inhibitory pathways in the spinal cord use NE as a neurotransmitter, TCAs are believed to increase the inhibitory influence on nociceptive transmitting neurons.[26] The selective serotonin reuptake inhibitors (SSRIs), such as fluoxetine, also have been used; although better tolerated than TCAs, they appear to be less efficacious.

16. When neuropathic pain is treated with antidepressants, what side effects should be monitored?

Significant anticholinergic side effects can result from the use of TCAs and should be monitored. Examples include dry mouth, constipation, sedation, and urinary retention. Orthostatic hypotension and arrhythmias also may occur. Do not use with monoamine oxidase inhibitors.

17. Can anticonvulsants be used concomitantly with antidepressants?

Phenytoin and carbamazepine have been used with varying degrees of success both alone and in combination with antidepressants. Gabapentin is highly efficacious in the treatment of a variety of neuropathic painful conditions, including postherpetic neuralgia and diabetic neuropathy.[27] Gabapentin has a favorable side-effect profile compared with phenytoin and carbamazepine and thus should be considered a first-line treatment for neuropathic pain.[28] Which mechanisms of action of anticonvulsants account for their analgesic efficacy is unknown. Some research shows that the primary effect of anticonvulsants on N-methyl-D-aspartate (NMDA) receptors is inhibition of high-frequency firing in neurons, which reduces ion flow. The result is a reduction in excitatory synaptic transmission, which can lead to an increase in the refractory period for the cell membrane and thus a slower rate of firing of action potentials in the damaged neuron.[26]

18. Why not simply use analgesics for the treatment of pain from peripheral neuropathy?

Simple analgesics, such as acetaminophen, aspirin, and nonsteroidal anti-inflammatory drugs (NSAIDs) may be used in conjunction with anticonvulsants and antidepressants but have poor response when used alone. Caution must be taken not to exceed the recommended daily dose because of renal or hepatic side effects, particularly in diabetics. The role of COX-2 inhibitors in the palliation of neuropathic pain has not been adequately studied. Narcotic analgesics also give a poor response for pain control. Because of the significant central nervous system and gastrointestinal side effects, coupled with problems of tolerance, dependence, and addiction, narcotic analgesics should be used rarely if ever. Focus should be on therapies with fewer side effects (e.g., gastrointestinal complications with chronic NSAID use), and preventive measures such as glycemic control and lifestyle changes should be emphasized.

19. How do electrical stimulators such as TENS or PENS help with neuropathic pain?

Electrical stimulation, ranging from transcutaneous electrical nerve stimulation (TENS)[29] to spinal cord stimulators,[30] has been used successfully to alleviate pain and discomfort associated with peripheral neuropathy. TENS portable units that generate a biphasic, exponentially decaying waveform (pulse width 4 ms, 25–35 V, > 2 Hz) are recommended for 30 minutes/day for 4 weeks. A recent study showed that percutaneous electrical nerve stimulation (PENS), in addition to decreasing pain, improves physical activity, sense of well-being, and quality of sleep while reducing the need for oral nonopioid analgesic medication.[31] PENS is similar to electroacupuncture, in which electrical stimulation is applied to disposable acupuncture-like needles, but differs in that it is delivered along the peripheral nerves innervating the region of neuropathic pain rather than at acupuncture points or following meridians. Although alternating low and high frequencies of 15 and 30 Hz at 30-minute intervals 3 times /week is recommended, the patient should be evaluated by a health care professional to adjust frequencies and time intervals as tolerated.

REFERENCES

1. Hamberg H: Diseases of the peripheral nervous system. In Wyngaarden JB, Smith LH Jr, Bennett JC (eds): Cecil Textbook of Medicine, 19th ed. Philadelphia, W.B. Saunders, 1992, pp 2240–2247.
2. O'Brian SP, Schwedler M, Kerstein MD: Peripheral neuropathies in diabetes. Surg Clin North Am 78:393–408, 1998.
3. Vinik AL: Diagnosis and management of diabetic neuropathy. Clin Geriatr Med15:294–303, 1999.
4. Vinik AL: Diabetic neuropathy: Pathogenesis and therapy. Am J Med 107(Suppl):17S–18S, 1999.
5. Diabetes Control and Complications Trial Research Group: The effect of intensive treatment of diabetes on the development and progression of neuropathy. Ann Intern Med 122:561–568, 1995.
6. Jablon SL, Nalifboff BD, Gilmore SL, Rosenthal MJ: Effects of relaxation training on glucose tolerance and diabetic control in type II diabetes. Appl Psychophysiol Biofeedback 22(3):155–169, 1997.
7. Rosenbaum L: Biofeedback-assisted stress management for insulin-treated diabetes mellitus. Biofeedback Self-Regul 8:519–532, 1983.
8. Weintraub MI: Magnetic bio-stimulation in painful diabetic neuropathy: A novel intervention. A randomized, double-placebo crossover study. Am J Pain Manage 9:8–17, 1999.
9. Tsigos C: Cerebrospinal fluid levels of beta endorphin in painful and painless diabetic polyneuropathy. J Diabetes Compl 9:92–96, 1995.
10. Han JS, Ding XZ, Fan SG: Cholescystokinin octapeptide (CCK-8) antagonism to electroacupuncture analgesia and a possible role in electroacupuncture tolerance. Pain 27:101–115, 1986.
11. Abuaisha BB, Costanzi JB, Boulton AJM: Accupuncture for the treatment of chronic painful peripheral neuropathy: A long-term study. Diabetes Res Clin Pract 39(2):115–121, 1998.
12. Ionescu-Targoviste C, Phleck-Khhayan A, Danciu V, et al: The treatment of peripheral polyneuritis by electroacupuncture. Am J Acupunct 9:92–96, 1981.
13. O'Connor J, Bensky D: Acupuncture: A Comprehensive Text. Chicago, Shanghai College of Traditional Medicine, Eastland Press, 1981.
14. Kishi Y, Schmelzer JD, Yao JK, et al: Alpha lipoic acid: Effect on glucose uptake, sorbital pathway, and energy metabolism in experimental diabetic neuropathy. Diabetes 48:2045–2051, 1999.
15. Nagamatsu M, Nicklander KK, Schmelzer JD, et al: Lipoic acid improves nerve blood flow, reduces oxidative stress, and improves distal nerve conduction in experimental diabetic neuropathy. Diabetes Care 18:1160–1167, 1995.
16. Ou P, Tritschler H J, Wolff SP: Thiotic (lipoic) acid: A therapeutic metal-chelating antioxidant? Biochem. Pharmacol 50:123–126, 1995.
17. Ruhnau KJ, Meissner HP, Finn JR, et al: Effects of 3-week oral treatment with the antioxidant thioctic acid (alpha-lipoic acid) in symptomatic diabetic polyneuropathy. Diabet Med 16: 1040–1043, 1999.

18. Ziegler D, Schatz H, Conrad F, et al: Effects of treatment with the anti-oxidant alpha-lipoic acid on cardiac autonomic neuropathy in NIDDM patients: A 4-month randomized controlled multicenter trial (DEKAN study). Diabetes Care 20:369–373, 1997.
19. Ziegler D, Reljanovic M, Mehnert H, Gries FA: Alpha-lipoic acid in the treatment of diabetic polyneuropathy in Germany: Current evidence in clinical trials. Exp Clin Endocrinol Diabetes 107(7): 421–430, 1999.
20. Schreeb KH, Freudenthaler S, Vormfelde SV, et al: Comparative bioavailability of two vitamin B1 preparations: benfotiamine and thiamine mononitrate. Eur J Clin Pharmacol 52:319–320, 1997.
21. Haupt E, Ledermann H, Kopcke W: Benfothiamine in treatment of diabetic polyneuropathy. Fourth International Symposium on Diabetic Neuropathy, July 15–19, 1997.
22. Barkai L, Kempler P, Kadar E, Feher A: Benfothiamine treatment for peripheral sensory nerve dysfunction in diabetic adolescents. Fourth International Symposium on Diabetic Neuropathy July15–19, 1997.
23. Tutuncu NB, Bayractar M, Varli K: Reversal of defective nerve conduction with vitamin E supplementation in type 2 diabetes: A preliminary study. Diabetes Care 21:1915–1918, 1998.
24. Lynn B: Capsaicin: Actions on nociceptive C-fibers and therapeutic potential. Pain 41:61–69, 1990.
25. Joss JD: Tricyclic antidepressant use in diabetic neuropathy. Ann Pharmocol 33:996–1000, 1999.
26. Ross EL: The evolving role of antiepileptic drugs in treating neuropathic pain. Neurology 55(5 Suppl 1): S41–S46, 2000.
27. Backonja M, Beydon A, Edwards KR, et al: Gabapentin for the symptomatic treatment of painful neuropathy in patients with diabetes mellitus. JAMA 280:1831–1836, 1998.
28. Backonja MM: Anticonvulsants (antineuropathics) for neuropathic pain syndromes. Clin J Pain 16:S67–S72, 2000.
29. Kumar D, Marshall H: Diabetic peripheral neuropathy; amelioration of pain with transcutaneous electrostimulation. Diabetes Care 20:1702–1705, 1997.
30. Tesfaye S, Watt J, Benbow SJ, et al: Electrical spinal-cord stimulation for painful diabetic peripheral neuropathy. Lancet 348:1696–1701, 1996.
31. Hamza M, et al: Percutaneous electrical nerve stimulation: A novel analgesic therapy for diabetic neuropathic pain. Diabetes Care 23:365–370, 2000.

54. INTEGRATIVE ONCOLOGY: GENERAL APPROACH

Matt Mumber, M.D.

OVERVIEW

1. Define integrative oncology.

Integrative oncology is the rational, evidence-based combination of conventional therapy with complementary and alternative interventions into an individualized therapeutic regimen that addresses the whole person with cancer.

2. How does integrative oncology differ philosophically from a strictly conventional approach?

Aside from the inclusion of complementary and alternative (CAM) methods, integrative oncology focuses on the whole person, including physical, mental, emotional, and spiritual concerns. Prevention of disease and supportive care are emphasized—for patient, family, and community. "Healing" is the goal of treatment, but it may or may not include curing the disease. For example, a patient may learn to heal a family conflict while facing a bleak cancer prognosis. Healing in this context is defined as personal growth, greater understanding, and acceptance of current events that leads to an improved quality of life.

An excellent definition of healing comes from Stephen Levine's *A Year to Live*: "If there is a single definition of healing it is to enter with mercy and awareness those pains, mental and physical, from which we have withdrawn in judgment and dismay."[7] A focus on healing gives the doctor and patient liberty to address long neglected issues and overcome unresolved problems.

3. Why should physicians embrace an integrative approach to the care of patients with cancer?

Patients with cancer demand an individualized approach to care and often seek out CAM practitioners and interventions in greater proportions than the general population. Studies show that up to 87% of patients with cancer under active conventional treatment use some form of CAM during their therapy.[15] Indeed, about 90% of the initial phone calls placed to the National Institute of Health's Office of Alternative Medicine were from cancer patients. Many patients do not tell their doctor about this use for fear of repercussions. Lack of communication is a double-edged sword: deleterious interactions may occur, or beneficial CAM therapies may go unrecognized and underutilized. A growing evidence base indicates that certain forms of complementary therapy may lessen side effects of conventional cancer treatments, possibly allowing patients to complete prescribed therapy in a timely manner and ultimately improving long-term outcomes.

Honest communication is a cornerstone of an ideal doctor–patient relationship. Subsequent integration requires education, literature research, contact with local practitioners, and thoughtful clinical application. Most major cancer centers, including Memorial Sloan Kettering in New York, MD Anderson Cancer Center in Houston, Stanford in California, and Massachusetts General Hospital in Boston have incorporated complementary care programs into their list of oncology services. These institutions are beginning to bridge the education gap between CAM and conventional practices while performing much needed research.

4. What causes cancer?

This question has plagued researchers for years. Certain types of cancers seem to have discrete causes: sun damage and skin cancer, *Helicobacter pylori* and one type of stomach lymphoma, mucosal damage and esophageal cancer, smoking and lung cancer, to name a few. However, not all of these irritants always result in cancer in exposed people. Certain types of cancer tend to run in families, making a case for genetic predisposition. It is more than likely true that the cause of cancer is multifactorial. People can have a genetic predisposition and, with the effects of a deleterious lifestyle and nutritional choices, environmental exposures, poor overall health, and poor immune status, may develop a malignancy.

5. What are the major treatment options in conventional oncology? What are the pros and cons?

Conventional oncology focuses on the elimination of cancer cells by three means: surgery, chemotherapy, and radiation. All three interventions aim to remove cancer from the body, but normal tissue structure and function can be significantly affected.

Surgery involves the local and regional removal of cancerous tissues. Normal tissue structure and function can be affected anatomically. There is no truth to the concept that opening the patient for surgery spreads the tumor.

Chemotherapy uses drugs that perfuse throughout the body. Both tumor cells and normal tissues are affected. Different agents are used for specific cancers, and all have varying mechanisms of action and side effects. One of the major side effects of chemotherapy is immune system suppression, which is more prevalent with some agents than others. The development of new growth factors has helped to lessen this acute problem. Long-term effects on the body's function are less well understood but may include the rare development of second malignancies, especially leukemia, after use of certain agents.

Therapeutic radiation uses high-energy x-rays generated from radioactive sources or machines to treat local and regional areas. The normal tissues surrounding the target receive the same dose of radiation as tumor cells, but the mechanism of radiation repair is believed to favor normal tissue. Late side effects from radiation are rare but possible and usually result from changes in small blood vessels, resulting in fibrosis or ulceration of affected tissue. It is also possible to see second malignancies as a result of radiation, but these are quite rare (on the order of 1 in 1000 patients for most disease presentations).

A large amount of data supports the use of these therapies, and the mortality rate from cancer has begun to show a decline, at least partly due to the effectiveness of these interventions. It is important to weigh the risks and benefits of each intervention in a specific patient as well as the patient's desires and concerns to come up with an individualized treatment plan.

6. Why is integrative oncology not the standard of care?

Major obstacles to overcome include the general mistrust of each field for the other. CAM practitioners label conventional therapy as unsuccessful, overly toxic, and, on a conspiratorial level, profitable for biomedicine. Allopathic practitioners argue that CAM therapies are unproven, dangerous, and sometimes expensive and toxic; they also claim that CAM therapies may cause harmful interactions.

The major reasons favoring an integrative approach in oncology include the growing evidence base that CAM practices have scientific merit; the generally high toxicity and cost profile of conventional oncology; and the growing consumer movement toward CAM options.

Another reason that conventional practitioners balk at integrating individualized treatment plans focused on the whole person is the lack of randomized data showing benefits to such an approach. It is nearly impossible to design a randomized trial testing specific individualized approaches; therefore, integrative oncology may be quite difficult to test. One reasonable method under current use is the best-case series approach sponsored by the National Cancer Institute (NCI). This study will analyze best-case scenarios from individual patients and look for common themes. Multiple anecdotes do not equal proof, but they do equal hypotheses, which can be confirmed by further observation.

7. What are the priorities of intervention in integrative oncology? How do they differ from conventional oncology?

It is helpful to think about three major categories of intervention: preventive, supportive, and antineoplastic. **Preventive therapies** include well-researched interventions such as nutrition, physical activity, lifestyle, and self-care issues that reduce the risk of developing cancer and probably also help to prevent recurrences. **Supportive therapies** help patients and families to address physical, emotional, social, and spiritual concerns. **Antineoplastic treatments** aim to kill cancer cells. Conventional oncology focuses almost exclusively on antineoplastic approaches with few resources directed toward preventive and supportive care.

By combining the best of CAM and conventional therapy, we can come up with an integrative model that addresses the whole person. Prevention must form the foundation of this approach, followed by supportive care and finally by antineoplastic therapies.

Most of the popular media coverage of CAM is focused on fringe antineoplastic therapies that completely reject conventional approaches. Very few CAM therapies have documented, well-researched outcomes in terms of eradication of cancer cells in humans. If solid data were available, they would be new standards of care.

The majority of CAM therapies mentioned in this book fit into the categories of preventive and supportive care. Most supportive and preventive therapies have very low toxicity; therefore, the risk-to-benefit ratio is favorable. It is certainly possible that through better support of the whole patients, cancer cure rates can be improved. Sound data indicate that when patients complete conventional therapy in a timely fashion, results are improved. This may be one possible mechanism by which CAM can be beneficial.

8. What is adjuvant therapy? How can its use in conventional oncology encourage consideration of CAM therapy?

Adjuvant therapy is defined as treatment given in addition to definitive management of the primary cancer to improve response rates, rid the individual of undetectable microscopic disease, and potentially improve local disease control or survival rates. For example, adjuvant radiation is given after lumpectomy to women with early-stage breast cancer to decrease the chance of local recurrence. In women with small, invasive tumors, adjuvant radiation decreases the chance of local recurrence from about 40% to about $\leq 10\%$. This increase in local control does not improve survival, but it does increase the chance that women will maintain breast form and function. Sixty percent of women treated with radiation would not have experienced recurrent disease without it, but it is impossible to determine who these patients are in advance.

Adjuvant therapy is given to almost all patients with breast cancer after lumpectomy—and not everyone benefits. But the risks associated with the treatment are seen as acceptable in light of the possible benefit. We can use the same general reasoning to recommend CAM therapies in an integrative fashion. Not everyone may benefit, but if the possible benefits outweigh the risks, adjuvant CAM therapy recommendations to certain groups of patients can be considered reasonable.

9. Should supplemental antioxidants be used concurrently with conventional cancer therapy?

This issue is highly controversial.[34,35] Some data support the theory that antioxidants, such as vitamins C and E, beta-carotene, selenium, and certain B vitamins, may improve both tolerance and results when given concurrently with chemotherapy and radiation. The major argument for the use of antioxidants is to protect normal cells, thus reducing toxic side effects of conventional therapies. Another argument for their use is the tumoricidal effect of certain supplements in vitro. However, few significant randomized human trials have investigated this issue. The major argument against their use is that simultaneous administration of antioxidants during conventional therapy may protect not only normal cells but also cancer cells.

Until definitive data decide the issue either way, it seems reasonable to withhold antioxidants during active treatment with chemotherapy or radiation. Supplemental antioxidants, like most nutritional interventions, have their greatest effect over the long term. This may be a likely explanation of why short-term changes in diet and supplementation have shown disappointing results in most studies. This issue is an ideal choice for future randomized trials.

10. Is there a cancer-prone personality type?

Various authors have postulated the existence of a type C personality, characterized by behavior that is appeasing, unassertive, unexpressive of negative emotions (especially anger), and socially compliant. Some authors theorize that these personality features may correlate with decreased immune function, resulting in deficient immunosurveillance and cancer progression. However, no clear evidence supports that this personality type, or any other, leads to the development or progression of cancer. Personality types generally categorize extreme examples of behavior that do not represent individual people with much accuracy.[4]

11. Can a positive attitude affect cancer prognosis?

Positive attitude, unfortunately, has been overemphasized as a major factor in the prognosis of patients with cancer. Well-meaning family members and friends "put on a happy face" and demand that their loved one with cancer do the same—for fear that expression of perceived negative emotions may result in worse treatment outcomes. The diagnosis and treatment of cancer are stressful, major life events. It is unrealistic to demand that anger, sadness, guilt, fear, and other perceived negative emotions be withheld, while only expression of joy, love, and peace are allowed. Maintaining a conspiracy of silence for the sake of being "positive" is certainly not an effective coping style for oncology-related stress. As a matter of fact, a good definition of healing includes bringing mindful awareness to what many perceive as negative attitudes and patterns.

12. Do coping styles affect cancer prognosis?

Evidence both supports and refutes the hypothesis that reaction to stress with passive coping styles—fatalism, anxious preoccupation with cancer, lack of fighting spirit, avoidance/denial, and helplessness hopelessness—are associated with poor outcome. Because of the complex nature of cancer diagnosis and treatment, there is no assurance that coping styles influence distress level—it well may be the other way around. That being said, a good supportive approach can include a focus on coping styles. The ways in which patients cope may be a critical factor in prognosis, but more prospective interventional studies are needed to help define appropriate therapy. Sound data indicate that, regardless of coping styles, psych-educational support can be helpful.[4]

13. What is the role of the placebo response in the treatment of patients with cancer?

Placebo effect is defined as a therapeutic result produced by belief in a treatment. Randomized trials often use a placebo as a control for comparison with an active intervention. In such studies, several patients receiving placebo have the exact same toxicities and benefits as patients receiving the active agent. One dramatic example is reported from a trial in gastric cancer in which patients either received chemotherapy or IV saline. About 30% of patients in the placebo group lost their hair and had nausea and vomiting. Belief that they were getting chemotherapy was enough to give them classic symptoms associated with active treatment.[18] This is an example of a placebo effect in the opposite direction (called a nocebo effect).

Conventional medicine views the placebo response as a nuisance. It cannot be explained mechanistically but must be controlled for in the testing of new agents. In general, responses to the natural medicines and lifestyle approaches that serve as the foundation for many CAM practices occur more gradually than responses to conventional pharmaceutical agents. A patient's belief in the value of an intervention, CAM or conventional, can help shape the course of therapy. It seems reasonable to put the power of the patient's belief system to work in a supportive way.

One criticism of CAM practices is that their success represents only a placebo response. An integrative approach recognizes the value of any response—regardless of the etiology, especially if the treatment is nontoxic, relatively inexpensive, and generally health-promoting; improves communication and trust in the doctor–patient relationship; and ultimately has benefits that outweigh risks. For further discussion on the placebo effect, see Chapter 4.

14. Can CAM therapies cure cancer? How about conventional oncology?

In *Choices for Healing: Integrating the Best of Conventional and Complementary Approaches to Cancer*, Michael Lerner states: "There is no cure for cancer among any of the alternative therapies."[6] This statement does not mean that alternative treatments have no value, but that they should not be used to the exclusion of known effective therapies. Conventional oncology has voluminous research data demonstrating that it can cure certain types, stages, and presentations of cancer. In the 1990s, the first overall reduction in cancer mortality was reported in the United States. Attitudes toward cancer diagnosis and treatment have shifted from pervasive fear and pessimism to optimism and concern for survivor quality of life. Integrative oncology is not defined by the domination by one system, belief, or individual over another but rather by the optimal use of all reasonable available resources.

ALTERNATIVE CANCER THERAPIES

15. Is there any merit to some of the more famous alternative cancer therapies? What are the facts about these systems? Is any research currently under way?

Systems of alternative cancer treatment share a few common features.[1-3] Most of them mandate adherence to a strict nutritional protocol and offer a substance—whether it be herbs, nutraceuticals, or products believed to have antineoplastic effects—-without significant toxicity. For patients in whom conventional oncology treatments have little to offer, they give hope, whether or not they are valid. Such therapies are often costly, both financially and in terms of patient dedication of time and resources, and are performed by a few practitioners at remote, single-treatment centers. These therapies, or their proponents, have had major clashes with conventional medicine, from local medical organizations to the NCI and Food and Drug Administration (FDA). Ultimately further research will determine the value of adding specific interventions to standard approaches.

16. Explain Hoxsey therapy.

Hoxsey therapy is based on a formulation of herbs developed by Harry Hoxsey, an herbal folk healer, using a recipe passed down to him from his great grandfather. Legend has it that the elder Hoxsey noted that horses with cancer that grazed on certain plants experienced remissions. The formula includes pokeweed, burdock root, licorice, barberry, buckthorn bark, stillingia root, red clover, prickly ash bark, potassium iodide, cascara, and sometimes other ingredients. These components were developed into a salve. Hoxsey treatment now consists of a mix of herbal preparations for both internal and external use, with an emphasis on diet, vitamin and mineral supplementation, and individual counseling. Some constituents of the herbal preparation have been studied separately and showed some anticancer activity, but no human studies have shown consistent value. No clinical trials are currently available, but the treatment is still offered in Mexico.

17. What are Burzynski's antineoplastons?

Stanislaw Burzynski, MD, PhD, isolated chemicals in the blood and urine of healthy people that he believed were natural forms of cancer protection called antineoplastons. Burzynski noted that people with chronic renal failure rarely developed cancer and proposed that this finding was due to an abundance of peptides within their blood. Antineoplastons are given either orally or intravenously. Several rounds of small trials have been approved by the NCI, but none has definitively demonstrated efficacy. The most interesting preliminary results have been in patients with brain tumors. Patients with aggressive brain tumors often have few treatment options, and antineoplaston therapy can benefit up to 50%, according to preliminary data. Patients may receive this therapy at Burzynski's clinic in Houston, where all of his patients are treated under investigational protocols. The clinic formulates an individual treatment plan, which also corrects nutritional deficiencies by using specific amino acids and vitamins.

18. Explain the basis of Gerson therapy.

Gerson therapy represents a nutritional approach that focuses on restoring the body through the use of ionized minerals, natural foods, and detoxifying enemas. Fresh fruits and vegetables, coffee enemas, and thyroid supplementation are the basics of the Gerson approach and have shown clinical responses in selected patients. Currently no clinical trials are testing this therapy.

19. What is the Gonzalez treatment?

Nicholas Gonzalez, MD, studied the work of William Donald Kelley, a Texas dentist who theorized that cancer was caused in part by the body's inability to metabolize proteins. Kelley used large doses of pancreatic enzymes with individually tailored dietary plans and detoxification with coffee enemas. Gonzalez adapted his treatments to formulate individualized regimens focusing on ingestion of pancreatic enzymes and specific diets and bowel cleansing in the form of coffee enemas. His treatment has been the most intriguing in patients with pancreatic cancer, in whom preliminary results compare favorably with largely inadequate conventional treatments. This therapy is currently being tested in a clinical trial sponsored by the National Center for Complementary and Alternative Medicine (NCCAM).

20. Are results from supportive CAM interventions generalizable?

If we use the same standards as those used to generalize conventional supportive therapies, the answer is yes. For example, cancer fatigue is a major problem. Its etiology is multifactorial. One of the factors contributing to cancer fatigue is loss of appetite and resultant weight loss. A synthetic progestin, megestrol (Megace), was investigated in patients with advanced cancer and found to stimulate appetite.[37] The results were then generalized to include use among all patients with all types and stages of cancer. The drug is widely used for this purpose despite the fact that it does not alter survival rates appreciably. Its risk-to-benefit ratio is favorable, and it results in improved appetite, weight gain, and improved quality of life in some patients.

Many studies have shown the benefit of supportive CAM measures such as mind-body interventions, acupuncture, diet, and physical activity in certain groups of patients (see questions below). Using the criteria set forth by conventional oncologists, coupled with clinical judgment, it seems reasonable to generalize these results.

21. What role does the immune system play in cancer development and treatment?

This issue is hotly debated, but most experts agree that somewhere in the cascade of development, promotion, and dissemination of cancer, there is some defect in the function of the immune system. The term *immune surveillance* refers to the natural defense process by which the immune system clears the body of dangerous particles, cells, and organisms. At any given time, cells in the human body can develop mutations that result in cancerous growth, but the immune system routinely rids the body of such cells. An imbalance in immunosurveillance can tip the scales toward the development of cancer. Certain immune system cells and products, such as natural killer (NK) cells and tumor necrosis factor (TNF), have been identified as important in cancer surveillance.[4] Furthermore, certain types of cancer can arise in people with defective immune function (e.g., skin cancers in immunosuppressed patient).

The picture is far from clear. Different types of cancer may be more immunogenic than others. Several types of cancer are known to be associated with viral exposure (e.g., cervical cancer and certain serotypes of human papilloma virus, nasopharynx cancer and Epstein Barr serotype A, non-Hodgkin's lymphoma and HIV). Considerable research in animal systems supports a role for immune surveillance, but definitive human data are lacking.

Epidemiologically, cancer develops with a relatively low incidence over a long time; therefore, it is difficult to correlate assessments of immune function in healthy people with the subsequent development of disease. However, some data reveal statistically significant relationships between various immune measures in patients with cancer and subsequent outcome. Many CAM therapies claim to help support the body's defense against cancer through an increase in the effectiveness of the immune system. The line between supportive and antineoplastic goals is blurred in this setting.

22. What general dietary measures help to prevent cancer?

Large-scale observational studies link a plant-based diet high in fiber to a lower incidence of several types of cancer throughout the body. Multiple mechanisms of action may explain this effect, including increased intake of vitamins and phytochemicals, decreased stool transit time, decreased fat intake, lowered insulin and related insulinlike growth factor release, and lower glycemic index (glycemic index refers to the speed at which foods are converted to useable sugar [glucose] in the body). Eating a diet that focuses on nutrient-rich fruits and vegetables is good medicine.

There is good reason to include foods containing omega-3 fatty acids. Examples include cold-water fish (e.g., salmon, sardines), walnuts, and flax seed. The two main components of fish oil—eicosapentanoic acid and doxahexanoic acid—also can be taken in supplement form. Mixed evidence supports the theory that omega-3 fatty acids are responsible for the lower rates of cancer found in people who eat large amounts of cold-water fish. One study showed that omega-3 oils can limit the recurrence of colon cancer.[27] Another study found that supplementation with fish oil resulted in weight gain and improved survival in severely ill patients.[21]

23. What foods should be avoided to reduce cancer risk?

Certain foods should be avoided because they are associated with increased cancer risk. Examples include salted, pickled, and smoked foods (associated with higher levels of cancers of the upper GI tract in Asian populations); tobacco (most types of cancer); alcohol (aerodigestive tract cancer); trans-fatty acids and processed and sugar-based foods (general cancer promotion); and grilled, fried, or charred meat (results in ingestion of heterocyclic amines, which are associated with cancer promotion).[40]

24. What general lifestyle measures help to prevent cancer?

Improved fitness level is significant and involves multiple mechanisms of action, including lowered obesity, improved cellular functioning, and improved immune system function.[24] Avoidance of exposure to environmental carcinogens is also important, including second-hand smoke and chemical carcinogens in the workplace. It appears that active participation in a loving social network is also protective.[4]

25. What is the most easily identified significant preventable cause of cancer? How can it be changed?

Abstention from tobacco and significant intake of alcohol. Multiple mechanisms of direct and indirect effect have proven links between tobacco use, in its many forms, and the development of cancer. Many methods have been proposed for tobacco cessation. It is clear that former smokers live longer than continuing smokers. People who quit before the age of 50 show a 50% reduction in risk for all causes of death in the subsequent 16 years, and by age 64 their risk is similar to people who have never smoked. Because the relative 5-year survival rate from cancer is now 56%, it is especially reasonable to counsel patients with cancer to quit smoking. Holland offers an excellent overview of current data about cessation techniques.[4] Chronic alcohol abuse (more than one alcoholic drink per day) also has been significantly associated with neoplasia.

26. Do any specific foods have cancer protective properties? How about broccoli?

Evidence indicates that some foods may aid in cancer prevention and have possible cancer-fighting effects. Cruciferous vegetables such as broccoli and other brassica vegetables (e.g., cabbage, cauliflower) are associated with a decreased risk for cancer. Broccoli contains several cancer inhibitory substances that are under investigation, such as sulforaphanes, which inhibit cancer development in animal studies, and indole-3-carbinol, which inhibits the growth of breast cancer cells in vitro.[1] These substances are highly concentrated in broccoli sprouts. Members of the allium family (e.g., garlic, onions) also may have some protective effects, though they are less well defined.

27. How about green tea?

Epidemiologic trials have shown significant reduction in cancer rates in societies that consume green tea (*Camellia sinensis*). This effect was first noticed as a possible explanation for why smokers in Japan had lower rates of lung cancer than American smokers. Green tea has a polyphenol, epigallotechin, that is believed to protect against cancer. It has also been shown to help maintain stable white blood cell counts in patients undergoing chemotherapy and may have some antineoplastic effects as well.[16] Green tea has few potential side effects when it is consumed with food (it contains small amounts of caffeine). Further research needs to be done to determine the optimal dosage, frequency, and mechanism of action, but it appears reasonable to incorporate moderate consumption of green tea into conventional supportive care. A good dosage of green tea is an 8-ounce cup of brewed tea with each meal. Patients should not go overboard because of some concern from animal studies and one small human trial that drinking more than 6 cups/day may cause anemia by inhibiting iron absorption.[33]

28. How can soy benefit patients with cancer?

Soybean products contain isoflavones, including genistein and daidzein, that act as weak estrogenic compounds in the body (phytoestrogens). They may both prevent and fight cancer. One proposed mechanism is competitive inhibition with more aggressive hormones for estrogen receptor sites (see Chapter 38). In addition to potential nutraceutical properties, soybean products are also believed to be a healthier protein source than meat and dairy products.[39] Lower risks of cancer in soy-eating populations may be due to decreased meat and dairy intake.

29. Discuss the role of mushrooms in patients with cancer.

Mushrooms, such as like maitake, reishi (*Ganoderma lucidum*), coriolus, and shiitake, have potential immunomodulatory effects that can help patients with cancer. Early clinical trials of mushroom extracts support a mechanism of action that includes immune system stimulation. There is no known risk to consuming mushrooms, except in allergic people.

A specific beta-D-glucan polysaccharide extract from maitake mushrooms, called D-fraction, is one of the few natural products to be given an investigational new drug (IND) number by the FDA. This compound is being studied for its supportive effects in patients receiving chemotherapy as well as possible immune stimulatory and antineoplastic action. Reasonable dosages of maitake extract are usually given by the manufacturer. Doses of 0.5–1.0 mg/kg have been used in early antitumor and immune stimulation studies.[38,42]

The mushroom *Coriolus versicolor* also contains an active polysaccharide compound called krestin or PSK (available as a product called VPS). This compound has been shown to improve overall survival when used in conjunction with radiotherapy in a small Japanese study of patients with stage I–III non-small cell lung cancer as well as to have beneficial effects in patients treated with chemotherapy after gastrectomy or surgery for colon cancer.[25,41,47]

Arabinoxylane isolated from reishi mushrooms, under the proprietary name of MGN 3, is a compound that contains rice bran and two other mushroom extracts. It is believed to have a similar immune-stimulating effect.[20]

Whether these nonspecific immune stimulants will help to decrease mortality and morbidity of various cancers is currently unknown, but preliminary data are encouraging.

30. What about intake of multivitamin supplements?

Low blood levels of various nutrients, especially antioxidants, are associated with increased incidence of certain types of cancer. It is currently unknown whether supplementation with vitamins can adequately ameliorate low levels due to poor dietary practices. Evidence indicates that supplementation can increase blood levels of specific nutrients,[12] but this increase may not be sufficient to show benefits in people with disease. Several randomized trials are under way to examine these questions, including the NIH-sponsored, multicenter SELECT trial (Selenium and Vitamin E Cancer Prevention Trial), which is designed to evaluate the use of vitamin E and selenium as cancer prevention. Although intake of single isolated nutrient supplements can be potentially dangerous (e.g., beta carotene in smokers[46]), eating a variety of nutrient-dense foods with naturally occurring antioxidants is heavily supported by observational data. These elements may interact within a food to provide a balanced, beneficial effect.[11] This line of reasoning also can be used to recommend a balanced multivitamin supplement instead of single nutrients.

31. Do any phytonutrients or nutraceuticals prevent or treat cancer?

As mentioned above, studies of mushroom extracts, such as maitake, reishi and shiitake, have shown some preliminary evidence pointing toward improved immune function. This finding may result in improvements in prevention and treatment, although the data are not firm.

Shark cartilage has been analyzed as a possible inhibitor of angiogenesis, which is a necessary step in tumor growth and spread. Data about its use are currently inconclusive, and its absorbability is questionable. FDA-sponsored trials are under way.[1,3]

Coenzyme Q-10 (CoQ10) is a vitamin-like substance that helps in cellular energy production. Several studies have shown improved outcomes and tolerance of conventional cancer treatment with CoQ10 supplementation.[26,30] CoQ10 also may have antineoplastic effects.

Melatonin, a hormone produced by the pineal gland, plays an important role in sleep-wake cycles. Preliminary data suggest that it can work as an adjunct to conventional treatments and has anticancer properties.[36] Trials investigating its clinical usefulness are under way. Recent information also suggests that night shift work and exposure to light at night may increase the risk of breast cancer.[14] It is believed that decreased melatonin levels may account for this effect. A good night's sleep in a dark room may help to prevent cancer.

Inositol hexaphosphate (IP6) is a natural compound found in beans, brown rice, corn, sesame seeds, wheat bran, citrus fruits, and other high-fiber foods. It has multiple known functions throughout the body, including the intracellular regulation of insulin and calcium and support of liver function. It is believed that inositol may be one of the key reasons that a high-fiber diet has protective effects against cancer. Some data from animal studies indicate that it may have antineoplastic activity, but not enough is known to make recommendations about supplementation. It seems reasonable, however, to recommend foods that contain IP6.[28]

32. Can any botanicals be used to prevent or treat cancer?

Several herbs have documented antineoplastic or cancer-inhibitory actions (mainly by in vitro studies). Many individual herbs can be combined and used for prevention and treatment. Essiac tea (promoted by nurse Rene Caisse in the 1920s) contains slippery elm, burdock root, Indian rhubarb, and sheep sorrel, all of which have antitumor activity in vitro. Studies of the combination, however, have failed to reveal positive results in humans. Excessive dosing of sheep sorrel can be nephrotoxic. The Hoxsey formula contains a mixture of eight herbs, some of which (burdock root, licorice root and red clover) have documented antineoplastic activity individually. But, as mentioned before, studies of this formula have been disappointing.

In various Chinese studies, Chinese herbal remedies have been shown to have possible beneficial actions as adjunctive therapy.[50] Panax ginseng inhibits tumor growth and also works as an adaptogen, helping to maintain overall strength and endurance. It is a component of multiple Chinese herbal preparations studied as cancer treatments. Unfortunately, herbal product quality is not guaranteed. A recent study showed that the herb *Aristolochia fangchi* contains toxins that cause urothelial cancer. This herb was inadvertently used in a diet formula in place of a different herb.[43] Herbs should not be used indiscriminately and optimally should be taken under the guidance of an experienced clinician.

33. What about mistletoe?

Mistletoe has a long history of use as a cancer treatment in Europe. The plant is poisonous when eaten, but a standardized injectable extract (Iscador) is available. Iscador has been shown to contain at least two different glycoproteins(substances with both sugar and protein components), called lectins. Lectin 1 is antineoplastic, and lectin 2 binds cancer-destroying immune cells to tumor receptors. Mistletoe is also a strong nonspecific immune activator. Animal studies have confirmed its effectiveness, and randomized human trials have shown that it stimulates the immune system, increases endorphin levels, and enhances quality of life.

Trials are under way to investigate the use of mistletoe as an antineoplastic agent. No definitive trials have shown reliable efficacy in humans, but some preliminary data are encouraging. A recent publication included prospective, controlled, nonrandomized and randomized matched pair studies nested within a cohort study of 10,226 patients with cancer treated with Iscador. Patients who received Iscador showed a significant improvement in survival time.[22]

There are appropriate concerns about the purity of all of the above-mentioned formulas—and most botanical preparations. More strict pharmaceutical control methods may be helpful in this regard (see Chapter 18).

34. Is body cleansing or detoxification useful in prevention or treatment of cancer?

Body cleansing is often an integral part of many alternative cancer therapies—whether through enemas, chelation therapy, or "parasite cleanses."[2] The proposed mechanism of action is the elimination of toxic substances or organisms, located in the large intestine, that are believed to cause cancer initiation or spread. This type of therapy was popular in the United States in the 1920s and 1930s, when colon irrigation machines were often found in hospitals and doctors' offices. No evidence supports the theory that this therapy has either preventive or antineoplastic benefits,[1] although clinical trials in which patients receive colonic enema as part of therapy (e.g, Gonzalez treatment in pancreatic cancer) are currently under way.

35. Do any useful CAM therapies gain therapeutic advantage because of the mind- body spirit connection?

Absolutely. Most of these interventions have proven supportive effect. Individual patients respond differently to different therapies and may seek out a good "match" based on their condition and preferences.[1,3,5]

36. Is aromatherapy effective?

Aromatherapy is the use of essential oils (fragrant substances distilled from plants). These oils are highly concentrated and can be inhaled or used in massage. Evidence suggests that aromatherapy can help reduce anxiety, depression, tension, and pain in patients with cancer as well as possibly alleviate some side effects of conventional treatment (e.g., treatment-related nausea).

37. What is the role of art therapy?

Art therapy uses creative activities to help people gain insight into their current situation, often at a deeper level than what can be expressed rationally and consciously. The credentialing board for art therapists is the American Art Therapy Association. Several case reports suggest benefits from this approach in patients with a variety of illnesses.

38. Is there any role for hypnosis or guided imagery?

Hypnosis is a state of restful alertness that can be self- or other-induced. It has been approved by the NIH as a useful complementary therapy in the management of chronic pain.[8] It also may help to decrease side effects of conventional cancer therapy[44] and may improve immune system function. There is a certifying board for hypnotherapists.

Guided imagery involves a combination of relaxation and visualization with the goal of positively influencing the experience and effectiveness of any treatment. Several studies and reviews document its effectiveness in reducing the side effects of chemotherapy and radiation.[9,10] Some studies suggest immune enhancement as well. These techniques are safe and should be taught by a trained professional. Several books and tape series provide instruction in this technique.

39. Can listening to music help?

Music therapy involves the use of music as a method to promote healing and enhance quality of life. It has documented effectiveness in helping to manage acute pain in patients with cancer (see Chapter 5). Music therapists can design specific music sessions for different individuals and groups.[31]

40. Can yoga be useful?

Yoga generally involves the use of movement, breathing exercises, and meditation to achieve a balance among body, mind, and spirit. There are many different types of yoga. The three most commonly used aspects are the postures of hatha yoga, the breathing techniques of pranayama yoga, and meditation. The NIH has endorsed yoga as an effective complementary method to decrease the side effects associated with conventional cancer treatments.[8]

Many other techniques can be useful in the supportive care of patients with cancer, including biofeedback, breath work, journaling, meditation, Native American ceremonies, psychotherapy, qi gong, and tai chi. Several of these therapies have been endorsed by the NIH as useful for the treatment of chronic pain and insomnia—symptoms often experienced by patients with cancer.[8]

41. Do support groups help patients with cancer?

Support groups have become a significant part of patient care. Several studies have shown that participating in a support group increased not only quality but also quantity of life in patients with cancer compared with patients with the same diagnoses who did not take part in a group. Patients with breast cancer, melanoma, leukemia, and lymphoma have been shown to benefit in terms of overall survival, although data about the specific issue of survival benefit are conflicting. Studies consistently demonstrate a significant benefit from support group participation in terms of improving quality of life, decreasing anxiety, and possibly improving treatment results.[13,45]

Several healing communities offer residential programs that focus on self-care, self-expression, and the use of the various supportive complementary interventions noted above. Commonweal in Bolinas, California (www.commonweal.org), Exceptional Cancer Patients (www.ecap-online.org), and Many Streams Healing Systems in Rome, Georgia (www.manystreamsheal.com) are excellent examples of resource and healing centers.

42. What about spiritual approaches, including prayer, spirituality, and faith healing?

Faith healing can involve prayer, visits to a religious shrine, or a strong belief in a higher power. Prayer can create changes. Significant developing literature indicates that prayer has a beneficial effect on disease outcomes. There are reports of spontaneous remissions of advanced cancer in people who visit certain healing shrines, such as Lourdes in France. Faith healing, however, can be a double-edged sword. One report showed that 90% of 172 cases of fatal illness among children treated only with faith healing could have been cured with conventional treatments. Many of these children had cancer.

Spirituality is defined as a personal relationship with a higher power and differs from religion, which is defined as a chosen method of worship. Certain religious groups have lower rates of cancer death due to dietary and lifestyle beliefs, such as Seventh Day Adventists, who abstain from alcohol and tobacco. Incorporating spirituality into standard health care is becoming a more standard practice and potentially benefits the patient by reducing anxiety and stress associated with cancer diagnosis and treatments.

43. Can acupuncture help patients with cancer?

Acupuncture is a part of traditional Chinese medicine that focuses on placing needles at specific points in the body, along meridians, to stimulate a healthy flow of chi, or life energy. It has been confirmed by the NIH as an acceptable method to reduce nausea associated with chemotherapy.[8] An over-the-counter product called "Sea Bands" is available for nausea prevention. It was initially developed as a method of preventing sea sickness. Preliminary reports suggest that acupuncture also can be used to control pain, to decrease hot flashes in patients on hormonal therapy, and to help reverse radiation-related xerostomia (dry mouth) in patients treated for head and neck cancer.[23,29]

44. What touch and energy therapies can benefit patients with cancer?

Bodywork includes several types of manual therapy, such as traditional Swedish massage, Rolfing, shiatsu, Feldenkrais method, Trager approach, and Alexander technique. Patients with cancer should speak with their physician before undergoing any bodywork to make sure that they have no contraindications (e.g., bony metastases).[1]

Bodywork therapies can involve manipulation, rubbing, and kneading of soft tissue and muscles. Massage can decrease stress, anxiety, depression, and pain. It has been shown to be helpful with general tolerance of conventional cancer therapies.[17] No documented scientific evidence supports the fear that massage can cause cancer to spread more rapidly.

Reiki is a Japanese word meaning "universal life energy." The Reiki practitioner is attuned to certain levels of energy that exist in and around the physical body and can help to resolve imbalances in these energy fields that may correspond to disease states. Preliminary evidence suggests that application of healing energy can help to alleviate pain and ease side effects of conventional cancer therapy.[1] Therapeutic touch works by the transmission of healing energy—much like Reiki. Therapeutic touch is taught in over 100 colleges and universities throughout the world. It may help to reduce anxiety and perceived stress in both patient and practitioner.[1,3]

45. What botanicals and supplements have shown benefit in patients with cancer?

A limited list of effective agents used to help decrease side effects of conventional cancer therapies includes the following:

Oral glutamine is used to help decrease digestive and general side effects in patients receiving taxol-based chemotherapy, radiation, or bone marrow transplant regimens.[32]

Aloe vera gel can be applied topically to help with radiation-induced skin damage.

Cayenne lotion can be used topically to help with postsurgical pain in the scar area. An over-the-counter formulation, Zostrix, was originally developed as a salve to help with postherpetic neuralgia due to herpes zoster infections.[49]

Panax ginseng and **Siberian ginseng** have been prescribed to help with fatigue, but data about their efficacy are conflicting.[48]

Ginger root, which can be made into a tea or used in a crystallized form, provides some help with nausea prevention and treatment.[1,11]

Some natural medicines may help symptoms often found in patients with cancer. For example, valerian can be used for insomnia or St. John's wort for anxiety and depression (see Chapter 18). It is extremely important to have an open dialogue with patients about these alternatives, because many patients hesitate to inform physicians about their use. Clear communication with other providers is critical. Some interactions can occur with medications commonly used in cancer patients. For example, use of the anticoagulant warfarin (Coumadin) with ginkgo, vitamin E, garlic, or fish oil can prolong bleeding times.

46. What about the medical use of marijuana in patients with cancer?

Marijuana has been used to ease anxiety, increase appetite, and prevent nausea. The active ingredient, delta 9 tetrahydrocannabinol (THC), has been available as a prescription drug (Marinol) since 1985 for the treatment of refractory nausea. Psychotropic side effects often limit patient use. There are at least 66 biologically active ingredients in marijuana, but Marinol contains only THC, which is believed to be the most potent. Use of the raw plant is illegal in the United States. The main risk to smoking marijuana lies in exposure to inhaled smoke. The long-term side effects of marijuana use are still debated hotly, and little is known about its effect on the immune system.[1]

47. How do I start to practice integrative oncology?

First, it is important to understand that integrative medicine should be practiced by everyone. It is a way of life—not just a way to use more CAM tools in patient interventions. The practice of integrative medicine positively affects the doctor–patient relationship. An organization that helps physicians set up onsite integrative practices can be researched at www.integrativeadvantage.com. This organization provides individualized, practical advice about how to implement integrative oncology services. General suggestions include the following:

1. Educate yourself about CAM therapies, such as those mentioned in this book. Many continuing medical education courses are available for practicing physicians. The Comprehensive Cancer Care (CCC) conference sponsored annually by the Center for Mind Body Medicine in Washington DC (director: James Gordon MD) is an excellent example. Consider exploring CAM therapies yourself, if appropriate.

2. Get to know some CAM practitioners. Ask them about their services. How are they provided? Who benefits? Who does not? How much does the service cost? What research is available? How did they receive training? How are they licensed and accredited in their field? Do they use progress notes? Will they send you copies for mutual patients?

3. Ask your patients about their use of CAM, including nutrition and exercise habits. Also ask what the disease means to them, how they are coping, and the role that they want their doctor to play in their life.

4. Decide on the goals of your treatment plan: preventive, supportive, or antineoplastic. If patients are interested, investigate CAM therapies that are reasonable and fit into each category. Decide on the level of evidence appropriate for each category so that you would feel comfortable making a referral. Understand the use of adjuvant therapy and how it relates to all recommended oncology care—both conventional and CAM practices.

5. Give hope. According to Bernie Siegel, MD, author of *Peace, Love and Healing* (Harper Perennial, 1989), healer, and surgical oncologist, "There is no such thing as false hope, only hope."

This is not to say that we should lie to our patients, but that we should tell them the absolute truth. We cannot predict what will happen in any individual patient, despite a pile of statisitics pointing in one direction or another. Siegel expresses concern about creating "false despair," when hope may be the only thing that gets a person out of bed in the morning. Find ways to be supportive. Turn up the care when we think that we can no longer cure.

6. Practice effective self-care. Model healthy behavior for your patients. Physicians who practice healthy behavior are better able to influence patient changes.[19]

REFERENCES

1. American Cancer Society's Guide to Complementary and Alternative Cancer Methods. Atlanta, American Cancer Society, 2000. A broad review of the full range of CAM methods in cancer care.
2. Diamond JW: An Alternative Medicine Definitive Guide to Cancer. Tiburon, CA, Future Medicine Publishing, 1997. A good overview of mostly alternative practices that claim antineoplastic effects.
3. Gordon JS, Curtain S: Comprehensive Cancer Care: Integrating Alternative, Complementary, and Conventional Therapies. Cambridge, MA, Perseus Publishing, 2000. An excellent review of the popular cancer conference with an extensive resource list included.
4. Holland JC (ed): Psycho-oncology. New York, Oxford University Press, 1998. An excellent resource concerning preventive and supportive therapy for cancer.
5. Labriola D: Complementary Cancer Therapies: Combining Traditional and Alternative Approaches for the Best Possible Outcome. Roseville,CA, Prima Publishing, 2000. A patient-directed book that provides an overview of both major conventional and CAM practices in cancer care.
6. Lerner M: Choices in Healing: Integrating the Best of Conventional and Complementary Approaches to Cancer. Cambridge, MA, MIT Press, 1994. A good overview of CAM practices in integrative oncology for both practitioner and patient.
7. Levine S: A Year to Live: How to Live This Year As If It Were Your Last. New York, Bell Tower, 1997. The title says it all—very insightful book.
8. Alternative Medicine: Expanding Medical Horizons. A Report to the National Institutes of Health on Alternative Medical Systems and Practices in the United States. Washington DC, U.S. Government Printing Office, 1994. National Institutes of Health publication 94-066.
9. Baider LF, et al: Psychological intervention in cancer patients: A randomized study. Gen Hosp Psychiatry 23:272–277, 2001.
10. Bridge LR, et al: Relaxation and imagery in the treatment of breast cancer. Br Med J 297: 1169–1172, 1988.
11. Brown J et al: Nutrition during and after cancer treatment: A guide for informed choices by cancer survivors. American Cancer Society Workgroup on nutrition and physical activity for cancer survivors. Cancer J Clin 51(3):153–187, 2001.
12. Cao G et al: Increases in human plasma antioxidant capacity after consumption of controlled diets high in fruits and vegetables. Am J Clin Nutr 68:1081–1087, 1998
13. Cunningham AJ, et al:A randomized controlled trial of the effects of group psychosocial therapy on survival in women with metastatic breast cancer. Psychooncology 7:508–517, 1998.
14. Davis S, et al: Night shift work, light at night, and the risk of breast cancer. J Natl Can cer Inst 93:1557–1562, 2001.
15. Downer SM, et al: Pursuit and practice of complementary therapies by cancer patients receiving conventional treatment. Br Med J 309:86–89, 1994.
16. Dufresne CJ, et al: A review of the latest research on the health promoting properties of tea. J Nutr Biochem 12:404–421, 2001
17. Ferrell-Torry AT, Glick OJ: The use of therapeutic massage as a nursing intervention to modify anxiety and the perception of cancer pain. Cancer Nurs 16(2):93–101, 1993.
18. Fielding JW et al: An interim report of a prospective, randomized, controlled study of adjuvant chemotherapy in inoperable gastric cancer. World J Surg 7:390–399, 1983.
19. Frank E, et al: Physician disclosure of healthy personal behaviors improves dredibility and ability to motivate. Arch Fam Med 9:287–290, 2000.
20. Ghoneum M, Jewett A: Production of tumor necrosis factor alpha and interferon gamma from human peripheral blood lymphocytes by MGN-3, a modified arabinoxylan from rice bran, and its synergy with interleukin 2 invitro. Cancer Detect Prev 24:314–324, 2000
21. Gogos CA, et al: Dietary omega-3 polyunsaturated fatty acid plus vitamin E restore immunodeficiency and prolong survival for severely ill patients with generalized malignancy. Cancer 82:395–402, 1998.
22. Grossarth-Maticek, R. et al: Use of iscador, an extract of European mistletoe (*Viscum album*), in cancer treatment: Prospective nonrandomized and randomized matched pair studies nested with a cohort study. Altern Ther Health Med 7:57–66, 68–72, 74–76, 2001.

23. Hammar M, et al: Acupuncture treatment of vasomotor symptoms in men with prostatic carcinoma: A pilot study. J Urol 161 853–856, 1999.
24. Hardman AE: Physical activity and cancer risk. Proc Nutr Soc 60:107–113, 2001
25. Hayakawa K, et al: Effect of Krestin (PSK) as adjuvant treatment on the prognosis after radical radiotherapy in patients with non small cell lung cancer. Anticancer Res 13:1815–1820, 1993.
26. Hodges S, et al: CoQ10: Could it have a role in cancer management? Biofactors 9:365–370, 1999.
27. Huang YC, et al: Omega three fatty acids decrease colonic epithelial cell proliferation in high risk bowel mucosa. Lipids 31:S313–S317, 1996.
28. Jariwalla RJ: Inositol hexaphosphate (IP6) as an anti-neoplastic and lipid lowering agent. Anticancer Res 19:3699–3702, 1999
29. Johnstone PA, et al: Acupuncture for pilocarpine-resistant xerostomia following radiotherapy for head and neck malignancies. IJROBP 50:353–357, 2001.
30. Jolliet P, et al: Plasma coenzyme Q-10 concentrations in breast cancer: Prognosis and therapeutic consequences. Int J Clin Pharmacol Ther 36:506–509, 1998.
31. Kerkvliet GJ: Music therapy may control cancer pain. J Natl Cancer Inst. 82:550–552, 1990.
32. Klimberg M: Glutamine, cancer, and its therapy. Am J Surg 172:418–424, 1996.
33. Kubota K, et al: Effect of green tea on iron absorption in elderly patients with iron deficiency anemia. Nippon Ronen Igakkai Zasshi 27:555–558, 1990.
34. Labriola D, Livingston R: Possible interactions between dietary antioxidants and chemotherapy. Oncology 13:1003–1012, 1999.
35. Lamson DW, Brignall MS: Antioxidants in cancer therapy: Their actions and interactions with oncologic therapies. Altern Med Rev 4:304–329, 1999.
36. Lissoni P, et al: A randomized study with the pineal hormone melatonin versus supportive care alone in patients with brain metastases due to solid neoplasms. Cancer:73:699–701, 1994.
37. Loprinzi CL, et al: Controlled trial of megestrol acetate for the treatment of cancer anorexia and cachexia. J Natl Cancer Inst 83:449–450, 1991.
38. Mazell M: Maitake extracts and their therapeutic potential. Altern Med Rev 6:48–60, 2001.
39. Messina M, Barnes S: The role of soy products in reducing risk of cancer. J Natl Cancer Inst 83:541–546, 1991.
40. Myrvik QN: Immunology and nutrition. In Shils ME, et al (eds): Nutrition in Health and Disease, 8th ed. Philadelphia, Lea & Febiger, 1994.
41. Nakazato H, et al: Efficacy of immunochemotherapy as adjuvant treatment after curative resection of gastric cancer. Lancet 343:1122–1126, 1994
42. Nanba H: Anti-tumor activity of orally administered "D-fraction" from maitaike mushroom (*Grifola frondosa*). J Naturopath Med 4:10–15, 1993.
43. Nortier JL, et al:Urothelial carcinoma associated with the use of a Chinese herb (*Aristolochia fangchi*). N Engl J Med 342:1686–1692, 2000.
44. Redd WH, et al: Hypnotic control of anticipatory emesis in patients receiving cancer chemotherapy. J Consul Clin Psychol 50:14–19, 1982.
45. Spiegel D, et al: Effect of psychosocial treatment on survival of patients with metastatic breast cancer. Lancet 2:888–891, 1989.
46. The effect of vitamin E and beta carotene on the incidence of lung cancer and other cancers in male smokers. The Alpha Tocopherol, Beta Carotene Cancer Prevention Study Group. N Engl J Med 330:1029–1035, 1994.
47. Torisu M, et al: Significant prolongation of disease free period gained by oral polysaccharide K (PSK) administration after curative surgical operation of colon cancer. Cancer Immunol Immunother 31:261–268, 1990.
48. Vogler BK, et al: The efficacy of ginseng: A systematic review of randomized trials. Eur J Clin Pharmacol 55:567–575, 1999.
49. Watson CPN, Evan RJ: The postmastectomy pain syndrome and topical capisacin: A randomized trial. Pain 51:372–379, 1992.
50. Wong R, et al: Integration of Chinese medicine into supportive cancer care: A modern role for an ancient tradition. Can Treat Rev 27:235–246, 2001.

55. APPROACH TO SPECIFIC CANCERS

Matt Mumber, M.D.

BREAST CANCER

1. What are the current screening recommendations for breast cancer?

Women aged 40 years and older should have an annual mammogram, an annual clinical breast exam, and monthly self-exams. Monthly self-exam was recently challenged by a large prospective trial which showed that self-exams were not necessarily beneficial; this issue, however, is controversial. Women aged 20–39 years should have exams yearly and do self-exams monthly, until further data become available.

2. Can a low-fat diet prevent breast cancer?

Breast cancer rates are much higher in countries with high-fat diets than in countries where fat intake is much lower, such as Japan and less developed countries. Exposure to excessive estrogen is one major risk factor for the development of breast cancer. Obesity can lead to increased estrogen exposure. A recent review that pooled the results of seven prospective studies from developed countries found no association between fat intake and breast cancer risk in adult women. These studies have several weaknesses, however, including the fact that few participants were on low-fat diets (i.e., there was not enough of a difference in fat intake to establish potential differences) and considerable error was made in the recording of fat intake on dietary questionnaires. There is also a trend for immigrants from countries with a low incidence of breast cancer to develop breast cancer at a rate similar to that of their new place of residence. For example, Japanese immigrants to the U.S. and their children have an incidence of breast cancer similar to that of U.S. citizens. Diet may play a role in this increased risk.

Population and animal studies have shown that fat intake greater than 20% of total calories was strongly associated with an increased incidence of breast cancer. Extensive evidence from animal and ecologic studies points toward a causative role of high-fat intake and breast cancer risk. These data are supported by basic science information about the biologic effect of fat on breast tissue, including information about hormone metabolism, oxidative damage, and immune function.[3]

3. Are all fats alike in regard to breast cancer prevention?

Data indicate that all fats are not alike (see Chapter 19). Omega-6 fatty acids, found in corn, sunflower oil, and safflower oil, have been shown in animal models to promote cancer growth and metastasis.[45] Trans-fatty acids, found in margarine and other highly unsaturated processed foods, also have been shown to lead to an increased risk of cancer.[50] On the other hand, omega-3 fatty acids, found in cold-water fish and flaxseed oil, and omega-9 fatty acids, found in monounsaturated fat sources such as olive oil, have been shown to have protective effects against cancer in both human and animal studies.

For a cancer-preventive diet, one can recommend a diet low in fat, emphasizing the use of olive oil instead of other vegetable oils, intake of omega 3 fatty acids from cold-water fish and flaxseeds, and avoidance of trans-fatty acids in margarine and processed foods.

4. Can a diet high in fruit, vegetables, and fiber prevent breast cancer?

The absolute benefits of a diet high in fruits, vegetables, and fiber relative to breast cancer risk are uncertain. Many studies show that increased intake results in lower risk, but other studies have found no such effect. Recently, an analysis of pooled results from a total of eight prospective cohort trials revealed no benefit to increased intake of fruits and vegetables in regard to breast cancer recurrence.[51] The American Institute for Cancer Research cautions that this study looked only at cohort trials; significant data from case control, correlational, intervention, and animal studies support the preventive role of fruits and vegetables. It is difficult to gather data about dietary influence, because the results usually rely on long-term habits but short-term ability to quantify actual intake.

Fruits and vegetables provide significant amounts of vitamins and phytonutrients (e.g., vitamins C and A, beta carotene, lycopene), which have been shown in various observational human studies to confer protective effects. Fiber intake may reduce intestinal reabsorption of estrogens, thus explaining the positive effect noted in some studies.[3]

A recent randomized Italian study showed that a diet low in animal fat and refined carbohydrates and rich in low glycemic index foods, monunstaturated and omega-3 fatty acids, and phytoestrogens significantly decreased the bioavailability of sex hormones in postmenopausal women selected on the basis of high serum androgen levels.[6]

The risk-to-benefit ratio of eating a plant-based diet is quite favorable—not only in regard to cancer prevention but also for many other health issues. It seems prudent to adopt the plant-based diet as a standard. Because cancer is a chronic disease that develops over time, we must focus on long-term dietary habits over the entire lifespan.

5. Can taking high doses of vitamins prevent breast cancer?

Significant data indicate that appropriate levels of certain nutrients, including vitamins A, C, and E, selenium, lycopene, folic acid, and coenzyme Q 10, may be protective against the development of breast cancer.[58,59] It is unknown whether these nutrients have the same activity when taken as supplements or whether they must be consumed in whole foods to maintain this benefit. As soil becomes depleted and the food supply is altered by modern farming techniques that include the use of toxic pesticides, fungicides, and growth hormones, it seems likely that supplementation will continue to emerge as a method to maintain adequate levels of certain nutrients.

6. Can soy products prevent breast cancer?

Countries in which women consume a great deal of soy products have significantly lower rates of breast cancer. Although genetics and environment play a role, some authors postulate that this lower incidence can be attributed to dietary factors. The effects of soy products are believed to be due to isoflavones (phytoestrogens or plant estrogens). Some laboratory data show that phytoestrogens bind to estrogen receptors in the human body—but weakly—or do not stimulate them. They may function, therefore, as competitive inhibitors and block other estrogens. The theory is that weak estrogens act as antiestrogens in breast cancer, although others suggest that this estrogenic activity may cause cancer to grow faster.

Clinical trials of chemoprevention in breast cancer are currently being sponsored by the National Cancer Institute. Until the results of these studies are available, it is wise for women with estrogen-responsive breast cancers (positive marker for estrogen and progesterone receptors) to avoid excessive intake of such foods and specifically to avoid concentrated isoflavone supplements. However, as part of a preventive plan, the addition of soy products to the diet, especially as a replacement for animal protein and fat, is entirely reasonable.[42,43]

7. Can fitness level influence the development of breast cancer?

Multiple studies suggest a role in fitness level and the development of breast cancer.[5,31] Obesity is a major influence on the conversion of circulating hormones into estrogen and may explain, at least in part, why increased fitness level appears protective. This effect appears to be especially pronounced in postmenopausal women, since sedentary aging tends to decrease lean muscle mass while increasing body fat percentage (see Chapter 21). A reasonable preventive prescription that can be followed by patients with breast cancer includes moderate aerobic exercise on a daily basis (e.g., at least 30 minutes of brisk walking 5 days per week, as tolerated). A recent trial in postlumpectomy patients showed that women who maintain their fitness level during treatments had an overall better performance status than those who did not.[49]

8. Can alcohol intake influence the development of breast cancer?

There are two distinct mechanisms by which alcohol intake may influence the development of breast cancer: direct and indirect. Alcohol is directly absorbed into breast tissue and may have a local cancer-promoting effect by increasing the dedifferentiation of cells. It also may have an indirect effect via increased exposure to estrogen. A recent study found that at any age even moderate consumption of alcohol was clearly associated with an increased risk of developing breast cancer.[21]

On the other hand, emerging data suggest that consumption of red wine, with its component resveratrol, may be protective. It is believed that this component may lessen the tumor-stimulatory effect of harmful substances in the standard American diet. Preliminary data also indicate that a substance in red wine may act in much the same way as aromatase inhibitors used in conventional medicine. Aromatase inhibitors inhibit the feeding of breast cancer cells by estrogen mainly through inhibiting the conversion of androgens into estrogens.[7] Moderate use of red wine (one glass on two days per week with a meal) seems like a reasonable preventive measure until further data are available. The greatest amount of resveratrol is found in wines from colder climates. Grape juice contains about half as much resveratrol as red wine.

9. Can hormone replacement therapy cause breast cancer?

No definitive data indicate that hormone replacement therapy after menopause causes breast cancer, although it can lead to an increased incidence.[14] The increased incidence may be simply a result of greater surveillance and early detection. Conjugated equine estrogens generally are used for hormone replacement. The most widely used product (Premarin) is derived from pregnant mare urine. Unopposed estrogen replacement can lead to an increased incidence of endometrial cancer but has beneficial effects on bone and possibly on the cardiovascular system. Using progesterone intermittently may help to prevent the increased cancer risk but also may mitigate the cardioprotective effects. The decision to undergo hormonal replacement should be made on a case-by-case basis, depending on specific individual and family history. Natural forms of estrogen are available (see Chapter 38) and may actually decrease cancer risks.

10. Can social support influence survival in breast cancer?

Substantial evidence indicates that social integration, as indicated by membership in organizations and frequency of social contacts, is associated with increased survival rate in patients with cancer. Of interest, studies of the beneficial effects of marital status and support network size have produced inconsistent findings. Involvement in a range of social activities predicts improved survival.[33]

11. Can support interventions, such as breast cancer support groups, influence survival?

Support groups for patients with cancer aim to provide emotional and informational assistance. In one trial, patients with metastatic breast cancer receiving standard care were randomized to support group intervention or controls. The author aimed to study the effect on quality of life but found that the quantity of life, or overall survival, was significantly improved in the treatment arm. Patients randomized to the support group survived an average of 18 months vs. 9 months in the control group.[54] Another randomized trial of patients with metastatic breast cancer found no overall survival benefit but did show improved quality of life.[16] Support groups run by trained professionals have little potential for harm. Many features of support group intervention require further study, including type, maximal content and duration, and optimal participant profile. It is reasonable to recommend inclusion in a local support group with the caveat that more intensive one-on-one assistance is available for referral (see also question 30 in Chapter 54.)

12. What supportive therapies can be used to help prevent and treat lymphedema?

Lymphedema is an accumulation of protein-rich fluid in soft tissues due to failure of normal lymphatic system drainage. In patients with breast cancer, the arm on the side of the cancer can be affected by surgery (axillary node dissection), chemotherapy, or radiation (sclerosis of lymphatics). Several studies have shown the benefit of massage and physical therapy of the upper extremity in the prevention of lymphedema.[57] This low-cost intervention can improve functional activity level and prevent life-threatening cellulitis. Women and their partners can be taught to do massage and exercises at home.

13. What herbal and nutraceutical therapies have been advised for support of patients with breast cancer?

Several herbs are thought to be supportive by lessening side effects or improving the activity of conventional treatments:

1. **Astragalus** (*Astragalus membranaceous*) was shown in one study to increase natural killer cell activity and lower the amount of chemotherapy requirement to attain a beneficial response.[2]

2. **Black cohosh** was recently investigated in a randomized trial to determine whether it can help with hot flashes in survivors of breast cancer survivors and was found to work no better than placebo.[36]

3. **Milk thistle** (*Silybum marianum*) has a documented effect on hepatocyte regeneration after injury by infectious processes such as hepatitis.[2] Some practitioners use these data to suggest that milk thistle can help the liver to recover from damage due to cytotoxic chemotherapy. No human trials have demonstrated this benefit specifically in patients with cancer who receive chemotherapy, but the herb is extremely safe. In patients with signs or symptoms of liver damage, a trial of milk thistle seems like a viable option.

4. **Slippery elm lozenges** and **aloe juice** help improve dysphagia and mucositis.

5. **Topical aloe** helps with radiation-associated skin damage.

6. **Ginger**, as either a tea or crystallized candy, can improve nausea.

No definitive data address the use of herbs in patients with breast cancer, and potential drug-herb interactions must be viewed with caution. Botanical therapy usually works best as a part of a comprehensive integrative approach rather than depending on herbs as a magic bullet.

14. What role does DHEA play in breast cancer development and treatment?

Dehydroepiandrosterone (DHEA) is the most abundant steroid hormone in the body and is produced by the adrenal glands. It is a four-ring precursor steroid that is converted into other steroid hormones, including estrogen and testosterone. DHEA production peaks at about age 30 and slowly declines, reaching about 5–15% of maximum levels by age 60. Research shows that low levels of DHEA are associated with breast cancer, but no definite causative link has been established. DHEA should not be supplemented in patients with cancer, especially those who are hormonally responsive, because of possible stimulation of the cancer.[1]

15. What types of complementary/alternative medicine (CAM) therapies have shown documented antineoplastic activity in studies of human breast cancer?

The Chinese herbal remedy **juzenthaito** (JT-48 or JTT) was shown to improve survival, tolerance of chemotherapy, and quality of life in patients treated for metastatic breast cancer in one study from Japan.[4]

Coenzyme Q10 has been examined in several small series of patients with breast cancer and may prevent some of the heart damage that can result from adriamycin-based chemotherapy regimens. It also may improve fatigue and antitumor efficacy.[37] Further studies of CoQ10 are currently under way.

16. Can a low-fat diet prevent progression in survivors of breast cancer?

Two large studies, Women's Intervention Nutrition Study (WINS) and Women's Healthy Eating and Living Study (WHEL), have been closed to accrual and are examining the role of a low-fat diet in patients with breast cancer. The results should be available in about 2004; until that time, it is reasonable to recommend a well-balanced, plant-based diet.[9]

PROSTATE CANCER

17. What are the screening recommendations for prostate cancer?

This issue is controversial. It is currently unknown whether measuring prostate-specific antigen (PSA) can detect prostate cancer at an earlier stage and affect overall survival. The low-grade, early-stage cancers found as a result of early biopsies may have little biologic significance. This issue is currently under study in national trials. The current recommendations include PSA and digital rectal exam annually for men over the age of 50 years. High- risk groups (men with two or more affected first-degree relatives and African Americans) should begin the protocol at age 45 years.

18. How do dietary factors influence the development of prostate cancer?

A consistent trend of increased death rates from prostate cancer is seen in men consuming higher levels of dietary fat. Epidemiologic studies have shown an increase in the development of prostate cancer with an increase in dietary fat or certain fatty foods, including meat-based diets. Eleven of 14 case-control studies have shown a positive association. Several case-control studies show a lower rate of prostate cancer with higher rates of fruit and vegetable intake, particularly cruciferous vegetables.[38] Increased intake of alcohol also has been associated with prostate cancer (> 10 drinks per week).[19]

A recent analysis of the association between dairy products, calcium, and prostate cancer risk supports the hypothesis that men who consume greater amounts of dairy products (and thus have higher amount of calcium intake) have a 32% higher risk of developing prostate cancer. It is believed that high calcium intake from dairy products may lower levels of vitamin D_3, a hormone thought to prevent prostate cancer. The exact mechanism of this effect is unknown.[11] Several in vitro and animal trials show that soy isoflavones may have a protective and antineoplastic effect.[42] It seems reasonable to limit intake of dairy products and use moderate amounts of soy substitutes until further information is available.

19. Can adequate vitamin levels prevent prostate cancer?

Some data indicate that low levels of selenium and lycopene (a carotenoid) are linked to a higher incidence of prostate cancer. **Vitamin E** also may be of some benefit, especially for smokers.

Selenium intake was tested in a prospective, double-blind, placebo-controlled trial, originally meant to examine the risks for recurrence of skin cancer. The researchers noted an increased number of cancers in the placebo arm, and added new endpoints. This analysis showed a significant decrease in the number of prostate, lung, colorectal, and total cancers in the group taking the selenium supplement at 200 µg/day.[13] The decrease in prostate cancer was the most pronounced. There was also a decrease in total cancer mortality. Patients who benefited most were those with low baseline selenium levels before the study. Other trials have supported this result. Currently a large randomized trial examining the effect of vitamin E and selenium supplementation—the NIH-funded Selenium and Vitamin E Cancer Prevention Trial (SELECT)—is under way. This study began accrual in 2001 and will randomize 32,400 men. It will help to examine the protective effects of short-term supplementation. Final results are anticipated in the year 2013.

Lycopene, the most potent of the carotenoids, has been shown in several large cohort and case-control studies to decrease the incidence of prostate cancer.[29] Lycopene is highly concentrated in processed tomato products, such as tomato sauce. Fifty seven of 72 studies showed an inverse association between lycopene levels or intake of tomato products with incidence of prostate cancer; 35 studies had statistically significant results.

Based on available evidence, patients with prostate cancer may take vitamin E (100 IU or more of mixed tocopherols) and selenium (200 µg), and consume a diet high in tomato-based products (at least 3 times per week).

20. What other lifestyle factors may affect the development of prostate cancer?

Obesity, fitness level, and intake of soy products may affect the development and progression of prostate cancer. Multiple epidemiologic studies support the theory that improved fitness levels and decreased obesity correlate with decreased incidence of prostate cancer, although some of the data are conflicting.[28,47] Some preliminary epidemiologic and basic science studies support the theory that soy isoflavones have activity in the prevention and possible treatment of prostate cancer.[42] The Preventive Medicine Research Institute is currently conducting a study of patients with prostate cancer using Ornish's successful lifestyle interventions for cardiac patients. Patients will be randomized to a lifestyle program including a low-fat vegetarian diet, aerobic exercise, stress reduction, and group support. More information about this program is available at www.pmri.org. Look for the prostate cancer lifestyle trial.

21. What supportive CAM therapies have proven useful in patients with prostate cancer?

Patients receiving hormonal therapy for advanced prostate cancer may experience significant hot flashes. **Acupuncture** has been shown to help decrease this problem.[30]

An interesting pilot trial showed a possible inhibitory effect on prostate cancer in men treated with **flaxseed** supplementation and **dietary fat restriction**.[18] Low-fat diets are certainly reasonable in this setting, because many men with prostate cancer also may be at risk for coronary artery disease.[38] Supplementation of flaxseed is still debated, mainly because it contains alpha-linolenic acid, a compound that is also found in animal fat sources, and has been associated with higher rates of prostate cancer. More than likely, the increased incidence is due to the other components of animal fat. Moderate use of flaxseed is more than likely safe and potentially beneficial. Until further data become available, it may be reasonable to get the bulk of dietary **omega 3-fatty acids** from fish oils (eicosapentaenoic acid and doxahexaenoic acid).

Support groups may help men with prostate cancer. National groups, such as Us Too and Man to Man, may help to provide resources and address family and patient psychosocial needs.[15]

22. Can saw palmetto benefit men with prostate cancer?

Several herbal therapies have been shown to improve urinary symptoms related to benign prostatic hypertrophy, the best known of which is saw palmetto (*Serenoa repens*) (see Chapter 41). One mechanism of action is as a 5-alpha reductase inhibitor, which blocks an active form of testosterone called dihydrotestosterone. Various studies have supported the use of saw palmetto to decrease urinary outlet obstruction. More clinical trials are ongoing in an attempt to confirm this benefit. Preliminary trials indicate that saw palmetto does not cause the same side effects of erectile dysfunction and libido loss as one of its pharmaceutical counterparts, finasteride. Saw palmetto is a component of PC-SPES (see below). However, saw palmetto is not considered an antineoplastic treatment for prostate cancer; rather, it treats the symptoms of prostate hypertrophy. Patients taking this herb should notify their physician, because it may affect PSA levels, which are routinely used as a marker of prostate cancer prognosis and progression. One small study, however, found no change in PSA levels.[26]

23. What is PC-SPES? Does it have a role in treatment of prostate cancer?

PC-SPES is a traditional Chinese preparation composed of eight herbs. Its use is steadily increasing worldwide. PC stands for prostate cancer; *spes* is the Latin word for hope. The herbs include chrysanthemum, isatis, licorice, *Ganoderma lucidum, Panax pseudoginseng, Rabdosia ruescens,* saw palmetto, and skullcap. Three recent studies confirm the ability of PC-SPES to stabilize the disease and improve quality of life in patients suffering from prostate cancer. The herbal preparation comes in capsule form, with doses varying among studies.[17] Patients with either hormonally sensitive disease or disease which is refractory to standard hormonal therapies respond to PC-SPES.

Toxicity of PC-SPES includes gynecomastia, hot flashes, and increased incidence of deep venous thrombosis, all of which point to its significant estrogenic activity. Conventional options for treatment of advanced, hormonally refractory prostate cancer are minimally efficacious; therefore PC-SPES has a relatively good toxicity profile and may be beneficial. Its side effects, like those of other effective cancer therapies, should be monitored by close follow-up. Liver function tests should be routinely checked because of some reports of hepatotoxicity. Recently concerns also have been raised about product purity (see Chapter 18).

LUNG CANCER

24. What are the screening recommendations for lung cancer?

There are currently no significant screening recommendations for the early detection of lung cancer, although this area is controversial. Previous studies examined the use of chest x-rays in smokers and found no benefit. They also showed that screening may detect tumors that never become life-threatening. The results of recent trials focused on CT scans of the chest are encouraging; there is some suggestion that lesions can be found at an earlier stage and treated for cure. Perhaps more importantly, the process of screening presents an educational opportunity during which smokers can be counseled to quit. Indeed, one study sponsored by the National Cancer Institute found that using CT scans to screen current and former smokers was better than chest x-rays and that 23% of those screened were convinced to quit smoking compared with a national annual cessation rate of 6%. Twenty-three percent were also convinced to reduce cigarette intake.[31] Currently a large trial is under way to evaluate screening in terms of cost-effectiveness.

25. What are the main preventive options for lung cancer?
1. Do not smoke.
2. Stop smoking.
3. Do not breathe second-hand smoke.

Smoking and alcohol are a significant "one-two" punch to the immune system; therefore, alcohol intake should be avoided. Dietary factors that have been shown to be beneficial for patients with lung cancer include a plant-based diet with less reliance on fat from meat products. This type of diet also focuses on foods with a low glycemic index; intake of dietary refined sugar has been shown in some studies to lead to an increased risk of lung cancer.[20]

26. What is known about vitamins and lung cancer?
Vitamin supplementation has shown variable results. Two studies reported that male smokers who took synthetic beta-carotene developed lung cancer 18% and 28% more often than those who did not use supplements.[48,55] In one of these studies the effect was reported in smokers, ex-smokers and men exposed to asbestos. Alcohol seemed to intensify this effect as well as heavy smoking. Another study found no significant increase or decrease in lung cancer rates with beta carotene supplementation.[34] Most reviewers point out that supplementation should include mixed carotenoids from natural sources, but until further data are available, it seems prudent to avoid supplementation with synthetic beta-carotene in smokers. Of interest, sound data also indicate that high levels of carotenoids and other nutrients (e.g., vitamin C) associated with whole foods confer a protective effect.[10,39]

27. What CAM-based therapies can help patients with lung cancer?
CAM interventions that help people to stop smoking and practice healthy lifestyle and nutritional habits should be strongly considered. Traditional Chinese medicine with its use of acupuncture and lifestyle counseling is one example. Lung cancer treatments are becoming more effective through the combination of various conventional modalities—namely, concurrent administration of chemotherapy and radiation. This combination is accompanied by significant toxicities, including increased dysphagia, fatigue, and immune suppression. It is important to provide as much help as possible during these treatments. The preventive and supportive therapies listed in the general section and throughout this book should be considered. One such intervention is the use of supplemental mushroom extract, *Coriolus versicolor*.[32] Support group participation also can have significant advantages.[41]

COLON CANCER

28. What are the current screening recommendations for colon cancer?
Most colon cancer develops from adenomatous (benign) polyps. It takes an average of 10 years for a 1-cm polyp to develop into a malignancy. Thirty percent of the population is considered to be at an increased risk because of family history of colon cancer, personal history of polyps, personal history of inflammatory bowel disease, or familial polyposis syndromes. The overall reduction in colon cancer mortality from flexible sigmoidoscopy done until age 80 is 45%. The American Cancer Society recommends that, beginning at age 50, men and women should have a fecal occult blood test yearly and flexible sigmoidoscopy every five years. Fecal blood tests should be done on the day after a meat-free diet, and the patient should collect three fecal occult blood slides. Samples collected from digital rectal exam have been shown to have high false-positive rates. If a positive test is found, the patient should have colonoscopy to visualize the entire colon. A colonoscopy also should be performed for people found to have a polyp greater than 1 cm in size on flexible sigmoidoscopy.

29. How does nutrition affect colon cancer?

Colon cancer has been shown to have a lower incidence in people who consume a significant amount of vegetables because of increased intake of either fiber or nutrients.[24,25,53] There are many similarities in risk factors for insulin resistance and colon cancer, and it is believed that insulin resistance may lead to colon cancer through the growth-promoting effects of elevated insulin, glucose, and triglyceride levels. Increased intake of saturated fat, especially fat from meat and polyunsaturated fat, has been shown to increase the incidence.[23] It is reasonable to recommend a plant-based diet focused on foods with a low glycemic index. Foods with omega-3 fatty acids also should be advised; examples include salmon, sardines, other cold-water fish, flaxseed, and walnuts.

30. Does fiber prevent colon cancer?

The role of increased dietary fiber as a preventive measure is debated, and study results are conflicting. Recent trials have shown that short-term increases in fiber intake in patients with previous adenomas do not reduce development of further polyps. However, long-term epidemiologic trials show a significant association between increased fiber intake and mortality from colon cancer. It may be that lifetime dietary choices are more important than later dietary changes. This theory emphasizes the need to counsel people at a young age about dietary choices.[53] Two recent trials showed that increased fiber did not affect recurrence of adenomas in patients placed on high-fiber diets. However, the level of fiber intake was significantly lower than in countries with a low incidence of colon cancer. It is also possible that once a patient has formed polyps, it is too late for diet to exert much of an influence on recurrence.

31. What nutrients need to be explored in prevention of colon cancer?

Some reports have associated increased iron levels with increased risk of colorectal cancer. Most experts agree that iron supplementation in nonanemic postmenopausal women and men is not indicated and may be dangerous for a variety of reasons, including possible increased risk of colon and other cancers.[46]

Calcium and folic acid are important in preventing the development of colorectal adenomas—a benign form of tumor that can evolve into a cancer over time. Results of the Women's Health Initiative trial, which included 64,500 postmenopausal women, will help to define the role of these two nutrients as well as the effect of a low-fat diet on cancer incidence in general.[27]

32. Do lifestyle factors play a role in prevention of colon cancer?

Decreased fitness level and obesity are risk factors for colon cancer. As a matter of fact, the evidence that high levels of physical activity are protective is the most consistent finding in prevention of colon cancer, which is reduced by 40–50% in the most active people compared with the least active.[31,40] Twenty to 30 minutes of walking per day—enough to elevate the heart rate—is a reasonable recommendation. Tobacco and alcohol intake also are associated with higher incidence rates of colon cancer.[53]

33. Is it true that anti-inflammatory medicines can lower the risk for colon cancer?

It appears so. Intake of 160 mg of aspirin per day has been related to a decreased incidence of colon cancer, and cyclooxygenase 2 enzyme (COX 2) inhibitors have been shown to reduce the formation of adenomas in families predisposed to their development. This new finding may help to explain the protective effect of aspirin and also opens the door to providing possible natural inhibitors of COX 2 (such as ginger and turmeric) and dietary fats that lead to less inflammatory products (e.g., omega-3 fatty acids). Some preliminary research is examining the role of COX-2 inhibitors as potential enhancers of tumor response to radiation therapy.[44]

34. What general supportive therapies can help patients with colon cancer?

Many patients with colon cancer are treated with a combination of surgery, chemotherapy, and radiation (radiation is added mostly in patients with rectal cancer). Significant body alterations often take place (e.g., colostomy); therefore, the use of mind-body therapies seems particularly appropriate. Biofeedback has been shown to help with liquid stool incontinence and severe urgency, which often follow treatment of rectal cancer.[12] One small trial showed a significant prolongation of disease-free period by supplementation with mushroom extract after curative surgery.[56] Other general supportive therapies may help to ease the side effects of therapy.

SKIN CANCER

35. What are screening recommendations for skin cancer?

Depending on sun exposure, skin type, and family history, a total body skin exam should be performed by a health professional at a frequency ranging from yearly to every 3 years. Any change in size, shape, color, or texture of a mole, especially if rapidly occurring, should be brought to the attention of a physician.

36. What are the major preventive strategies for skin cancer?

Limiting the amount of significant overexposure to sunlight is an important way to minimize risk for both melanomatous and nonmelanomatous skin cancer. The general recommendation is to limit sun exposure at midday (between 10 AM and 4 PM). During exposure one should apply a sunscreen with a sun protection factor (SPF) of 15 or higher, which blocks about 93% of the burning ultraviolet (UV) rays. There is no truth to the belief that sunscreens cause skin cancer. A sunscreen should block both UVA and UVB rays. Newer sun blocks physically deflect sunlight, whereas sunscreens chemically absorb rays. Sun blocks that contain micronized titanium dioxide offer substantial UVA and UVB protection and are less conspicuous on the skin than previous sun blocks, such as zinc oxide. Be careful of reflective surfaces, and wear hats, sunglasses, and protective clothing.

A plant-based diet, high in antioxidant vitamins, is also important. Because some botanical products, such as St. John's wort, can increase photosensitivity, extra caution is necessary. Recent data show that smoking is also a significant risk factor.[52] Animal and epidemiologic studies have shown that both black and green tea may be helpful in prevention of skin cancer due to sun exposure. Studies of the appropriate amounts are ongoing.[8]

37. What CAM supportive and treatment options can help patients with skin cancer?

Conventional treatment for skin cancer may result in surgical or radiation-related skin damage, and local application of moisturizers such as aloe vera can promote repair. Common folk remedies to help repair damaged skin include calendula and diluted essential lavender oils, although no significant data support their use. Some alternative practitioners recommend tea tree oil for the treatment of actinic keratosis (benign precancerous skin growths), but no data support its use. A group of escharotic herbs (compounds that destroy superficial tissue) may be appropriate treatment options for premalignant lesions, although further research is necessary.

One study revealed that structured support groups improve survival rates and increase natural killer cell activity in patients with melanoma.[22] Because melanoma is known to be responsive to immunotherapy, these results are quite important. Various supportive regimens that boost immune system function deserve further research.

REFERENCES

1. Fugh-Berman A: Alternative Medicine: What Works. Baltimore,Williams & Wilkins, 1997. A good overview of scientific evidence for CAM practices.
2. Pelletier KR: The Best Alternative Medicine: What Works? What Does Not? New York, Simon & Schuster, 2000. A good overview of CAM and multiple health applications.
3. AICR response to 2/14/01 JAMA review on vegetables, fruits and breast cancer (press release). American Institute for Cancer Research, 2001.
4. Adachi I: Role of supporting therapy of Juzenhaiho-to (JTT) in advanced breast cancer patients. Japanese J Cancer Chemother 16(4 Pt 2-2):1533–1537, 1989.
5. Bernstein L, et al: Physical exercise and reduced risk of breast cancer in young women. J Natl Can Inst 86:1403–1408, 1994.
6. Berrino F, et al: Reducing bioavailable sex hormones through a comprehensive change in diet: The Diet and Androgens (DIANA) randomized trial. Cancer Epidemiol Biomark Prev 10:25–33, 2001.

7. Bhat KP. et al: Estrogenic and antiestrogenic of resveratrol in mammary tumor models. Cancer Res 61:7456–7463, 2001.

8. Bickers DR, Athar M: Novel approaches to chemoprevention of skin cancer. J Dermatol 11:691–695, 2000.

9. Brown J, et al: Nutrition during and after cancer treatment: A guide for informed choices by cancer survivors. American Cancer Society Workgroup on nutrition and physical activity for cancer survivors. Cancer J Clin 51:153–187, 2001.

10. Cao G, et al: Increases in human plasma antioxidant capacity after consumption of controlled diets high in fruits and vegetables. Am J Clin Nutr 68:1081–1087, 1998

11. Chan JM, et al: Dairy products, calcium, and prostate cancer risk in the Physicians Health Study. Am J Clin Nutr 74:549–554, 2001.

12. Ciarioni G, et al : Liquid stool incontinence with severe urgency: Anorectal function and effective biofeedback treatment. Gut 34:1576–1580, 1993.

13. Clark LC, et al: Decreased incidence of prostate cancer with selenium supplementation: Results of a double blind cancer prevention trial. Br J Urol 81:730–734, 1998.

14. Colditz GA, et al: Relationship between estrogen levels, use of hormone replacement therapy, and breast cancer. J Natl Cancer Inst 90:814–823, 1998.

15. Coriel J, Behal R : Man to Man prostate cancer support groups. Cancer Pract 7(3):122–129, 1999.

16. Cunningham AJ, et al :A randomized controlled trial of the effects of group psychosocial therapy on survival in women with metastatic breast cancer. Psychooncology 7:508–517, 1998.

17. Darzynkiewicz A, et al: Chinese herbal mixture PC-SPES in treatment of prostate cancer (Review). Int J Oncol 17:729–736, 2000.

18. Denmark-Wahnefried W, et al: Piolt study of dietary fat restriction and flaxseed supplementation in men with prostate cancer before surgery: exploring the effects on hormonal levels, prostate specific antigen, and histopathologic features. Urology 58:47–52, 2001.

19. Dennis LK, Hayes RB: Alcohol and prostate cancer. Epidemiol Rev 23:110–114, 2001.

20. De Stefani E, et al: Dietary sugar and lung cancer: A case control study in Uruguay. Nutr Cancer 31:132–137, 1998.

21. Ellison RC, et al: Exploring the relation of alcohol consumption to risk of breast cancer. Am J Epidemiol 154:740–747, 2001.

22. Fawzy I, et al : Malignant melanoma: Effects of an early structured psychiatric intervention, coping, and affective state on recurrence and survival 6 years later. Arch Gen Psychiatry 47:720–735, 1993.

23. Franceschi S, et al: Dietary glycemic load and colorectal cancer risk. Ann Oncol12:173–178, 2001.

24. Fuchs CS, et al: Dietary fiber and the risk of colorectal cancer and adenoma in women. N Engl J Med 340:169–176, 1999.

25. Garay CA, Engstrom PF: Chemoprevention of colorectal cancer: dietary and pharmacologic approaches. Oncology 13:89–97, 1999.

26. Gerber GS, et al: Saw palmetto (*Serenoa repens*) in men with lower urinary tract symptoms: Effects on urodynamic parameters and voiding symptoms. Urology 15:1003–1007, 1998

27. Giovannucci E, et al: Multivitamin use, folate, and colon cancer in women in the Nurses Health Study. Ann Intern Med 129:517–524, 1998.

28. Giovannucci E, et al: A prospective study of physical activity and prostate cancer in male health professionals. Cancer Res 58:5117–5122, 1998.

29. Giovannucci E: Tomatoes, tomato based products, lycopene, and cancer: Review of the epidemiologic literature. J Natl Cancer Inst 91:317–331, 1999.

30. Hammar M, et al: Acupuncture treatment of vasomotor symptoms in men with prostatic carcinoma: A pilot study. J Urol 161:853–856, 1999.

31. Hardman AE : Physical activity and cancer risk. Proc Nutr Soc 60:107–113, 2001.

32. Hayakawa K, et al: Effect of Krestin (PSK) as adjuvant treatment on the prognosis after radical radiotherapy in patients with non small cell lung cancer. Anticancer Res 13:1815–1820, 1993.

33. Helgeson VS, et al: Social ties and cancer. In Hollnd J (ed): Psycho-Oncology. Oxford, Oxford University Press, 1998.

34. Hennekens CH, et al: Lack of effect of long term supplementation with beta carotene on the incidence of malignant neoplasms and cardiovascular disease. N Engl J Med 334:1145–1149, 1996.

35. Henschke CI, et al: Early lung cancer action project: A summary of the findings on screening. Oncologist 6:147–152, 2001.

36. Jacobsen JS, et al: Randomized trial of black cohosh for the treatment of hot flashes among women with a history of breast cancer. J Clin Oncol 19:2739–2745, 2001.

37. Jolliet P, et al: Plasma coenzyme Q-10 concentrations in breast cancer: Prognosis and therapeutic consequences. Int J Clin Pharmacol Ther 36:506–509, 1998.

38. Kolonel LN, et al: Dietary fat and prostate cancer: current status. J Natl Cancer Inst 91:414–428, 1999.

39. Lee IM, et al: Antioxidant vitamins in the prevention of cancer. Proc Assoc Am Physicians 111:10–15, 1999.

40. Martinez ME, et al: Leisure time physical activity, body size and colon cancer in women. J Natl Cancer Inst 89:948–955, 1997.
41. McCarthy MM, et al: The benefits of support group participation to lung cancer survivors-an evaluation. ClinLung Cancer 1:110–117, 1999.
42. Messina M, Barnes S: The role of soy products in reducing risk of cancer. J Natl Cancer Inst 83(8):541–546, 1991.
43. Messina MJ, Loprinzi CL: Soy for breast cancer survivors: A critical review of the literature. J Nutr 131:3096S–3108S, 2001.
44. Milas L: Cyclooxygenase-2 (COX-2) enzyme inhibitors as potential enhancers of tumor radioresponse. Semin Radiat Oncol 4:290–299, 2001.
45. Myrvik QN: Immunology and nutrition. In Shils ME, et al (eds): Nutrition in Health and Disease, 8th ed. Philadelphia, Lea & Febiger, 1994.
46. Nelson RL: Iron and colorectal cancer risk: Human studies. Nutr Rev 59:140–148, 2001
47. Oliveria SA, et al: The association between cardiorespiratory fitness level and prostate cancer. Med Sci Sports Exerc 28:97–104, 1996.
48. Omenn GS, et al : Effects of a combination of beta carotene and vitamin A on lung cancer and cardiovascular disease. N Engl J Med 334:1150–1155, 1996.
49. Segal R, et al: Structured exercise improves physical functioning in women with stages I and II breast cancer: Results of a randomized controlled trial. J Clin Oncol 19:657–665, 2001.
50. Simopoulos AP : Is insulin resistance influenced by dietary linoleic acid and trans fatty acids? Free Radic Biol Med 17:367, 1994.
51. Smith-Warner SA, et al: Intake of fruits and vegetables and risk of breast cancer—A pooled analysis of cohort studies. JAMA 285:769–776, 2001.
52. Sofie AE, et al: Relation between smoking and skin cancer. J Clin Oncol 19:231–238, 2001.
53. Slattery ML: Diet, lifestyle and colon cancer. Semin Gastrointest Dis 11(3):142–146, 2000.
54. Spiegel D, et al : Effect of psychosocial treatment on survival of patients with metastatic breast cancer. Lancet ii:888–891, 1989.
55. The effect of Vitamin E and beta carotene on the incidence of lung cancer and other cancers in male smokers. The Alpha Tocopherol, Beta Carotene Cancer Prevention Study Group. N Engl J Med 330:1029–1035, 1994.
56. Torisu M, et al: Significant prolongation of disease free period gained by oral polysaccharide K (PSK) administration after curative surgical operation of colon cancer. Cancer Immunol Immunother 31:261–268, 1990.
57. Zanolla R, et al : Evaluation of the results of three different methods of post-mastectomy lymphedema treatment. J Surg Oncol 26:210–213, 1984.
58. Zhang S, et al : Dietary carotenoids and vitamins A, C and E and risk of breast cancer. J Natl Cancer Inst 91(6):547–556, 1999.
59. Zhang S, et al: A prospective study of folate intake and the risk of breast cancer. JAMA 281:1632–1637, 1999.

56. PEDIATRIC ABDOMINAL PAIN

Joy A. Weydert, M.D., FAAP

1. Define recurrent abdominal pain (RAP) in children.

Apley and Naish define RAP as at least three episodes of pain over a 3-month period severe enough to interfere with normal activities but for which no underlying organic disease is found. During the interval between the pain episodes, the child is well.[1]

2. If no organic disease is present, why worry about it?

RAP is one of the most common reasons that parents seek medical attention for their children. It affects 10–15% of all school-aged children and is responsible for 2–4% of all pediatric outpatient visits.[2] Significant health care costs are associated with this disorder as parents and physicians try to "get to the root of the problem" through multiple and repeated laboratory and x-ray investigations.

3. Besides the expense, what other problems are associated with RAP?

Children with RAP miss, on average, 26 days of school per year compared with 5 days per year in children without RAP.[3] This problem affects not only the child's school performance but also the family's psychosocial and economic balance. Long-term follow up finds that 30% of children with RAP become adults with chronic recurrent abdominal pain (frequently diagnosed as irritable bowel syndrome).[4] Lastly, children with RAP have higher indices of anxiety and depression that continue throughout adulthood.[5]

4. Did children with RAP have colic as infants?

Studies have concluded that there is no relationship between infantile colic and subsequent childhood RAP.[6]

5. What causes RAP?

The cause and pathogenesis are not known, but there are three prevailing theories:

1. **Visceral hyperalgesia.** The brain-gut axis, with its shared neuropeptides, has bidirectional communication. Alterations in gut wall sensory receptors, modulation of sensory transmission along these pathways, cortical perceptions, and pain memories may have an effect on the viscera, causing the perceived pain.[7]

2. **Gastrointestinal (GI) motility.** No specific motility disturbance has been identified, but it is thought that children with RAP may have an abnormal GI motor response to various stimuli such as stress, meals, or abdominal distention (gas).[8]

3. **Psychosocial issues.** Some children with RAP exhibit anxiety, depression, or low self-esteem, and often the family structure is characterized by parental depression, enmeshment, overprotectiveness (vulnerable child), or rigidity. Any of these factors can influence how the disorder is experienced.[9]

6. Describe the three classic clinical presentations of RAP.

1. **Isolated paroxysmal abdominal pain** (functional abdominal pain)
   - Usually periumbilical in location
   - Variable severity and duration
   - Rare association of pain to meals, activity, or bowel habits
   - May have associated autonomic symptoms (i.e. nausea, dizziness, headache, pallor, fatigue)
2. **Nonulcer dyspepsia** (functional dyspepsia)
   - Pain localized to epigastrium or either upper abdominal quadrant
   - Ulcer-type pain, early satiety, nausea, vomiting, indigestion, belching, bloating, or oral regurgitation may be present.
   - Temporal relationship between pain and meals

3. **Abdominal pain associated with altered bowel patterns** (irritable bowel syndrome)
   - Pain localized to lower abdomen that may be relieved with defecation
   - Onset of pain associated with change in frequency of stool or form of stool
   - May have feeling of straining or urgency, incomplete passage of stool, bloating, or abdominal distention
   - Alternating diarrhea and constipation with passage of mucous

7. What is the best way to approach the work-up of a child with RAP?

Rather than a diagnosis of exclusion, present RAP to the family as a positive diagnosis because it is the *most common* cause of chronic abdominal pain in children. Of all children diagnosed with RAP, only about 10% are found to have serious disease. Organic disease can be ruled out by systematically obtaining a thorough history and physical exam. The work-up can be streamlined to the most specific of the diagnoses based on the history and physical exam, thus saving time and money.

In addition to the past medical, social, and family histories and information about the child's diet, the history should consist of questions about the nature of the symptoms. Ask about location, severity, quality, timing (in relation to food, menstrual cycle, or bowel movements), and radiation of the pain as well as the course of pain episodes (i.e., start of pain, changes in location or severity). It is also helpful to know whether the pain has been experienced before and, if so, how frequently, what measures relieve or exacerbate it, and the extent to which the pain disrupts the child's normal activities. Other specific questions should include:
   - Does the pain wake the child from sleep?
   - Has the pain been associated with a change of appetite, weight loss, or growth delay?
   - Does the child have fevers, chills, jaundice, vomiting, rashes, joint involvement, or perianal disease?
   - Does the child report changes in color of the stools or urine, bile-stained emesis, blood in the stool, or urinary symptoms?
   - What is the pattern of stool frequency and consistency?
   - What is the child's sexual history? Is abuse suspected?
   - Is there a family history of peptic ulcer disease, inflammatory bowel disease, lactose intolerance, or significant psychosocial disorders?
   - Does the child have a previous history of any abdominal surgeries or bowel disease (necrotizing enterocolitis [NEC] as a newborn)?

There should be a higher index of suspicion for serious organic disease if pain is located away from the umbilicus, radiates to other locations, or wakes the child from sleep. Weight loss, fever, persistent vomiting, a change in the color of stool or urine, blood in the stool, or bile stained emesis also should be red flags. In children younger than 5 years of age, pain should be considered organic until proved otherwise.

8. Describe the important components of the physical examination.

Consistent with the principles of any good physical exam, inspection, auscultation, palpation, and percussion should be performed and carefully described. Assessing for abdominal masses, localized tenderness, or evidence of inflammation is of great importance. A rectal examination is imperative to assess not only for the above entities but also for occult blood, perianal disease, and constipation. In sexually active adolescents, a thorough genitourinary exam, including a pelvic exam for females, is warranted. Evidence of skin rashes or joint inflammation may indicate inflammatory bowel disease.

9. Which differential diagnoses for acute abdominal pain in children can be potentially serious, requiring swift intervention?

The differential diagnosis depends somewhat on the age and gender of the patient.[10]

Infants: intussusception, volvulus, malrotation, intestinal infection (e.g., NEC)

Children: appendicitis, ovarian torsion, GI bleeding, pancreatitis, cholecystitis, pneumonia

Adolescents: all of the above plus ectopic pregnancy, pelvic inflammatory disease, pyelonephritis, inflammatory bowel disease

If a history of abdominal trauma is elicited, consider pancreatic pseudocyst, intra-abdominal hemorrhage, or ruptured viscus.

10. What laboratory investigations should be obtained in the work-up of abdominal pain?

The initial work-up should include a complete blood count to evaluate for anemia or infection, sedimentation rate to assess for inflammatory processes, stool for occult blood, and urinalysis to rule out urinary tract infection. If warranted by the history, obtain a serum amylase, hepatic enzymes, beta human chorionic gonadotropin, appropriate stool or genitourinary cultures, or *Helicobacter pylori* serology. Other considerations include a chest x-ray to rule out pneumonia or abdominal plain films to assess for intestinal obstruction, stool retention, renal stones, or pancreatic calcifications. Abdominal ultrasound is useful to rule out hydronephrosis, ectopic pregnancy, and appendicitis and to evaluate any abdominal masses. Upper GI endoscopy may be indicated in patients with significant epigastric distress and hemoccult-positive stools. If an acute abdomen is apparent, immediate consultation with a surgeon is warranted.

11. What is the best complementary/alternative medicine treatment for RAP in children?

Because RAP is a multidimensional disorder, a biopsychosocial approach to its treatment is necessary. An integrative approach is best taken by using interventions tailored to the individual patient's needs. These interventions may be allopathic and derived from conventional medical knowledge or alternative, utilizing modalities recognized for their therapeutic effects.

12. Does a change in diet help?

It can, especially if certain foods are known to trigger problems (e.g., milk in lactose-intolerant children). Highly processed foods with refined sugars (e.g., snack foods, cookies, candy) frequently are not fully digested. The sugars ferment, causing increased gas formation. Sorbitol, found in sugar-free gum, and high-fructose corn syrup, found in sweetened beverages and bottled fruit juices, may lead to the same digestive problems. Caffeine frequently increases GI motility and also should be avoided.

13. What about fiber?

Studies have shown a reduction or complete resolution of pain episodes in children with RAP when they are given an additional 10 grams of insoluble fiber per day.[11] This finding applied to children with or without underlying constipation. Dietary fiber can be obtained through fruits and vegetables (1–4 gm/serving), legumes (3–6 gm/serving), whole wheat or bran products (2 gm/serving), or psyllium powder (1 tsp = 2 gm). When increasing fiber, also increase water intake to prevent constipation.

14. What else can be used, especially during a pain episode?

Progressive muscle relaxation, biofeedback, and hypnosis have been used successfully in both clinical studies and clinical practice.[12] These interventions, based on the knowledge of the brain-gut axis, are effective by stopping the reflex response to pain, calming the patient and thus reducing the perception of the pain experience. These interventions are considered mind-body therapies.

15. Which herbs may be helpful?

Chamomile tea, peppermint tea, and ginger have been used for centuries to ease abdominal pain and calm stomachaches. The active ingredients in chamomile work on receptors in the GI tract to relax the smooth muscle[13] and on the benzodiazepine receptors in the central nervous system to reduce anxiety.[14] Peppermint works by blocking calcium channels and inhibiting smooth muscle contractions in the GI tract.[15] One study in children found it to be effective treatment for irritable bowel syndrome.[16] Ginger exerts antispasmodic effects by antagonism of serotonin receptor sites.[17] These herbs can be given safely as teas, by capsule, or by elixir. Chamomile, on rare occasion, has been linked to allergic reaction in people with allergy to ragweed, asters, or chrysanthemums. Peppermint, with its calcium channel-blocking effects on the lower esophageal sphincter, may cause increased dyspepsia unless taken as an enteric-coated capsule.

16. What about prescription medications?

Many drugs are prescribed for pediatric abdominal pain, but no controlled studies document efficacy or safety. Common side effects include:

- Metoclopramide: dystonic reactions, irritability
- Cisapride: arrhythmia, adverse outcomes in prolonged QT syndrome
- Anticholinergics: constipation, blurred vision, sedation
- Tricyclic antidepressants: sedation, agitation, lowered seizure threshold, death with untreated overdose.

No studies in children support the use of H_2 receptor antagonists or proton pump inhibitors. They are relatively safe, however, especially with short-term use (6–8 weeks) in patients whose primary symptom is dyspepsia.

17. What other modes of alternative therapies have been used to treat RAP?

No published studies support the use of acupuncture, traditional Chinese medicine, homeopathy, osteopathy, or cranial-sacral manipulation for treatment of RAP. Much like prescription drugs, these therapies are probably used despite the lack of studies. Unlike the prescription drugs, the safety profiles of these therapies are excellent; the risk of using them through qualified practitioners is minimal.

18. What can be done in the long term to help patients and families cope?

Pain behavior often is reinforced unknowingly but with good intent. Help families recognize that special attention or treatment during pain episodes (e.g., staying home from school, dismissal from chores or responsibilities, personal attention from a parent) may foster ongoing pain behavior and diminish the child's self-reliance. Encourage school attendance as well as completion of personal responsibilities. Physicians can facilitate a return to a normal lifestyle by offering a thorough explanation of the diagnosis and pathophysiology, reassurance, and options for management and adaptation.

In children or families with significant psychosocial dysfunction, counseling by a child psychiatrist or clinical psychologist may be the best therapy. Cognitive-behavioral family intervention therapy, which often includes teaching specific, coping skills, social skills, and relaxation, has been shown to be efficacious in studies of children with RAP.[18]

REFERENCES

1. Apley J, Naish N: Recurrent abdominal pains: A field survey of 1000 school children. Arch Dis Child 33:165–170, 1958.
2. Starfield B, Katz H, Gabriel A: Morbidity in childhood-a longitudinal view. N Engl J Med 310:824–829, 1984.
3. Stone RT, Barbero GJ: Recurrent abdominal pain in childhood. Pediatrics 45:732–738, 1970.
4. Walker LS, Guite JW, Duke M, et al: Recurrent abdominal pain: A potential precursor of irritable bowel syndrome in adolescents and young adults. J Pediatrics 132:1010–1015, 1998.
5. Campo JV, DiLorenzo C, Bridge J, et al: Adult outcomes of pediatric recurrent abdominal pain: Do they just grow out of it? Pediatrics 108(1):E1, 2001.
6. Barr RG, Rappaport L: Infant colic and childhood recurrent abdominal painsyndromes: Is there a relationship? Devel Behav Pediatr 20:315–317, 1999.
7. Hyams JS, Hyman PE: Recurrent abdominal pain and the biopsychosocial model of medical practice. J Pediatr 133:473–438, 1998.
8. Youssef NN, DiLorenzo C: The role of motility in functional abdominal disorders in children. Pediatr Ann 30:24-30, 2001.
9. Boyle JT: Recurrent abdominal pain: An update. Pediatr Rev 18:310–321, 1997.
10. Barr R: Abdominal pain. In Hoekelman R: Primary Pediatric Care, 2nd ed. St. Louis, Mosby, 1992.
11. Feldman W, McGrath P, Hodgeson C, et al: The use of dietary fiber in the management of simple, childhood, idiopathic, recurrent abdominal pain. Am J Dise Child 9:1216–1218, 1985.
12. Humphreys PA, Gevirtz RN: Treatment of recurrent abdominal pain: Components analysis of four treatment protocols. J Pediatr Gastroenterol Nutrition 31:47–51, 2000.
13. Forster HB, Niklas H, Lutz S: Antispasmodic effects of some medicinal plants. Planta Medica 40:309–319, 1980.
14. Viola H, Wasowski C, Levi De Stein M, et al: Apigenin, a component of maricaria recutita flowers, is a central benzodiazepine receptor ligand with anxiolytic effects. Planta Medica 61:213–216, 1995.
15. Hills JM, Aaronson PI: The mechanism of action of peppermint oil in GI smooth muscle. Gastroenterology 101:55–65, 1991.
16. Kline RM, Kline JJ, DiPalma J, et al: Enteric coated, pH dependent peppermint oil capsules for the treatment of irritable bowel syndrome in children. J Pediatr 138:125–128, 2001.
17. Murray MT: Healing Power of Herbs. Rocklin, CA., Prima Publishing, 1995.
18. Finney JW, Lemanek KL, Cataldo MF, et al: Pediatric psychology in primary health care: Brief targeted therapy for recurrent abdominal pain. Behav Ther 20:283–291, 1989.

57. INFANT COLIC

Joy A. Weydert, M.D., FAAP

1. Define infant colic.

The most widely accepted definition comes from Wessel: colic is unexplained or uncontrollable crying in infants 3 weeks to 3 months of age for more than 3 hours/day on more than 3 days /week for 3 weeks or more (rule of 3s).[1] The crying is usually at the same time every day in the afternoon and evening hours.

2. What are the symptoms of colic?

Crying is the most common symptom. Others include flexing of the knees up to the abdomen, clenching of the fists, reddening of the face, or slight distention of the abdomen. Despite many interventions, such as feeding, holding, or walking with the infant, nothing seems to provide consolation.

3. What causes colic?

Many physicians have theorized that colic is due to an underdeveloped digestive tract, leading to poor digestion, gas, bloating, and abdominal pain. Others speculate possible food allergies. Still other theories have pointed to an immature nervous system that makes infants more sensitive to their environment. This last theory has been questioned because premature infants usually do not develop symptoms of colic until 1–3 months corrected age (the age of the child calculated from its due date rather than the delivery date). Pediatric developmentalists now believe that colic is a behavior, not a condition, which is at the upper end of the spectrum of normally developing infants. Compared to infants without colic, colicky infants do not cry more often—rather, they cry longer, indicating a longer transition from a crying state to a quiet state.[2]

4. Does any factor during pregnancy or delivery contribute to colic?

Studies show that mothers who smoked 15 or more cigarettes per day during pregnancy or in the postpartum period doubled the infant's risk of developing colic.[3] The causative mechanism of this relationship is not fully understood. Other considerations include birth trauma, forceps delivery, or vacuum extraction, which may lead to a higher incidence of colic. Formal studies, however, have not been conducted to determine this relationship.

5. Is colic harmful to the infant?

Colicky infants may be at increased risk of abuse at the hands of exhausted and frustrated caregivers. From a physiologic standpoint, however, they are usually a picture of health, showing good growth and normal development.

6. What is the best approach in evaluating an infant suspected of having colic?

Start with a good history about the crying episodes:
- At what age did the excessive crying begin?
- How many episodes of crying occur in a day?
- When does the crying occur: with or after feedings? at certain predictable times each day?
- Are other problems associated with crying, such as vomiting, fever, diarrhea, weight loss, or poor weight gain?

Also ask abut the following:
- Maternal smoking during and after pregnancy
- History of pregnancy and delivery
- Use of forceps or vacuum extraction
- Measures of comfort already tried

Always obtain the infant's weight to evaluate for losses, and perform a thorough physical examination to assess neurologic development, organomegaly, or other abnormalities. Urinalysis and culture as well as stool for occult blood help rule out certain disorders.

Listen to the caregivers' stories of frustration and empathize with their fatigue. Assess the family support systems, and decide whether social intervention is necessary to help the caregivers cope.

7. What other disorders are in the differential diagnosis? What symptoms are associated with each?

Intussusception. Although rare under the age of 3 months, intussusception is the most common gastrointestinal obstruction in children 3 months to 6 years of age. Typically the infant has a sudden onset of severe pain that recurs at frequent intervals throughout the day and night. The infant may be comfortable and play normally between paroxysms but with each episode demonstrates crying, straining behaviors, and likely vomiting. If the disorder is not recognized, the infant becomes progressively weaker and lethargic. Only two-thirds of patients have the classic currant jelly stools (blood mixed with mucous). This medical emergency needs prompt intervention.[4]

Gastroesophageal reflux disease (GERD). The behavior most commonly associated with GERD is crying with each feeding. The infant may act hungry but upon sucking and swallowing, pulls away from feeds, cries, and arches the back. Feedings may become frustrating for the caregiver as well as the infant because they take a long time to finish. Patients may be "spitty babies" but between feedings often arch, gasp, or cough from the reflux with no apparent vomiting. This disorder can be treated with reflux precautions (e.g., keeping the infants head elevated 30° for feedings and for 1 hour after feeds, frequent burping with feeds, thickening feeds) and H_2 blockers (ranitidine).

Pyloric stenosis (PS). PS most typically develops around 6 weeks of age and seems to have a propensity for first-born males. Another risk factor is a mother who had PS as an infant—she is more likely to have offspring who also develop PS. This disorder is characterized by nonbilious vomiting with each feeding. The vomiting becomes more forceful or projectile with time. The classic physical sign of an olive-sized midepigastric mass is found in 80% of infants with PS.[5] Infants cry because they are hungry but unable to maintain proper nourishment because of the vomiting. They can quickly dehydrate and develop significant electrolyte abnormalities if not diagnosed and treated promptly both medically and surgically.

Milk protein intolerance. This disorder can occur in both bottle-fed infants taking cow's milk formula and breast-fed infant whose mother ingests dairy products. Frequently affected infants are also "spitty" but vomit curdled milk. They may have loose, watery stools. If the problem is prolonged, they can develop bloody stools and, in the worst scenario, edema from a protein-losing enteropathy. Changing to a soy or hydrolyzed casein or whey formula for bottle-fed babies can treat this disorder.[6] In breast-fed infants, instruct the mother to eliminate all cow milk protein from her diet (e.g., milk, cheese, ice cream, creamer, sour cream, yogurt).

8. How do I help families deal with a colicky infant?

Explain that colic is a self-limiting manifestation of normal infant behavior, albeit at the extreme end of the spectrum. Try not to label the infant as "a difficult child" because labels can become self-fulfilling prophesies over the long term. Help caregivers see the infant's positive behaviors and focus on those rather than the momentary colic, which will eventually pass.

Explain that many infants have trouble with self-regulation, which means that once crying starts, it is hard for them to stop. Early response to the crying infant with feeding, holding, or rocking may stop the progression to prolonged crying. Early interventions will not spoil the child.[7] Other comfort measures include bundling, white noise, vibrating chairs, infant massage, warm bath, womb-simulation tape recordings, or glucose water. Give permission for parents to take breaks and encourage assistance from neighbors, friends, and family for respite. This approach promotes bonding between infant and caregivers in the short and long terms.

9. Do dietary changes help?

Dairy products should be avoided in infants with possible milk protein intolerance. If the infant is breastfed, consider what else in the mother's diet may contribute to problems. Gas-forming foods (e.g., broccoli, cauliflower, cucumbers, beans, legumes), citrus foods and juices, caffeine, and chocolate have been implicated as possible culprits.

Another consideration for breast-fed infants is to make sure that they fully empty the first breast to get the rich hind milk before starting on the second breast. Infants are more content after receiving this fuller milk.

Probiotics (*Lactobacillus acidophilus* or *bifidus*) improve digestion and may help in colic, especially if there was a history of antibiotic use during pregnancy or after birth (to rule out sepsis or treat mastitis in breast-feeding mothers). Antibiotics can disrupt the normal flora of the intestines, causing problems with digestion. Probiotics help restore that normal balance and can safely be taken by breast-feeding mothers or dissolved in formula for bottle-fed infants.

The addition of fiber or lactase enzymes has not been shown to help.[8]

10. What herbal remedies have been used for colic?

Calma-Bebi, an herbal tea that contains chamomile, vervain, licorice, fennel, and lemon balm, was used in a study of infants with colic and eased symptoms in more than half of infants when given 1–3 times/day.[9] Chamomile is a well-known soother and relaxant that has been used for centuries by mothers for these reasons. Fennel, peppermint, and ginger have been used historically, although no clinical studies in infants have been conducted to date. The German Commission E approves yarrow, garden angelica, and cardamom for use in infants and breast-feeding mothers.[10] Herbs should be used under the supervision of a qualified expert. Gripe water is a combination of minute amounts of dill seed oil, caraway oil, cinnamon-bark oil, clove bride oil, and cardamom, blended in deionized water, which is used orally for infant colic. Nonalcohol preparations are safest for use in infants.

11. Are any risks associated with using herbal teas in infants?

If herbal products are obtained from reputable companies and distributors, there should no danger of contaminated or unsafe products. One report described two infants who developed fulminant liver failure after ingesting a home-brewed mint tea for calming purposes. It was later discovered that the homegrown plants contained pennyroyal oil, a known hepatotoxin.[11]

Herbal remedies are apparently far safer than conventional drugs, as indicated by information from the Poison Control Center. Herbal remedies are accidentally ingested by children but rarely with harmful results.

Any tea brewed for use in infants should be cooled to room temperature before administration to prevent accidental scalds or burns.

12. What other complementary/alternative therapies can be used for infants with colic?

Homeopathy has a variety of remedies that can be prescribed to infants, depending on their individual nature and constellation of symptoms[12] (see Chapter 13).

- Chamomilla is recommended for infants who are very irritable, draw in their legs, and cry no matter what the caretaker does. Symptoms are worse in the evening and often improve when the infant is carried.
- Colocynthis is for infants who are extremely irritable and seem to have pain that comes in waves. Frequently they double up with the crying. Such infants seem better when firm pressure or warmth is applied to the abdomen.
- Magnesia phosphorica is often used in combination with colocynthis for colicky infants with bloating and gas who get some relief from warmth or bending over. Such infants may appear weak, tired, and exhausted.

Acupressure can be used to activate the digestive system, improve circulation, and relax the nervous system in infants.

Cranial-sacral manipulation can be used in colicky infants with a history of forceps or vacuum extraction at delivery. It is theorized that this type of force on the cranium at the time of birth leads to abnormal pressure on the intracranial nerves, causing nerve irritation. Realigning the cranial sutures and removing the pressure via gentle hands-on therapy can restore normal nervous system activity.

In one study, **chiropractic manipulation** in infants with colic produced a reduction in the number of hours of crying compared with those who did not receive manipulation.[13] These results were not duplicated in another study.[14]

13. Can pharmaceuticals be prescribed for treatment of colic?

Simethicone is widely used but in clinical studies was found to be no better than placebo.[15] Dicyclomine showed some effectiveness but also had worrisome side effects, such as respiratory difficulties, seizures, apnea, syncope, and asphyxia.[16] Methylscopolamine had no benefits but significant side effects.[17]

14. Do infants with colic have recurrent abdominal pain as children or adults?

No.[18]

REFERENCES

1. Wessel MA, Cobb JC, Jackson EB, et al: Paroxysmal fussing in infancy, sometimes called "colic." Pediatrics 14:421–434, 1954.
2. Barr RG: Colic and crying syndromes in infants. Pediatrics 102(5):1282–1286, 1998.
3. Sondergaard C, Henrickson TB, Obel C, et al: Smoking during pregnancy and infant colic. Pediatrics 108:342–346, 2001.
4. Behrman RE, Kliegman R, et al (eds): Nelson Textbook of Pediatrics, 16th ed. Philadelphia, W.B. Saunders, 2000.
5. McMillan JA, De Angelis CD, Feigin RD, et al (eds): Oski Pediatrics, 3rd ed. Philadelphia, Lippincott Williams & Wilkins, 1999.
6. Lucassen PL, Assendelft WJ, Gubbels JW, et al: Infantile colic: Crying time reduction with a whey hydolysate. A double blind randomized placebo-controlled trial. Pediatrics 106: 1349–1354, 2000.
7. Taubman B: Clinical trial of the treatment of colic by modification of parent-infant interaction. Pediatrics 74: 998–1003, 1984.
8. Garrison MM, Christakis DA: A systematic review of treatments for infant colic. Pediatrics 106:184–190, 2000.
9. Weizman Z, Alkrinawi S, Goldfarb D, et al: Efficacy of herbal tea preparation in infantile colic. J Pediatr 122:650–652, 1993.
10. Schilcher H: Phytotherapy in Pediatrics. Stuttgart, Medpharm Scientific Publishers, 1997.
11. Bakering JA, Gospe SM, Dimand RJ, et al: Multiple organ failure after ingestion of pennyroyal oil from herbal tea in two infants. Pediatrics 98:944–947, 1996.
12. Jonas WB, Jacobs J: Healing with Homeopathy. New York, Warner Books, 1996.
13. Wiberg JM, Nordsteen J, et al: The short-term effect of spinal manipulation in the treatment of infantile colic: A randomized controlled clinical trial with a blinded observer. J Manip Physiol Ther 22:517–522, 1999.
14. Olafsdottir E, Forshei S, Fluge G, et al: Randomized control trial of infantile colic treatment with chiropractic spinal manipulation. Arch Dis Child 84:138–141, 2001.
15. Metcalf TJ, Irons TG, Sher LD, et al: Simethicone in the treatment of infant colic: A randomized placebo controlled, multicenter trial. Pediatrics 94: 29–34, 1994.
16. Williams J, Watkins-Jones R: Dicyclomine: Worrying symptoms associated with its use in some small babies. Br Med J 288:901, 1984.
17. Illingsworth RS: Three months colic: Treatment by methylscopolamine nitrate. Acta Paediatr 44: 203–208, 1995.
18. Barr RG, Rappaport L: Infant colic and childhood recurrent abdominal pain syndrome: Is there a relationship? Devel Behav Pediatr 20:315–317, 1999.

58. OTITIS MEDIA

Marcey Shapiro, M.D.

1. Why are children so susceptible to otitis media?
  In children, otitis media (OM) is especially common because the eustachian tube is small and narrow. It is easily closed in the presence of inflammation, preventing drainage of fluids. OM is the most frequently diagnosed illness in children under 15 years of age. In fact, OM is the second most common reason for a child to visit a physician (after well-child check-ups).

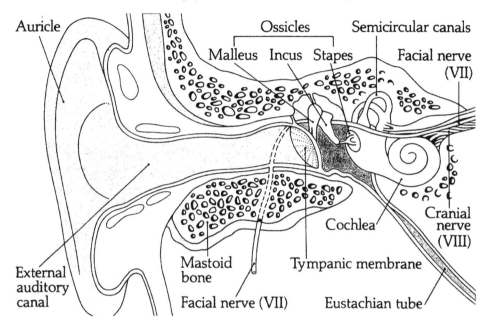

Important structures in the middle ear. (From Zitelli BJ, Davis HW: Atlas of Pediatric Physical Diagnosis, 3rd ed. St. Louis, Mosby–Year Book, 1997/)

2. What common factors indicate uncomplicated OM?
  • Unilateral disease
  • Mild fever or no fever
  • No perforation of eardrum
  • Little or no bulge in tympanic membrane
  • Little or no erythema of tympanic membrane
  • Presence of some movement of tympanic membrane with insufflation (if other favorable factors are noted, absence of this finding alone should not rule out uncomplicated OM)
  • Well appearance
  • Mild pain

3. Which bacterial pathogens are commonly implicated in OM?
  Common bacterial pathogens implicated in acute otitis media include *Haemophilus influenzae, Streptococcus pneumoniae,* and *Brahnamella catarrhalis.*[1] Some studies, however, have found no bacterial pathogen in up to 62% of cases.

4. Why does breast-feeding decrease the risk of acute OM?

Breast-feeding for over 4 months decreases the risk of acute OM for several reasons.[2] Passive immunity is conferred by immune-enhancing constituents of breast milk, such as secretory IgA and lactoferrin,[3] and breast-fed infants also experience later introduction of more allergenic cow's milk (on which most formulas are based). Breast-feeding apparently enhances protection against acute OM for years after it has ceased.[4] Breast-feeding protects infants even in the day-care setting.

5. How can cranial osteopathy aid in the treatment of OM?

A fundamental tenet of osteopathic philosophy is that structure affects function. Obstruction of the eustachian tube contributes significantly to the pathogenesis of OM. In children the eustachian tube is narrow and relatively straight and horizontal. It lies in a space between the temporal and sphenoid bone, opening into the pharynx at the medial pterygoid plate of the sphenoid bone. Osteopaths note that molding of the bones through the compressive forces of the birth process, as well as later trauma, can affect the patency of the eustachian tube because of its anatomic position.[5] Compression of the cranial bones, affecting the function of underlying structures such as the eustachian tube, is termed a cranial osteopathic lesion.

Most cranial osteopaths consider more than one episode of acute OM in a child under 12 months of age to be diagnostic of a cranial osteopathic restriction. Because the cranial bones have some mobility at the sutures, gentle manipulation by a trained practitioner can improve the anatomic relationship of the bones and relieve compression that contributes to stricture of the eustachian tube. A study sponsored by the National Institutes of Health to examine the role of osteopathic manipulation in treatment of pediatric OM is currently under way at the University of Arizona. A referral for a qualified cranial osteopath can be obtained from the Cranial Academy of the American Academy of Osteopathy (AAO) [www.cranialacademy.org].

6. Why is it particularly important to treat a child osteopathically at as young of an age as possible if restriction is present?

In infants, many of the bones of the head are not fused. At birth, for example, the occiput is composed of four separate bones, which partly fuse by 6 months of age and fully fuse by 2 years of age. All bones of the head are more or less set in the adult configurations by about age 7. An infant or child with a strain pattern in the cranium (often caused in the birth process) can be spared much suffering if treated by a qualified cranial osteopath as early as possible. Primary prevention consists of osteopathic assessment of all infants, along with well-infant check-ups, by age 2 months. Children also should be assessed after any fall in which the head is struck.

7. What is the most common cause of cranial injury in young children?

The most common cause of cranial injury in children is falling from tricycles.

8. When is lymphatic drainage appropriate in the management of acute or recurrent OM?

Lymphatic drainage is an important adjunct in treatment of OM. Both osteopaths and some specially trained massage therapists provide this type of treatment. A trained practitioner gently massages to stimulate fluid movement in the lymphatics. Because all lymph eventually flows into the circulatory system, areas closest to the heart are drained first so that blocked flow will have an unobstructed avenue toward the heart. Lymph drainage may be helpful in the acute setting, assisting the body to clear excessive waste products and inflammatory mediators of infection. Its greatest value, however, is in the resolution of chronic or serous otitis and in the prevention of recurrent otitis. In persons, including children, for whom this gentle technique is most appropriate, palpation of anterior, posterior cervical, or posterior auricular lymph nodes reveals congestion or "shotty" adenopathy.

9. How do flavonoids help prevent OM?

A diet high in bioflavonoids helps decrease allergic and inflammatory responses. Often OM is triggered by mucous build-up in an allergic patient. Especially in small children, whose eustachian tube is narrow (< 2 mm), only a small plug of mucous or a small amount of inflammation can close off normal anatomic drainage. Daily consumption of a variety of fresh fruits and vegetables, which contain natural immune-enhancing substances such as bioflavonoids, proanthocyanidins, and antioxidants, allows the body to develop maximal natural resistance to a variety of illnesses.

10. What is the association between day care and development of acute OM?

Infants who attend day care at early ages (< 6 months of age) have an increased risk of acute OM, whereas infants cared for at home have a decreased risk. Of note, infants in day care who are formula-fed are twice as likely as breast fed infants to develop acute OM.[6]

11. What are some of the most commonly chosen homeopathic remedies[7] in OM and the main indications of each[8]?

Belladonna is the appropriate homeopathic remedy when OM frequently affects the right ear. The patient also may have a cold with fever and flushed face. Other typical symptoms include scant thirst and restlessness; light or noise may disturb the patient.

Chamomilla is appropriate when patients are irritable and cranky and cannot be appeased for long. Hot compresses typically exacerbate the pain. Of note, one cheek may be red while the other is pale.

Ferrum phosphoricum is the most commonly used remedy for early OM. Typical findings include dislike of noise and stimulation, gradual onset of symptoms, flushed face, and desire to lie still.

Kali muraticum is appropriate in patients with an earache and a feeling of fullness and congestion in the ear. Hearing may be impaired. Patients may hear popping and cracklings when they swallow or blow the nose. This remedy is also commonly used to clear the eustachian tubes when serous fluid persists after acute OM.

Pulsatilla is used for ear aches associated with colds, especially with white nasal drainage. The pain in the ears is throbbing. The patient wants emotional consolation and may be clingy, weepy, or fidgety or have rapidly changing moods. Heat tends to aggravate the symptoms, and patients have decreased thirst.

12. How does the U.S. compare with other nations in use of antibiotics for acute OM?

The Netherlands has the lowest overall use of antibiotics (only 31% of cases).[9] In Germany, physicians who practice complementary and alternative medicine (CAM) usually treat only 5–10% of cases with antibiotics.[10] In the United States, up to 98% of cases of acute OM are treated with antibiotics. In Britain, most journals now discourage practitioners from using antibiotic treatment in routine upper respiratory tract ailments, including OM.[11]

Although the use of extended courses of antibiotics in OM with effusions is common, it is no longer advised. The Pediatric Upper Respiratory Consensus Team of the American Academy of Family Physicians has advised limiting use of antibiotics to episodes of acute OM.[12]

13. What is the role of second-hand smoke in the pathogenesis of OM?

Parental or caregiver smoking is strongly associated with increased risk of numerous upper respiratory conditions in people, including children, who are exposed to the smoke. Rates of asthma, upper respiratory infections, and OM, both acute and serous, are dramatically increased in children exposed to second hand smoke.[13] Parents and caregivers should not smoke when children are present.

14. Is the smoke from wood fires or stoves safe for children with OM?

No. Burning wood contains many toxins that become airborne when wood fireplaces and stoves are used. These toxins contribute to allergies, which can narrow respiratory pathways and lead to ongoing or acute OM.

15. When are alternative therapies most appropriately used in treating OM?

CAM modalities can be the initial treatment of choice in uncomplicated OM. A review of the evidence indicates that the benefit of antibiotic treatment for all cases of acute OM is minimal; in fact 17 children must receive early antibiotic treatment to prevent one child from experiencing pain at 2–7 days.[14] CAM therapies also seek to address the underlying nutritional, anatomic, and immunologic imbalances that predispose a child to OM.

16. Many children enjoy the taste of chamomile tea. Is it useful for treatment of OM?

Chamomile is a familiar herb used throughout the world by children and adults for over 2000 years. *Matricaria chamomilla, Matricaria recutita,* and *Anthemus nobile* are similar species, all of which are known commonly as chamomile. The German form, *Matricaria chamomilla,* is the best studied for its anti-infective activity and is the preferred variety.

Chamomile is a particularly versatile and gentle herb with a wide range of beneficial actions. In acute OM it is a useful antiviral, anti-inflammatory, and anti-infective agent; it also is soothing to colic and digestive upsets. The essential oil fraction, flavenoids, and sesquiterpene lactones contribute substantially to chamomile's pharmacology. Components of the essential oil fraction, including chamazulene and the spiroethers, are particularly responsible for the anti-infective properties. The flavenoids, particularly apigenin and luteolin, have demonstrated significant anti-inflammatory activity. and the essential oil azulene (chamazulene) is antiseptic, anti-inflammatory, and pain-relieving. All of these qualities make chamomile tea or infusion an excellent first-line remedy for children with acute or ongoing OM.

For tea, which is popular with children, pour 1 cup boiling water over 1 heaping tablespoon of flowers. Cover and steep for 10 minutes; strain and drink once it is cooled.

Occasional allergies to chamomile have been noted, most commonly in people allergic to asters and chrysanthemums. A small test dose should be administered to see if allergies are present in persons unfamiliar with the herb.

17. How is echinacea used in the treatment of OM?

Echinacea angustifolia and *Echinacea purpurea* are native North American plants, known commonly as echinacea. They are used extensively as medicine by Native American tribes and were one of the most popular and widely used herbal anti-infectives in the U.S. before the discovery of antibiotics. Echinacea has demonstrated efficacy as an antibiotic, antiviral, antiseptic, and immunostimulant. Its mechanism of action is considered to be nonspecific activation of the immune system. Research has shown that echinacea activates natural killer cells, increases circulating levels of alpha-interferon, stimulates fibroblasts, and activates macrophages, thus increasing phagocytosis. Pharmacologically significant constituents of echinacea include polysaccharides, caffeic esters, anthocyanins, and alkylamides. Echinacea is fairly well studied and is used for prevention and treatment of colds and flu.[15–17] It is useful in treatment of both acute and serous OM, because it stimulates host defenses and helps clear debris from congested lymphatic passages.

Echinacea is generally used as tincture (1:5). Both water and alcohol extraction yield a full-spectrum echinacea. Glycerites are available for small children and infants. Tablets, capsules, and whole herb taken as tea or infusions are also used orally. Echinacea generally is avoided in people with autoimmune disorders (e.g., systemic lupus erythematosus).

18. Which botanicals help to loosen mucous congestion?

Plants known traditionally as mucilages, such as marshmallow (*Althea officinalis*), slippery elm bark (*Ulmus fulva*), and mullein (*Verbascum thapsus*), can used to loosen and moisten thick mucus that blocks delicate passages such as the eustachian tube. They are considered safe, gentle herbs, useful in soothing inflamed mucous membranes. Marshmallow is also immunostimulating, and mullein has the greatest anti-inflammatory effect. Slippery elm is an endangered species because of Dutch elm disease; until the elms recover, it is best used sparingly. Mucilages are generally given as teas or lozenges, but tinctures and glycerinates are also effective. If marshmallow or slippery elm is taken with prescription medications, the medications should be taken at least 1 hour before or 2 hours after marshmallow root, because the herb may decrease absorption of drugs.

19. When is elder flower useful in treatment of OM?

Elder is an ancient herb that is mentioned frequently in Greek and Roman texts. The botanical names for elder are *Sambucus nigra* (European alder) and *Sambucus canadensis* (American elder). It has over 2000 years of documented use in Eurasia and a strong tradition among Native Americans as well. When OM presents with flu or colds, elder dries mucous and cools inflammation. It is an excellent decongestant. Recent research has shown powerful immunostimulating properties in elderberry extracts. This research supports the traditional use of elder as a tonic for people, including children, who get frequent respiratory infections. The immunostimulant action is attributed, at least in part, to sambucin. Elder is acknowledged as a good herbal antibacterial, antiseptic, antiviral, and anti-inflammatory. For acute OM, it is most appropriate when mucous. allergies, sinusitis, or upper respiratory tract infections (colds) are present.

Important constituents of elder flower include flavenoids, tannins, mucilage, essential oil, and C14-31 n-alkanes, of which sambucin, sambunigrin, and sambucine are notable examples. Elder flower is taken as a tea or tincture and occasionally as a syrup.

20. How is ginger root used in treatment of OM?

Zingiber officinalis, commonly known as ginger, is used as anti-inflammatory and anti-infective for upper respiratory tract infections. Its significant constituents include shogoals and gingeraols, which are anti-inflammatory. Ginger is an important herb in Western, Chinese, and ayurvedic medicine and cuisine; it is recognized worldwide for its warming, decongestant, and soothing properties. It is best used in OM accompanying a cold, especially the type with a lot of clear, watery mucous. It usually is avoided if thick, green mucous or high fever is present. Ginger can be taken as a tea, tincture, candy, or capsule.

21. How is astragalus helpful in preventing incidences of acute OM?

Astragalus membranaceus is one of the most renowned of the traditional Chinese medicinal herbs. It also has been widely studied because of its ability to enhance the immune system. Astragalus is an herb used specifically to strengthen resistance to infections. It is often used in infants, children, and adults who get frequent colds, flus, or ear infections.

Research has discovered that both the polysaccharides and saponins in astragalus are responsible for its immunostimulating properties. Astragalus has been shown to increase the cytotoxicity of natural killer cells in a manner similar to that of alpha-interferon.[18] It also activates macrophages and increases production of interluekin-2, thus enhancing splenic lymphocyte activity.

Astragalus is usually given as a tincture or decoction. There are no known precautions or contraindications.

22. Why is goldenseal *not* a good choice in acute OM?

Goldenseal (*Hydrastis canadensis*) is an excellent antifungal and antibacterial herbal, but it is not highly regarded as an antiviral. Its antimicrobial activity is largely due to berberine alkaloids in direct contact with bacterial or fungal pathogens. Because it is not well absorbed systemically, it is not a good choice for oral administration in acute OM. In addition. large doses may interfere with B vitamin metabolism, and even moderate doses can cause digestive upset, especially in children.

23. What is an allergy rotation diet? How can it be used to discover food allergies that may contribute to OM?

Although there are many methods for determining the foods to which a person is sensitive, the best method is probably an allergy rotation or elimination diet. The patient or caregiver writes down all of the foods that are consumed each day as well as all of the symptoms experienced on that day. No food may be consumed more frequently than every 4 days, and every 7 days is an even better spacing. On its assigned day, a food may be eaten more than once. Symptoms of allergy or sensitivity are not always immediate; in fact, the initial symptoms of food sensitivity may not appear until 24 hours after a food is consumed. If a person has many allergies, a simplified diet at the onset of the allergy rotation protocol is advised, with foods slowly added as they are shown to be tolerable.

Allergy rotation diet can be used in conjunction with other methods of allergy testing, such as skin scratch testing and serum antibody testing. By eliminating offending foods from the diet, as well as correcting intestinal permeability deficits, many people have healed chronic OM.

The most common food allergies include wheat, cow's milk, soy, corn, and strawberries.

24. Describe a good diet for a child who suffers from recurrent OM.

After food allergies are identified and offending foods eliminated, a diet high in nutritious foods such as fresh fruits, vegetables, whole grains, beans, lean meats, and fish is advisable. The diet should be low in processed foods, and consumption of sweets should be minimized. Common foods such as wheat, dairy products, and orange juice are mucous-forming and should be avoided during episodes of upper respiratory infection or acute OM.

25. Can acupuncture be helpful for OM?

Acupuncture is approved by the World Health Organization for treatment of acute OM, and in China acupuncture is used widely for this condition. Although the concept of needles may be quite scary for children, the needles themselves are usually well tolerated. For young or frightened children, acupressure or laser acupuncture may be an appropriate therapeutic choice instead of needling. Acupuncture should be administered only by people with appropriate training.

26. Are pacifiers a good idea for children prone to OM?

No. One study found that children who attend day care and use pacifiers regularly[19] have a significantly increased risk of upper respiratory infection and OM compared with other children in day care. At-risk children should avoid using a pacifier.

27. Which essences in aromatherapy may be useful in OM?

Both practitioners and patients should be especially careful with essential oils, almost all of which are toxic in large doses. They should not be used directly on children's skin. Advise parents to store oils, as they would any medicine, out of reach of children. Ingestion of essential oils can be toxic,and even fatal. Below is a list of relatively safe oils used in treatment of OM as diluted inhalations.

Chamomile (*Matricaria chamomilla*) is used as an anti-inflammatory and antiseptic. It also helps colic, diarrhea, and insomnia associated with acute OM. Chamomile is a gentle oil that is popular worldwide in all age groups. It is used frequently in children because it addresses many problems and is well liked and quite safe. A few drops of chamomile are often used in a bath. The only known contraindication is allergy to chamomile. Be careful that the oil is not introduced into the eye.[20]

Eucalyptus (*Eucalyptus aetheroleum*) is used as an analgesic, anti-inflammatory, antibacterial, antiseptic, antiviral, and expectorant in bronchitis, colds, cough, flu, headache, and sinusitis. It is a well-known oil and flavoring, found in cough drops and chest rubs. It makes an excellent steam inhalation for all sorts of upper respiratory ailments, including OM, because it is antiseptic as well as anti-inflammatory. Its major constituent is cineol. It must be used with caution on mucous membranes. Eucalyptus induces the p 450 system and may decrease efficacy of other drugs.[21] Eucalyptus is contraindicated for use on sensitive, diseased, or damaged skin. It should not be used in children younger than 2 years old and should not be applied to the face of children under age 5.

Helichrysum (*Helichrysum angustifolium*) is among the most frequently used children's oils. It is distilled from the waxy daisy-like flower immortelle (everlasting), which is popular with florists. Helichrysum is not irritating to sensitive skin and is used in baths and skin massages (diluted, of course) even for infants. In treatment of OM it is used as an anti-inflammatory and expectorant and for treatment of allergies. It is also helpful for cough and stomachache. It blends well with other children's' oils (e.g., chamomile, lavender, mandarin). There are no known contraindications to external use.

Rosemary oil (*Rosmarinus officinalis*) has been appreciated as a medicinal plant for at least 2000 years and was known throughout the ancient Mediterranean region. The essential oil fraction of rosemary contributes most to its culinary and medicinal virtues, specifically the phenolic acids such as rosmarinic acid. In treatment of OM, it is used as an analgesic, anti-inflammatory, and antiseptic and helps clear the sinuses. A few drops of the oil are often used in the bath. Rosemary must be used with caution in the presence of a seizure disorder,[22] because it may lower seizure threshold. Do not use the oil directly on sensitive or damaged skin

28. What resources are available for more information about herbal treatments?

- James A. Duke: *Handbook of Medicinal Herbs.* Orlando, FL, CRC Press, 1985.
- Aviva Romm: *Natural Healing for Babies and Children.* Freedom, CA, Crossing Press, 1996.

- Heinz Schilcher: *Phytotherapy in Paediatrics*. Stuttgart, Medpharm Scientific Publishers, 1997.
- Varro E. Tyler: *The Honest Herbal*. New York, Haworth Press, 1993.

REFERENCES:

1. Bluestone CD, Stephenson JS, Martin LM: Ten year review of otitis media pathogens. Pediatr Infect Dis J 11(Suppl 7):1–8, 1992.
2. Duncan B, Ey J, Holberg CJ, et al: Exclusive breast feeding for at least four months protects against otitis media. J Pediatr 120:856, 1992.
3. Qui J, Hendrixson DR, Baker, EN, et al: Human milk lactoferrin inactivates two putative colonization factors expressed by Haemophilus influenzae. Proc Natl Acad Sci USA 95:12641–12646, 1998.
4. Hanson LA: Breastfeeding provides passive and likely long-lasting active immunity. Ann Allergy Asthma Immunol 81:522–533, 1998.
5. Mills et al: Cranial Osteopathic Manipulation in Recurrent Otitis Media. Prototcol for Oklahoma State University College of Osteopathic Medicine Study. Oklahoma State University College of Osteopathic Medicine Study, 1999.
6. Duffy LC, Faden H, Wasielewski R, et al: Exclusive breast-feeding protects against bacterial colonization and day care exposure to otitis media. Pediatrics 100:E7, 1997.
7. Freise KH, et al: Acute otits media in children: Comparison of conventional and homeopathic Treatment. CITY, Hals-Nasen-Oren, 1996, pp 462–466.
8. Panos M, Heimlich J: Homeopathic Medicine at Home. New York, Houghton Mifflin 1980.
9. Glasziou PP, Hayem M, Del Mar CB: Antibiotics for otitis media in children. Cochrane Database System Review (2):CD000219, 2000.
10. Lohman M: Treatment of otitis media: An interdisciplinary interview of experts. ENT J Germany Oct:1-4, 1998.
11. Damoiseaux RA, van Balen FA, Hoes AW, de Melker RA: Antibiotic treatment of acute otitis media in children under two years of age: Evidence based? Br J Gen Pract 48:1861–1864, 1998.
12. Dowell SF, Schwartz B, Phillips WR: Appropriate use of antibiotics for URI's in children. Part 1: Otitis media and acute sinusitis. Am Fam Physician 58:1113–1123, 1998.
13. Owen MJ, Baldwin CO, et al: Relation of Infant feeding practices, cigarette smoke exposure, and group childcare to the onset and duration of otitis media with effusion in the first two years of life. J Pediatr 123:702–711, 1993.
14. Del Mar C, Glasziou P, Hayem M: Are antibiotics indicated as initial treatment for children with acute otitis media? A meta-analysis. Br Med J 314:1526–1529, 1997.
15. Melchart D, Linde K, Worku F, et al: Immunomodulation with echinacea: A systematic review of controlled clinical trials. Phytomed 1:245–254, 1994.
16. Braunig B, Dorn M, Limburg E, Knick E: *Echinacea purpurea* root for strengthening the immune response in flu-like infection. Zeitschr Phytother 13:7–13, 1992.
17. Schoneberger D: The influence of immune stimulating effects of pressed juice of echinacea purpurea on the course and severity of colds. Forum Immunolog 8:2–12, 1992 .
18. Tang W, Eisenbrand G: Chinese Drugs of Plant Origin. Frankfort, Springer-Verlag 1992.
19. Niemela M, Uhari M Mottonen M: A pacifier increases the risk of recurrent acute otitis media in children in day care centers. Pediatrics 96:884–888, 1995.
20. Davis P: Aromatherapy: An A-Z. CITY, C.W. Daniel, 1995.
21. Blumenthal M, et al (eds):. The German Commission E Monographs American Botanical Council. Boston, Integrative Medicine Communications,1998.
22. Tisserand R, Balacs T: Essential Oil Safety: A Guide for Health Professionals. Churchill Livingstone, 1998.

59. ALLERGIC RHINITIS

James Nicolai, M.D.

1. Define allergic rhinitis. How is it classified?

Also known as seasonal allergies or hay fever, allergic rhinitis is an allergic response to pollen, molds, or other microscopic substances found in the environment. It is a typical allergic response in which the immune system incorrectly identifies a normally harmless substance as a threat. Allergies are learned responses of the immune system and can be unlearned and influenced in the right direction with proper lifestyle and environmental modifications.

Allergic rhinitis can be classified as seasonal or perennial. **Seasonal** allergic rhinitis occurs when particular plants, trees, or grasses release pollen during their reproductive cycles. In the springtime, it is usually caused by pollinating trees, whereas during the summer grasses and weeds are the culprits. Autumn brings out ragweed; most molds release their spores during the wet conditions of rainy seasons, usually from late March until November.

Perennial allergic rhinitis usually results from year-round exposure to allergens. Molds that occur in damp indoor areas, dust mites, animal dander, and feathers are typical agents. Usually these irritants can be found in pillows, down clothing, draperies, upholstery, thick carpeting, bedding, shower curtains, and basements. In addition, people are often allergic to more than one agent—a fact that makes change of residence a difficult strategy for escaping allergies.

2. Describe the characteristic allergic reaction.

The allergic response is characterized by three separate reactions that occur in succession:

1. The immune system develops a sensitization to a particular substance, called an allergen. Common allergens are noted in question 1; other examples include latex and various foods (e.g., eggs, nuts, fish, shellfish, dairy products, wheat). First-time exposure to the allergen causes the formation of large amounts of allergic antibodies known as immunoglobulin E (IgE), which are specifically "tagged" to recognize the particular substance.

2. A second exposure causes the allergic reaction. Particles of the substance bind specifically to IgE molecules located on mast cells. Mast cells are a type of white blood cell found mostly in connective tissues, such as the skin and tongue, mucous membranes of the nose and mouth, and lining of the intestinal tract, lungs, and upper airways.

3. Activation of these antibodies causes the mast cell to degranulate, releasing inflammatory chemicals into the blood stream. These chemicals lead to swelling of tissues; itching; dilation, distention, and leakage of blood vessels into surrounding tissue; increased secretions; and tightening of muscles that surround airways. Some of these chemicals attract other white blood cells, known as eosinophils, which contribute to the allergic response.

3. Describe the typical clinical presentation of a patient with allergic rhinitis.

Although the term *rhinitis* specifically refers to inflammation of the nasal passages, allergic rhinitis typically causes inflammation and irritation of the mucous membranes of the nose, upper respiratory tract, and eyes. The condition is characterized by nasal congestion; rhinorrhea; sneezing; itchy, watery eyes with conjunctival injection; and fatigue. A patient may present with allergic shiners—swollen eyelids with slight discoloration, especially of the lower lids. Others may present with nasal polyps or severely inflamed nasal passages. Nasal mucosa can vary from pale and boggy to erythematous and excoriated. Turbinates can be swollen, and patients may complain of sinus pressure or tenderness. The oral mucosa can be injected, and in some cases mild anterior cervical lymphadenopathy is present. Posterior auricular lymph nodes also may be mildly enlarged with tympanic membrane swelling and injection.

4. What can patients do to reduce environmental allergens in their home?

Of the several ways to intervene in the treatment of allergic symptoms, avoidance of the potential allergen seems to be the easiest option (at least on the surface). Basic recommendations include prohibition of smoking in the home, use of a high-efficiency particulate air (HEPA) filter, keeping pets outside, keeping house (and basement) humidity below 50% to prevent mold growth, and routine but thorough house cleaning (to control cockroach debris). For more ways to reduce home environment allergens, there are well-published strategies to follow.[1]

5. What is the differential diagnosis of allergic rhinitis?

Look for structural abnormalities of the nasopharynx, exposure to environmental or occupational irritants, upper respiratory infection, or pregnancy with prominent nasal mucosal edema. Other etiologies to exclude are prolonged use of alpha-adrenergic agents in over-the-counter nasal sprays (rhinitis medicamentosa) or herbal products such as rauwolfia and topical ephedra preparations. Beta-adrenergic antagonists and estrogens also can cause rhinitis-like symptoms.[2] Food allergies can cause similar clinical presentations as classic environmental allergies and should be considered as part of the clinical work-up.

6. Do many people use complementary and alternative therapies to treat allergies?

Allergic rhinitis is the most common allergic disorder in the United States; an estimated 50 million people are affected annually. Allergies are also one of the primary chronic conditions for which people seek alternative therapies, second only to back pain.[3] According to Ziment, U.S. physicians must be "aware that many patients do use alternative medicines for asthma and allergies."[4] Because conventional treatments other than immunotherapy focus on management of symptoms, alternative therapies may offer cheaper, more effective treatment without causing as many side effects.

7. What are the most common pharmacologic options for treatment of allergic rhinitis?

1. **Antihistamines** are the largest group of drugs on the market for the treatment of allergic rhinitis. They help relieve symptoms by blocking H_1 histamine receptors, which are located mainly in the nose and sinus membranes as well as in the lining of the stomach and intestines. First-generation antihistamines readily cross the blood-brain barrier, which partly explains their sedative effects. Second-generation antihistamines, which do not cross the blood-brain barrier, do not cause as much sedation, fatigue, or anticholinergic effects. However, they can have significant side effects (e.g., torsades de pointes) when given with other commonly prescribed medications, such as macrolides, antifungals, or even antidepressants.[5]

2. **Decongestants** are available as nasal sprays, eye drops, and oral preparations in liquid and pill form. Nasal sprays and eye drops can cause a rebound worsening effect and are therefore recommended for only short periods of use (no more than 1 week). Oral decongestants take longer to work and are contraindicated in people with heart disease, hyperthyroidism, glaucoma, and diabetes mellitus.[5]

3. **Nasal sprays and eye drops** are available in four forms:
   - Salt-water solutions relieve mild congestion, loosen mucus, and prevent excess irritation.
   - Decongestants work quickly but are potentially dangerous if used longer than 3–7 days.
   - Corticosteroids reduce inflammation but have local side effects, including nasal irritation, bleeding, and even risk of septal perforation. They are absorbed into the systemic circulation, but concentrations in blood are minimal with proper use.
   - Cromolyn sodium is available as a nasal and eye preparation. It reduces inflammation by keeping mast cells from degranulating but may take weeks to become effective.

4. **Immunotherapy** (allergy shots) may be the most effective form of treatment for long-term allergies. These injections offer gradual exposure to particularly sensitive allergens and help the immune system develop a tolerance. Immunotherapy is a process that requires several years (at least 3–5) and is thought to reduce sensitivity to allergens but not to cure the allergy.

8. Why should we consider alternative therapies for allergic rhinitis?

Although conventional treatments work for many people, a large subset of patients find that they are neither effective nor desirable. Desensitization shots are expensive, can be painful, and are risky.

Antihistamines often reduce itching and calm symptoms but can cause drowsiness and depression. The newer antihistamines are more effective but do not work for everyone and are not cheap. Decongestants and steroids are also effective but have their share of potentially damaging side effects. A recent evaluation of current therapeutic strategies for the management of allergic rhinitis revealed that only 26% of the reported population suffering from hay fever believed their symptoms to be "well-controlled" or "completely controlled," whereas 52% believed that effective treatments were available.[6]

The challenge with conventional drugs is that they suppress or obstruct the allergic process but perpetuate the disease by merely blocking symptoms. Regular use also may interfere with the reeducation of the immune system that must occur for allergic response to be muted. The goal is peaceful coexistence with the common allergens with which the patient comes into contact. Some alternative therapies, such as homeopathy, traditional Chinese medicine, and lifestyle modification, focus on the potential root of the problem as opposed to the symptoms. Other botanicals and supplements work on lessening symptoms but may be cheaper and, in some patients, more effective remedies without the dangerous side effects of over-the-counter or prescription drugs

9. What are the main botanical treatments for allergic rhinitis?

The main botanicals used for allergic rhinitis are stinging nettles, quercetin, and bromelain; their use is supported by the best evidence. Some herbalists combine botanical preparations to create synergistic formulas and include lesser known herbs.

10. How effective are stinging nettles in controlling seasonal allergies?

The leaves of the stinging nettles plant (*Urtica dioica*) have been shown to be quite effective in treating symptoms of hay fever. The recent development of freeze-drying allows stinging nettles to work much like antihistamines without the sedative side effects. A recent randomized, double-blind study in patients with allergic rhinitis reported that almost 50% of patients found freeze-dried stinging nettles (300 mg) to be equally as or more effective than previous medication in treating symptoms.[7] The recommended dose (300 mg/day) should be taken with food. Side effects are rare and typically allergic or gastric in nature, especially if the herb is taken on an empty stomach.

11. How does quercetin work?

Quercetin is a bioflavonoid found in buckwheat, a wide variety of herbs and vegetables, and citrus fruits. It inhibits inflammatory processes, mainly by its action on membranes of specific immune cells. This membrane stabilization prevents mast cells and basophils from degranulating and releasing inflammatory mediators. A Japanese study of mast cells from nasal mucosa of people with perennial allergic rhinitis found quercetin to be almost twice as effective as sodium cromoglycate in inhibiting antigen-stimulated histamine release.[8] Recommended dosages range from 250 to 600 mg 2 or 3 times/day, taken 5–10 minutes before a meal. It should be taken regularly, allowing 6–8 weeks for maximal effect. In addition, the effectiveness of quercetin may be enhanced when it is taken with bromelain.

12. Describe how bromelain is used for allergic rhinitis.

Bromelain, a proteolytic enzyme derived from the stem of the pineapple plant (*Ananas comosus*), has been found to be an effective mucolytic agent, as well as an anti-inflammatory mediator. It reduces platelet aggregation, edema (from decreased vascular permeability), and other prostaglandin-related phenomena.[9] The therapeutic dose for allergic rhinitis ranges from 400 to 500 mg 3 times/day of bromelain with a potency of 1800–2000 milk-clotting units (mcu). Most authorities recommend taking bromelain on an empty stomach, but no comparison data have evaluated its effects when taken with or between meals. Toxicity has been shown to be quite low, and although allergic reactions may occur in patients who are sensitive to pineapple, other side effects, such as gastrointestinal symptoms and menstrual changes, are rare.

13. What other botanicals may be useful?

A recent European study suggested that an extract of butterbur (*Petasites hybridus*), an herbal supplement grown in Europe, Asia, and Africa, offers relief of hay-fever symptoms similar to that of the second-generation antihistamine cetirizine (Zyrtec).[11] There are questions, however, about the study's design, and further research into the efficacy of butterbur extract should be encouraged before it is recommended by conventional physicians.

Other botanicals without large randomized trials but with well-established traditional use for allergic rhinitis include chamomile, elder flower, eyebright, garlic, goldenrod, feverfew, yarrow, and hydrangea root.

14. Are antioxidants useful for the treatment of allergic rhinitis?

Some authorities believe that some of the increase in the rates of asthma and allergy over the past 20 years can be explained by the reduced intake of antioxidant nutrients. Mainly found in fresh fruits and vegetables, antioxidants include beta-carotene, vitamins A, C, and E, and the mineral cofactors essential for antioxidant defense mechanisms (e.g., zinc, selenium, copper). Antioxidants are thought to provide important defense mechanisms for the respiratory tract. In addition, they seem to reduce bronchoconstriction and increased reactivity to other agents caused by free radicals and other oxidizing agents.[12] Specific recommendations include a good high-potency multivitamin with at least 200 mg of vitamin C, 25,000 IU of beta-carotene (preferably with mixed carotenoids), 400–800 IU of vitamin E, and 200 mg of selenium.

15. How has vitamin C been used in the treatment of seasonal allergies?

Vitamin C is especially important to the respiratory tract, because it is the major antioxidant in the mucosal lining of the upper and lower respiratory epithelium. Vitamin C intake in the general population seems to correlate inversely with occurrence of allergy and asthma.[13] Moreover, vitamin C appears to prevent the secretion of histamine from white blood cells, and there seems to be an inverse relationship between histamine levels in the blood and plasma ascorbic acid concentrations. Vitamin C is nontoxic and virtually free of side effects, although gastric disturbances may result from doses greater than 3000 mg. Studies have recommended doses of 2000 mg/day for treatment of allergic rhinitis.[14] More recent data, however, suggest that tissues become saturated at doses of 120–200 mg.[15]

A study in the early 1990s examined the effectiveness of intranasal vitamin C in patients with perennial allergic rhinitis. Subjects sprayed ascorbic acid solution or placebo into the nose 3 times/day. After 2 weeks almost 75% of the treatment group reported decreased nasal symptoms. In addition, the baseline pH of nasal secretions seemed to be more alkaline (7.0–8.0) in patients with allergies. Use of the ascorbic acid solution restored pH to normal ranges (5.5–7.0) and was especially effective for patients with extreme alkaline secretions.[16]

16. Are omega-3 fatty acids important in relieving allergic symptoms?

Several clinical studies have shown that increased intake of omega-3 fatty acids improves airway response to allergens, as well as respiratory function as a whole.[12] These benefits are related to increasing the ratio of omega-3 to omega-6 fatty acids in cell membranes, thereby reducing the production of arachidonic acid. This reduction leads to a shift in synthesis from the extremely inflammatory to the less inflammatory leukotrienes. This shift is directly linked to improvement in symptoms. The effects may take as long as 1 year to become evident as cell membranes incorporate omega-3 fats into their structure. The usual dose is 1–3 gm of omega-3 fatty acids, although higher doses are often recommended.

17. Is acupuncture effective in the treatment of allergic rhinitis?

Acupuncture and traditional Chinese medicine (TCM) tailor the treatment to the individual patient; there are no specific "allergy" points per se (see Chapters 11 and 12). An example of how TCM pathogenic patterns of disease fit the Western diagnosis of allergic rhinitis include **kidney qi deficiency**, which is characterized by cold aversion, facial edema, pale tongue, and "wind-cold type" (associated with nasal obstruction and frequent sneezing).[17]

Although the use of acupuncture for allergic rhinitis has not been verified in western literature, studies are available in the traditional Chinese medicine journals. Two such studies show positive effects with significant decreases in subjective clinical ratings (decreased nasal congestion, discharge, and eye itchiness) as well as laboratory measures.[17,18] The studies, however, have small sample sizes and use less-than-gold-standard techniques for data collection and analysis. Nonetheless, acupuncture is indicated as highly effective in the treatment of allergic rhinitis to the traditional Chinese doctor. It is used either alone or in combination with herbs, meditation, and Chinese massage.

18. What dietary modifications can help reduce susceptibility to environmental allergens?

Dietary changes can influence immune reactiveness profoundly. Foods can either trigger or ameliorate allergic symptoms. Food allergies have been underrecognized as a cause of perennial allergies. The gastrointestinal tract is the largest immune-reacting surface in the body[19] and may be exposed to more potential allergens than the respiratory tract. Complex proteins, such as cow's milk, are suspected of triggering immune reactions because of their highly antigenic nature, especially in sensitive people. On the other hand, beneficial foods fight inflammation and boost natural defense mechanisms. The following specific recommendations are targeted to reduce the immune response to potential allergens:

1. Eat fewer foods and additives that are likely to cause inflammation and allergic reactions, such as saturated fats (specifically animal protein and dairy products), hydrogenated fat in refined or processed food, eggs, citrus, bananas, chocolate, peanuts, shellfish, food coloring, preservatives, caffeine, alcohol, tobacco, and sugar.

2. Eat foods with omega-3 fatty acids, such as cold-water fish (salmon, tuna, sardines, mackerel, herring), flax oil or seeds, and walnuts.

3. Eat more fresh fruits and vegetables, whole grains, nuts, and seeds. Also think about avoiding wheat (another complex possible antigenic protein).

4. Drink plenty of water and fresh juices.

19. What role does the mind/body connection have in the treatment of allergic rhinitis?

Although allergies reflect a biologic oversensitivity of the immune system, it is thought that psychological factors also play a part in the response. Studies evaluating the mind's role in illness have demonstrated the dynamic interplay between belief and immune response. Specifically, evidence suggests that harmless, nontoxic substances can trigger allergic reactions, whereas the same allergic response in the presence of the actual allergen can be blunted. Japanese physicians Ikemi and Nakagawa hypnotized allergic volunteers and told them that a leaf applied to their skin was toxic, similar to poison ivy. The leaf caused patients' skin to become red and irritated. Conversely, when the researchers told the hypnotized subjects that a toxic leaf was harmless and then applied it to the skin, the allergic response was dramatically reduced.[20]

In addition, it has been shown that hives can result from a true allergic reaction or be triggered directly by emotions with no evidence of exposure to a physical allergen. Similar hypnosis experiments have found that hives can be treated successfully with suggestion alone; in addition, symptoms can be recreated either by giving patients direct suggestions of skin irritation or by bringing to mind situations that arouse anger.

By recognizing that the allergic response is a learned reaction of the body's immune system, it is intriguing to realize that these processes can possibly be unlearned or uncoupled. Because the mind can exert a powerful influence on physiologic mechanisms, we can begin to explore ways to modify allergic responses.

20. Does homeopathy work for allergic rhinitis?

Reilly and colleagues at the University of Glasgow recently completed a series of four trials comparing the use of homeopathically prepared allergens (as treatment) with placebo. The purpose of their studies was to determine whether homeopathic dilutions differ from placebo. All four studies used allergy as a model, evaluating effects in atopic patients with hay fever, asthma, and perennial allergic rhinitis. Their findings showed that in all four cases, compared with placebo, homeopathy showed a trend toward a therapeutic effect independent of the placebo response.[21]

The studies by Reilly, et al. were not done for clinical purposes but to prove or disprove the validity of homeopathy as a viable option in general. The facts that allergy was used as a model and that results indicate that homeopathic dilutions differ from placebo suggest that homeopathy may be a viable option for treating symptoms in atopic patients. The specific homeopathic dosage used in these four studies was 30C (30 stages of 1-in-99 serial agitated dilutions) of original standard allergen material (the principal allergen of a particular patient). Their work is the only attempt in western allopathic literature to study homeopathy for the treatment of allergic rhinitis, but the results look promising.

21. What specific homeopathic remedies are used to treat allergic rhinitis?

Another study in the German literature found that a homeopathic nasal spray (brand name: Luffa.comp.-Heel) was as effective and as well tolerated as intranasal cromolyn sodium therapy. The homeopathic dosage was 0.14 ml per application (4 times/day in each naris).[22] Other common remedies for the treatment of allergic rhinitis are listed below. The usual dose is 12X to 30C every 1–4 hours for 2–3 days, with caution to stop if no improvement occurs after 3–4 doses. Treat until symptoms improve.

• Allium cepa for copious irritating nasal discharge and tearing eyes
• Euphrasia for bland nasal discharge with stinging irritating eyes
• Sabadilla for sneezing with watery discharge from nose and eyes
• Wyethis for an itchy nose, throat, and soft palate

If symptoms are not as clear-cut as indicated by these remedies, refer to a licensed homeopathic practitioner.

REFERENCES

1. Economides A, Kaliner MA: Allergic rhinitis. In Kaliner MA (ed): Current Review of Allergic Diseases. Philadelphia, Current Medicine, 2000, pp 227–243.
2. Thornhill SM, Kelly AM: Natural treatment of perennial allergic rhinitis. Altern Med Rev 5:448–454, 2000.
3. Spiegelblatt LS: Alternative medicine: Should it be used by children? Current Probl Pediatr 25(6):180–188, 1995.
4. Ziment I: Alternative therapies for asthma. Curr Opin Pulm Med 3:61–71,1997.
5. Milgrom H, Bender B: Adverse effects of medications for rhinitis. Ann Allergy Asthma Immunol 78:439–444, 1998.
6. Storms MD, Meltzer EO, Nathan RA, Seiner JC: Allergic rhinitis: The patient's perspective. J Allergy Clin Immunol 99:825–828, 1997.
7. Mittman P: Randomized, double blind study of freeze dried Urtica dioica in the treatment of allergic rhinitis. Planta Med 56:44–47, 1990.
8. Otsuka H, Inaba M, Fujikura T, Kunitomo M: Histochemical and functional characteristics of metachromic cells in the nasal epithelium in allergic rhinitis: Studies of nasal scrapings and their dispersed cells. J Allergy Clin Immunol 96:528–536, 1995.
9. Taussig S: The mechanis of the physiological action of bromelain. Med Hypothesis 6:99–104, 1980.
10. Kelly GS: Bromelain: A literature review and discussion of its therapeutic applications. Altern Med Rev 1:243–257, 1996.
11. Schapowal A: Randomised controlled trial of butterbur and cetirizine for treating seasonal allergic rhinitis. Br Med J 324:144, 2002.
12. Murray MT, Pizzorno J: Asthma and hay fever. In Murray MT, Pizzorno J (eds): Encyclopedia of Natural Medicine, 2nd ed, Rocklin, CA, Prima Publishing, 1998, p 266.
13. Clemetson CA: Histamine and ascorbic acid in human blood. J Nutr 110:662–668, 1980.
14. Bucca C, Rolla G, Olivia A, Farina JC: Effect of vitamin C on histamine bronchial responsiveness of patients with allergic rhinitis. Ann Allergy 65:311–314, 1990.
15. Levine M, Rumsey SC, Daruwala R, et al: Criteria and recommendations for vitamin C intake. JAMA 281:1415–1423, 1999.
16. Podoshin L, Gertner R, Fradis M: Treatment of perennial allergic rhinitis with ascorbic acid solution. Ear Nose Throat J 70:54–55, 1991.
17. Lingling T: A clinical observation on therapeutic effects of acupuncture for allergic rhinitis. J Trad Chin Med 19(2):129–131, 1999.
18. Lau BH, Wong DS, Slater JM: Effect of acupuncture on allergic rhinitis: Clinical and laboratory evaluations. Am J Chin Med 3:263–270, 1975.
19. Barrie S: Food allergies. In Pizzorno JE, Murray JT (eds): Textbook of Natural Medicine, 2nd ed. Edinburgh, Churchill Livingstone, 1999, p 456.
20. Grossbart TA: The skin: Matters of the flesh. In Goleman D, Gurin J (eds): Mind/Body Medicine: How to Use Your Mind for Better Health. New York, Consumer Reports Books, 1993, pp 157–158.
21. Taylor MA, Reilly D, Llewellyn-Jones RH, et al: Randomised controlled trial of homeopathy versus placebo in perennial allergic rhinitis with overview of four trials. Br Med J 321:471–476, 2000.
22. Weiser M, Gegenheimer LH, Klein P: A randomized equivalence trial comparing the efficacy and safety of Luffa comp.-Heel nasal spray with cromolyn sodium spray in the treatment of seasonal allergic rhinitis. Forsch Komplementarmed 6:142–148, 1999.

60. ASTHMA

John D. Mark, M.D.

1. What is asthma?

Asthma is a chronic inflammatory process involving the airways of the lungs. Its many components include excessive mucus production due to increased goblet cells, bronchial smooth muscle hypertrophy with increased interstitial collagen, and damaged epithelial cells with cellular leakage. Untreated, this chronic inflammatory process can lead to irreversible changes involving fibrosis and remodeling of the airways. Asthma is thought to have a strong genetic predisposition along with environmental factors that trigger the typical symptoms of cough, wheeze, and shortness of breath. About 6–7.5 % of children and 5% of adults suffer from asthma.[1]

2. Describe the conventional approach to treating asthma.

The National Institutes of Health and the National Heart, Lung, and Blood Institute formed a National Asthma Education and Prevention Program in 1997.[2] This panel of experts formulated guidelines for diagnosing, categorizing, and treating both children and adults with asthma. Recommendations include the following:

- The use of objective measures of lung function (such as peak flow meters and spirometers) to assess the severity of asthma and to monitor the course of treatment
- Environmental control measures to avoid or eliminate factors that trigger asthma symptoms or flare-ups
- Medication therapy for long-term management to reverse and prevent airway inflammation as well as therapy to manage asthma flare-ups (the most common medications are inhaled corticosteroids for chronic use and beta agonists for exacerbations)
- Patient education to foster a partnership of patient, family, and health care providers

3. What are the six goals for the effective management of asthma?

1. Prevent chronic and troublesome symptoms.
2. Maintain near-normal breathing.
3. Maintain normal activity levels, including exercise.
4. Prevent recurrent asthma flare-ups, and minimize the need for emergency department visits or hospitalizations.
5. Provide optimal medication therapy with no or minimal adverse effects.
6. Meet patients' and families' expectations of satisfactory asthma care.

4. Is asthma in children different from asthma in adults?

Although asthma may present at any age, it is common in childhood in association with viral illnesses, such as bronchiolitis (from respiratory syncytial virus) and the common cold. One study showed an 80–85% correlation with viral upper respiratory infection and asthma exacerbation in school-age children.[3] There is also a high association with atopic dermatitis. Some children simply wheeze with certain infections, primarily in the first 3 years of life as the immune system is building itself. Often, with subsequent growth of the airway width, they no longer have this respiratory symptom.

5. How does a child "grow out" of their asthma?

If the person does not have wheezing due simply to small airways (see previous question), the term "grow out of asthma" has a different meaning. Some children and adults have highly sensitive airways with asthma exacerbations triggered by weather change, emotional outbursts, exposure to dust or perfume, exercise, and mild viral respiratory illnesses (common colds). If the asthma is well-treated—i.e., controlled with anti-inflammatory medications and suppression of environmental triggers (bedding encased, pets outdoors)—some children appear to "outgrow" asthma. They have asthma by spirometry if induced by methacholine challenge or exercise but in daily life may not have any symptoms or require medication.

6. What factors are common triggers of asthma symptoms?
- Allergens
- Viral or sinus infections
- Exercise
- Gastroesophageal reflux disease (potential cause of airway irritation and inflammation)
- Medications or foods
- Emotional anxiety

7. How do irritants differ from triggers? Give examples of common irritants.
Some substances do not trigger allergies but can nonetheless aggravate the airways. These substances, called irritants, can also cause asthma symtoms:
- Air pollutants, such as tobacco smoke, wood smoke, chemicals in the air, and ozone
- Occupational exposure to allergens, vapors, dust, gases, or fumes
- Strong odors or sprays, such as perfumes, household cleaners, cooking fumes (especially from frying), paints, or varnishes
- Other airborne particles, such as coal dust, chalk dust, or talcum powder
- Changing weather conditions, such as changes in temperature and humidity, barometric pressure, or strong winds

8. How are anxiety and emotions related to asthma symptoms?
Asthma exacerbations can be triggered by emotional stress. One study[4] suggests that 35–40% of asthmatic patients may respond to stress or suggestion of stress with bronchoconstriction. But certainly wheezing, chest tightness, and inability to get enough air into the lungs can create anxiety. Asthmatic patients score high on depression scales and accordingly have worse quality of life. But do the depression and anxiety cause the asthma, or are asthma patients depressed because of their disease? Airway reactivity, shortness of breath, and increased respiratory resistance have been reported after an emotional challenge in asthmatic patients.[5] Psychosocial factors also contribute to the persistence of infantile asthma into childhood.[6]

Learning to control anxiety and enhance relaxation may benefit patients with asthma. Biofeedback specifically aimed to help patients relax, or to take slow, deep breaths has been shown to improve lung function, reduce severity of symptoms, and decrease medication use and emergency department visits.[7,8] A recent study showed that expressive writing about stressful life experiences significantly improved the health status of patients with asthma, including improvement in forced expiratory volume in one second (FEV_1), compared with matched controls.[9]

9. What botanicals are commonly used for asthma?
Use of botanicals is the oldest traditional treatment for asthma worldwide. Some of these therapies have been used effectively for thousands of years, but little scientific research proves efficacy and safety. Some of the more common examples include:
- Gingko (*Gingko biloba*): active ingredients are ginkgolides, which inhibit platelet-activating factor and thus decrease airway inflammation and allergic reaction.[10]
- Coleus (*Coleus forskohlii*): thought to act much like theophylline by increasing cyclic adenosine monophosphate (cAMP); studied for its effect as a bronchodilator.[11]
- Ma huang (*Ephedra sinica*): ephedrine, the active ingredient in ma huang, is a potent bronchodilator but unfortunately also stimulates cardiac activity. Improper use has led to adverse side effects, including tachyarrhythmias and even death.[12]
- Licorice (*Glycyrrhiza glabra*): has an anti-inflammatory effect and enhances endogenous steroids; also thought to be an expectorant, aiding in the expulsion of mucus in the bronchial passages. Because the glycyrrhizin component of licorice can increase blood pressure, it must be used with caution in people with hypertension.[13]

10. What dietary supplements are used in the treatment of asthma?

Antioxidants theoretically fight the oxygen radicals released from inflamed bronchial cells. Higher **vitamin C** intake has been associated with 30% lower incidence of bronchitis and wheezing,[14] but studies of vitamin C supplementation have been mixed. **Vitamin B$_6$** (pyridoxine) is found in lower concentrations in asthmatic patients,[15] and supplementation at doses of 50–100 mg 2 times/day has shown some reduction in wheezing, exacerbations, and medication use.[15,16] Patients taking theophylline may have lower serum levels of B$_6$ because its active form may be depleted in theophylline metabolism.

Magnesium has been shown in both epidemiologic studies and acute intervention trials to play an important role in treatment of asthma. Lower levels of magnesium have been directly correlated with severity of asthma.[17,18] Dietary intake of magnesium has been correlated with significantly higher FEV$_1$ and lowered airway hyper-reactivity,[19] although magnesium supplementation has had mixed results. Intravenous magnesium sulfate, given to adults and children presenting with severe asthma or status asthmaticus, results in rapid improvements in pulmonary status.[20–22]

Fish oils are rich sources of **omega-3 fatty acids**. In adequate amounts in the diet, omega-3 oils may limit leukotriene synthesis, block arachidonic acid metabolism, and thus improve asthma symptoms. Because regular amounts of cold-water oily fish (mackerel, sardines, herring, salmon, and cod) are not standard in most western diets, the use of fish oil capsules has become more popular.

11. Can any dietary supplements or botanicals interfere with conventional medications for asthma?

Ma huang, a plant with natural ephedrine compounds that has been used for thousands of years, has been reported to cause palpitations, tachycardia, headache, anxiety, and even seizures when used in combination with medications such as beta agonists (albuterol, salmeterol) and theophylline preparations.

Licorice poses theoretical problems when used with conventional therapy. True licorice (not the common anise-flavored candy) may enhance endogenous steroids. If the patient is using either inhaled or oral steroid medications, blood pressure, edema, and other signs of aldosteronism should be monitored.

None of the listed vitamins and minerals should interfere with conventional asthma medications, although high-dose vitamin C (> 5 gm/day) has caused renal problems, high doses and prolonged use of vitamin B$_6$ have caused peripheral neuropathy, and high-dose magnesium has caused diarrhea.

12. What role does nutrition play in the development of asthma?

Diet therapies or nutritional advice is the most common alternative therapy given by conventional physicians to patients with asthma. Eliminating certain allergenic foods and decreasing exposure to such foods as dairy products (associated with increased mucus production) may help reduce chronic symptoms and severity.[23] The biogenic amines in yeast and cheese have occasionally been implemented in the pathophysiology of bronchoconstriction.[24] Other common food triggers for asthma are eggs, artificial coloring, and wheat.[25] Some epidemiologic studies suggest that populations with an increased polyunsaturated fatty acid intake have an increased prevalence of asthma, eczema, and allergic rhinitis.[26]

13. List common nutritional recommendations for patients with asthma.

1. Eliminate potential food allergens, especially if the patient has a history of food intolerance or eczema. Sulfites, to which asthmatics may be sensitive, are found in many food substances, including dried fruits. Additives such as aspartame, benzoates, and food colorings should be avoided.[27]

2. Decreasing or eliminating dairy products is recommended, but no study supports this strategy for all asthmatics. It may be worth trying the elimination of all dairy products for 3–4 weeks and then reintroducing them to evaluate symptom progression.

3. Increase intake of fruit and vegetables, which are rich in antioxidants that have been shown to be low in patients with chronic lung problems such as asthma.

4. Increase omega-3 fatty acid intake by eating cold-water fish (e.g., sardines, herring, salmon); decrease omega-6 fatty acids found in corn and safflower oils, and use olive oil in its place.

5. Breast-feed infants (especially with strong family history of atopy) to reduce the risk of asthma during childhood.[28]

14. What can be done to the patient's environment to improve asthma?

Reducing exposure to dust mites, *Dermatophagoides pteronyssinus*, and cockroaches may help reduce the antigenic load in sensitive patients. House dust mites are ubiquitous microscopic insects that live off dead skin flakes. Studies correlate dust mite exposure with asthma symptoms.[29] To reduce exposure to dust mites, especially in the bedroom where they are most often found, enclose pillows and mattress in airtight polyurethane covers, or use fiberfill products instead of down or foam pillows; remove carpeting (hardwood or linoleum is better) and curtains; wash sheets and stuffed toys (for pediatric patients) in hot water every week; and clean bedrooms 2–3 times/week with a vacuum with an added HEPA filter. Cockroaches and their feces are another trigger for asthma[30,31]; cleanliness is important to decrease cockroach debris.

15. Does hypnosis help decrease symptoms of asthma or only make the person "feel better"?

Hypnosis has been successfully used in asthma management.[32] It has been also used for achieving relaxation, relieving pain, and helping with physical discomfort. Because it is multidimensional, it aids patients in developing a heightened concentration of an idea or image. Hypnosis has been shown to be effective in patients with mild asthma, especially if their symptoms have an emotional component. If the asthmatic patient is motivated, symptoms and medication use often decrease and pulmonary function improves.[34]

Guided imagery is a form of self-hypnosis in which patients use an image of their own creation after an initial relaxation period to help decrease asthma symptoms. This technique is especially effective in children who enjoy an active and vibrant imagination. They often can be taught guided imagery in less than 30 minutes, and their asthma symptoms improve after a few practice sessions.

16. Since exercise can cause asthma symptoms, should it be avoided in patients with asthma?

Although exercise can induce symptoms in patients with asthma, numerous studies have shown that asthma can be better controlled in patients who exercise regularly.[35] It has been assumed that swimming may be more beneficial then other types of exercise because the environment is moist, whereas cold dry air may exacerbate asthma symptoms. Adequate fluid intake to prevent dehydration during exercise is also important. Any exercise that the patient will do on a regular basis and that does not cause increase symptoms should be encouraged.

Older patients (over 50 years old) seem to do better than younger age groups if they follow an exercise regimen. This finding may be due in part to a better self-image and overall improved health. Yoga is a form of exercise that helps many patients with asthma. The cardiovascular component involves regulated breathing exercises (pranayama) and, in many yoga practices, a mind-body component using relaxation and meditation. In one study of asthmatic adults, yoga helped decrease medication use and anxiety.[35]

17. What is the role of homeopathy in treating asthma?

Several studies have shown the efficacy of homeopathic remedies in the treatment of both asthma and allergies.[36] The remedies depend on the patient's symptom pattern and should be selected on individual basis by an experienced homeopath (see Chapter 13). Some of the commonly used homeopathic remedies include:

- *Arsenicum album*: used for asthma with restlessness and anxiety.
- Ipecac: used for chest constriction and cough.
- Pulsatilla: used for chest pressure and air hunger.
- Sambuscus: used for asthma symptoms that awaken the patient during the night.

18. Does acupuncture help asthmatics?

Acupuncture and other forms of traditional Chinese medicine can be beneficial in the treatment of asthma. Clinical observations suggest that acupuncture and individually mixed Chinese herbs are effective, although clinical trials have not supported these observations. The National Institutes of

Health 1997 Consensus Development Conference recommended acupuncture for many conditions, including asthma. One review demonstrated modest improvement in asthma symptoms using acupuncture,[37] whereas another study suggested that acupuncture before exercise protected against exercise-induced symptoms.[38]

19. Do massage therapy and other manipulative modalities help in treating asthma?

Massage therapy is an ancient treatment, dating back to the second century in China. It was called the "art of rubbing" and was common until the time of large use of pharmaceutical agents starting in the 1950s. Current studies in children with asthma have shown that daily massage improves airway caliber and control of asthma,[39] decreases anxiety, and improves attitude toward the condition.

Other manipulative therapies, such as chiropractic and osteopathic manipulation, are adjunctive treatments for patients with asthma. Although data are minimal, manipulative therapies have been reported to be safe and helpful in many asthmatic adults. Applying manual therapy to reduce musculoskeletal restriction of ribcage function in patients with chronic airway disease appears to improve lung ventilation through changes in posture and deep breathing instructions.

20. Can combinations of different modalities of complementary/alternative medicine (CAM) be used in treating asthma?

It is important to discuss the use of different types of CAM therapies with a health care practitioner. At times some of the modalities may enhance and complement each other well. For example, using massage in addition to exercise and nutritional changes may give a person with asthma the extra support and improved airway function to allow gradual improvement in symptoms. However, if a patient with asthma is taking a traditional Chinese herbal mixture, caution should be exercised in regard to dietary supplements and botanicals because of possible overlapping, herb–herb interactions, or adverse side effects.

21. Should regular medications, such as inhaled steroids and albuterol, be stopped if CAM therapies are used in treating asthma?

In general, conventional medications such as cromolyn, steroid inhalers, beta$_2$ agonists, and leukotriene receptor modifiers should be continued even if the patient is using CAM therapies. It is important to discuss with both the CAM practitioner and the conventional practitioner what medications the patient is taking because several drug–herbal interactions have been recently described. Some botanicals and supplements also may have side effects that are wrongly attributed to the conventional medications. If an integrative approach is taken, the patient is given a care plan that best suits his or her symptom complex. The risk of problems using these different modalities even with conventional therapies diminishes dramatically.

22. Why is asthma increasing worldwide if conventional treatment and CAM therapies are better than ever?

Many experts worldwide have been trying to answer this question. In general, it is believed that, although the genetic predisposition is the same, stronger environmental influences may cause the greater incidence and prevalence of asthma. Environmental exposure may include both prenatal and postnatal exposure to such triggers as air pollution, environmental toxins, and diet. There has been speculation that the dramatic increase throughout the past century in the dietary intake of omega-6 fatty acids (vegetable oils) and the decrease in omega-3 fatty acids (flax seed, natural grasses, cold-water fish) may contribute to proinflammatory cellular conditions.

Another theory is that routine childhood immunizations and subsequent decrease in certain viral infections (e.g., measles) has caused a shift from the usual immune response in early childhood to a response that is more cellular and more prone to illnesses such as asthma. These observations also have become important in directing treatment of asthma. Long-term therapy is necessary to suppress chronic airway inflammation and should include not only medications but also changes in diet, lifestyle, and environment for optimal management and well-being.

REFERENCES

1. Miller AL: The etiologies, pathophysiology, and alternative/complementary treatment of asthma. Altern Med Rev 6:20–47, 2001.
2. National Institutes of Health: Guidelines for the diagnosis and management of asthma: Expert Panel Report 2. Bethesda, MD, NIH Publication No. 97-4051, 1997.
3. Johnston SL, Pattemore PK, Sanderson G, et al: Community study of role of viral infections in exacerbations of asthma in 9–11 year old children. Br Med J 310:1225–1229, 1995.
4. Isenberg SA, Lehrer PM, Hochron S: The effects of suggestion and emotional arousal on pulmonary function in asthma: A review and a hypothesis regarding vagal mediation. Psychosom Med 54:192–216,1992
5. Miller AL: The etiologies, pathophysiology, and alternative/complementary treatment of asthma. Altern Med Rev 6:20–47,2001.
6. Klinnert MD, Nelson HS, Price, MR, et al: Onset and persistence of childhood asthma: Predictors from infancy. Pediatrics 108(4):e69, 2001 [http://www.pediatrics.org/].
7. Kern-Buell CL, McGrady AV, Conran PB, Nelson LA: Asthma severity, psychophysiological indicators of arousal, and immune function in asthma patients undergoing biofeedback-assisted relaxation. Appl Psychphysiol Biofeedback 25:79–91, 2000.
8. Peper E, Tibbetts V: Fifteen-month follow-up with asthmatics utilizing EMG/incentive inspirometer feedback. Biofeedback Self Regul 17:143–151,1992.
9. Smyth JM, Stone AA, Hurewitz A, Kaell A: Effects of writing about stressful experiences on symptom reduction in patients with asthma or rheumatoid arthritis: A randomized trial. JAMA 281:1304–1309,1999.
10. Review of Natural Products: Gingko. St. Louis, Facts and Comparisons, 1998.
11. Pizzorno J, Murray M: Coleus forskohlii. In Murray M (ed): Textbook of Natural Medicine, 2nd ed. London, Harcourt Brace, 1999.
12. Haller CA, Benowitz NL: Adverse cardiovascular and central nervous system events associated with dietary supplements containing ephedra alkaloids. N Engl J Med 343:1833–1838, 2001.
13. Brinker F: Herb Contraindications and Drug Interactions. Sandy, OR, Eclectic Medical Publications, 1998.
14. Schwartz J, Weiss ST: Dietary factors and their relation to respiratory symptoms. The Second National Health and Nutrition Examination Survey. Am J Epidemiol 132:67–76, 1990.
15. Reynolds RD, Natta CL: Depressed plasma pyridoxal phosphate concentrations in adult asthmatics. Am J Clin Nutr 41:684–688,1985.
16. Collipp PJ, Goldzier S, Weis N, et al: Pyridoxine treatment of childhood bronchial asthma. Ann Allergy 35:93–97,1975.
17. Alamoudi OS: Hypomagnesemia in chronic, stable asthmatics: Prevalence, correlation with severity and hospitalization. Eur Respir J 16:427–431, 2000.
18. Hashimoto Y, Nishimura Y, Maeda H, Yokoyama M: Assessment of magnesium status in patients with bronchial asthma. J Asthma 37:489–486, 2000.
19. Britton J, Pavord I, Richards K, et al: Dietary magnesium, lung function, wheezing, and airway hyperactivity in a random adult population sample. Lancet 344:357–362, 1994.
20. Harari Mm, Barzillai R, Shani J: Magnesium in the management of asthma: Critical review of acute and chronic treatments, and Deutsches Medizinsches Zentrum's (DMZ's) clinical experience at the Dead Sea. J Asthma 35:525–536, 1998.
21. Schiermeyer RP, Finkelstein NA: Rapid infusion of magnesium sulfate obviates need for intubation in status asthmaticus. Am J Emerg Med 12:164–166,1993.
22. Gurkan F, Haspolet K, Bosnak M. et al: Intravenous magnesium sulfate in the management of moderate to severe acute asthmatic children nonresponding to conventional therapy. Eur J Emerg Med 6:201–205, 1999.
23. Ziment I: How your patients may be using herbalism to treat their asthma. J Respir Dis 19:1070–1081, 1998.
24. Baker GJ, Collett P, Allern DH: Bronchospasm induced by metabisulphite-containing food and drugs. Med J Aust 2:614–616, 1981.
25. Lewith GT, Watkins AD: Unconventional therapies in asthma: An overview. Allergy 51:761–769, 1996.
26. Haby M, Peat J, Marks G, et al: Asthma in preschool children: Prevalence and risk factors. Thorax 56:589–595, 2001.
27. Wraith DG, Merrett J, Roth A, et al: Recognition of food allergic patients and their allergens by the RAST technique and clinical investigation. Clin Allergy 9:25–36, 1979.
28. Haby MM, Peat JK, Marks GB, et al: Asthma in preschool children: Prevalence and risk factors. Thorax 56:589–595, 2001.
29. Sporik R, Holgate ST, Platts-Mills TAE, Cogswell JJ: Exposure to house-dust mite allergen (Der p 1) and the development of asthma in childhood: A prospective study. N Engl J Med 323:502–507, 1990.

30. Call RF, Smith TF, Morris E. et al: Risk factors for asthma in inner city children. J Pediatr 121:862–866, 1992.

31. Rosenstreich DL, Eggleston P, Kattan MM, et al: The role of cockroach allergy and exposure to cockroach allergen in causing morbidity among inner-city children with asthma. N Engl J Med 336:1356–1363, 1997.

32. Ewer TC, Stewart DE: Improvement in bronchial hyperresponsiveness in patients with moderate asthma after treatment with a hypnotic technique: A randomised controlled trial. Br Med J 293:1129–1132, 1986.

33. Kohen DP, Wynne E: Applying hypnosis in a preschool family asthma education program: Uses of story-telling, imagery and relaxation. Am J Clin Hypnosis 39:169–181, 1997.

34. Hallstrand TS, Bates PW, Schoene RB: Aerobic conditioning in mild asthma decreases the hyperpnea of exercise and improves exercise and ventilatory capacity. Chest 118:1460–1469, 2000.

35. Vedanthan PK, Kesavalu LK, Murthy KC, et al: Clinical study of yoga techniques in university students with asthma: A controlled study. Allergy Asthma Proc 19:3–9, 1998.

36. Taylor MA, Reilly D, Llewellyn-Jones, et al: Randomised controlled trial of homoeopathy versus placebo in perennial allergic rhinitis with overview of four trial series. Br Med J 321:471–476, 2000.

37. Jobst KA: Acupuncture in asthma and pulmonary disease: An analysis of efficacy and safety. J Altern Complement Med 2:179–120, 1996.

38. Fung KP, Chow OK, So SY: Attenuation of exercise-induced asthma by acupuncture. Lancet 2:1419–1422, 1986.

39. Field T, Henteleff, T, Hernandez-Reif M, et al: Children with asthma have improved pulmonary functions after massage therapy. J Pediatr 132:854–858, 1998.

IV. Special Topics

61. DRUG–HERB INTERACTIONS

Monica J.Stokes, M.D., FACOG

1. What are the key differences between botanical medicines and drugs?

The World Health Organization estimates that 80% of the world's population relies on botanicals for primary healthcare needs. The use of botanicals from many traditions has increased dramatically in the U.S. in the past 10 years.

Most herbs are less concentrated, have a more gradual onset of action, and reach therapeutic levels at lower serum concentrations than the average prescription drugs, which have a narrow therapeutic range and reach peak concentrations far above that range. Herbs are known to have a much lower incidence of side effects and generally cost much less than drugs. Whole herb preparations (e.g., dried herb, teas, decoctions, tinctures, other solutions, powders, freeze-drying) as opposed to single, isolated products (e.g., pure salicylic acid) contain multiple, even hundreds of naturally occurring constituents. Whole herbs have multiple active compounds that act synergistically, inert ingredients and constituents with unknown properties.

Extracts of herbs are concentrated preparations. Different herbs may require different and/or sequential extraction procedures, depending on the specific constituents that one is interested in preserving, concentrating, or removing from the crude herb.

2. How important is standardization of botanicals?

For the health care provider accustomed to using a specific dosage to achieve a specific effect, standardization is very important. The standardization process guarantees a uniform concentration (bottle to bottle and capsule to capsule) only of the constituent to which the product is standardized (a marker compound or the one constituent believed to be the most active based on available research), but it usually remains a whole herb product. For example, the active ingredient in St. John's wort was thought to be hypericin, and good manufacturers standardized their products to guarantee 0.3 hypericin. Recent data showed that another ingredient, hyperforin, may be more important, and St. John's wort is commonly standardized to 4% hyperforin as well. The quality of market herbal products varies widely, although industry standards for quality do exist (American Herbal Products Association and Good Manufacturing Practice Guidelines).

3. Why doesn't the FDA regulate herbal products in the United States?

The Dietary Supplements Health and Education Act of 1994 (DSHEA) changed the legal status of botanical medicines in the U.S. Although it clarified some issues, application of the DSHEA is a work in progress. The act places the burden of proof on the Food and Drug Administration (FDA) to show (in court) that an herb or dietary supplement is unsafe before it can be involuntarily removed from the market. Although the FDA cannot establish or regularly enforce standards of quality for botanicals, it may investigate products that make disease treatment claims or those against which complaints have been lodged. DSHEA allows a label to claim only how an herb or a constituent helps maintain body structure or function ("support" claims). For example, the phrase "supports immune function" is allowed, but not the phrase "supports the body's ability to resist infection."

Botanical products that choose to engage in the extensive and expensive FDA approval process, which includes considerable documentation and clinical research, can make disease claims just as over-the-counter drugs do.

4. What benefit may whole herbs have over isolated pure components?

Constituents in whole herb products may provide early warning signs of toxicity that allow discontinuance of use before a serious, potentially life-threatening situation arises. An excellent example is the crude preparation of the foxglove (*Digitalis* species) leaf vs. digoxin, which is the isolated constituent drug derived from the foxglove plant. The whole leaf product gives early signs of toxicity, such as nausea and vomiting, when taken to excess, but the first sign of digoxin toxicity is often cardiac dysrhythmia. Protective constituents in the whole foxglove plant apparently are left behind when only pure digoxin is isolated.

5. What benefits and problems do pharmaceutical drugs have compared with botanicals?

Pharmaceutical products, in general, have a more rapid onset of action, a narrow therapeutic range, and increased risk of toxicity. The physiologic potency can be measured in terms of weight of the isolated constituent. The benefits include easier identification, consistency of expected dosing, convenience of administration, purity, and FDA oversight of production, safety, and efficacy. Drugs have strong and sometimes long-lasting effects, which often affect non-target systems in the body and may lead to a much larger catalog of undesired short- and long-term side effects than the majority of botanicals. According to Lazarou et al., the fourth to sixth leading cause of death in U.S. hospitals is adverse effects from properly administered pharmaceutical drugs—not overdoses or drug errors. Anything that has the power to heal also has the power to harm; this effect is greatly magnified with isolated constituent substances.

6. What is the prevalence of herb–drug interactions?

The full extent of drug–drug interactions is unknown, but conservative estimations from emergency department admission and inpatient hospital records reveal that they occur quite frequently. This problem may be compounded if health care providers fail to ask patients about the use of herbs and supplements. The full extent of adverse drug–herb interactions is even less well elucidated, and there are no widely recognized reporting policies, procedures, or agencies with adequate authority or staffing for proper investigation of reports of possible interactions. The scope of possible interactions between complex herbal formulations from different herbal traditions has not even begun to be explored.

7. If a patient has an adverse reaction while taking an herb, is the herb itself always to blame?

Any noted reaction may be due to issues that contribute to poor herb product quality. Reputable botanical companies adhere to good manufacturing practices for all their products and ensure impeccable quality control. However, not all companies have such high standards and their products vary widely in quality.

Minimal amounts or none of the stated herb in the product; misidentified plant (or plant part) or mislabeling that results in ingestion of a different herb altogether; improper processing; substitution of a cheaper herb for a more expensive one in a product without labeling that reflects the change; adulteration with an herb that grows near the identified herb in the collection process; or alcohol in the alcoholic or hydroalcoholic tinctures also may be the offender in an interaction scenario. A more disturbing problem occasionally seen with low-quality companies is the addition of pharmaceutical drugs without disclosure on the label and even contamination with heavy metals, such as arsenic, lead, or mercury, that may cause illness when the herb is taken in the recommended doses. Huang et al. and Ko noted this problem in a recent random sampling of imported Chinese herbal preparations. Therefore, it is best to work with a qualified herbalist or a medical provider knowledgeable in botanicals or to choose standardized or guaranteed potency products from reputable companies. (http://news.bmn.com/hmsbeagle/120/notes/feature4).

8. What is the difference between toxicity reaction, allergic reaction, and drug–herb interaction?

Toxicity is rare with botanical medicines. It may occur if patients have a medical problem (occult or known) that increases sensitivity to a particular herb, if they take excessive doses, or if they take the proper dosage for too long (accumulation). The reference data about toxicity of botanical medicines is based mostly on in vitro or animal studies of constituents that, in isolation (and often administered intraperitoneally or intravenously), exhibit toxicity. Data about oral administration are limited. Most published human data are in the form of case reports. With most botanical medicinals and pharmaceuticals, mild gastrointestinal upset does not qualify as a toxicity reaction. The simple fact that a product is "natural" does not indicate that large amounts (too much) are safe.

An idiosyncratic reaction occurs when any substance provokes an unpredictable negative response in a sensitive person.

Allergic or hypersensitivity reactions are more likely with plant families with a high degree of allergenicity such as the Asteraceae (cumin found in curry and chilis) and Apiaceae (sunflower; e.g., echinacea, arnica, chamomile) families. Contact dermatitis may occur on the skin. Some plant parts from an otherwise widely used (and carefully extracted and concentrated) herbal product may have warnings against oral use. Essential oils are volatile compounds and should not be placed undiluted on the skin or taken internally because of the potential for chemical burns and central nervous system effects.

Drug–herb interactions, with few exceptions, take longer to manifest. Assuming that the patient is taking no more than the recommended dose, the average time required to notice a problem is 7–14 days after the patient begins the combined regimen. For a drug that is reported to take longer to achieve maximal response in most people (e.g., ginkgo biloba), the interval may be longer. If the herb and the drug have the same potential adverse reaction or organ toxicity profile, increased caution should be exercised.

9. Are all interactions that occur between herbs and drugs adverse?

No. In fact, some herbs have been found to potentiate the actions of some drugs that have undesirable side effects associated with higher therapeutic dosing. Concurrent use of the herb allows reduced dosing schedules without loss of therapeutic effect. For example, a patient may successfully lower the dose of antihypertensive medication if a garlic supplement is effective enough in lowering blood pressure—a synergistic effect between botanical and pharmaceutical drug. Other herbs help protect against toxicity reactions caused by drugs that must be used for treatment of a particular disease. For example, milk thistle (*Silybum marianum*) is a liver-protecting compound proven to protect against viral- and chemical-induced liver damage. It may be useful in conjunction with drugs whose use is limited by derangement of liver function. For example, some patients taking an antifungal medication with hepatotoxic side effects may choose to take milk thistle to decrease these known side effects.

10. How are interactions between drugs and herbs classified?

Pharmacokinetic interactions

- *Absorption.* An herb may reduce or enhance a drug's absorption in the gut. Examples include laxatives, soluble fibers, or bulk-forming agents (e.g., psyllium) taken in close temporal proximity with the drug. Reducing transit time in the gut may result in reduced absorption and therefore lower serum concentrations of the drug. Black pepper and ginger may increase drug absorption by causing vasodilatation in the gut mucosa. St. John's wort inhibits the P-glycoprotein drug transport system in the intestine, possibly resulting in reduced absorption.
- *Displacement.* An herb may displace a drug that is highly protein-bound in the serum, resulting in increased bioavailable serum levels. For example, plant salicylates may displace warfarin, resulting in increased bioavailability and therefore increased anticoagulation effect.
- *Metabolism.* An herb may induce or inhibit hepatic enzyme systems affecting the metabolism of drugs metabolized by that system (e.g., 3A4 isoenzyme pathway of the cytochrome p450 system [CYP3A4], resulting in unexpectedly high or low serum concentrations of the drug). For example, grapefruit or its juice inhibits a system resulting in enhanced drug bioavailability. St. John's wort induces CYP3A4, causing precipitous reductions in serum levels of indinivir, cyclosporine, and many other drugs

Pharmacodynamic interactions

- *Additive effects* due to synergistic or similar mechanisms of action or effect. For example, ginkgo biloba and warfarin result in a greater anticoagulant effect not predictable by prothrombin time measurement, and valerian combined with benzodiazepines causes prolonged

sedation and other additive effects. In addition, if the herb and the drug have the same reported potential adverse reaction or organ toxicity profile, increased caution should be exercised.
- *Antagonistic effects.* One of the known actions of the herb opposes what the provider is trying to achieve with the drug in question. Examples include the combination of licorice (which has water-retaining properties) with a diuretic or hyperglycemic herbs (e.g., stinging nettles) with hypoglycemic agents.

11. Which botanicals may possibly interact with the anticoagulant warfarin?

Botanical interaction with warfarin may be due to platelet aggregation inhibition, fibrin formation inhibition, increased fibrinolytic activity, or presence of coumarin-like constituents in the herb. Little clinical evidence supports additive anticoagulant potential. The potential increases dramatically, however, if combinations of potential coagulation-affecting herbs or large amounts of any one are used or if any herb is used for prolonged periods.

Increased anticoagulation effects are found with ginkgo biloba, garlic, feverfew, Panax ginseng, ginger, papaya, devil's claw, danshen, dong quai, *Trametes versicolor* (turkey tail), *Ganoderma lucidum* (reishi), wintergreen leaf oil and sweet birch bark oil (sources of methyl salicylates), licorice, sweet clover, and possibly others.

Decreased anticoagulation effects are found with St. John's wort. There is one case report involving Panax ginseng.

12. Which other herbs should be avoided before surgical procedures? For how long?

All of the herbs and mushrooms that may effect coagulation by *any* mechanism are best avoided, even though the risk of increased bleeding is low in most people. Abstinence for at least 5–7 days is recommended for ginkgo biloba; 10–14 days is a safer recommendation before any elective or semielective surgical procedure.

The following botanicals do not affect coagulation but should be avoided before surgery because of potential interactions:

POSSIBLE EFFECT	BOTANICAL
Increased sedation or muscle relaxation	Valerian, St. John's wort, kava kava
Tachycardia and blood pressure elevation	Ephedra (ma huang)
Blood pressure elevation and possible hypokalemia	Licorice
Slower anesthetic or analgesic agent metabolism (prolonged duration of effect)	Goldenseal, cat's claw, echinacea, St. John's wort, marijuana, wild cherry

13. How should I counsel a patient about the use of herbs while they are taking a pharmaceutical drug (prescription or over the counter)?

First, assess whether the patient has a medical condition for which the proposed herb is contraindicated. Next, recommend that the patient choose a standardized preparation whenever possible. Patients should write down the brand name, specifications of the product, and the actual dosage and frequency with which they use it. It is also good to encourage patients to bring botanical bottles to the office along with prescription medications. The patient also should keep a written record of response and lab test results (as applicable). Encourage patients to familiarize themselves with the expected response and response time frame.

14. What else should patients be taught?

They also should be aware of the signs and symptoms of adverse reactions and toxicity as well as possible interactions between the herb and the drug (which may affect the decision-making process). Adverse (or positive) responses may first reveal themselves with alterations in lab values, as with cholesterol-lowering or glycemic-modulating herbs.

To make informed decisions about health care, patients should be made aware that the amount of evidence from studies (or evidence of traditional response or adverse reaction) may be small or nonexistent. Encourage open lines of communication about responses, positive or negative. This approach helps you to develop a level of comfort over time. Review the current literature sources, such as those listed at the end of this chapter, to help familiarize yourself with the individual herbs as patients in your practice bring up issues. If you do not feel comfortable acting as a reference source, some pharmacists provide this service free of charge. However, they may provide more theoretical risk information than clinical information to the patient. In addition, it may be helpful to develop a relationship with an experienced local herbalist to whom you may address questions or refer the patient for more extensive discussion.

15. How should I interpret the emerging literature about drug–herb interactions?

Be aware of the level of evidence used to support the claim of an interaction. Most human data are supported only by case reports. Recognized traditional mechanisms of action and side effects should be considered. The majority of current articles and reference books report primarily theoretical information based on possible pharmacokinetic or pharmacodynamic interactions gleaned from in vitro and animal studies rather than large trials in humans. These theoretical interactions may not apply to your patient but should be considered and/or monitored (e.g., liver damage from kava kava).

Herb–drug interactions are typically less severe than drug–drug interactions. Few case series or controlled trials are available, but more should be forthcoming as appropriate systems are established to monitor for such effects.

16. What websites are helpful for exploring more information about herb–drug interactions?

www.hermed.org: well-organized, evidence-based database for herbal information with hyperlinks to clinical and scientific publications; published by the Alternative Medicine Foundation.

www.herbalgram.org: read-only format, unless you subscribe. Good introductory information; look under Herbal Information section. Phone: (800) 373-7105

www.mcp.edu/herbal: Longwood Herbal Task Force, based at the Massachusetts College of Pharmacy. Helpful herb information resource, still in development. In-depth monographs available on some herbs.

www.naturaldatabase.com: subscription service updated weekly with excellent cross-referencing.

www.fda.gov/oc/oha/default.htm: FDA's "Information for Health Professionals" includes a homepage with links to relevant federal websites. Updates on adverse event reporting are available.

17. What are the potential interactions with pharmaceuticals for the 14 top-selling herbs in the U.S.?

1. **Black cohosh:** decreased supplemental iron absorption; potential emmenagogue effect.
2. **Echinacea:** nonspecific immune stimulation.
3. **Ephedra:** stimulant and hypertensive effects; tachycardia.
4. **Feverfew:** inhibition of nonsteroidal anti-inflammatory drug effect; anticoagulation; inhibition of supplemental iron absorption.
5. **Garlic** (high purified doses): hypoglycemic and anticoagulation effects; gastric irritation.
6. **Ginger:** may increase absorption of oral drugs and potentiate effect of warfarin.
7. **Ginkgo biloba:** vasodilatation; anticoagulation; potentiation of monoamine oxidase inhibitors. May lower seizure threshold.
8. **Ginseng (Panax):** hypoglycemic and anticoagulation effects; increased coagulation; blood pressure elevation and central nervous system hyperstimulation; inhibition of loop diuretic effect; estrogen-like effects on breast and endometrium.
9. **Grapefruit juice:** inhibition of GI tract wall metabolism (CYP3A4 isoenzyme system) of many oral drugs, leading to enhanced drug bioavailability.
10. **Kava kava:** depression; dermatosis with prolonged use.
11. **Milk thistle:** hepatoprotective effect; increases liver cell regeneration; may partially counteract hepatotoxic effect of drugs.
12. **Saw palmetto:** antiandrogenic and antiestrogenic activity.
13. **St. John's wort:** may decrease bioavailability of numerous drugs; serotonin reuptake inhibition.

14. **Valerian:** prolongation of the effect of drugs with sedative effects; inhibition of supplemental iron absorption

REFERENCES

1. Blumenthal M, Goldberg A, Brinkmann S: Herbal Medicine: Expanded Commission E Monographs. Newton, MA, Integrative Medicine Communications, 2000.
2. Brinker F: Herb Contraindications and Drug interactions, 2nd ed. Sandy, OR, Eclectic Medical Publications, 1998.
3. DerMarderosian A, Beutler J (eds): The Review of Natural Products, 2nd ed. St. Louis, Facts and Comparisons, 2001.
4. Eskinazi D (ed): Botanical Medicine: Efficacy, Quality Assurance, and Regulation. Larchmont, NY, Mary Ann Liebert, Inc., 1999.
5. Foster D: Herbs for Your Health. Loveland, CO, Interweave Press, 1996.
6. Huaug WF, Wen KC, Hsiao ML: Adulteration by synthetic therapeutic substances of traditional Chinese medicines in Taiwan. J of Clin Pharm 37:344–350, 1997.
7. Ko RJ: Adulterants in Asian patent medicines. N Engl J Med 339:847, 1998.
8. Lazarou J, Pomeranz BH, Corey PN: Incidence of adverse drug reactions in hospitalized patients -a meta-analysis of prospective studies. JAMA 279:1200–1204, 1998.
9. Lininger S, Gaby A, et al: A-Z Guide to Drug-Herb-Vitamin Interactions. Roseville, CA, Prima Publishing, 1999.
10. McGuffin M, Hobbs C, Upton E, Goldberg A (eds): American Herbal Products Association's Botanical Safety Handbook. New York, CRC Press 1997.
11. Mills S, Bone K: Principles and Practice of Phytotherapy: Modern Herbal Medicine. London, Churchhill Livingstone, 2000.
12. Murray M: The Healing Power of Herbs, 2nd ed. Rocklin, CA, Prima Publishing 1995.
13. Robbers J, Tyler VE: Tyler's Herbs of Choice: The Therapeutic Use of Phytomedicinals. New York, Hawthorne Herbal Press, 1999.
14. Schulz V, Hansel R, Tyler VE: Rational Phytotherapy: A Physicians Guide to Herbal Medicine, 3rd ed. New York, Springer, 1997.

62. THE BUSINESS OF COMPLEMENTARY AND ALTERNATIVE MEDICINE

Nancy Schulman, M.S.B., and Michael J. Stuart-Shor, M.P.H.

1. Define reimbursement.
Reimbursement is the term which describes payment from a third-party payer or patient for services rendered.

2. Can physicians bill for complementary/alternative medicine (CAM) services?
Yes, in certain circumstances. Physicians as well as all other health care practitioners can bill third-party payers for services rendered assuming three requirements are met:
1. The practitioner's CAM service is within the state scope of practice laws.
2. The practitioner is contracted with the payer.
3. The CAM service is eligible for coverage within the payer's fee schedule.

For example, a physician in California appropriately trained in acupuncture can bill for services if the payer reimburses for them.

3. Why is the state scope of practice law so important?
The laws are highly significant because they dictate what services a practitioner is legally allowed to perform within a specific state. A practitioner practicing outside of the state scope is not considered to be in compliance with the regulations, which is punishable by law. The challenge with CAM modalities is that each state has its own rules and interpretations with no national organization or board. Physician's scope of practice does not vary much from state to state. A good practice is to keep apprised of all modifications on a regular basis. The following two examples show the variations for the same types of practitioner in 2001:

1. A California acupuncture license authorizes the holder to perform nutritional services and to administer herbs as dietary supplements to promote health, whereas in Illinois the scope of practice does not include herbal preparations and nutritional supplements.

2. A licensed chiropractor in New Jersey is not allowed to administer acupuncture needles, whereas in Colorado a chiropractor is allowed to administer acupuncture needles with 100 additional hours of acupuncture training and 25 case studies.

4. How are CAM services reimbursed?
Although the vast majority of CAM services continue to be reimbursed on a cash only basis, interest among insurers in covering these services is growing. Each type of insurer has differing goals and objectives for providing coverage. The basic types of insurers are as follows:
- Group health, which reimburses for illness, injury, and defined preventive services that are not work-related.
- Workers' Compensation, which pays for illness or injury during the course of and/or as result of employment.
- Auto insurance, which pays for health services arising from an auto accident.

5. What types of plans are included in group health? How do I know what is covered?
- Health maintenance organizations (HMOs), which cover care that is provided by or appropriately referred by affiliated doctors and hospitals.
- Preferred provider organization (PPOs), which offer one level of coverage if the member uses affiliated doctors and hospitals and less coverage for care provided by others.
- Traditional indemnity plans, which provide the same level of coverage regardless of the doctor or hospital used.

If there is a question about specific coverage or eligibility, all group health plans have a member relations department that is an excellent resource for specific information. Their number is usually printed on the membership card. Each type of group health plan also has what is called a subscriber benefit description (SBD), which outlines eligible services and how and when they are to be covered. The SBD also specifies what is excluded. The patient has a copy of the SBD or access to it.

6. Discuss the types of CAM reimbursement programs.

Current CAM reimbursement programs fall into three distinct categories

1. Discounted fee for service/affinity programs
2. Covered benefits
3. No coverage

A discounted fee for service/affinity program is an arrangement whereby groups of CAM practitioners agree to provide a discount to members of a particular health plan or association. An example of a discounted program is Naturally Healthy Rewards, which is offered to members of Blue Cross Blue Shield of Massachusetts. Members receive a 20% discount from participating acupuncturists, massage therapists, and other selected types of providers.[1] Another example is the Aetna Natural Alternatives Program, which offers a negotiated fee schedule for CAM therapies paid out of pocket by Aetna members. The fees are published on the program's website.[2]

An example of a covered benefit is Progressive Health Care, a Massachusetts-based organization that has a negotiated fee schedule and a benefit structure determined by the specific diagnosis. Coverage is provided for acupuncture, massage, mind-body medicine, and homeopathy. Acupuncturists, massage therapists, and homeopaths contract directly with the organization and receive an agreed upon fee schedule.

Many insurers are developing CAM riders for their policies. A rider is an additional benefit that an employer can purchase to cover benefits that are not part of the basic plan.

Although the number of insurers beginning to cover CAM services is growing, at present the majority of plans do not. However, over the next few years if research demonstrates clinical efficacy and cost-effectiveness, coverage may grow steadily.

7. What are potential pitfalls of accepting insurance coverage?

Although insurance reimbursement broadens the market for services, a number of potential financial risks are involved:

1. Because insurers typically represent large employee populations, they usually expect a discount off of existing rates in exchange for patient referrals or listing in their directory of "preferred providers." Discounts can range from 15% to 30%.

2. In addition to accepting a discounted fee, significant additional costs are associated with the billing and collections process. These costs typically represent between 10–20% of collections to pay for staff time in processing claims, collections, denials and communication with the insurance companies and clients.

3. Cash flow can be a major problem. With third-party reimbursement, actual payment for services may be received from 30 to upward of 100 days after claims submission. Although "clean claim laws," stating a claim must be paid in 30 days, have been enacted in most states, some insurers are still negligent in paying promptly. It is a good practice to make sure that any agreement with an insurer has a performance clause that requires practitioners to be paid within a certain number of days from actual receipt of a clean claim.

Conversely, CAM practitioners who accept cash only may have to spend more time and financial resources in aggressive marketing to attract new patients. However, all-cash practices generally have lower overhead costs and better cash flow.

8. What are the potential benefits of accepting insurance coverage?

Benefits depend on the particular provider and clinic situation. For patients who would not otherwise have been able to afford CAM therapies, it is an obvious benefit. Some CAM clinicians believe that insurance reimbursement may be the key to long-term financial viability and clinical success because it broadens the market to a wider population who would not pay out of pocket for CAM services. Another benefit of the arrangement is that it may increase awareness of CAM services among patients who may have never considered its use. Offering financial accessibility to a more diverse patient population may be more congruent with the healing philosophy of the provider. Most plans tend to promote CAM programs heavily to appeal to patients' desire for a whole-person approach to care. The result may be a steady influx of new patients.

From an overall social policy perspective, one of the risks of not participating in third-party reimbursement is that CAM will will remain inaccessible for clients without the ability to pay. However, because of the pitfalls mentioned above, altruistic CAM clinics may find themselves in the dilemma of not being able to serve the very patients they wish to serve because of the business demands of a practice.

9. What criteria are insurers likely to use to determine CAM coverage?

Group health insurers primarily make coverage decisions based on what is considered medically necessary (is it necessary to help relieve the patient's condition?) and acceptable medical practice (is it considered part of normal medical services?). They do not cover services that are considered experimental, that are not accepted medical practice, or that are viewed as "comfort measures." Insurers are increasingly interested in medical efficacy, which means an accepted body of clinical evidence that a therapy or service is effective. This requirement can be challenging for CAM because studies of CAM therapies acceptable to most medical authorities are just beginning to be published in mainstream journals.

One of the real challenges to CAM coverage is that, more often than not, the scope of coverage is determined by a panel of conventional physicians with little appreciation or understanding of complementary therapies. In addition, coverage decisions are heavily influenced by the culture of the local medical community.

Workers Compensation insurers are interested in many of the same issues as group health insurers but have a bit more flexibility. Because of their interest in reducing wage replacement expenses, which are generally higher than medical costs for this population, they are more likely to cover CAM services if they believe that they will result in a more rapid return to work or avoidance of expensive or equivocal surgery.

10. Are CAM services eligible for reimbursement through medical savings accounts (MSAs)?

Some are; for others the answer is less clear. Many employers now provide MSAs, which enable employees and their dependents to use pretax dollars to pay for a wide variety of medical services that are approved by the Internal Revenue Service (IRS), but not covered by the employer's insurance plan. According to IRS rules, acupuncture, chiropractic treatment, and "therapy" received as part of medical treatment are eligible expenses. For a detailed list, refer to IRS Form 502.[3]

11. What are the barriers to incorporating CAM into mainstream health care?

1. Probably of greatest importance is the perception that most CAM interventions have not been submitted to the same type of randomized, controlled clinical trials that are currently the gold standard for evaluating clinical efficacy. The irony of this argument is that studies show that only 20%[4] to 37%[5] of accepted current practices in conventional medicine have been subjected to this same standard.

2. Lack of a good communication and a common nomenclature for CAM and conventional medicine.[6] CAM providers and conventional providers have a limited history of working collaboratively, and there is often a strong reluctance to initiate dialog from either side.

3. Doctors' lack of CAM knowledge. To providers who are not educated in CAM, its therapies may seem "fringe." For example, considerable data support the benefits of nutrition and exercise, yet most medical school curricula are inadequate in these areas. As a result, these therapies are not recommended as broadly as they should be.

4. Patients' level of education and access. Many patients are unaware of the clinical benefits of most complementary modalities. Lack of awareness on the part of patient and physician creates a double-sided barrier.

5. Lack of traditional referral patterns. Conventional practitioners often find it challenging to identify appropriate complementary care resources. Few CAM providers have active relationships

with conventional practitioners. As a result, even if a physician or nurse practitioner has an interest in referrals, they often are not sure where or to whom they should refer.

12. Why is the definition of "medically necessary" important for billing third-party payers?

For payers to reimburse, services must be considered medically necessary. Many integrative programs have found the supposedly objective definition of "medical necessity" to be inflexible and creates undue restrictions on delivering care.

What may be considered necessary to a practitioner may not be considered necessary to the payer. For example, the patient and physician may agree that six osteopathic treatments are important to ensure recovery from a particular injury, but the insurance company may believe that fewer visits are warranted. It is in the payer's best interest to limit coverage to certain treatments and not to pay for experimental and excessive treatments.[7] To some payers and regulatory agencies, CAM therapies are not considered necessary. Check with local and state regulations for exact definitions.

13. What are current procedural terminology (CPT) codes? Are codes available for integrative medicine?

The American Medical Association (AMA) owns and approves CPT codes. The coding system is used nationally as the mechanism for describing services to private and government health care payers for claims submission. According to an AMA spokesman, the CPT approval panel is made up of 16 members: 11 are conventional medical doctors, four represent the insurance industry, and one represents the American Hospital Association and the Centers for Medicare and Medicaid. This composition does not leave much room for CAM or integrative representation. Many insurers believe that the AMA will not add CAM codes in the near future.[9] Thus far, the CAM codes have not been adequate to describe the CAM services.

This inflexibility has caused some clinics to choose CPT codes that may not identically fit the service so that the service will qualify for payment by insurers. Valid CPT codes for 2001 include acupuncture, massage, biofeedback, psychotherapy, hypnotherapy, nutrition ,and osteopathic manipulation. Integrative and CAM programs have been successfully reimbursed for these codes, assuming that the services are supported by proper documentation.

14. Is there a specific coding system for CAM therapies?

Actually, there is. Alternative Link developed a coding system for CAM practitioners so that they would not be at risk of filing fraudulent claims. The ABC system, which is available at www. alternativelink.com, includes a greater range of CAM coding options than the CPT codes. The codes include five alpha characters, whereas the CPT codes include five numeric characters. For example the acupuncture CPT code is 97780, and the ABC code is CABAE.

Alternative Link is in the process of applying for recognition as a national coding system. To date, however, few payers are reimbursing for ABC codes because some believe that the system will drain resources during an implementation and training phase, whereas other payers believe that it is not necessary to have two coding systems.

15. Is the current coding and payment system effective for integrative services?

Not really. The current system does not take into account the patient's history and unique situation for whole-person services. The actual service time and complexity are not reflected in the current CPT and ICD-9 coding systems. The current payment system creates financial incentives for physicians to see more patients with shorter visits versus fewer patients with longer visits. The dollar- per-minute reimbursement increases substantially if a physician in Seattle sees three patients at 15 minutes each vs. one patient at 45 minutes. This payment system is not conducive to longer, whole-person centered services.[10] Quantity—but not always quality—is rewarded.

16. How does a clinic collect what is equitably owed to them?

Before a physician or other clinician signs any insurance contract, he or she should check the specific wording in the agreement about covered services, reimbursement rates, fees or discounts, and time from claim submission to claim payment. Some contracts can be quite complicated, and it may make sense to contract an attorney for assistance. This step may prevent legal and financial problems down the road.

Before submitting a claim, make sure that a Health Care Finance Administration(HCFA) form 1500 or other appropriate document is used with the correct ICD-9 and CPT codes. Insurers will deny payment for any errors. It can be quite painful to a clinic's bottom line for the money to sit in the insurers' bank account. This problem makes it difficult to pay clinic staff, clinic expenses, and yourself. Next to excellent care and patient satisfaction, consider the billing and collections process one of the most important parts of your practice.

A helpful techniques to improve cash flow is to submit claims more frequently. Many medical practices bill on a 30-day cycle. Reducing the cycle to 14 days can increase your cash flow by decreasing the delay in days from claim submission to payment.

Also, make sure that you understand the terms of the agreement with the insurer. Before participating in any HMO, PPO, or other plan, make sure that you understand exactly which of your services is covered, how much you will be paid for them, and when you will be paid. The agreement should contain specific details about the turnaround time for payment and a description of fees or discounts. Some contracts can be quite complicated. If several practitioners are considering a specific plan, it may make sense to pool financial resources and retain a contract attorney familiar with health care to review the agreements. Although attorneys are a bit expensive, you will learn a lot and avoid some ugly financial consequences.

17. What is the simplest way to ensure coding compliance?

The safest approach is to consult directly with the local payer. Coding requirements can change quickly, and it is important to keep apprised of the changes. The major layers of compliance include the following:

- Local payer rules (e.g., the insurance carriers with which you contract and Medicare)
- American Medical Association CPT rules
- State scope of practice laws
- State rules
- Federal regulations through Centers for Medicare and Medicaid Services (CMS), formerly known as the Health Care Financing Administration (HCFA)

Some communities are developing associations in which experiences can be shared and potential problems avoided. However, it is crucial that shared information be checked by an attorney or authority to ensure accuracy and to avoid creation of more problems.

18. What CAM modalities have the highest revenue potential?

The answer varies by geographical area and local competitive conditions. Typically, practitioners of massage and psychotherapy see one patient per hour, whereas chiropractors and acupuncturists can see multiple patients simultaneously, thus increasing revenue. A chiropractor's contribution to the bottom line of an integrative clinic can be quite positive because of consumer familiarity and the likelihood of insurance coverage. Although many integrative and CAM clinics have resisted adding chiropractors, as noted in a national Integrative Clinic Benchmarking study, the chiropractor can turn a clinic's bottom line from red to black.[11]

19. What is "incident-to" reimbursement?

Incident-to billing allows a clinic to charge the physician's full rate when a nonphysician performs the service. Be aware the national Medicare policy can be different from local carrier policy, therefore. The local payer should be contacted directly for the reimbursement fee schedule and rules.[12] The 2001 Medicare rules include the following:

- The service must be an integral part of the physician's services.
- The service must be commonly rendered and included in the physician's bill.
- The service must be commonly supplied in physicians' offices or clinics.
- The service must be supplied under the physician's direct personal supervision.

Incident-to reimbursement has increased tremendously, according to a 2001 Office of the Inspector General (OIG) study, thus making these claims on a potential radar screen. Knowledge of the rules decreases the chance of compliance problems in the future.

20. Is "incident-to" billing legal for CAM modalities?

Yes—if the service falls within the physician's scope of practice, the nonphysician is licensed to practice the modality within the state, and all other rules are followed. The best practice is to get assurance from the payer before the services are rendered.

Numerous court cases have involved incident-to billing by chiropractors. Chiropractic care is not included within a physician's scope of practice, and a physician cannot supervise a chiropractor. This practice is in violation of the incident-to rules. On the other hand, massage therapists have successfully been billed incident-to physicians and chiropractors when the services were in compliance with the rules.

21. Are lifestyle change programs reimbursed by third-party payers?

In certain cases. Lifestyle Advantage currently offers the Dean Ornish Program for Reversing Heart Disease, a lifestyle-based program emphasizing nutrition, exercise, psychological support, and stress reduction for patients with cardiovascular disease. In 2001, roughly 40 insurers reimbursed the program to some degree, and roughly 500 people received third-party reimbursement. Highmark reimburses the program at 100%, whereas other payers reimburse at 80% on average.[13] In 2001, Medicare began a pilot program for paid demonstration of the Ornish program to 1,800 people.

22. Why did a payer begin to reimburse for the Ornish program?

Mountain States Blue Cross Blue Shield (MSBCBS), headquartered in West Virginia, offers 100% reimbursement to their members for the Ornish program as of January 2002. A spokesman states that the program is a cost-effective way to improve the physical and emotional well-being of its members. MSBCBS has partnered with 10 hospitals in the state to offer the Ornish program to patients. They are attempting to make the Ornish program a "community initiative." An Ornish study showed that for every dollar invested, the payer saved five dollars through prevention of a costly procedures.[14]

23. Can lifestyle change services be reimbursed by third-party payers?

Some insurers now pay for risk reduction visits directly or as brief medical visits. The medical visits are allowable if the patient has a billable diagnosis (high blood pressure, high cholesterol, diabetes, heart disease, and in certain cases overweight and/or obesity) and if all components of a brief medical visit are met.

For example, credible evidence indicates that nonpharmacologic interventions contribute to the reduction of blood pressure, high cholesterol, weight, and symptoms of depression and improve glycemic control as an adjunct to medication or as a stand-alone intervention. Thus, a patient with any of these conditions may be entered into a risk reduction program and monitored for progress toward the medical goal with a treatment plan focused on both pharmacologic and nonpharmacologic interventions.

The Roxbury Heart Center in Boston created a multiple risk reduction and prevention program in the inner city. All patients are seen individually at the beginning of the visit and assessed for progress toward goal. Visits are billed as a short medical visit for the treatment of a medical condition and cover only the brief individual component of the group program.[15]

24. Do employer benefit programs cover CAM services?

They are starting to do so. The result of a Price Waterhouse Coopers study that interviewed 30 employers covering 1.3 million people found that 76% of employers offer some type of CAM reimbursement, with chiropractic services the most frequently covered.

Modality	% Covered	Modality	% Covered
Chiropractic	76	Biofeedback	10
Acupuncture	48	Herbal therapies	3

| Nutritional counseling | 17 | Energy work | 3 |
| Massage therapy | 14 | Other | 10 |

The study noted that the main reason for covering CAM therapies was employee demand—a close description for coverage of CAM by other insurers, being market demand.[9] Another survey of 382 employers suggests that 82% currently cover chiropractic treatment and 19% offer an alternative health benefit other than chiropractic treatment. Forty-two percent of the respondents cited as their reason for not offering CAM benefits the lack of sufficient proof of efficacy.[16]

A study from Natural Business Communications estimated that nearly $31 billion was expected to be spent on CAM care in 2000.[17] However, to date no studies have shown how much of this amount is cash business versus insurance or employer reimbursement.

25. Are CAM services cost-effective?

Yes, when used prudently. For example, compelling evidence indicates that St. John's wort is as effective as the popular antidepressants imipramine and fluoxetine for the treatment of mild to moderate depression at less than 20% of the cost and with far fewer side effects.[18] Saw palmetto has been shown to be clinically equivalent to the pharmaceutical finasteride for the treatment of benign prostatic hypertrophy (BPH) at a fraction of the price and with fewer side effects.[19]

A Scandinavian study demonstrated that acupuncture was an effective modality for reducing pain in patients awaiting knee surgery—so effective that 24% of patients elected not to have the surgery, saving an estimated $9000 per patient.[20]

A cohort study of the effects of massage on preterm neonates demonstrated weight gains 47% higher than the control group and substantially reduced durations of stay for an average cost savings of $3000 per infant.[21]

26. What are the unique characteristics of employers who are likely to cover CAM benefits?

Experience from a few CAM clinic managers suggests that certain types of employers are more likely to offer CAM services as benefits. The typical profile is a self-insured, medium-to-large company or union trust fund that is culturally progressive and financially successful. These employers place a high value on their workforce and have an interest in attracting and retaining highly skilled employees. Employee groups at high risk for repetitive motion injuries, physical injuries, and accidents (e.g., construction and manufacturing workers) also may be receptive to CAM benefits because they see CAM services as an alternative to medications and equivocal surgeries.

27. How can patients encourage coverage of CAM therapies?

1. Consumer demand is the single most powerful vehicle for creating systemic and organizational change. Patients can encourage coverage of CAM therapies by sharing both successful and unsuccessful experiences with their primary care physicians, employer, and insurance company. Studies have shown that most patients do not share this information.

2. Patients can request that the CAM provider and physician share notes and coordinate their approach to care.

3. Another successful strategy has been through legislation. Several states have "mandated benefits" laws that require coverage of certain types of benefits. Such laws result result from legislative lobbying by interested groups. In 1984, the Massachusetts Society for Cardiac Rehabilitation (MSCR) successfully worked with its state representatives to frame legislation that mandates cardiac rehabilitation as a basic benefit. The law became effective on March 26, 1986.[22]

28. Do other countries offer CAM reimbursement?

Perhaps the most important lesson to be appreciated is that modalities considered complementary in U.S. society are considered conventional care in other societies. For example, France has a history of providing coverage for spa visits for a variety of conditions. Mounting scientific evidence by French researchers, however, indicates that this benefit is ineffective both financially and clinically.[23]

The types of services covered by different countries cover vary considerably. The National Health Service in the United Kingdom and private insurers in Germany cover homeopathic care if it is prescribed by a medical doctor.[24] The Japanese National Health Service includes coverage for a number of herbal remedies.[25]

The difference in the types of services covered in other countries speaks volumes to the impact of cultural and historic experience as a driver of social policy. In U.S. society, well-organized conventional medicine continues to be the most dominant force in determining accepted clinical practice.

Although we have tried to portray the current business issues surrounding CAM, perhaps its real future will be determined by consumer behavior. As patients and conventional practitioners become more familiar with CAM and have their own experiences, their advocacy may become the most powerful agent of change.

REFERENCES

1. www.ahealthyme.com/nhsearch/ (accessed 2/25/02).
2. www.aetna.com/products/natural_alt_99.html (accessed 11/15/01).
3. www.irs.gov/forms_pubs/pubs/p50205.htm (accessed 11/10/01).
4. www.shef.ac.uk/~scharr/ir/percent.html (accessed 1/15/02).
5. Imrie R: The evidence for evidence-based medicine. Complement Therap Med 8:123–126, 2000.
6. Caspi O: The Tower of Babel: Communication and medicine. An essay on medical education and complementary-alternative medicine. Arch Intern Med 160:3193–3195, 2000.
7. Cohen MH: Complementary and Alternative Medicine: Legal Boundaries and Regulatory Perspectives. Baltimore, Johns Hopkins University Press, 1998.
8. Reference deleted.
9. Pelletier KR, et al: Current trends in the integration and reimbursement of complementary and alternative medicine by managed care, insurance carriers and hospital providers. Am J Health Promot 12(2):112–123, 1997.
10. Weeks J: Coding time and complexities in health creation. Integr Med Consult 4(1), January, 2002.
11. Schulman N, Novey D: Chiropractors and integrative clinics: Credentialing and revenue projections. Integrator Novermber, 2000, pp 1, 4, and 5.
12. Gosfield AG: The ins and outs of "incident to" reimbursement. Fam Pract Manage Nov/Dec:23–27, 2001.
13. Silberman A, President, Highmark Advantage, Pittsburgh, PA, private discussion, December 10, 2001.
14. Waring, N: Dr. Dean Ornish's Low-Tech Approach to CAD. Hippocrates Jan:34, 2001.
15. Stuart E, The Roxbury Heart Center, Boston Massachusettes, private discussion, January, 2002.
16. Health Benefits and Alternative Medicine: Is There a Fit? Census of Certified Employee Benefit Specialists, Survey Results 1999.
17. Emerich M: LOHAS means business. Available at lohasjournal.com, 2000.
18. Schrader E: Equivalence of St. John's wort extract (Ze 117) and fluoxetine: A randomized, controlled study in mild-moderate depression. Int Clin Pyschopharmacol 15(2):61–68, 2000.
19. Wilt T: Saw palmetto extracts for the treatment of benign prostatic hyerplasia: A systematic review. JAMA 280:Nov. 11 (18), pp 1604-1609, 1998.
20. Christensen BV: Acupuncture treatment of severe knee osteoarthritis: A long term study. Acta Anaesthesiol Scand 36:519–525, 1992.
21. Field T, et al: Tactile/kinesthetic stimulation effects on preterm neonates. Pediatrics 77:654, 1986.
22. Massachusetts Society for Cardiac Rehabilitation: Guidelines for Cardiac Rehabilitation. Executive Committee Report, April 1986.
23. Allard P: Is spa therapy cost effective in rheumatic disorders? Rev Rhumatisme(English edition) 65:600–602, 1998.
24. Jorgenson L, Director of Administration and Human Resources, Cathnet-Sciences, Paris France, e-mail communication, Jan. 15, 2002–Feb. 4, 2002.
25. Tsutani K: The evaluation of herbal medicines: An East Asian perspective. In Lewith GT, Aldridge D (eds): Clinical Research Methodology for Complementary Therapies. London, Hodder & Stoughton, 1993.

INDEX

Page numbers in **boldface type** indicate complete chapters.

Abdominal pain, recurrent, in pediatric patients, **388–391**

Abortion, as violation of physician's moral code, 51

Absorption, of drugs, 419

Academy of Medical Acupuncture, 78

Accreditation Commission for Acupuncture and Oriental Medicine, 77

Acetaminophen, contraindication in hepatitis, 242

N-Acetyl-cysteine (NAC), 140, 242, 353

Acetyl-l-carnitine (ALC), as Alzheimer's dementia therapy, 342

Achillea millefolium. See Yarrow

Acne, **205–209**

   premenstrual, 205, 208, 265

Acne rosacea, 206–207

Acquired immunodeficiency syndrome (AIDS), relationship with the human immunodeficiency virus (HIV), 284

Acquired immunodeficiency syndrome (AIDS) patients, prayer interventions for, 49

Acupressure, 154, 349, 394

Acupuncture, **74–78**

   acceptance of, 7–8

   as allergic rhinitis treatment, 406–407

   use in allopathic medicine, 90

   applications of, 77

   as asthma treatment, 412–413

   basic concept of, 74

   as cancer treatment, 373

   chiropractors' use of, 103

   cost-effectiveness of, 429

   discomfort associated with, 75

   as energy medicine, 154

   as fibromyalgia treatment, 334, 335

   five element, 70–71

   as hepatitis treatment, 241, 242

   as HIV infection treatment, 284

   introduction into United States, 3

   as low back pain treatment, 318

   in menopausal women, 257

   meridians in, 74

      energy transmission through, 156, 157

   as multiple sclerosis treatment, 355

   needle insertion points in, 74, 76

   needles used in, 74–75

   as neuropathic pain treatment, 220, 359

   effect on neurotransmitter levels, 177–178

   as osteoarthritis treatment, 327

   as otitis media treatment, 401

   as pain treatment, 310

   as peptic ulcer disease treatment, 256

   placebo use in, 72

   as prostate cancer adjunct treatment, 382

   safety of, 75

   as stroke treatment, 188

   as tension headache treatment, 349

   as weight loss technique, 225

Acupuncture Efficacy (Birch and Hammerschlag), 72

Acupuncture practitioners, licensing and certification of, 77–78

Adams, Patch, 16

Adaptogen-acting herbs, as attention-deficit hyperactivity disorder treatment, 171

Addiction, definition of, 308

Addiction withdrawal, acupuncture treatment for, 78

S-Adenosyl methionine (SAM-e), 176, 325

Adjustment, chiropractic, 103, 104

Adolescents, acute abdominal pain in, 389–390

Adrenaline, music-induced reduction in, 33

Aerobic capacity ($\dot{V}O_2$max), 146–147

Aescin, 188

Aesculus hippocastanum (horse chestnut), 120, 188

Agency for Health Care Policy and Research, 103

Aggravation, homeopathic, 81–82

Aging. *See also* Elderly persons

   effect of exercise on, 144

Agitation/psychosis suppression therapy, for Alzheimer's dementia, 343

Agrimony, as irritable bowel syndrome treatment, 250

Aikido, as energy medicine, 154

Air, optimal, 292

Albuterol, 413

Alcohol dependence, as suicide risk factor, 177

Alcohol use

   anxiety-inducing activity of, 165

   carcinogenicity of, 369, 378–379, 384

   cardioprotective effects of, 184–185

   contraindications to

      depression, 177

      hepatitis, 244

      pregnancy, 273

   as gastroesophageal reflux cause, 234

   as migraine headache cause, 345

   moderate, 184–185

      by hypertensive patients, 200

   by physicians, 87

Alexander technique, 114

Alfalfa, as "superfood," 140

Alkanet, contraindication during lactation, 275

Allergens

   as asthma triggers, 410

   reduction of, 404

Allergic reactions, 403

   to herbal remedies, 119, 390, 399, 419

   to milk, 124

Allergy rotation diet, 400

Allium cepa. See Onions

Allium sativum. See Garlic

Allopathic medicine, **84–91**

   cultural differences in, 84–85

   definition of, 84

   evidence-based, 6–7, 87–88, 91, 309

   effect of managed care on, 89

Allopathic medicine (*cont.*)
  medical care discrepancies in, 88–89
  origin of, 84
  relationship with pharmaceutical industry, 89
Aloes
  chemotherapy patients' use of, 380
  contraindication during lactation and pregnancy,
    272, 275
Aloe vera, 236
  as chemotherapy side effects treatment, 374
  contraindication during lactation, 275
  as fibromyalgia treatment, 334–335
  as peptic ulcer disease treatment, 256
  as skin cancer adjunct treatment, 385
Aloin, 236
Alpha-linoleic acid, 126
Alpha-lipoic acid, 219, 242, 353, 359
Alternative medicine, 1. *See also* Complementary and
    alternative medicine
Althea officinalis (marshmallow), 235–237, 399
Aluminum
  as Alzheimer's disease risk factor, 339
  antacid content of, 255
  antiperspirant content of, 339–340
Aluminum poisoning, as attention-deficit
    hyperactivity disorder cause, 171
Alzheimer's disease, dementia of, **338–344**
Amalaki (*Emblica officinalis*), 251
American Academy of Ayurvedic Medicine, 65
American Academy of Osteopathy, 98
American Academy of Pediatrics, 170
American Art Therapy Association, 34
American Association of Physicians of Indian Origin,
    65
American Board of Holistic Medicine, 19
American Board of Homeotherapeutics, 83
American Chiropractic Association, 101
American College of Sports Medicine, 143, 202
American Diabetes Association, 223
American Holistic Nursing Association, 3–4
American Institute for Cancer Research, 377–378
American Massage Therapy Association, 113
American Medical Association, 2, 38, 85
American Osteopathic Association, 98
American Osteopathic Board
  of Neuromusculoskeletal Medicine, 98
  of Special Proficiency in Osteopathic Manipulative
    Medicine, 98
American Psychological Association, 41
American School of Osteopathy, 92
American Society of Clinical Hypnosis, 41
Amino acid supplements, 139–140
  as Alzheimer's disease treatment, 341
4-Aminopyridine, as multiple sclerosis treatment, 355
Amitriptyline, 72, 333
Analgesia, placebo, 28
Analgesic injections, as osteoarthritis treatment, 323
Analgesics
  caffeine-containing, as migraine headache rebound
    phenomenon cause, 347
  as low back pain treatment, 317

Analgesics (*cont.*)
  as neuropathic pain treatment, 360–361
Anandamide, 132
Anatomy, energetic, 157
Anatomy of an Illness, As Perceived by the Patient
    (Cousins), 32
Anemia, tea consumption-related, 369
Angelica, 236, 394
Angelica sinensis. See Don quai
Angell, Marsha, 89–90
Angina, lifestyle modification treatment for, 181
Angiotensin-converting enzyme inhibitors, 181, 193,
    203
Anorectal disorders, kshara sutra surgical treatment
    for, 62
Antacids, 255
Anthocyanins, 185
Anthraquinones, 236
Anthroposophically-extended medicine, definition of,
    3
Antibiotics
  as acne treatment, 207
  bacterial resistance to, 287
  as multiple sclerosis treatment, 354
  as otitis media treatment, 398
  as sinusitis treatment, 296
  topical, as dermatitis cause, 211
  as upper respiratory tract infection treatment, 287
  as urinary tract infection treatment, 302
Anticholinergics, 391
Anticonvulsants, as neuropathic pain treatment, 360,
    361
Antidepressants, 174. *See also* St. John's wort
  as acne cause, 206
  as fibromyalgia treatment, 333
  as low back pain treatment, 317
  as neuropathic pain treatment, 360–361
  as premenstrual syndrome treatment, 269
Antifungal therapy, for chronic sinusitis, 296
Antihistamines, 278, 286, 404, 405
Antihypertensive agents, 200, 203, 204
Antimonium crudum, as gastroesophageal reflux
    disease treatment, 237
Antineoplastons, 367
Antioxidants, 138–139
  adverse effects of, 139
  as allergic rhinitis treatment, 406
  antiatherosclerotic activity of, 183–184
  as asthma treatment, 411
  as cancer treatment, 365
  chocolate as, 132
  use in detoxification, 249
  as HIV infection treatment, 282
  as multiple sclerosis treatment, 353
  in red wine, 185
  as sinusitis treatment, 293, 295
Antiparkinsonian agents, herbal, 65
Antiperspirants, aluminum content of, 339–340
Antiretroviral therapy, for HIV infection, 282–283
Antiseptic herbs, as postpartum perineal discomfort
    treatment, 274–275

Anxiety, **163–167**
  as arteriosclerosis risk factor, 186
  asthma-exacerbating effect of, 410
  definition of, 163
  depression-associated, 165
  energy medicine treatment for, 160
  meditation-related, 44
  meditation therapy for, 43, 48
  premenstrual syndrome-related, 265, 267
  yoga therapy for, 56
Apiaceae family, allergic reactions to, 419
Apoproteins, 180
Appendicitis, in children, 389
Arabinogalactans, 141
Arabinoxylane, 370
Aralia racemosa (spikenard), as partus preparator, 273
Arctium lappa, as eczema treatment, 212
Arctostaphylos uva ursi (Uva ursi), as urinary tract infection treatment, 298, 302
Ardhrakam (*Zingiber officinale*), 251
Argentum nitricum, 203, 252
L-Arginine, 140
Aricept (donepezil), 343
Arishta (*Azairachta indica*), 251
Arnica, as low back pain treatment, 317
Aromatherapy, 64, 311, 372, 401
Arsenicum album, 412
Artemesia absinthium. See Wormwood
Artemesia vulgaris (mugwort), 76, 272
Artichoke, bitterness of, 243
Artistry of the Mentally Ill, 34
Art therapy, 31, 34, 341, 372
Art Therapy Credentials Board, 34
Arya Vaidya Sala, 66
Asafoetida/asafetida, 252
Asbestos exposure, 383
Ascorbic acid. *See* Vitamin C
Ashtanga Hrdaya, 59
Ashtanga Sangraha, 59
Aspirin
  as colon cancer preventive, 384
  as coronary artery disease treatment, 181
  as peptic ulcer disease risk factor, 254
  white willow bark as source of, 134
Assisted suicide, as violation of physician's moral code, 51
Associated Bodywork and Massage Professionals, 113
Asteraceae family, allergic reactions to, 419
Asters, allergic reactions to, 390, 399
Asthma, **409–415**
  as atopic disorder, 210
  herbal remedies for, 410–411
  milk allergy-related, 124
  triggers of, 410, 412
  yoga therapy for, 56
Astragalus, 141, 380, 400
Astringent herbs, as postpartum perineal discomfort treatment, 274–275
Atherosclerosis, **180–190**

Athletic performance, effect of imagery on, 38
Atkins Diet, 127
Atopy, 210
Atrial natriuretic peptide, 33
Attention-deficit hyperactivity disorder, **168–173**
  energy medicine treatment for, 160
  milk allergy-related, 124
Auras, 156, 157, 345
Aurum metallicum, 203
Australia, use of complementary and alternative medicine in, 4
Avena sativa (wild oats), as attention-deficit hyperactivity disorder treatment, 171
Avocado/soybean unsaponifiables, as osteoarthritis treatment, 326
Ayurveda medicine, 8–9, **59–66**
  branches of, 60
  definition of, 59
  diagnostic applications of, 62–63
  as fibromyalgia treatment, 335
  as irritable bowel syndrome treatment, 251–252, 253
  as osteoarthritis treatment, 327
  as peptic ulcer disease treatment, 256
  three doshas of, 60–61
  treatment modalities of, 64
  yoga as component of, 54
Ayurvedic Institute, 63, 65, 66
Ayurvedic practitioners, certification, registration, and licensing of, 65–66
Azairachta indica (arishta), 251
Azelaic acid, as acne treatment, 207, 208

Bach flower crabapple, as acne treatment, 207
Bacitracin, as contact dermatitis cause, 211
Back, musculature of, 313
Back injuries, exercise therapy for, 149
Baldrinals, 164
Baraka, 154
Barberry, contraindication during pregnancy, 272
Barley grass, 140
Barrett's esophagitis, 234
Basal metabolic rate, aging-related decrease in, 148
Basil, contraindication during lactation, 275
Beach, Wooster, 2
Becker, Robert O., 157, 161
Bee pollen, 140
Beer, as migraine headache cause, 345
Bee sting therapy, for multiple sclerosis, 355
Behavioral interventions
  for attention-deficit hyperactivity disorder, 170
  for migraine headaches, 348
Being In Movement, 111
Belladonna, as otitis media treatment, 398
Benaras Hindu University, 66
Benign prostatic hypertrophy, 120, **276–280**, 382
Benny, Jack, 322
Benzocaine, 211
Benzoyl peroxide, 207
Berberis, as sinusitis treatment, 295

Beta amyloid proteins, as Alzheimer's' disease cause, 33
Beta blockers, 181, 203
Beta carotene, 295, 383, 406
Beta sitosterol, 277, 278
Bhavaprakasha, 59–60
Bifidobacterium bifidum, 139
Bilberry, anticoagulant/antithrombolytic activity of, 188
Bile production, circadian rhythm of, 241–242
Bilirubin lights, 159
Binge eating, 130, 131
Biodynamics, 3
Bioelectromagnetics (BEM), 153, 160
Biofeedback
    as migraine headache treatment, 348
    as peripheral neuropathy treatment, 358
    as rectal cancer treatment, 384–385
    as recurrent pediatric abdominal pain treatment, 390
    as tension headache treatment, 348
Bioflavonoids, 136, 138, 208, 256
Biomedicine. *See* Allopathic medicine
Biotin, as diabetes therapy, 218, 219
Bismuth subsalicylate, 235
Bitter melon (*Momordica charantia*), 220
Bitters
    definition of, 243
    as hepatitis treatment, 243
    as hydrochloric acid stimulants, 235
    as irritable bowel syndrome treatment, 250
Black cohosh (*Cimicifuga racemosa*)
    as breast cancer treatment, 380
    contraindication during lactation, 275
    drug interactions of, 421
    as hot flushes treatment, 259
    as partus preparator, 273
Black currant oil, as dermatitis treatment, 212
Black elder (*Sambucus nigra*), 288–289
Bladderferwrack, contraindication during lactation, 275
Blood-letting, 2, 79, 84
Blood root, contraindication during pregnancy, 272
Blood type, diet based on, 128
Blueberry juice, as urinary tract infection preventive and treatment, 301
Blue cohosh (*Caulophyllum thalictrodes*), 272, 273
Blueprint for Immortality: The Electric Patterns of Life (Burr), 158–159
Board of the American College of Anthroposophically Extended Medicine, 3
Body, energy anatomy of, 156
Body cleansing, 371–372
Body fat
    aging-related increase in, 148
    ideal percentages of, 145–146
    measurement of, 146
Body mass index (BMI), 145, 147
Body purification, by Native Americans, 4

Bodywork
    as cancer treatment, 373
    as osteoarthritis treatment, 327
    as tension headache treatment, 348
    in traditional Chinese medicine, 67
Boldo (*Peumus boldus*), 245
Bone density, 228
Bone growth, 228
Bone health, dietary guidelines for, 230
Bone quality, 228
    Z-score of, 229
Bone remodeling, 228
Bone strength, 228
Bonnie Pruden myotherapy, 114
Borage, contraindication during lactation, 275
Borage oil, as dermatitis treatment, 212
Borderline personality disorder, as contraindication to meditation, 44
Boron, 230, 326
Boswellia, as low back pain treatment, 317
Botanical medicine, **116–122**. *See also* Herbal remedies
Botanical products, definition of, 117
Botanical Safety Handbook (McGuffin et al.), 272, 275
Bouchard nodes, 323
Bovine colostrum, immune-enhancing properties of, 141
Boxwood, as HIV infection treatment, 283
Braid, James, 37
Brain-gut connection, 247
Brain Longevity (Khalsa), 339
Breast cancer, 377–380
Breast-feeding, 3, 393, 397, 412
Breast milk, effect of herbs on, 275
Breech presentation, moxibustion treatment for, 72
Bright light therapy. *See also* Phototherapy
    for fibromyalgia, 334
Bristol Myers Squibb, 137
British Society of Medicine, 38
Broccoli, cancer preventive properties of, 369
Bromelain, as allergic rhinitis treatment, 405
Bruyere, Rosalyn, 158
Buckthorn, purging, contraindication during lactation, 275
Buckwheat, 405
Buddhism, 32, 43, 48
Bugleweed, contraindication during lactation, 275
Burnheim, Hippolyte, 38
Burnout, of physicians, 87
Burns
    energy medicine treatment for, 160
    hypnosis treatment for, 40
Burr, Harold Saxton, 158–159
Burzynski's antineoplastons, 367
Butterbur (*Petasites hybridus*), as allergic rhinitis treatment, 405

Caffeine
    anxiety-inducing activity of, 164–165

Caffeine (*cont.*)
  contraindications to
    benign prostatic hypertrophy, 278
    depression, 177
    hypertension, 203
    premenstrual syndrome, 268
  effect on migraine headaches, 345
  as pediatric abdominal pain cause, 390
  pregnant women's consumption of, 273
Calcarea carbonica, 203
Calcium
  antacid content of, 255
  antihypertensive effects of, 201–202
  cardioprotective effects of, 184
  colon cancer protective effects of, 384
  dietary sources of, 231
  in osteoporosis, 230–231
  as prostate cancer risk factor, 381
Calcium carbonate, as premenstrual syndrome
    treatment, 268
Calcium deficiency, attention-deficit hyperactivity
    disorder-associated, 170
Calcium deposits, 111
Calendula
  as acne treatment, 207
  as dermatitis treatment, 212
  as postpartum perineal discomfort treatment,
    274–275
  as skin injury treatment, 385
California College of Ayurveda, 66
Calma-Bebi, 394
Calomel, 2
Calorie-restricted diets, 123
CAM. *See* Complementary and alternative medicine
Camellia sinensis. See Green tea
Campbell, Don, 33
Camphor, effect on homeopathic remedies, 82
Cancer, **377–387**. *See also* specific types of cancer
  causes of, 363–364
  dietary prevention of, 124, 127
  treatment for
    adjuvant, 365
    alternative, 367–375
    hypnosis, 39–40
    integrative oncology, **363–376**
    mushroom extracts, 141
    placebo effect in, 366
    vegetarians' reduced risk of, 124
Cancer-prone personality, 365–366
Candida, overgrowth of, as gastroesophageal reflux
    cause, 234, 236
Candidiasis, as sinusitis risk factor, 291, 293, 294,
    296
Capsaicin cream, as neuropathic pain treatment, 360
Carbohydrates
  diabetics' intake of, 216–217
  glycemic index of, 124
  as obesity cause, 222
  as reactive hypoglycemia cause, 169
Carbo vegatalis, as gastroesophageal reflux disease
    treatment, 238

Cardamon, as infant colic treatment, 394
Cardiac rehabilitation, standard, 187
Cardiorespiratory endurance, exercise-related increase
    in, 147
Cardiovascular system, effect of aerobic exercise on,
    143–144
Carnegie Foundation, 2
Carnitine, as congestive heart failure treatment,
    194
L-Carnitine, 140, 282
β-Carotene, 295, 383, 406
Carotenoids, 138, 383
Carpal tunnel syndrome, yoga therapy for, 55, 56
Cartier, Jacques, 4
Cascara sagrada, 273, 275
Case studies, 9–10
Cassia senna (senna), contraindication during
    pregnancy and lactation, 272, 273, 275
Catechins, 132, 138
Catnip, sedative and muscle relaxant properties of,
    261
Cauda equina syndrome, chiropractic manipulation-
    related, 104, 105
Caulophyllum thalictrodes (blue cohosh), 272, 273
Cayenne lotion, as chemotherapy side effects
    treatment, 374
Cayenne pepper, 119, 188, 254
Cayenne pepper tea, 254
CD4 counts, 48, 49, 281
Center for Mind Body Medicine, 374
Centers for Disease Control and Prevention, 75,
    144
Cerebrovascular disease, 180, 188, 189. *See also*
    Stroke
Cernilton, 279
Cetirizine (Zyrtec), 405
Chakras, 156
Chalice of Repose, The (Shroeder-Shaker), 32
Chamomile
  allergic reactions to, 399
  as allergic rhinitis treatment, 406
  as gastroesophageal reflux disease treatment,
    237
  as infant colic treatment, 394
  as irritable bowel syndrome treatment, 252
  as otitis media treatment, 399, 402
  as pediatric abdominal pain treatment, 390
  as peptic ulcer disease treatment, 255–256
  sedative and muscle relaxant properties of, 261
Chamomilla, 238, 394, 398
Chance, role in evidence-based medicine, 88
Chanting, 4, 32, 33, 155
Chaparral, 243
Charaka Samhita, 59, 60, 61
Charcot, Jean, 38
Chaste berry tree (*Vitex agnus-castus*), 259, 260, 269
Cheese
  aluminum content of, 339
  as migraine headache cause, 345
Chelation therapy, 188–189, 371
Chemicals, as hepatitis cause, 240

Chemotherapy, 364
  antioxidant use with, 139
  hypnosis use with, 39–40
  side effects of, herbal remedies for, 373–374, 380
Chi, 154
Chicken soup, as common cold treatment, 288
Children
  art therapy for, 34
  asthma in, 409–410
  chiropractic use in, 106–107
  diabetes in, 150
  faith healing-related deaths of, 373
  heart disease risk factors in, 150
  herbal remedies use by, 120
  music therapy for, 33
  physical inactivity of, 150
  recurrent abdominal pain in, **388–391**
  resistance strength training by, 150
Chinese club moss (*Huperzia serrata*), 342
Chinese red yeast rice (*Monascus purpureas*), 120–121, 182–183, 283
Chinese rhubarb, contraindication during lactation, 275
Chinese traditional medicine, **67–73**
  as acne treatment, 208
  approach to the common cold in, 288
  as asthma treatment, 412
  as cancer treatment, 371
  comparison with Western medicine, 203
  as dermatitis treatment, 213
  diagnosis in, 67–68
  eight principles of, 69
  five elements of, 69–71
  as HIV infection treatment, 284
  as hypertension treatment, 203
  as irritable bowel syndrome treatment, 250–251, 253
  as osteoarthritis treatment, 327
Chippewa, 52
Chiropractic, **101–109**
  as asthma treatment, 413
  comparison with osteopathy, 95
  definition of, 101
  differentiated from massage, 113–114
  as fibromyalgia treatment, 334
  as infant colic treatment, 395
  as low back pain treatment, 319
  mechanical assessment procedures in, 102
  as pain treatment, 310
  philosophy of, 107–108
  terminology of, 103–104
Chiropractic schools, 85
Chitosan, 225
Chlamydia pneumoniae, 180, 354
Chlorella, 140
Chlorine, as water sanitizer, 130
Chocolate
  health benefits of, 132
  as migraine headache cause, 345

Choices for Healing: Integrating the Best of Conventional and Complementary Approaches to Cancer (Lerner), 366
Cholagogue, 241
Cholecalciferol. *See* Vitamin D
Cholecystitis, in children, 389
Choleretic, 241
Cholesterol
  as atherosclerosis risk factor, 180
  as benign prostatic hypertrophy risk factor, 277
  dietary control of, 182
  as prostate cancer risk factor, 277
Cholesterol-lowering agents, 182–183
Cholestin, 120–121, 182–183
Chondroitin, as osteoarthritis treatment, 325
Chopra, Deepak, 63–64
Chopra Center for Well-Being, 66
Christianity, use of meditation in, 43
Christian Scientists, 47
Chromium, 208–209, 218
Chromium picolinate, 224, 295
Chronic immune dysfunction syndrome (CFIDS), 331
Chronic pain syndrome, **304–312**
Chrysantheums, 382
  allergic reactions to, 390, 399
Cimetidine (Tagamet), 236
Cimicifuga racemosa. See Black cohosh
Cisapride, 391
Citrate salts, 298
Claviceps purpura, 65
Coagulation, effect of herbal remedies on, 420
Cockroaches, 412
Coenzyme Q10, 183–184
  antihypertensive effects of, 201
  antioxidant activity of, 138
  as cancer preventive or treatment, 370, 378
  use by chemotherapy patients, 380
  as congestive heart failure treatment, 193–194
  as multiple sclerosis treatment, 354
Coffee. *See also* Caffeine
  contraindication during homeopathic treatment, 82
  hepatic effects of, 243
Cognex (tacrine), 343
Cognitive-behavioral therapy, 187, 335
Cognitive enhancement therapy, for Alzheimer's dementia, 342–343
Colchicine, autumn crocus as source of, 134
Cold remedies, contraindication in benign prostatic hypertrophy, 2770278
Coleus, as asthma treatment, 410
Coleus forskolii, as eczema treatment, 212
Colic, infant, 388, **392–395**
Colocynthis, 252, 394
Colon cancer, 125, 383–385
Colon irrigation machines, 372
Color, sound, and light therapy, as energy medicine, 155
Coltsfoot, 243
  contraindication during pregnancy and lactation, 272, 275

Comfrey, contraindication during pregnancy and lactation, 272, 275

Commiphora mukul (guggul), 183, 188

Common cold, **286–289**
sinusitis associated with, 290, 291

Communication, in physician-patient relationship, 18, 91
in pain management, 305

Communication skills, in pain management, 305

Comparison groups, 10

Complementary and alternative medicine (CAM)
use in allopathic medicine, 89–90
alternative terms for, 1
business of, **423–430**
cost-effectiveness of, 420
definition of, 1
history of, in the United States, **1–5**
prevalence of use, 1, 4, 6
reimbursement for, 5, 423–430
trends in, 4–5
worldwide use of, 4

Compresses, 118

Computed tomography, 158
use in chiropractic, 102

Congestive heart failure, **191–199**
chronic systolic, 191, 193
classification of, 192

Conservatism, therapeutic, as chiropractic principle, 108

Consortium of Academic Health Centers for Integrative Medicine, 19

Contraception. *See also* Oral contraceptives
for perimenopausal women, 261

Controls, in research, 10
placebos as, 28

Convallaria majalis (lily of the valley), contraindication during pregnancy, 272

Conventional medicine. *See* Allopathic medicine

Coping strategies/styles
effect on cancer prognosis, 366
spirituality/religiousity as, 48

Copper, as osteoarthritis treatment, 326

Coriolus versicolor, 370, 383

Coronary artery disease, 180
antioxidant therapy for, 183–184
chelation therapy for, 189
cholesterol-lowering therapy for, 182–183
dietary therapy for, 125, 181
relationship with Alzheimer's disease, 339
risk factors for, 180
somatic dysfunction associated with, 96

Coronary heart disease, estrogen deficiency as risk factor for, 2572–58

Corpus luteum insufficiency, 267, 269

Corticosteroids, as acne cause, 206

Cortisol, 33, 111

Council for Homeopathic Certification, 83

Counterstrain, 319

Cousins, Norman, 32

Cramp bark, 269

Cranberry, 120

Cranberry juice, as urinary tract infection preventive and treatment, 273, 300, 301

Cranial injury, in children, 397

Cranial osteopathy, 94–95
as otitis media treatment, 397

Cranial-sacral manipulation, 114, 159, 394

Crataegus laevigata or *monogyna* or *oxyacantha* (hawthorne), 185, 194–195

C-reactive protein, 180

Creatine, exercise performance-enhancing properties of, 151

Creative arts therapy, **31–36**

Critical rationalism, as chiropractic principle, 108

Cupping, use with acupuncture, 76

Curanderas, 4

Current procedural terminology (CPT) codes, 426

Cyanocobalamin. *See* Vitamin B_{12}

Cyclooxygenase-2 enzyme inhibitors, 384

Cystitis, 298
relationship with urinary tract infections, 299

Cytochrome P450 3A4, 175

Cytomegalovirus, 240

Dairy foods, 124
as asthma risk factor, 411
contraindication during premenstrual syndrome, 268
as migraine headache cause, 345
as prostate cancer risk factor, 381

Damiana (*Turnera aphrodisiaca*), contraindication during pregnancy, 272

Dance therapy, 31, 35

Dandelion (*Taraxacum officinale*), 212, 244, 250

Dan-shen (*Salvia miltiorrhiza*), 185
drug interactions of, 420

Da quing ye (*Isatis indigotica*), as prostate cancer treatment, 279

DASH (Dietary Approaches to Stop Hypertension) diet, 200

Datura stramonium, 65

David (biblical figure), 32

Day care, as otitis media risk factor, 398, 401

Dean Ornish Program for Reversing Heart Disease, 125, 181, 187, 381
health insurance reimbursement for, 428

Death and dying
ayurvedic medicine's approach to, 64
fear of, hypnosis therapy for, 40
use of music during, 32

de Broglie wavelength, 155

Decision-making, medical, 88

Declaration of Helsinki, 28

Decongestants, 286, 404, 405

Defibrillators, 159

Degenerative joint disease. *See* Osteoarthritis

Dehydration, massage-related, 111–112

Dehydroacetic acid/dehydroascorbate, 127, 138, 212–213, 293

Dehydroepiandrosterone (DHEA), 140–141
as acne treatment, 205
as breast cancer risk factor, 380

Dehydroepiandrosterone (DHEA) (*cont.*)
  contraindication in benign prostatic hypertrophy,
    278
  as multiple sclerosis treatment, 354
De Materia Medica (Dioscorides), 116
Dementia
  Alzheimer's, **338–344**
  definition of, 338
Demulcents, 235–236
Dendrantherma (Chrysanthemum) morifolium, 279
Dental fillings, as multiple sclerosis risk factor,
    354–355
Depo-Provera, use by perimenopausal women, 261
Depression, **174–179**
  anxiety-associated, 165
  as arteriosclerosis risk factor, 186
  electroshock therapy for, 159
  integrative treatment approach in, 174–175
  meditation-related, 44
  meditation therapy for, 43
  in multiple sclerosis patients, 353
  pathophysiology of, 174
  in physicians, 87
  premenstrual syndrome-related, 265, 269
  St. John's wort treatment for, 7–8, 120, 137,
    175–176, 417
  traditional Chinese medicine treatment for, 71, 72
  yoga therapy for, 56
Dermatitis, 210, 211, 212, 213
Dermatologic disorders, meditation therapy for, 43
"Designer" food, 129–130
Detoxification, 249, 371–372
Detoxification pathways, phases 1 and 2, 241
Devils' claw, 327, 420
Dextroamphetamine, as attention-deficit hyperactivity
    deficit treatment, 169, 171
D-fraction, 370
DHEA. *See* Dehydroepiandrosterone
Diabetes mellitus, **215–221**
  as atherosclerosis risk factor, 180
  in children and adolescents, 150
  definition of, 215
  dietary factors in, 123
  insulin therapy for, 215, 216
  low-fiber diet as risk factor for, 125
  milk allergy-related, 124
  peripheral neuropathy associated with, 358
  type 1, 124, 215, 216
  type 2, 215–216
  urinary tract infections associated with, 299
Diabetes Prevention Program, 217
*Diagnostic and Statistical Manual of Mental
    Disorders (DSM)*, 168, 174
Diarrhea, herbal remedies for, 250
Dicylomine, 395
Diet. *See also* Dietary supplements; Nutritional
    factors; Nutritional therapy
  effect on health, 86
  for weight loss, 223
Diet aids, contraindication in benign prostatic
    hypertrophy, 2770278

Dietary Approaches to Stop Hypertension (DASH)
    diet, 200
Dietary Health Supplement Health and Education Act,
    117, 120, 417
Dietary reference intakes (DRIs), 134–135
Dietary Supplement and Health Education Act, 134,
    137
Dietary supplements, **134–142**. *See also* Nutritional
    therapy
  definition of, 134
  delivery systems for, 141
  for enhanced exercise performance, 151
  as fibromyalgia treatment, 334–335
  labeling of, 137
  as premenstrual syndrome treatment, 268
  quality of, 137
  as urinary tract infection treatment, 302
Diet for a Small Planet (Moore), 131
Digitalis purpurea (foxglove), 193, 418
Digoxin, 193, 418
Dihydrotestosterone, 276, 277
Dioscorea, as fibromyalgia treatment, 334–335
Dioscorides, 116
Diosgenin, 258
Disease
  ayurvedic medicine's concept of, 59, 60, 62–63
  Native Americans' concept of, 4
  traditional Chinese medicine's concept of, 67–68
Dissociation, in massage clients, 111
Diuretics, 193, 203
Doctors of osteopathy, 92–93
  certification of, 98–99
  differentiated from medical doctors, 95
  manual and medicine training of, 98
Donepezil (Aricept), 343
Dong quai
  anticoagulant/antithrombolytic activity of, 188
  contraindication during pregnancy, 272
  drug interactions of, 420
  as hot flushes treatment, 259
  as premenstrual syndrome treatment, 269
Dopamine, St. John's wort-induced reduction in, 175
Doshas, 60–61
Double-blinding, 25, 72, 82, 88
Doulas, 274
Doxycycline, as acne treatment, 207
*Drawing on the Right Side of the Brain: A Course in
    Enhancing Creativity and Artistic Confidence*
    (Edwards), 31–32
Drug abuse, by physicians, 87
Drug dependence, definition of, 308
Drug interactions, of herbal remedies, 117, 119,
    417–422. *See also* specific herbs
Drugs. *See also* specific drugs
  as acne cause, 206
  definition of, 117
  as hepatitis cause, 240
  laboratory synthesis of, 134
  as neuropathy cause, 357
  plant-derived, 90, 134
  potency of, 418

Drug use, definition of, 307–308
Duke University, 19
Dust mites, 412
Dutch elm disease, 236
Dysmenorrhea, yoga therapy for, 56
Dyspepsia, 388, 390

Ear disorders, acupuncture treatment for, 77
Eating disorders, 131
"Eat Right for Your Blood Type" diet, 128
Echinacea, 120, 137
    as common cold preventive and treatment, 287
    drug interactions of, 421
    immunostimulatory activity of, 141, 287
    long-term use of, 287–288
    as otitis media treatment, 399
    preparations and dosages of, 116–117, 288
    safety of, 287
    side effects of, 119
    as sinusitis treatment, 293, 295
Eclectic medicine, 2
Eczema, **210–214**
Edema, pulmonary, 192–193
EDTA (ethylenediamine tetraacetic acid) chelation
    therapy, 189
Eggplant, as osteoarthritis aggravant, 326
Eicosapentaenoic acid, 127, 201, 212–213, 293
Einstein, Albert, 155
Elder flower (*Sambucus*), 399–400, 406, 412. *See
    also* Black elder
Elderly persons
    chiropractic use in, 107
    creatine supplementation in, 151
    exercise by, 144, 145
        contraindications to, 148
    exercise testing in, contraindications to, 148
    religious beliefs of, 48
Elecampane, contraindication during lactation, 275
Electrical muscle stimulation. *See also* Percutaneous
    electrical stimulation (PENS); Transcranial
    electrostimulation (TCES); Transcutaneous
    electrical stimulation (TENS)
    chiropractors' use of, 103
Electric eels, 154
Electroacupuncture, 72, 76, 178
Electrocardiography, 158
Electroencephalography, 158
Electromagnetic fields, 153
    as pain therapy, 310
    pulsed, 160–161, 327
Electromagnetic modalities, as osteoarthritis
    treatment, 327
Electromagnetic radiation, effect on homeopathic
    remedies, 82
Electromyographic feedback, as tension headache
    treatment, 348
Electromyography, 158
Electrons, 157–158
Electroshock therapy, for depression, 159
Elements, traditional Chinese medicine's theory of,
    69–71

Eleutherococcus senticosus, 116, 171
Elimination diet, 131
Emblica officinalis (amalaki/Indian gooseberry), 251
Emotional disorders, acupuncture treatment for, 77
Emotions, asthma-exacerbating effect of, 410
Empathy, 18
Empiricism, 6
Empowerment, 19–20
End-of-life care, religious beliefs about, 47, 52
Endorphins, music-induced release of, 33
Endothelial dysfunction, 180
Endurance training, 146–147, 148–149
Energy, human, measurement of, 157–158
Energy cultivation (qi-gong), 72, 154, 159
Energy fields
    measurement of, 158
    perception of, 161
Energy medicine, **153–162**
Energy therapy/work
    for cancer, 373
    in traditional Chinese medicine, 67
Ephedra
    adverse effects of, 137
    as asthma treatment, 410, 411
    contraindications to
        benign prostatic hypertrophy, 278
        hypertension, 203
        lactation, 275
        pregnancy, 272
    drug interactions of, 421
    side effects of, 224
    as weight loss aid, 224
Epicatechins, 132
Epoxycholesterols, 277
Epstein-Barr virus, 240, 354
Equisetum arvense (horsetail), 232
Ergosterol. *See* Vitamin D
Erickson, Milton, 38
Eritadenine, 186
Erythromycin, as acne treatment, 207
Esophageal cancer, 363
Esophagitis, Barrett's, 234
Essential fatty acids
    deficiency of
        attention-deficit hyperactivity disorder-related,
            170
        vegetarianism-related, 124
Essential fatty acids. *See also* Omega fatty acids
    adequate intake of, 127
    as gastroesophageal reflux disease treatment, 237
    metabolism of, in atopic dermatitis, 212
    as migraine headache treatment, 348
    as sinusitis treatment, 293, 296
    as "superfood," 140
Estrogen
    effect on benign prostatic hypertrophy, 278
    excess levels of, 267–268
    food content of, 277
    interaction with St. John's wort, 117
    natural, use by menopausal women, 257, 258
    role in premenstrual syndrome, 266, 267–268

Estrogen deficiency, 257–258
Estrogen replacement therapy, 257, 259, 261–262
    as breast cancer risk factor, 379
    as depression treatment, 178
    as osteoporosis prophylactic and treatment, 230
    soy phytoestrogens as alternative to, 184
Ethinyl estradiol, 259
Ethylenediamine tetraacetic acid (EDTA) chelation
        therapy, 189
Eucalyptus, as otitis media treatment, 402
Euphrasia, 408
Euthanasia, as violation of physician's moral code,
        51
Evening primrose oil, 212, 259
Evidence-based medicine, 6–7, 87–88, 91, 309
Evidence-based Medicine, 13
Excedrin Migraine, 347
Exelen (rivastigmine), 342
Exercise, **143–152**
    aerobic
        cardiovascular benefits of, 143–144
        definition of, 143
    by Alzheimer's disease patients, 340
    anaerobic, definition of, 143
    as anxiety treatment, 165
    by asthma patients, 412
    as attention-deficit hyperactivity disorder treatment,
        172
    ayurvedic medicine's emphasis on, 62, 64
    cardioprotective effects of, 187
    as chronic pain treatment, 308
    as chronic sinusitis treatment, 293
    definition of, 143
    as depression treatment, 176
    by diabetics, 217
    effect on health, 86
    as fibromyalgia treatment, 334
    flexibility, 144
    as hypertension treatment, 200, 202
    as low back pain treatment, 317–318
    by multiple sclerosis patients, 354
    as osteoarthritis treatment, 324
    for osteoporosis preventive, 232
    during pregnancy, 150
    psychological benefits of, 151
    role in weight loss, 223, 224
    as urinary tract infection preventive, 300
    warm-ups and cool-downs in, 144
Exercise testing, in elderly persons, contraindications
        to, 148
Experience, role in evidence-based medicine, 88
Extracts
    solid, 118
    standardized, 118–119
Eyebright, as allergic rhinitis treatment, 406
Eye disorders, acupuncture treatment for, 77
Eye drops, as allergic rhinitis treatment, 404

FACT, 13
Faith Assembly, 49
Faith healing, 373

Falls
    by children, 397
    by elderly people, 228, 229–230
Faraday, Michael, 155
Fasting, by Islamic patients, 52
Fat, dietary, 125–127. *See also* Fatty acids; Essential
        fatty acids
    as Alzheimer's disease risk factor, 340
    diabetics' intake of, 216–217
    "good" and "bad," 182
    hydrogenated, 127
    as prostate cancer risk factor, 381
    restriction of. *See* Low-fat diet
    role in weight loss, 225
    as satiety indicator, 125
Fatigue
    premenstrual syndrome-related, 265
    sinusitis-related, 290
    yoga therapy for, 56
Fatty acids
    monounsaturated, 125–126, 201
    polyunsaturated, 125, 126, 127, 182, 201, 411
    saturated, 125, 126, 182
    trans, 127, 182, 377
Fatty acid supplementation, during pregnancy and
        breast-feeding, 275
Fecal occult blood test, for colon cancer, 383
Feeding the Hungry Heart (Roth), 131
Feingold diet, 169–170
Fennel, as irritable bowel syndrome treatment, 252
Fenugreek (*Trigonella foenum graecum*), 220
Fermented foods, as migraine headache cause, 345
Ferrum phosphoricum, as otitis media treatment, 398
Fever, common cold-associated, 288
Feverfew
    as allergic rhinitis treatment, 406
    contraindication during pregnancy, 272
    drug interactions of, 420, 421
    as migraine headache treatment, 347
    as osteoarthritis treatment, 327
Fiber, dietary
    antihypertensive effects of, 201
    cholesterol-lowering effects of, 182
    as colon cancer preventive, 384
    diabetics' intake of, 216
    dietary sources of, 217
    effect on estrogen levels, 268
    health benefits of, 125
    irritable bowel syndrome patients' intake of, 248
    low intake of, as peptic ulcer disease risk factor,
        254
    mushroom content of, 186
    as recurrent pediatric abdominal pain treatment,
        390
    role in weight loss, 223, 224
Fibrinogen, 180
Fibromyalgia, 56, 112, **330–337**
    as somatoform disorder, 332
    tender points in, 332–333
Fibromyalgia syndrome, 330
Fields of Life, The (Burr), 158–159

Fish oil. *See also* Omega fatty acids
  drug interactions of, 374
Fit for Life, 131
Fitness, **143–152**
  cancer preventive properties of, 369, 378
  definition of, 143
Flavonoids, as otitis media preventive, 397–398
Flax consumption, cholesterol-lowering effects of, 182
Flaxseed oil, 126, 127
  anticoagulant/antithrombolytic activity of, 188
  as eczema treatment, 212–213
  as prostate cancer adjunct treatment, 382
  as sinusitis treatment, 296
Flexner, Abraham, 2, 85
Flexner Report, 2, 85
Fluoride, water content of, 130
Fluoride poisoning, as attention-deficit hyperactivity disorder cause, 171
Fluoxetine (Prozac), 269
Folic acid, 136, 341, 378, 384
Folic acid deficiency, 177, 184
Folk medicine, 4
Follicle-stimulating hormone, 258
Food
  cancer preventive properties of, 369
  carcinogenic, 369
  "designer," 129–130
  emotional need for, 131
  estrogenic hormone content of, 277
  as migraine headache trigger, 345
  organic, 129
    chronic hepatitis patients' consumption of, 242
  spicy, effect on peptic ulcer disease, 254
Food additives, as migraine headache trigger, 345
Food allergies
  attention-deficit hyperactivity disorder-related, 171
  as eczema cause, 213
  elimination diet in, 131
  as gastroesophageal reflux disease cause, 236
  as otitis media risk factor, 400, 401
  as peptic ulcer disease risk factor, 254
  sinusitis-related, 293
  trigger foods for, 131
  as urinary tract infection risk factor, 298
Food and Drug Administration, 137, 417
Food and Nutrition Board, 135
Food colorings, artificial, 169–170
Food combining, 131
Food cravings, premenstrual syndrome-related, 265
Food intolerance, as depression cause, 177
Food Pyramid Guide, 130
Food sensitivity, irritable bowel syndrome-related, 249
Food servings, 130
Forskolin, as eczema treatment, 212
Four Vedas, 59
Foxglove (*Digitalis purpurea*), 193, 418
Fractures
  energy medicine treatment for, 160–161
  of the hip, osteoporosis-related, 228, 229–230

Fragrances, as contract dermatitis cause, 211
Franklin, Benjamin, 37
Free radicals, 138, 249
"Free weights," 144, 145
"French paradox," 185
Freud, Sigmund, 38
Fringe medicine, 1
Fructooligosaccharides, 139
Functional medicine
  definition of, 248
  as irritable bowel syndrome treatment, 248–249
Fungal infections, as sinusitis risk factor, 291

Galen, 84, 175
Gamma-linoleic acid (GLA), 127, 212, 219–220, 268
Gan cao, as prostate cancer treatment, 279
Ganoderma lucidum (ling shi, reishi), 279, 370, 382, 420
Garcinia, 224–225
Gardenia formula, as dermatitis treatment, 212, 213
Garlic (*Allium sativum*), 120
  as allergic rhinitis treatment, 406
  anticoagulant/antithrombolytic activity of, 188
  antihypertensive effects of, 202–203
  cholesterol-lowering effects of, 182
  contraindication during homeopathic treatment, 82
  contraindication during lactation, 275
  drug interactions of, 374, 420, 421
  side effects of, 119
  as sinusitis treatment, 293, 295
  as "superfood," 140
  topical application of, as contact dermatitis cause, 211
  as urinary tract infection treatment, 298
Gastroesophageal reflux disease (GERD), **234–239**
  differentiated from infant colic, 393
  as sinusitis risk factor, 291
Generalized anxiety disorder, 163, 164, 165
General practitioners, 85
Gentian, 235, 243, 250
GERD. *See* Gastroesophageal reflux disease
Germ theory, 84
Gerson therapy, 367
Gibran, Kahlil, 304
Ginger/ginger root (*Zingiber officinale*), 185
  anticoagulant/antithrombolytic activity of, 188
  as chemotherapy side effects treatment, 374, 380
  drug interactions of, 419, 420, 421
  as gastroesophageal reflux disease treatment, 237
  as low back pain treatment, 317
  as osteoarthritis treatment, 327
  as otitis media treatment, 400
  as pediatric abdominal pain treatment, 390
  as premenstrual syndrome treatment, 269
Gingko biloba, 120, 188
  as Alzheimer's dementia treatment, 341–342
  anticoagulant/antithrombolytic activity of, 188
  as asthma treatment, 410
  drug interactions of, 374, 419–420, 421
  as multiple sclerosis treatment, 354

Ginkgolides, 342
Ginseng (*Panax*), 120
    American, 116
    as chemotherapy side effects treatment, 374
    Chinese/Korean, 116, 374
    contraindication in hypertension, 203
    drug interactions of, 420, 421
    Siberian, 374
    species of, 116
    as vaginal dryness treatment, 260
Glucosamine sulfate, as osteoarthritis treatment,
    324–325
Glutamine, 252, 374
L-Glutamine, 140, 282
Glutathione, 140, 282
L-Glutathione, 140
Glycemic control, 215, 216, 220
Glycemic index, 124
Glycerites, 118, 120
Glycyrrhiza glabra. See Licorice
Glycyrrhiza uralensis (gan cao), 279
Glycyrrhizin, 236
Glycyrrhizinic acid, 236
God, belief in, 47, 49, 52
Goldenrod, as allergic rhinitis treatment, 406
Goldenseal (*Hydrastis canadensis*), 236
    contraindication during pregnancy, 272
    as otitis media treatment, 400
    as sinusitis treatment, 295
    as urinary tract infection treatment, 298, 301–302
Gonzalez treatment, for cancer, 367–368
Gotu kola, 171, 301
Grapefruit, drug interactions of, 243, 419, 421
Grapefruit seed extract, as sinusitis treatment, 295
Grape juice, 379
Grape seed extract, 138, 184, 293, 295
Green, Elmer, 158
Green tea
    antioxidant activity of, 138
    cancer protective properties of, 369
    cardioprotective effects of, 184
    hepatic effects of, 243
Grifola frondosa (maitake) mushrooms, 141, 370
Gripe water, as infant colic treatment, 394
Group support, cardioprotective effects of, 187
Growth hormone, 226, 278
Guggul (*Commiphora mukul*), 183
Gugulipid, 188
Guided imagery, 37, 38, 186, 372, 412
Gujarat Ayurved University, 66
Gymnema sylvestre, 220
Gynecologic disorders, acupuncture treatment for, 77

Hahnemann, Samuel, 2, 79, 80, 84
Hajj, 52
Hakomi integrative somatics, 111
Haloperidol, 343
Haritaki (*Terminalia chebula*), 251
Harmony, as traditional Chinese medicine concept, 67
Harvard Mastery of Stress study, 158
Harvard University, 19

Harvey, William, 84
Hawaiian massage, 114
Hawthorne (*Crataegus laevigata* or *monogyna* or
    oxyacantha), 185, 194–195
Hawthorne effect, 28
Headache diary, 345, 346
Headaches, **345–351**
    chiropractic manipulation-related, 105
    cluster, 350
    migraine, 345, 347–348
    premenstrual, 265, 268
    sinusitis-related, 290
    tension, 348–349
    yoga therapy for, 56
Healing
    definition of, 16
    differentiated from the placebo effect, 24
Healing with Homeopathy (Jonas and Jacobs),
    165–166
Health
    ayurvedic concept of, 60
    definition of, 16
    traditional Chinese medicine's concept of, 67
Health food, as psoriasis treatment, 210
Health food stores, 141
Health insurance reimbursement
    for chiropractic services, 105
    for complementary and alternative medicine
        services, 5, 423–430
Health maintenance evaluations (HMEs), 86–87
Healthy Pleasures (Ornstein and Sobel), 32
Heart attack. *See* Myocardial infarction
Heart disease
    low-fiber diet as risk factor for, 125
    meditation therapy for, 43
    vegetarians' reduced risk of, 124
Heart disease patients, weight-lifting by, 149
Heart rate, during aerobic training, 147
Heart transplant recipients, religiosity in, 48
Heat therapy, 67, 103, 333
Heaven's Gate Cult, 49
Heavy metal poisoning, 171, 188
Heberden nodes, 323
Heel spurs, 111
Helichrysum, as otitis media treatment, 402
Helicobacter pylori
    as abdominal pain cause, 390
    as cancer cause, 363
    as gastroesophageal reflux cause, 234, 235, 238
    as peptic ulcer disease cause, 254
    as rosacea cause, 207
"Hello-goodbye effect," 27
Hepatitis, **240–245**
Hepatotoxicity, kava-related, 164
Herbalism
    in China, 4
    Thomsonian, 85
Herbalists, Native American, 52
Herbal remedies, 90
    for acne, 207
    with anticoagulant/anithrombolytic activity, 188

Herbal remedies (*cont.*)
  antihypertensive effects of, 203
  for asthma, 410
  for atherosclerosis, 188
  for attention-deficit hyperactivity disorder, 171
  ayurvedic, 64, 65
  for cancer therapy side effects, 371, 373–374
  cardioprotective effects of, 185–186
  contraindications to
    lactation, 275
    pregnancy, 271–273
    surgery, 420
  definition of, 117
  differentiated from drugs, 417
  drug interactions of, 117, 119, **417–422**
  for eczema, 212
  forms of, 118
  for glycemic control, 220
  history of, 116, 134
  for HIV infection, 283, 284
  immune-enhancing properties of, 141
  for infant colic, 394
  menopausal women's use of, 257
  of Native Americans, 4
  for osteoarthritis, 327
  photosensitizing effect of, 385
  for postpartum perineal discomfort, 274–275
  potency of, 121
  use during pregnancy, 271–273
  for premenstrual syndrome, 269
  for prostate cancer, 279–280
  quality of, 117–118
  for recurrent pediatric abdominal pain, 390
  safety of, 119–120
  sales of, 134
  side effects of, 119
  as sleep aids, 309
  standardization of, 417
  ten top-selling, 120
  traditional Chinese, 71–72
  as weight loss aids, 224–225
Herniated discs, chiropractic manipulation-related, 104
Hesoeridin, 136
High-density lipoprotein (HDL) cholesterol, 143
High-protein diet, 127–128
High-velocity, low-impact thrust, 93, 94
"Highway hypnosis," 37
Hip, osteoporotic fractures of, 228, 229–230
Hippocrates, 84, 90, 123, 154, 175
Histamine2 receptor inhibitors, 236, 255, 391
Holism
  of chiropractic, 108
  of traditional Chinese medicine, 67
Holistic health movement, 3
Holistic medicine, 1
Holy Spirit, 154
Holy thistle, bitterness of, 243
Home births, 274
Homeopathic aggravation, 81–82
Homeopathic Materia Medica, 79, 81

Homeopathic remedies, 79–80, 81
  for allergic rhinitis, 407–408
  for anxiety, 165–166
  for asthma, 412
  for atopic dermatitis, 210
  for attention-deficit hyperactivity disorder, 172
  for fibromyalgia, 335
  for gastroesophageal reflux disease, 237–238
  for hypertension, 203
  for infant colic, 394
  for irritable bowel, 252, 253
  for otitis media, 398
  for peptic ulcer disease, 256
  use during pregnancy, 271
  for urinary tract infections, 302
Homeopaths, credentialing of, 83
Homeopathy, 2, 3, **79–83**
  classic, 81
  definition of, 79, 84
  as energy medicine, 155
  legal status of, 82
  origin of, 79
  serial dilution and succussion method in, 80
  side effects and complications of, 81
Homocysteine, 180, 184
Hops, 235, 250
Horehound, 236
Hormones. *See also* specific estrogens
  meat content of, 243
  natural, 258
  synthetic, 259
Hormone testing, in premenstrual syndrome patients, 269
Horse chestnut (*Aesculus hippocastanum*), 120, 188
Horsetail (*Equisetum arvense*), 232
Hot flashes/flushes, 257, 259–260, 262
  in breast cancer survivors, 380
Hoxsey therapy, 367
Huang Di Nei Jing (The Yellow Emperor's Inner Classic), 67, 110, 116
Huang qin (*Scutellaria baicalensis*), as prostate cancer treatment, 279
Huang Ti, 110
Hull, Clark, 38
Human herpesvirus 6, association with multiple sclerosis, 354
Human immunodeficiency virus (HIV)-infected patients, religiosity of, 48
Human immunodeficiency virus (HIV) infection, **281–285**
Humanism, as chiropractic principle, 108
Humor, 32
Hunger, body versus emotional, 131
Hunt, Valerie, 158
Huperzia serrata (Chinese club moss), 342
Huperzine-A, 342
"Hurry sickness," 186
Hydrangea root, as allergic rhinitis treatment, 406
Hydrastis canadensis. See Goldenseal

Hydration
  in common cold and influenza patients, 2
  as urinary tract infection treatment, 300
Hydrochloric acid, 235
Hydropathy, 2
3-Hydroxy-3-methylglutaryl coenzyme A (statins), 181, 277
5-Hydroxytryptophan, 177, 225
Hyperbaric oxygen therapy, for multiple sclerosis, 355
Hyperforin, 175
Hypericin, 175, 417
Hypertension, **200–204**
  as atherosclerosis risk factor, 180
  effect of religiosity on, 48
  in vegetarians, 201
  yoga therapy for, 56
Hypertension Control Program, 200
Hypnosis, **37–42**
  use in allopathic medicine, 90
  as asthma treatment, 412
  as cancer treatment, 372
  as eczema treatment, 213
  as irritable bowel syndrome treatment, 248
  myths about, 40
  as pain treatment, 310
  as recurrent pediatric abdominal pain treatment, 390
  side effects and complications of, 40
  trance induction in, 38–39
Hypnotherapists, reputable, 41
"Hypnotic death rehearsal," 40
Hypoglycemia
  chelation therapy-related, 189
  reactive, 169
Hypomagnesemia, diabetes-related, 218

Ice water ingestion, as weight loss technique, 224
Ignatia, as gastroesophageal reflux disease treatment, 238
Illness, energetic basis for, 158–159
Imagery, guided, 37, 38, 186, 376, 412
Immune surveillance, in cancer, 368
Immune system function
  effect of acupuncture on, 75
  effect of dietary supplements on, 141
  effect of hypnosis and imagery on, 39–40
  effect of sugar on, 286
Immunotherapy, for allergic rhinitis, 404
Incontinence, urge, 257
India
  ayurvedic medicine in, 59, 63, 66
  Department of Indian Systems of Medicine and Homeopathy, 65–66
  traditional medicine in, 59
Indian gooseberry (*Emblica officinalis*), 251
Indinavir, 117
Indoor air, optimal, 292
Infants
  colic in, 388, **392–395**
  massage in, 114

Infants (*cont.*)
  therapeutic touch-induced weight gain in, 159
Influenza, 82, 288–289
Inositol hexaphosphate, 141, 371
Insomnia
  in cancer patients, 374
  melatonin treatment for, 140
  perimenopausal and menopausal, 260–261
  yoga therapy for, 56
Institute for Functional Medicine, 248
Institute of Medicine, 135
Insulin resistance, 218, 222, 384
Integrative medicine, 1, **16–21**
  definition of, 16
  intuition in, 17–18
  principal tenets of, 16–17
  self-care in, 17
Interferon beta 1A and 1B, 352
Interleukin-6, 48, 175, 180
International Chiropractors Association, 101
International Massage Association, 113
Interval training, 146–147
Intestines, bacterial colonization of, 139
Intuition, in integrative medicine, 17–18
Intussusception, 389
  differentiated from infant colic, 393
Ipecac, 412
  contraindication during pregnancy, 272
Ireland Cancer Center, 32
Iron deficiency, attention-deficit hyperactivity disorder-related, 170
Iron supplements
  as colon cancer risk factor, 384
  contraindication in hepatitis, 244
  effect on glycemic control in diabetes, 220
Irrigation, nasal, 292–293
Irritability, premenstrual, 265, 267
Irritable bowel syndrome, **246–253**
  4-R program for, 250
  milk allergy-related, 124
  pediatric, 389
  yoga therapy for, 56
Irritants, as asthma triggers, 410
Isatis, 382
Isatis indigotica (da quing ye), as prostate cancer treatment, 279
Iscador, 371
Islam, use of meditation in, 43
Islamic patients, 52
Isoflavones, 184

Jefferson, Thomas, 37
Jehovah's Witnesses, 47
Jesus, 154
Jewish patients, 52
Jin shin do, 111
Joe pye, contraindication during lactation, 275
Joint injections, as osteoarthritis treatment, 323
Journaling, 31, 35
Journal of Family Practice, 88
Journal of the American Medical Association, 13, 35

Journals, in complementary and alternative medicine, 13
Judaism
  kabalistic tradition of, 154
  use of meditation in, 43, 44
Judith (Walker) Delaney neuromuscular therapy, 114
Jung, Carl, 34, 47, 161
Juniper berries (*Juniperis communis*), contraindication during pregnancy, 272
Juzenthaito, 380

Kali muraticum, as otitis media treatment, 398
Kava ceremonies, 4
Kava (*Piper methysticum*), 120, 164
  as anxiety treatment, 164
  drug interactions of, 421
  hepatotoxicity of, 164
  muscle relaxant properties of, 261
Kegel exercises, 300
Kelley, William Donald, 367–368
Kelp, 140
Keratosis, actinic, 385
Ki, 154
Kirksville College of Osteopathic Medicine, 92
Krestin, 370
Kshara sutra surgery, 62

Labor and delivery
  breech presentation in, moxibustion treatment for, 274
  partus preparator use during, 273
  perineal discomfort after, 274–275
Labyrinth meditations, 44
Lactation, 275
Lactobacillus, 252
Lactobacillus acidophilus, 207, 394
Lacto-ovovegetarian diet, 123
Lactose intolerance, 124, 390
Lad, Vasant, 63
Lafayette (Marie Joseph), Marquis de, 37
Lane, Deforia, 32
Lanolin, as contract dermatitis cause, 211
Larch (*Larix occidentalis*), 141
Laser therapy, low-level, for osteoarthritis, 327–328
Laughter, 32
Lavastatin, 120
Lavender, 250, 385
Laxatives
  drug interactions of, 419
  herbal, contraindication during pregnancy, 273
Lead poisoning, as attention-deficit hyperactivity disorder cause, 171
Learning disorders, energy medicine treatment for, 160
Lectins, 128
Ledum palustre, 82
Left-brain activities, 31–32
Lemon balm (*Melissa officinalis*), 171, 250, 261
Lenticus edodes polyporaceae (shiitake mushroom), 141, 186
Leptin, 222–223

Leukotrienes, in benign prostatic hypertrophy, 277
Licorice (*Glycyrrhiza glabra*)
  as asthma treatment, 410, 411
  contraindications to
    hypertension, 203
    lactation, 275
    pregnancy, 272
  deglycerizinated, as gastroesophageal reflux disease treatment, 235–237
  drug interactions of, 420
  as eczema treatment, 212
  as hepatitis treatment, 244
  as irritable bowel syndrome treatment, 250, 252
  as peptic ulcer disease treatment, 255
  as premenstrual syndrome treatment, 269
Lifestyle, effect on health, 86
Lifestyle Heart Trial, 86, 181
Lifestyle modifications
  as coronary artery disease treatment, 181
  as hypertension treatment, 200
Light therapy. *See* Phototherapy
Lily of the valley (*Convallaria majalis*), contraindication during pregnancy, 272
Ling zhi. *See* Reishi
Linoleic acid, 126
  alpha, 126
  conjugated, 225
  gamma (GLA), 127, 212, 219–220, 268
Lipid profiles, effect of exercise on, 143
Lipoic acid
  alpha, 219, 242, 353, 359
Lipoprotein a, 180
Listening skills, of physicians, 18, 91
Liver pain, hepatitis-related, 245
Lobelia, contraindication during pregnancy, 272
Lodestone, 160
Lomilomi, 114
Lost Art of Healing, The (Lown), 17
Lovastatin, 183
Low back pain, **313–321**
  causes of, 313
  chiropractic treatment for, 102, 104
  classification of, 314
  "dirty half-dozen" diagnoses of, 319
  exercise therapy for, 149
Low-density lipoprotein (LDL) cholesterol, 143, 180
Low-fat diet, 125
  for breast cancer patients, 380
  for breast cancer prevention, 377
  as prostate cancer adjunct therapy, 382
Lubricants, intravaginal, 260
Lumbar manipulation, under anesthesia, 104
Lung cancer, 363, 382–383
Lutein, antioxidant activity of, 138
Lycopene, 138, 381
Lycopodium, 238, 252
Lymphatic drainage, as otitis media treatment, 397
Lymphedema, in breast cancer patients, 379
Lymph nodes, manual drainage of, 238
Lyon Diet Heart study, 86, 181
L-Lysine, 140

Macular degeneration, estrogen deficiency-related, 257–258
Madhava Nidana, 59–60
Magnesia phosphorica, as infant colic treatment, 394
Magnesium
 as Alzheimer's disease treatment, 341
 antihypertensive effects of, 202
 as asthma treatment, 411
 effect on bone health, 230
 cardioprotective effects of, 184
 as diabetes treatment, 218
 as fibromyalgia treatment, 334
 as migraine headache treatment, 348
 muscle relaxant properties of, 261
 in osteoporosis, 231
 as premenstrual syndrome treatment, 268
 as sinusitis treatment, 295
Magnesium deficiency, attention-deficit hyperactivity disorder-associated, 170
Magnetic fields, static, as fibromyalgia treatment, 335
Magnetic resonance imaging, 158
 use in chiropractic, 102
Magnetoencephalography, 158
Magnets, 160–161
 as chronic pain treatment, 310–311
 as osteoarthritis treatment, 327
 as peripheral neuropathy treatment, 359
Maharishi Ayurved University, 63, 65
Maharishi Mahesh Yogi, 63
Ma huang. *See* Ephedra
Maitake (*Grifola frondosa*) mushrooms, 141, 370
Male fern, contraindication during lactation, 275
Maltic acid, as fibromyalgia treatment, 334
Mammography, 377
Managed care, effect on allopathic medicine, 89
Manganese, 230, 326
Manipulation therapies. *See also* Chiropractic; Osteopathic medicine
 for asthma, 413
Manual medicine, 97. *See also* Chiropractic; Osteopathic medicine
 non-chiropractic, differentiated from chiropractic, 105–106
 as pain treatment, 310
Manual trigger point release, 114
Mao Tse-Tung, 4
Marijuana, medical use of, 374
Marinol, 374
Marshmallow (*Althea officinalis*), 235–237, 399
Marx Brothers, 32
Massage, **110–115**
 as anxiety treatment, 166
 as asthma treatment, 413
 as attention-deficit hyperactivity disorder treatment, 172
 ayurvedic, 64
 as cancer therapy, 373
 chiropractors' use of, 103
 contraindications to, 110–111
 cost-effectiveness of, 429
 definition of, 110

Massage (*cont.*)
 differentiated from chiropractic, 113–114
 as fibromyalgia treatment, 310, 333
 as HIV infection therapy, 283–284
 in infants, 114
 as low back pain treatment, 310, 318
 orthopedic, 113
 physical and emotional benefits of, 111
 types of, 114–115
Massage therapists, qualifications of, 113
Mastic gum, 235
Materia Medica (Cullen), 79
Materia Medica (Dioscorides), 116
Maximal heart rate (MHR), 147
Maxwell, James Clerk, 155
McGuide, Charlotte, 3–4
MCI (mild cognitive impairment), 338, 340
McKenzie exercises, for back pain, 318
Meals, timing of, 130
Meat
 grilled, fried, or charred, carcinogenicity of, 369
 hormone-free, 243
Medical Education in the United States and Canada (Flexner), 2, 85
Medical Herbalism, 13
Medical history, bio-psycho-social model of, 306
Medical savings accounts, 425
Medical schools
 complementary and alternative course work in, 4
 non-allopathic, 85
Medicare, 86, 105
Medicine and Culture (Payer), 84
Medicine men, 52
Meditation, **43–46**
 by Alzheimer's disease patients, 340–341
 as anxiety treatment, 164
 cardioprotective effects of, 186
 definition of, 43
 formal, 44, 45–46
 informal, 44
 psychological effects of, 43–44
Mediterranean diet, 126, 127, 181, 201, 223
Medroxyprogesterone acetate, 259
Megavitamin therapy, contraindication during pregnancy, 273
Megbe, 154
Melaleuca alternifolia (tea tree oil), 207, 208, 211, 385
Melanoma, 385
Melatonin, 140–141, 371
Melissa officinalis (lemon balm), 171, 250, 261
Mellaril (thioridazine), 343
Memory impairment, age-associated, 338
Menadione. *See* Vitamin K
Menominee, 52
Menopause, **257–264**
Menstrual bleeding, during perimenopause, 259
Mentha pulegium (pennyroyal), contraindication during pregnancy, 272
Merck and Company, 120

Mercury dental fillings, as multiple sclerosis risk factor, 354–355
Mercury poisoning, as attention-deficit hyperactivity disorder cause, 171
Meridians, 74, 156, 157
Mesmer, Franz Anton, 2, 37, 160
Mesmeric societies, 37–38
Mesmerism, 2
Meta-analysis, 12
L-Methionine, 140
Methylcobalamin. *See* Vitamin B$_{12}$
Methylphenidate, 169, 171
Methylsulfonylmethane, 325
Metoclopramide, 391
Metronidazole, 207
Metzger, Deena, 31
Mevacor, 121, 183
MGN-3, 141, 370
Middle ear, anatomy of, 396
Midwifery, 274
Mild cognitive impairment (MCI), 338, 340
Milk
    as calcium source, 231
    nondairy, 124
Milk protein intolerance, 124, 393–394
Milk thistle
    chemotherapy patients' use of, 380
    drug interactions of, 421
    as hepatitis treatment, 244
    as HIV infection treatment, 283
    as irritable bowel syndrome treatment, 250
Mind-body relationship, 3
    Cartesian, 26
    effect on immune system function, 39–40
    in Native American medicine, 4
Mind-body therapy, 309–310
    for anxiety, 165
    for cancer, 372
    cardioprotective effects of, 186
    for gastroesophageal reflux disease, 238
    for HIV infection, 284
    for hypertension, 202
    for irritable bowel syndrome, 246–252
    for low back pain, 318
    for multiple sclerosis, 355
Mineral deficiency, in attention-deficit hyperactivity disorder, 170
Mineral supplements
    prevalence of use, 134
    as weight loss aids, 226
Minocycline, as acne treatment, 207
Mint, effect on homeopathic remedies, 82
Miracles, 50
Mistletoe (Viscum album), 272, 371
Mitchella repens (partridge berry), 273
Mobilization, chiropractic, 103, 104
Momordica charantia (bitter melon), 220
Monacolin K, 120, 121
Monascus purpureas (Chinese red yeast rice), 120–121, 182–183, 283
Monoamine oxidase, 175, 176

Monosodium glutamate, 335, 345
Monounsaturated fatty acids, 125–126
Morning sickness, during pregnancy, 273
Morphine, 75
Mountain States Blue Cross Blue Shield, 428
Movement therapy, 31
Moxibustion, 67, 72, 76, 274
Mozart, Wolfgang Amadeus, 33
"Mozart effect," 33, 155
Mucilages, plants as, 399
Mucous membranes, healing of, 292–293
Mucuna pruriens, 65
Mugwort (*Artemesia vulgare*), 76, 272
Mullein (*Verbascum thapsus*), 399
Multiple sclerosis, **352–356**
Multiple Sclerosis Diet Book, The (Swank), 353
Multivitamin supplements, as cancer therapy, 370
Muscle energy, 319
Muscle mass, aging-related loss of, 148
Muscle relaxants, as low back pain treatment, 317
Musculoskeletal disorders, acupuncture treatment for, 77
Mushrooms
    as cancer therapy, 370
    immune-enhancing properties of, 141
    maitake, 141, 370
    shiitake, 141, 186, 188
Music, physiologic effects of, 33
Music therapists, 33
Music therapy, 31, 32–33
    for Alzheimer's disease, 341
    for anxiety, 166
    for cancer, 372
    cardioprotective effects of, 187
    as energy medicine, 155
    history of, 32
Myocardial infarction
    annual number of, 180
    in women, 181
Myocardial infarction patients, music therapy for, 33
Myofascial release techniques, 94
Myrrh, as postpartum perineal discomfort treatment, 274–275

NAC (n-acetyl-cysteine), 140, 242, 353
Narigenin, 243
Nasal sprays, 292, 404
National Acupuncture Detox Association, 78
National Association of Music Therapy, 33
National Center for Complementary and Alternative Medicine (NCCAM), 4, 9, 309, 368
National Certification Board for Therapeutic Massage and Bodywork, 113
National Certification Commission for Acupuncture and Oriental Medicine, 72–73, 77
National Institutes of Health, 4, 9, 65
National Osteopathic Board of Medical Examiners, 98
Native American medicine, 4
Native Americans
    religious beliefs of, 52
    shamans of, 90

Natural therapeutics, 134
Nature's Way, 342
Naturopathy, definition of, 3
Nausea
  chemotherapy-related, 374, 380
  migraine headache-related, 345
  premenstrual, 265
Navajo, 52
NCCAM. *See* National Center for Complementary
  and Alternative Medicine
Needles, use in acupuncture, 74–75
Neglect, medical, religion-based, 47, 49
Neomycin, as contract dermatitis cause, 211
Nerve injury, acupuncture-related, 75
Nettle leaves. *See also* Stinging nettle
  as osteoarthritis treatment, 327
Neurodegenerative disorders, magnetic stimulation
  therapy for, 161
Neuroleptics, as fibromyalgia treatment, 333
Neurologic disorders, acupuncture treatment for, 77
Neuromuscular therapy, 113, 114
Neuropathy, peripheral, **357–362**
  diabetic, 160, 219–220, 358
  toxic, 357
Neurotransmitters, effect of acupuncture on, 177–178
New England Journal of Medicine, The, 89–90
Newton, Isaac, 155
New York Heart Association, heart failure
  classification system of, 192
Niacin. *See* Vitamin B$_3$
Niacinamide. *See* Vitamin B$_3$
Nicotine, effect on chronic pain, 308
Nightshades, as osteoarthritis aggravant, 326
Nixon, Richard M., 3
Nocebo effect, 24–25
Nonspecific effect, 25
Nonsteroidal anti-inflammatory drugs (NSAIDs)
  complications of, 105
  as fibromyalgia treatment, 333
  as low back pain treatment, 317
  as migraine headache treatment, 347
  as osteoarthritis treatment, 323
  as peptic ulcer disease risk factor, 254
  as premenstrual syndrome treatment, 268
Noradrenaline, music-induced reduction in, 33
Norepinephrine, St. John's wort-induced reduction in,
  175
North American Society of Homeopaths, 83
Nosodes, 80
Nuclear magnetic resonance, 158
Nurses, touch therapy use by, 160
Nursing, role in complementary and alternative
  medicine, 3–4
Nutraceuticals, 134. *See also* Dietary supplements
  as cancer prophylactic or treatment, 370–371
Nutrition, **123–133**
  during pregnancy, 273
  in traditional Chinese medicine, 67
Nutritional counseling, by chiropractors, 103
Nutritional factors
  in allergic rhinitis, 407

Nutritional factors (*cont.*)
  in chronic pain, 308
  in multiple sclerosis, 353
  in premenstrual syndrome, 268
Nutritional therapy
  for Alzheimer's disease, 340
  for attention-deficit hyperactivity disorder, 170,
    171, 172
  ayurvedic medicine's emphasis on, 62, 64–65
  for coronary artery disease, 181
  for diabetes, 216
  for hepatitis, 243–244
  for HIV-positive patients, 281
  for hypertension, 200
  for infant colic, 393–394
Nux vomica, 238, 252

Obesity, **222–227**
  abdominal, 147
  cause of, 222
  as colon cancer risk factor, 384
  definition of, 146, 222
  as diabetes risk factor, 216, 217
  excessive estrogen production in, 267
  as prostate cancer risk factor, 381
Obsessive-compulsive disorder, 166
Obstetric patients. *See also* Pregnancy
  music therapy for, 33
Occupational Safety and Health Administration,
  acupuncture safety standards of, 75
Office ergonomics, 349
Office of Alternative Medicine, 4, 9
Office of Technology Assessment, 88
Office visits, average duration of, 18
Oil detoxification therapy, ayurvedic, 62, 64
Ojibwa, 52
Okinawa, calorie-restricted diet in, 123
Okra, as demulcent, 236–237
Olive oil, 125–126, 340, 377
Omega fatty acids, as paleolithic-type diet
  component, 128
Omega-3 fatty acids, 126–127
  as allergic rhinitis treatment, 406, 407
  Alzheimer's disease patients' consumption of, 340
  antihypertensive effects of, 201
  as asthma treatment, 411
  as benign prostatic hypertrophy treatment, 277
  cancer patients' consumption of, 368–369
  cancer preventive properties of, 377
  cardioprotective effects of, 182
  deficiency in, as depression risk factor, 177
  as eczema treatment, 212–213
  flax content of, 182
  as prostate cancer adjunct treatment, 382
  as recurrent colon cancer preventives, 369
  role in weight loss, 225
  as sinusitis treatment, 293, 296
Omega-6 fatty acids, 126, 127
  carcinogenicity of, 377
Omega-9 fatty acids, 126, 377
Omega-3/omega-6 fatty acids ratio, in depression, 177

Oncology, integrative, **363–376**. *See also* specific
types of cancer
Oneida, 52
Onions
as allergic rhinitis treatment, 408
as urinary tract infection treatment, 298
Opiates, endogenous, acupuncture-induced release of,
75
Opium, 2
Optimism, in coronary artery disease patients, 186
Oral contraceptives, 205, 261, 269
Oral disorders, acupuncture treatment for, 77
Oral glucose tolerance test, 215
Oranges, vitamin C content of, 134
Orenda, 154
Organic foods, 129
Ornish Program for Reversing Heart Disease, 125,
181, 187, 381
health insurance reimbursement for, 428
Oscillococcinum, 82
Osha (*Ligusticum porten*), contraindication during
pregnancy, 272
Osler, William, 18, 47, 84
Osteoarthritis, **322–329**
energy medicine treatment for, 160
homeopathic remedy for, 82
yoga treatment for, 56
Osteopathic medicine, 2, **92–100**
as asthma treatment, 413
comparison with chiropractic, 95
cranial, 94–95
definition of, 92
as gastroesophageal reflux disease treatment, 238
as low back pain treatment, 318–319
use in pediatric patients, 99
schools of, 85
as upper respiratory tract infection treatment, 288
Osteopenia, estrogen deficiency-related, 257–258
Osteoporosis, **228–233**
definition of, 228
effect of exercise on, 148
risk factors for, 229
Otitis media, 98, 99, **396–402**
Out-of-body experiences, yoga-related, 57
Ovarian torsion, in children, 389
Over-the-counter drugs
aluminum-containing, 339
contraindication in hepatitis, 242
Oxalates, 231
Oxidative stress, 138, 249
Oxygen consumption, 147

Pacemakers, 159
Pacifiers, as otitis media risk factor, 401
Pain
behavioral components of, 307
prevalence of, 304
psychosomatic, 304
Pain diary, 310
Pain management, 304–312
boundary setting in, 307

Pain management (*cont.*)
in diabetic neuropathy, 220
with energy medicine, 160
inadequate, 304
with massage, 111
with meditation, 43, 48
physician's communication skills in, 305
with yoga, 56
Paleolithic-type diets, 128
Palliative treatment, osteopathic manipulative, 98
Palmer, Daniel, 101
Palmer School of Chiropractic, 101
Panax. *See* Ginseng
Panax notoginseng, 185
Panax pseudoginseng (san qi), 279, 382
Panchakarma, 64
Pancreatitis, in children, 389
Panic disorder, 43, 163, 165
Pantothenic acid. *See* Vitamin B$_5$
Papaya, drug interactions of, 420
Parabens, as contract dermatitis cause, 211
Paracelsus, Philippus, 154, 160
"Parasite cleanses," 371
Parathyroid hormone, 188–189
Partridge berry (*Mitchella repens*), as partus
preparator, 273
Partus preparators, 273
Passionflower, as attention-deficit hyperactivity
disorder treatment, 171
Pasteur, Louis, 84, 286
Patient education, 19
Patients, negative stereotyping of, 87
PC-SPES herbal regimen, for prostate cancer,
279–280, 382
Peace, Love and Healing (Siegel), 374–375
Pediatrics. *See also* Children; Infants
osteopathic principles in, 99
Pelvic floor exercises, 300
Penicillin, discovery of, 2
Pennyroyal (*Mentha pulegium*), contraindication
during pregnancy, 272
Pepper (black). *See also* Cayenne pepper
drug interactions of, 419
Peppermint, 237, 250, 252, 390
Peppers, as osteoarthritis aggravant, 326
Peptic ulcer disease, **254–256**
Percutaneous electrical stimulation (PENS), 319,
361
Perimenopause, 257, 258
menstrual bleeding during, 259
Perineal discomfort, postpartum, 274–275
Peripheral vascular disease, 180, 188, 189
Personality, cancer-prone, 365–366
Petasites hybridus (butterbur), as allergic rhinitis
treatment, 405
Peumus boldus (boldo), 245
Phantom limb phenomenon, 156
Pharmaceutical industry, relationship to allopathic
medicine, 89
Pharmanex, 120, 121
Phenylethylamine, 132

Phenylpropanolamine, contraindication in benign prostatic hypertrophy, 278
Phenytoin, as acne cause, 206
Phobias, 163
Phoenix Rising Yoga Therapy, 111
Phosphatidylserine, 342, 354
Photons, 155
Photophobia, migraine headache-related, 345
Photosensitivity, herbal remedies-related, 385
Phototherapy, 159
    for depression, 178
    for fibromyalgia, 334
Phyllanthus, as hepatitis treatment, 244
Phylloquinone, 138
Physical activity. *See also* Exercise
    as attention-deficit hyperactivity disorder treatment, 172
Physical inactivity, of children, 150
Physician office visits, average duration of, 18
Physician-patient relationship, communication in, 18, 91
    in pain management, 305
Physicians
    "crisis of meaning" among, 17
    generalist vs. specialist, 85
    job dissatisfaction among, 87
    listening skills of, 18, 91
    moral code of, violations of, 51
    same-sex, for Muslim patients, 52
    spiritual beliefs of, 50–51
    support for complementary and alternative medicine by, 1
    training in complementary and alternative medicine, 9
Physics, Newtonian, 155
Phytochemicals, 134
Phytodolor, 327
Phytoestrogens, 184, 257, 258, 260
Phytonutrients, as cancer preventives or treatment, 370–371, 378
Picrorrhiza, as hepatitis treatment, 244
Pima Indians, diabetes prevalence in, 123, 217
Piper methysticum. See Kava
Pistacia lentiscus, 235
Placebo, 10, 11, **23–30**
    active, 24
    in acupuncture studies, 72
    definition of, 23
    ethical use of, 28–29
Placebo effect, 23, 24
    in cancer treatment, 366
    comparison with nonspecific effect, 25
    as conditioned response, 28
    cultural factors in, 28
    expectation-induced, 27
    misattribution of patient outcome to, 26–27
Planck, Max, 155
Planetree system, 90
Plantain banana, 235–237
Plantain herb, 235–236
Plantar fasciitis, 112

Plant sterols, 185, 278
Play, 32
Pleasure, 32
Pneuma, 154
Pneumothorax, acupuncture-related, 75
Poetry, 31, 35
Polarity therapy, 154, 159
Polyphenols, 138, 184, 185
Polyps, colonic, 383
Polyunsaturated fatty acids, 125, 126, 127, 182, 201
Positive attitude, effect on cancer prognosis, 366
Positron emission tomography, 158
Posttraumatic stress disorder, 163
Potassium, 184, 202
Potassium citrate, 298
Potassium:sodium ratio, in healthful diets, 201
Potatoes, as osteoarthritis aggravant, 326
Pot marigold. *See* Calendula
Poultices, 118
Powerful Placebo, The (Beecher), 26
Prana, 63, 154
Pranayama, 55
Prayer, 4, 44, 48, 49, 50, 155, 187, 373
Pregnancy, **271–275**. *See also* Labor and delivery
    exercise during, 150
    herbal remedies use during, 271–273
    homeopathic remedies use during, 271
    smoking during, 392
    urinary tract infections during, 299
    yoga during, 57
Premarin, 258, 379
Premenstrual syndrome (PMS), **265–270**
Preventative Medicine Research Institute, 181
Preventive medicine
    allopathic, 86–87
    ayurvedic, 62
    traditional Chinese, 73
Primary respiratory mechanism, 94
Principle of similars, 79
Pritikin diet, 125
Proanthocyanidins, 138, 185
Proanthocyanins, 293, 295
Probiotics, 139, 238, 282, 394
Procarin, 355
Process acupressure, 111
Procyanidolic oligomers, 184
Progesterone, in premenstrual syndrome, 266, 267
Progesterone therapy
    in postmenopausal women, 262
    topical, 260, 261, 269
Propionibacterium acnes, 205
Propolis, 140
Prospective descriptive case study, 10
Prospective experimental case study, 10
Prostaglandins, 212, 268, 277, 353
Prostate cancer, 277, 279–280, 380–382
Prostate-specific antigen, 279, 380–381
Protein, dietary
    diabetics' intake of, 216–217
    in high-protein diets, 127–128
    optimal intake of, 129

Protein, dietary (*cont.*)
  in osteoporosis, 231
Protein supplements, 139
Proton pump inhibitors, 236, 255, 391
Provac (fluoxetine), 269
Pseudoaddiction, 308
Pseudoephedrine, contraindication in benign prostatic
  hypertrophy, 278
Pseudofolliculitis barbae, 206
PSK, 370
Psoriasis, 210
Psychoneuroimmunology, 18–19
Psychophysical integration, Trager, 115
Psyllium, 182
Publication bias, in complementary and alternative
  medicine, 8
Pulsatilla, 238, 398, 412
Pulsed electromagnetic field therapy, 160–161, 327
Pulse diagnosis, in traditional Chinese medicine,
  68–69
Pumpkin seed extract, as benign prostatic hypertrophy
  treatment, 278
Purging, 2, 79, 84
Purging buckthorn, contraindication during lactation,
  275
Purification, internal, in ayurvedic medicine, 64
Pycnogenol, antioxidant activity of, 138
Pygeum bark, as benign prostatic hypertrophy
  treatment, 278, 279
Pyloric stenosis, differentiated from infant colic, 393
Pyridoxine. *See* Vitamin B$_6$
Pythagoras, 154
Pythagoreans, 154

Qi, 67, 68, 74, 75, 154
  defensive, 288
Qiging, as diabetes therapy, 217–218
Qi-gong, 72, 154, 159
Quackery, 1, 2
Quanta, 155
Quantum Healing (Chopra), 63–64
Quantum therapy, 155
Quercetin, 136, 212–213, 405
Quinine, 79

Rabdosia ruescens, 382
Radiation therapy, side effects of, 364, 374
Radiography, chiropractic, 102
Ragweed, allergic reactions to, 390
Ramadan, 52
Randomization, 12
Randomized trials, 25
  controlled, 6, 8, 10, 11, 12, 13
  controlled, double-blinded, 88
Ranitidine (Zantac), 236
Rebound phenomenon, 347
*Reclaiming Our Health: Exploding the Medical Myth
  and Embracing the Source of True Healing*
  (Robbins), 84
Recommended daily allowances (RDA), 134–135
Rectal cancer, 384–385

Red clover (*Trifolium pratense*), 259, 260
Red wine, 185, 345, 379
Red yeast rice (*Monascus purpureas*), 120–121,
  182–183, 283
Reflexology, 115
Reiki, 155, 159, 373
Reishi (*Ganoderma lucidum*), 279, 370
  drug interactions of, 420
Relativity, theory of, 155
Relaxation training, 45, 178, 247, 335
Religious beliefs, 47–53, 187
Reporatory, homeopathic, 81
Research, in complementary and alternative medicine,
  6–15
Resistance strength training, 144, 147, 148–149
  in children, 150
Resperdal (respiridine), 343
Respiratory disorders, acupuncture treatment for, 77
Respiridine (Resperdal), 343
Rest, as common cold treatment, 288
Resveratrol, 379
Retinoids, as acne treatment, 207
Retinol, 183, 208. *See also* Vitamin A
Reumalex, 327
Rexall, 137
Rhabdosia rubescens, 279
Rheumatoid arthritis, prayer interventions for, 48
Rhinitis, allergic, 210, **403–408**
Rhubarb (*Rheum palmatum*), contraindication during
  pregnancy, 272
Rhus toxicodendron, 82, 335
Riboflavin. *See* Vitamin B$_2$
Right-brain activities, 31–32
Ritual healing, 4
Rituals, of allopathic medicine, 90
Rivastigmine (Exelon), 342
Rolf, Ida, 115
Rolfing, 113, 115
Rosemary oil, as otitis media treatment, 402
Rosen method, of massage, 111
Royal jelly, 140
Rubenfield synergy massage, 111
Rutin, 136
Rye grass pollen, as benign prostatic hypertrophy
  treatment, 278, 279

Sabadilla, 408
Saccharomyces boulardii, 141
S-adenosylmethionine (SAM-e), 176
Sage (*Salvia officinalis*), 272, 274–275
St. John's wort, 7–8, 120, 175–176
  cost-effectiveness of, 429
  drug interactions of, 117, 419, 420, 421
  hyperforin content of, 417
  hyperium content of, 175, 417
  interaction with antiretroviral medications, 283
  photosensitizing activity of, 385
Salix alba (white willow bark), 317, 327
Salt restriction, 193, 200, 268
Salvia miltiorrhiza (dan-shen), 185
  drug interactions of, 420

Sambucol, 288–289
Sambucus. See Elder flower
Sambucus nigra (black elder), 288–289
SAM-e (S-adenosylmethionine), 176, 325
Sample size, 9
San qi, as prostate cancer treatment, 279
Saponins, 185, 188
Sarafem, 269
Sarcopneia, 147
Saturated fatty acids, 125, 126, 182
Saw palmetto (*Serenoa repens*), 120
    as benign prostatic hypertrophy treatment, 120,
        278–279, 382
    drug interactions of, 421
    as prostate cancer treatment, 279
Schizandra, as hepatitis treatment, 244
Scientific method, 2
Scurvy, Native-American treatment for, 4
Scutellaria baicalensis (huang qin), as prostate cancer
    treatment, 279
Sea Bands, 373
Seasonal affective depression (SAD), 140, 178
Second-hand smoke, as otitis media risk factor, 398
Selective serotonin reuptake inhibitors, 174, 175, 269,
    333
Selenium
    as acne treatment, 209
    as Alzheimer's disease treatment, 341
    antioxidant activity of, 138
    cancer preventive effects of, 378, 381
    cardioprotective effects of, 184
    as fibromyalgia treatment, 334
    as HIV infection therapy, 282
    immune-enhancing properties of, 141
    effect on liver function, 242
    as osteoarthritis treatment, 326
    as sinusitis treatment, 293, 295
    toxicity of, 242
Self-care, in integrative medicine, 17
Self-hypnosis, 41
Serenoa repens. See Saw palmetto
Serial dilution and succusion, 80
Serotonin, 75, 175, 177
Serotonin syndrome, 176
Sertraline (Zoloft), 176
Seventh Day Adventists, 123, 373
Sex hormones, as multiple sclerosis treatment, 354
Sham controls, 10
Shark cartilage, 370
Sharngadhara Samhita, 59–60
Shaving, as acne cause, 206
SHEN physio-emotional release therapy, 111
Shiatsu, 67, 15, 159
Shiitake (*Lenticus edodes polyporaceae*) mushrooms,
    141, 186, 188
"Sick role," 1
Sigmoidoscopy, flexible, 383
Silicon, effect on bone health, 230
Silvers, William, 296
Silver sulfadiazine, as contract dermatitis cause, 211
Simethicone, 395

Similars, principle of, 79
Similia, 79
Singing, physiologic effects of, 33
Sinuses, anatomy and function of, 290
Sinusitis, **290–297**
Sinus survival (Ivker), 294
Sinus Survival Program, 294
β-Sitosterol, 277, 278
Skin cancer, 363, 385
Skullcap, 171, 250, 382
Sleep, as sinusitis treatment, 294
Sleep deprivation, as diabetes risk factor, 218
Sleep disturbances
    hepatitis-related, 241–242
    in perimenopausal and menopausal women,
        260–261
Sleep hygiene, 308–309
Slippery elm bark (*Ulmus fulva*), 235–237, 255, 256,
    380, 399
SmithKLine Beecham, 137
Smoke, as otitis media risk factor, 398
Smoking
    as atherosclerosis risk factor, 180
    carcinogenicity of, 369
    contraindication in depression, 177
    as lung cancer cause, 363, 383
    maternal, as infant colic risk factor, 392
    as peptic ulcer disease risk factor, 254
    as sinusitis risk factor, 291
Smoking cessation, preoperative, 308
SOAP (subjective, objective, assessment, and plan)
    notes, 19
Social isolation, as arteriosclerosis risk factor, 186
Society for Clinical and Experimental Hypnosis, 41
Sodium citrate, 298
Soft drinks, deleterious effect on bone growth, 230
Solid extracts, 118
Somatic dysfunction, 95, 96, 97
Somatic experiencing, 111
Somatoemotional release, 111
Somatosynthesis, 111
Soy, 184
    antihypertensive effects of, 201
    as benign prostatic hypertrophy preventive and
        treatment, 277, 278
    cancer preventive properties of, 370, 378, 381
    as hot flushes treatment, 259
    as osteoporosis preventive, 231–232
    as phytoestrogen source, 258
Spicy foods, effect on peptic ulcer disease, 254
Spikenard (*Aralia racemosa*), as partus preparator,
    273
Spinal manipulation, chiropractic, 102, 103, 104,
    105–106
Spinal stimulation, electrical, 159
SPIRIT questionnaire, 50
Spirituality, **47–53**
Spirulina, 140
Sports drinks, 151
Stanford University, 19
Statins, 181, 277

Steiner, Rudolf, 3
Steroid hormones, as acne cause, 206
Steroid injections, as osteoarthritis treatment, 323
Steroids
  inhaled, as asthma treatment, 413
  topical, as dermatitis cause, 211
Sterols, plant-based, 185, 278
Stevia, 220
Stevoside, 220
Still, Andrew Taylor, 92
Stillingia, contraindication during lactation, 275
Stillman Diet, 127
Stinging nettle, 120, 278, 405
Stomach, stretch receptors in, 123
Storytelling, 35
Strain-counterstrain technique, 94
Stress
  as arteriosclerosis cause, 186
  as common cold risk factor, 286
  dermatitis-exacerbating effects of, 210, 212
  irritable bowel syndrome-exacerbating effects of, 247
  meditation-related, 44
  as migraine headache cause, 347
  as peptic ulcer disease risk factor, 254, 256
  as sinusitis risk factor, 291
Stress hormones, music-induced reduction in, 33
Stress management, 247–248, 256, 349
Stroke, 189, 257–258
Structural integration, 113
Subluxation, 95
Substance abuse, 43, 48
Sufi tradition, 154
"Sugar buster," 220
"Sugar-Busters" Diet, 127
Sugar/sugar-based foods
  anxiety-inducing activity of, 165
  effect on attention-deficit hyperactivity disorder symptoms, 169
  carcinogenicity of, 369
  contraindication in depression, 177
  contraindication in premenstrual syndrome, 268
  diabetics' intake of, 216
  effect on immune system function, 286
  as pediatric abdominal pain cause, 390
  as urinary tract infection risk factor, 298
Suicide, 87, 177, 205, 353
Sulfa drugs, discovery of, 2
Sunscreens, 385
Superconducting quantum interference, 158
"Superfoods," 140
Superoxide dismutase, antioxidant activity of, 138
Support groups, for cancer patients, 372–373
  for breast cancer patients, 379
  for prostate cancer patients, 382
Surgery
  ayurvedic, 64
  as cancer treatment, 364
  herbal remedies contraindicated prior to, 420
  kshara sutra, 62
  surgeons' musci listening during, 33–34

Sushruta Samhita, 59, 60
Sweat lodges, 4
Swedish massage, 115
Sweet birch bark oil, drug interactions of, 420
Sweet clover, drug interactions of, 420
Symphytum officinale, 82
Syringes, Native Americans' invention of, 4
Systemic reviews, 12

Tacrine (Cognex), 343
Tagamet (cimetidine), 236
Tai chi, 154, 187
Tang-gui, as dermatitis treatment, 212, 213
Taoism, 67
Taraxacum officinale (dandelion), 212, 244, 250
Tastes, in ayurvedic diets, 64–65
Tau protein, as Alzheimer's disease cause, 339
Taxol, 134
Taylor, Charles F., 110
Taylor, George H., 110
TCM. *See* Chinese medicine, traditional
Tea. *See also* Green tea
  as anemia cause, 369
  herbal, 118
Tea tree oil (*Melaleuca alternifolia*), 207, 208, 211, 385
Telangiectasia, acne rosacea-related, 206
Tender point injections, as fibromyalgia treatment, 335
Tender points, 112, 332–333
Terminalia chebula (haritaki), 251
Testosterone, in benign prostatic hypertrophy, 276, 278
Testosterone replacement therapy, in postmenopausal women, 262–263
Tetracycline, as acne treatment, 207
Tetrahydropapaveroline, 267
Thai massage, 115
Thermal injury, hypnosis therapy for, 40
Thiamine. *See* Vitamin B$_1$
Thimerisol, 211
Thioridazine (Mellaril), 343
Thomasonianism, 2
Thomson, Samuel, 2
Thrusts, high-velocity, low-impact, 93, 94
Thuja, contraindication during pregnancy, 272
Thyroid products, contraindication as weight loss aids, 226
Tibetan medicine, relationship with ayurveda medicine, 61–62
Tibetan monks, 33
Tinctures, 118
Tobacco. *See also* Smoking
  anxiety-inducing activity of, 165
  as osteoarthritis aggravant, 326
α-Tocopherol, antiatherosclerotic activity of, 183
Tomatoes, as osteoarthritis aggravant, 326
Tongue diagnosis, in traditional Chinese medicine, 68
Tormentil, as irritable bowel syndrome treatment, 250
Touch
  healing, as energy medicine, 155, 159

Touch (*cont.*)
  therapeutic, 154, 159, 373
Touch Research Institute, 110, 114
Toxicity reactions, 418–419
Toxins, as hepatitis cause, 240
Traction, chiropractors' use of, 103
Traditional medicine, non-Western, 84
Traditional (Western) medicine. *See* Allopathic medicine
Trager psychophysical integration, 115
Trametes versicolor (turkey tail), drug interactions of, 420
Trance induction, 38–39
Transcendental meditation, 3, 4, 63
Transcranial electrostimulation (TCES), 159
Transcranial magnetic stimulation (TMS), 178
Transcutaneous electrical stimulation (TENS), 159, 310, 319, 324, 361
Transdermal histamine and caffeine therapy, for multiple sclerosis, 355
Trans-fatty acids, 127, 182, 377
Tricyclic antidepressants, 174, 175, 278, 391
Trifolium pratense (red clover), as hot flushes treatment, 259, 260
Trigger points, 112, 114, 316
Trigonella foenum graecum (fenugreek), 220
Triphala powder, 252
Triptans, 3347
Tryptophan-containing beverages, 261
Tui-na, 67
Turkey tail (*Trametes versicolor*), drug interactions of, 420
Turmeric, 188, 237, 317, 327
Type A behavior, 186
L-Tyrosine, 140

Ulmus fulva (slippery elm bark), 235–237, 255, 256, 380, 399
Ultrasound, therapeutic, 159
U. S. Department of Health and Human Services, 309
U. S. Preventive Health Services Task Force, 86–87
United States Pharmacopoeia, 134
  Native American drugs included in, 4
University Hospitals of Cleveland, 32
University of Arizona, 19, 158
University of Basil, 160
University of California, Los Angeles, 158
University of California, San Francisco, 19
University of Edinburgh, 79
University of Massachusetts, 19
University of Miami, Touch Research Institute of, 110, 114
University of Minnesota, 19
University of Poona, 66
Upper respiratory tract infection (URI), 286–289
Urinary incontinence, urge, 257
Urinary tract infections, **298–303**
  during pregnancy, 273
  urine pH in, 28
Urine, acidification of, 298
Uva ursi, as urinary tract infection treatment, 298, 302

Vaginal dryness, 260
Vaginitis, atrophic, 257
Valerian, 119, 120, 164, 250, 261
  drug interactions of, 422
Valpotriates, 164
Vanadium, as diabetes therapy, 218, 219
Varicose veins, 188
Vegetarian diet, 3, 15, 123–124
  as fibromyalgia treatment, 334
Vegetarians, hypertension in, 201
Venous insufficiency, 188, 211
Verbascum thapsus (mullein), 399
Vertebral artery dissection, yoga-related, 57
Vertebral column, anatomy of, 314
Vertebrobasilar reactions, chiropractic manipulation-related, 104, 105
Vicia faba, 65
Viscum album (mistletoe), 272, 371
Vis medicatrix naturae, 154
Visual analog pain scales, 306
Visualization, 38, 213
Vitalism, 108
Vitamin A
  as acne treatment, 208
  as Alzheimer's disease therapy, 341
  antiatherosclerotic activity of, 183
  antioxidant activity of, 138
  cancer preventive properties of, 378
  characteristics of, 135
  deficiency of, as AIDS progression risk factor, 281
  as diabetes treatment, 218, 219
  as eczema treatment, 212–213
  excessive doses of, 135, 139
  as peptic ulcer disease treatment, 255
  teratogencity of, 273
  toxic dose of, 135
Vitamin B_1, 135, 268, 341, 359
Vitamin B_2, 135, 348
Vitamin B_3, 135, 268, 326, 341, 354, 359
Vitamin B_5, 135, 208
Vitamin B_6
  as acne treatment, 208
  as Alzheimer's disease treatment, 341
  antihypertensive effects of, 202
  as asthma treatment, 411
  deficiency of, plasma homocysteine levels in, 184
  as morning sickness treatment, 273
  as multiple sclerosis treatment, 354
  as peripheral neuropathy treatment, 359
  as premenstrual syndrome treatment, 268
  side effects of, 359–360
  toxic dose of, 135
Vitamin B_{12}
  as Alzheimer's disease therapy, 341
  deficiency of, 124, 177
  as HIV therapy, 282
  as multiple sclerosis treatment, 353
  as peripheral neuropathy treatment, 359
Vitamin B complex
  contraindication during premenstrual syndrome, 268

Vitamin B complex (*cont.*)
  as hepatitis treatment, 244
Vitamin C, 136
  as acne treatment, 208
  as allergic rhinitis treatment, 406
  as Alzheimer's disease therapy, 341
  antiatherosclerotic activity of, 183
  antihypertensive effects of, 202
  antioxidant activity of, 138
  as asthma treatment, 411
  cancer preventive properties of, 378
  as common cold preventive and treatment, 287
  as diabetes therapy, 218, 219
  excessive doses of, 139
  as HIV infection therapy, 282
  as multiple sclerosis treatment, 354
  as neonatal rebound scurvy cause, 273
  as osteoarthritis treatment, 325
  as peripheral neuropathy treatment, 360
  as premenstrual syndrome treatment, 268
  as sinusitis treatment, 293, 295
  toxic dose of, 136
Vitamin D
  as multiple sclerosis treatment, 354
  as osteoarthritis treatment, 326
  as osteoporosis preventive, 232
Vitamin E, 136
  as acne treatment, 208, 209
  as allergic rhinitis treatment, 406
  as Alzheimer's disease treatment, 341
  antiatherosclerotic activity of, 183
  antioxidant activity of, 138
  cancer preventive properties of, 378, 381
  as diabetes treatment, 218, 219
  drug interactions of, 374
  as eczema treatment, 212–213
  egg content of, 134
  as gastroesophageal reflux disease treatment, 238
  as hemostasis impairment cause, 360
  as hepatitis treatment, 245
  as osteoarthritis treatment, 325
  as peptic ulcer disease treatment, 255
  as peripheral neuropathy treatment, 360
  as premenstrual syndrome treatment, 268
  selenium-related potentiation of, 184
  as sinusitis treatment, 293, 295
Vitamin K, 136
Vitamin K_1, 138
Vitamin K_3, 138
Vitamins
  as Alzheimer's disease treatment, 341
  cancer preventive properties of, 378
  characteristics of, 135–136
  definition of, 135
  for HIV-positive patients, 281
  natural compared with synthetic, 137–138
  prevalence of use, 134
  as weight loss aids, 226
Vitex agnus-castus (chaste berry tree), 259, 260, 269
Volatile oils, effect on homeopathic remedies, 82

Volvulus, 389
$\dot{V}O_2$max (aerobic capacity), 146–147
VPS, 370
Vulnerary herbs, as postpartum perineal discomfort treatment, 274–275

Wakan, 154
Waldorf Schools, 3
Walking, as peripheral vascular disease therapy, 188
Warfarin, 374
Warfarin, interaction with herbal remedies, 419–420
Washington, George, 37
Water
  bottled, 130
  I_E structures in, 80
  inadequate consumption of, 130
Water intake
  in hepatitis patients, 244
  of urinary tract infection patients, 300
Watermelon, diuretic activity of, 298
Wegman, Ita, 3
Weight, ideal, 145
Weight-lifting, by heart disease patients, 149
Weight loss
  as chronic pain treatment, 308
  as diabetes treatment, 216
  difficulty of, 222–223
  as hypertension treatment, 200, 202
Wellness behaviors, effect of religious beliefs on, 48
Wennberg, John, 88
Western medicine. *See* Allopathic medicine
Wheatgrass, 140
White House Commission on Complementary and Alternative Medicine Policy, 9
White oak bark, 274–275
White willow bark (*Salix alba*), 317, 327
Wild oats (*Avena sativa*), 171
Wintergreen leaf oil, drug interactions of, 420
Witch hazel, 274–275
Withania somnifera, 171
Withdrawal, acupuncture treatment for, 78
WomenHeart, 181
World Health Organization, 4, 16, 84
Wormwood (*Artemesia absinthium*)
  bitterness of, 243
  contraindication during pregnancy and lactation, 272, 275
Writing, therapeutic, 34–35
Wyethis, 408

Xenobiotics, 276–277
Xenoestrogens, 277
X-rays, use in chiropractic, 102

Yarrow (*Achillea millefolium*), 272, 394, 406
Yashtimadha, 252
Year to Live, A (Levine), 363
Yeast, brewer's (nutritional), 140
Yeast Connection, The (Crook), 294
Yellow Emperor's Inner Classic, The (Huang Di Nei Jing), 67, 110, 116

Yesod, 154
yGyud-bzhi (gyu-shi), 62
Yin and yang, 67, 68
  of food, 123
Yoga, **54–58**
  as asthma treatment, 412
  ayurvedic, 61, 64
  as cancer treatment, 372
  cardioprotective effects of, 187
  as energy medicine, 154
  integrative, 111
  as Phoenix Rising Therapy, 111

Zantac (ranitidine), 236
Zinc
  as acne treatment, 208
  as Alzheimer's disease therapy, 341

Zinc (*cont.*)
  attention-deficit hyperactivity disorder-related
    deficiency of, 170
  as benign prostatic hypertrophy treatment, 278
  effect on bone health, 230
  cardioprotective effects of, 184
  as common cold treatment, 287
  as eczema treatment, 212–213
  effect on glycemic control in diabetes, 220
  as hepatitis treatment, 245
  as osteoarthritis treatment, 326
  as peptic ulcer disease treatment, 255
  as premenstrual syndrome treatment, 268
Zingiber officinale. See Ginger/ginger root
Zoloft (sertraline), 176
"Zone" diet, 128
Zyrtec (cetirizine), 405